Orthopaedic Physical Therapy SECRETS

Orthopaedic Physical Therapy SECRETS

Second Edition

JEFFREY D. PLACZEK, MD, PT
Hand and Upper Extremity Surgery
Michigan Hand & Wrist, PC
Novi, Michigan

Providence Park Medical Center
Novi, Michigan

Associate Clinical Professor
Department of Physical Therapy
Oakland University
Rochester, Michigan

DAVID A. BOYCE, PT, EdD, OCS, ECS
Assistant Professor
Bellarmine University Physical Therapy Program
Louisville, Kentucky

MOSBY
ELSEVIER

MOSBY
ELSEVIER

11830 Westline Industrial Drive
St. Louis, Missouri 63146

ORTHOPAEDIC PHYSICAL THERAPY SECRETS ISBN-13: 978-1-56053-708-3
ISBN-10: 1-56053-708-6

Previous edition copyrighted 2001

ISBN-13: 978-1-56053-708-3
ISBN-10: 1-56053-708-6

Acquisition Editor: Kathy Falk
Publishing Services Manager: Patricia Tannian
Project Manager: Jonathan M. Taylor
Design Direction: Bill Drone

Printed in the United States of America

Last digit is the print number: 9 8 7 6

To my wife, Laura, my best friend, my soul mate, my rock, my inspiration.
To my four angels, Alexis, Bailey, Lily and Addison, my life's true joy,
my deepest love, my serenity, my peace.

JDP

To my mother and father, for instilling in me a strong work ethic. To my wife, Marcia Boyce, and my children, Elizabeth, Emily, and Cole, for your constant love and support. Finally, to my students and patients—thank you for teaching me so much over the years.

DAB

In loving memory of Dr. Edward G. Tracy (November 2, 1941 - March 3, 2004) who devoted himself to educating health professionals for three decades. It is hoped that the presentation of his contribution to this book provides a window into his humor, kindness, compassion, and enthusiasm. Dr. Tracy brought joy into his classroom and made a heavy burden seem light. Generations of students remember him in the same way they remember the material he taught—with affection.

Contributors

Jeffrey E. Balazsy, MD
Attending Trauma Surgeon
Department of Orthopaedic Surgery
William Beaumont Hospital
Royal Oak, Michigan

Judith L. Bateman, MD
Oakland Arthritis Center
Bingham Farms, Michigan

Turner A. "Tab" Blackburn, Jr., PT, MEd, ATC
Vice President, Corporate Development
Clemson Sports Medicine and Rehabilitation
Seneca, South Carolina
Clinical Director
SportsPlus Physical Therapy of Manchester
Manchester, Georgia
Adjunct Assistant Professor
Physical Therapy School
Belmont University
Nashville, Tennessee

David A. Boyce, PT, EdD, OCS, ECS
Assistant Professor
Bellarmine University Physical Therapy Program
Owner, Physical Therapy Plus
Louisville, Kentucky

Douglas Boyce, MD, RPh
Associate Clinical Professor
Wayne State University
Detroit, Michigan

Kathleen A. Brindle, MD
Chief, Musculoskeletal Radiology
Assistant Professor of Radiology
George Washington University
Washington, D.C.

Timothy J. Brindle, PT, PhD, ATC
Post Doctoral Research Physical Therapist
Physical Disabilities Branch
National Institutes of Health
Bethesda, Maryland

Joseph A. Brosky, Jr., PT, MS, SCS
Associate Professor
Bellarmine University Physical Therapy Program
Louisville, Kentucky

Judith M. Burnfield, PT, PhD
Director, Movement Sciences Center
Clifton Chair in Physical Therapy and Movement Science
Institute for Rehabilitation Science and Engineering
Madonna Rehabilitation Hospital
Lincoln, Nebraska

Mark A. Cacko, PT, MPT, OCS
Physical Therapy Specialists, PC
Troy, Michigan

Charles D. Ciccone, PT, PhD
Professor
Department of Physical Therapy
Ithaca College
Ithaca, New York

George J. Davies, PT, DPT, MEd, SCS, ATC, LAT, CSCS, FAPTA
Professor
Armstrong Atlantic State University
Department of Physical Therapy
Savannah, Georgia

Michael Dohm, MD, FAAOS
Rocky Mountain Orthopaedic Associates
Grand Junction, Colorado

Susan Dunn, PT
Dunn & Associates Physical Therapy, PLLC
Lecturer, Bellarmine University
Louisville, Kentucky

Christopher J. Durall, PT, DPT, MS, LAT, SCS, CSCS
Clinical Research Director
Director of Physical Therapy
Student Health Center
University of Wisconsin–La Crosse
La Crosse, Wisconsin

Beth Ennis, PT, EdD, PCS
Assistant Professor
Bellarmine University Physical Therapy Program
Louisville, Kentucky

John L. Echternach, PT, DPT, EdD, ECS, FAPTA
Professor and Eminent Scholar
School of Community Health Professions and Physical Therapy
Old Dominion University
Norfolk, Virginia

Richard Erhard, PT, DC
Assistant Professor
Department of Physical Therapy
University of Pittsburgh
Pittsburgh, Pennsylvania

Sean P. Flanagan, PhD, ATC, CSCS
Assistant Professor
Department of Kinesiology
California State University Northridge
Northridge, California

Tracey M. Fleck, PT, MPT
Instructional Assistant
Department of Physical Therapy
Wayne State University
Detroit, Michigan
Physical Therapist
Maines and Dean Physical Therapy
Howell, Michigan

Timothy W. Flynn, PT, PhD, OCS, FAAOMPT
Associate Professor
Department of Physical Therapy
Regis University
Denver, Colorado

Julie M. Fritz, PT, PhD, ATC
Assistant Professor
Division of Physical Therapy
University of Utah
Salt Lake City, Utah

Kathleen Galloway, PT, MPT, DSc, ECS
Assistant Professor
Department of Physical Therapy
Oakland University
Rochester, Michigan

Teri L. Gibbons, PT, MPT, OCS
Physical Therapy Specialists, PC
Troy, Michigan

Patricia Douglas Gillette, PT, PhD
Associate Professor
Bellarmine University Physical Therapy Program
Louisville, Kentucky

David G. Greathouse, PT, PhD, ECS
Director, Clinical Electrophysiology Services
Texas Physical Therapy Specialists
New Braunfels, Texas
Adjunct Professor
U.S. Army–Baylor University Doctoral Program in Physical Therapy
Fort Sam Houston, Texas

Darren Gustitus, OTR, CHT
Director of Rehabilitation Services
Michigan Hand and Wrist Rehabilitation Center
Novi, Michigan

Robert "Cliff" Hall, PT, MS, SCS, ATC
Deputy Director of Health and Fitness
National Defense University
Washington, D.C.

John S. Halle, PT, PhD
Associate Professor
School of Physical Therapy
Belmont University
Nashville, Tennessee

Craig T. Hartrick, MD, DABPM
Director, Anesthesiology Research
Department of Anesthesiology and Perioperative Medicine
William Beaumont Hospital
Royal Oak, Michigan

Harry N. Herkowitz, MD
Chairman, Department of Orthopaedic Surgery
William Beaumont Hospital
Royal Oak, Michigan

James Robin Hinkebein, PT, OCS, ATC
Director, Bardstown Rehab Services
Kentucky Orthopedic Rehab Team
Bardstown, Kentucky

Sally Ho, PT, DPT, MS
Adjunct Assistant Professor
Department of Biokinesiology and Physical Therapy
University of Southern California
Los Angeles, California
Owner and Director
Ho Physical Therapy
Beverly Hills, California

Todd R. Hockenbury, MD
Assistant Clinical Professor of Orthopedic Surgery
University of Louisville
Bluegrass Orthopedic Group
Louisville, Kentucky

Susan J. Isernhagen, PT
DSI Work Solutions
Duluth, Minnesota

Jay D. Keener, MD, PT
Assistant Professor
Department of Orthopaedic Surgery
University of North Carolina
Chapel Hill, North Carolina

Matthew A. Kippe, MD
Department of Orthopedic Surgery
William Beaumont Hospital
Royal Oak, Michigan

Patrick H. Kitzman, PT, PhD
Department of Rehabilitation Sciences
Division of Physical Therapy and the Rehabilitation Sciences Doctoral Program
University of Kentucky
Lexington, Kentucky

John R. Krauss, PT, PhD, OCS, FAAOMPT
Assistant Professor
School of Health Sciences
Program in Physical Therapy
Assistant Professor
OMPT Program Coordinator
Oakland University
Rochester, Michigan

Kornelia Kulig, PT, PhD
Associate Professor of Clinical Physical Therapy
Department of Biokinesiology and Physical Therapy
University of Southern California
Los Angeles, California

EDWARD M. LICHTEN, MD, FACS, FACOG
Department of Obstetrics and Gynecology
Providence Hospital
Southfield, Michigan
(Retired)

M. ELAINE LONNEMANN, PT, DPT, MSc, OCS, MTC, FAAOMPT
Assistant Professor
Bellarmine University Physical Therapy Program
Louisville, Kentucky
Instructor
University of St. Augustine
St. Augustine, Florida

JANICE K. LOUDON, PT, PHD, ATC
Department of Physical Therapy Education and Rehabilitation Sciences
University of Kansas
Kansas City, Kansas

TERRY R. MALONE, PT, EDD, ATC, FAPTA
Professor and Director
Division of Physical Therapy
University of Kentucky
Lexington, Kentucky

JAMES W. MATHESON, PT, MS, SCS, CSCS
Clinical Research Director
Therapy Partners, Inc.
Maplewood, Minnesota
Staff Physical Therapist
Minnesota Sport and Spine Rehabilitation
Burnsville, Minnesota

JOSEPH M. MCCULLOCH, PT, PHD, CWS, FAPTA, FCCWS
Dean, School of Allied Health Professions
Louisiana State University Health Sciences Center
Shreveport, Louisiana

ANDREA LYNN MILAM, PT, MSED
Assistant Professor
Division of Physical Therapy
University of Kentucky
Lexington, Kentucky

ARTHUR J. NITZ, PT, PHD, ECS, OCS
Professor
Division of Physical Therapy
Department of Rehabilitation Sciences
College of Health Sciences
University of Kentucky
Lexington, Kentucky

JOHN NYLAND, PT, EDD, SCS, ATC, CSCS, FACSM
Assistant Professor
Division of Sports Medicine
Department of Orthopaedic Surgery
University of Louisville
Adjunct Professor
School of Physical Therapy
Bellarmine University
Louisville, Kentucky

BRIAN T. PAGETT, PT, MPT
Physical Therapy Specialists, PC
Troy, Michigan

JOHN J. PALAZZO, PT, DSC, ECS
Director, Neurolabs
Waterford, Michigan

STANLEY V. PARIS, PT, PHD
President and Professor
Department of Physical Therapy
University of St. Augustine
St. Augustine, Florida

SARA R. PIVA, PT, MS, OCS, FAAOMPT
Department of Physical Therapy
School of Health and Rehabilitation Sciences
University of Pittsburgh
Pittsburgh, Pennsylvania

JEFFREY D. PLACZEK, MD, PT
Hand and Upper Extremity Surgery
Michigan Hand & Wrist, PC
Novi, Michigan
Providence Park Medical Center
Novi, Michigan
Associate Clinical Professor
Department of Physical Therapy
Oakland University
Rochester, Michigan

Fredrick D. Pociask, PT, PhD, OCS, FAAOMPT
Assistant Professor
Physical Therapy Program
College of Pharmacy and Health Sciences
Wayne State University
Detroit, Michigan

Christopher M. Powers, PT, PhD
Associate Professor
Department of Biokinesiology and Physical Therapy
Co-Director
Musculoskeletal Biomechanics Research Laboratory
University of Southern California
Los Angeles, California

Michael Quinn, MD
Bloomfield Hand Specialists
Bloomfield Hills, Michigan

Stephen F. Reischl, PT, DPT, OCS
Adjunct Assistant Professor of Clinical Physical Therapy
Department of Biokinesiology and Physical Therapy
University of Southern California
Los Angeles, California

Susan Mais Requejo, PT, DPT
Department of Physical Therapy
Mount St. Mary's College
Assistant Adjunct Professor of Clinical Physical Therapy
University of Southern California
Los Angeles, California

Robert C. Rinke, PT, DC, FAAOMPT
Puget Orthopedic Rehabilitation
Everett, Washington

T. Kevin Robinson, PT, DSc, OCS
Associate Professor
School of Physical Therapy
Belmont University
Nashville, Tennessee

Matthew G. Roman, PT, OMPT
Senior Physical Therapist, Department of Physical and Occupational Therapy
Duke University Medical Center
Durham, North Carolina

Paul J. Roubal, PT, PhD
Owner and Director
Physical Therapy Specialists, PC
Troy, Michigan

Robin Saunders Ryan, PT, MS
Chief Operating Officer
The Saunders Group, Inc.
Chaska, Minnesota

H. Duane Saunders, PT, MS
Chief Executive Officer and President
The Saunders Group, Inc.
Chaska, Minnesota

Edward Schrank, MPT, DSc, ECS
Assistant Professor of Physical Therapy
Shenandoah University
Winchester, Virginia
Physical Therapist in Private Practice
Colorado Springs, Colorado

Robert A. Sellin, PT, DSc, ECS
Director
Electrophysiologic Testing
Professional Rehabilitation Associates
Lexington, Kentucky

Amanda L. Simic, MS, OTR, CHT
Milliken Hand Center
Barnes-Jewish Hospital
St. Louis, Missouri

Paul Simic, MD
Southern California Orthopedic Institute
Van Nuys, California

Britt Smith PT, MSPT, OCS, FAAOMPT
S.O.A.R. Physical Therapy
Grand Junction, Colorado

LeAnn Snow, MD, PhD
Assistant Professor
Department of Physical Medicine and Rehabilitation
University of Minnesota
Minneapolis, Minnesota

Tracy Spigelman, MEd, ATC
Division of Athletic Training
University of Kentucky
Lexington, Kentucky

Rebecca G. Stephenson, PT, DPT, MS
Coordinator of Women's Health Physical Therapy
Department of Rehabilitation Services
Brigham and Women's Hospital
Boston, Massachusetts
President
International Organization of Physical Therapists in Women's Health
Subgroup of the World Confederation for Physical Therapy

Susan W. Stralka, PT, MS
Baptist Rehabilitation Hospital
Germantown, Tennessee

LaDora V. Thompson, PT, PhD
Associate Professor
Program in Physical Therapy
Department of Physical Medicine and Rehabilitation
University of Minnesota
Minneapolis, Minnesota

David Tiberio, PT, PhD, OCS
Associate Professor
Department of Physical Therapy
University of Connecticut
Storrs, Connecticut

†Edward G. Tracy, PhD

Eeric Truumees, MD
Attending Spine Surgeon
Department of Orthopaedic Surgery
William Beaumont Hospital
Royal Oak, Michigan
Orthopaedic Director
Harold W. Gehring Center for Biomechanical Research
Adjunct Faculty
Bioengineering Center
Wayne State University
Detroit, Michigan

Tim L. Uhl, PT, PhD, ATC
Associate Professor
Division of Athletic Training
Director of Musculoskeletal Laboratory
College of Health Sciences
University of Kentucky
Lexington, Kentucky

Frank B. Underwood, PT, PhD, ECS
Professor of Physical Therapy
Department of Physical Therapy
University of Evansville
Evansville, Indiana

Victoria L. Veigl, PT, PhD
Assistant Professor
Division of Natural Science and Math
Jefferson Community and Technical College, Downtown Campus
Louisville, Kentucky

Brady Vibert, MD
Fellow in Spine Surgery
UCSD Medical Center
University of California–San Diego
San Diego, California

Michael L. Voight, PT, DHSc, OCS, SCS, ATC
Associate Professor
School of Physical Therapy
Belmont University
Nashville, Tennessee

†Deceased

BARRY L. WHITE, PT, MS, ECS, CNIM, DABNM
Director of Neurophysiological Services
Human Performance and Rehabilitation Centers, Inc.
Columbus, Georgia
(Retired)

J. MICHAEL WIATER, MD
Attending Shoulder and Elbow Surgeon
Department of Orthopaedic Surgery
William Beaumont Hospital
Royal Oak, Michigan
Beverly Hills Orthopaedic Surgery
Beverly Hills, Michigan

MARK WIEGAND, PT, PHD
Program Director/Department Chairperson
Bellarmine University Physical Therapy Program
Louisville, Kentucky

PATRICIA WILDER, PT, PHD
Professor Emeritus
Department of Health Professions
Program in Physical Therapy
University of Wisconsin–La Crosse
La Crosse, Wisconsin

ERIC WINT, PT, OCS
Regional Director
Physical Therapy Plus Orthopedic Clinic
Prospect, Kentucky
Lecturer in Orthopedics
Bellarmine University
Louisville, Kentucky

First Edition Contributors*

JEFF BALAZSY, MD
Chapter 77

HUGH L. BASSEWITZ, MD
Chapter 54

ALAN L. BIDDINGER, MD, PHD
Chapter 46 and 48

TURNER A. "TAB" BLACKBURN, JR, MED, PT
Chapter 71

PIERO CAPECCI, MD
Chapter 64 and 66

LISA DEPASQUALE, MS, PT
Chapter 53

MATTHEW DOBZYNIAK, MD
Chapter 44

GREGORY P. ERNST, PHD, PT
Chapter 69

ANNE HODGES, PT
Chapter 51

DAVID N. JOHNSON, MPT
Chapter 18

JOSEPH KAHN, PHD, PT
Chapter 11

TIM MCCARTHY, PT
Chapter 33

MAJOR MICHAEL PATRICK O'BRIEN, MD
Chapter 50 and 52

GREG RASH, EDD
Chapter 2

ROBERT A. WARD, MD, MS
Chapter 73

THOMAS W. WOLFF, MD
Chapter 51

*Material presented in this text includes questions from the first edition that were prepared by the contributors listed below.

Preface

We are pleased that the first edition of *Orthopaedic Physical Therapy Secrets* has become a standard study guide for the orthopaedic certification specialty examination. This text provides condensed, high-quality, preprocessed information that gets to the heart of orthopaedic examination, intervention, and outcomes. *Orthopaedic Physical Therapy Secrets* promotes the concept of efficient and effective practice and thus has also become a widely used, quick, and well-organized clinical resource guide.

We have included new, extremely detailed chapters covering differential diagnosis and radiology. These chapters are a direct reflection of the direction in which contemporary physical therapy practice is moving. Likewise, we have added significant detail to the chapters covering anatomy, orthopaedic neurology, pharmacology, and the evaluation of medical laboratory tests. As always, we have emphasized questions founded on sound outcome-based and evidence-based research.

Orthopaedic Physical Therapy Secrets has gathered experts from a wide variety of disciplines, including orthopaedic physical therapy, occupational therapy, orthopaedic surgery, radiology, rheumatology, spine surgery, sports medicine, exercise physiology, anesthesiology, and obstetrics/gynecology. This vast array of experts has made this text an exceptional, well-rounded quick reference and study guide for not only physical therapists, but also occupational therapists, athletic trainers, and primary care physicians.

We hope this text provides its readers insight into the rapidly advancing field of orthopaedic physical therapy, and ultimately, benefits and improves the quality of life in those so important to us . . . our patients.

Jeffrey D. Placzek, MD, PT
David A. Boyce, PT, EdD, ECS, OCS

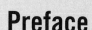

Contents

Section I

Basic Science

Chapter 1

Muscle Structure and Function

LeAnn Snow, MD, PhD, and
LaDora V. Thompson, PT, PhD

1. What is the organizational hierarchy of skeletal muscle?

- Muscle fascicles
  - Muscle fibers or cells
    - Myofibrils (arranged in parallel)
      - Sarcomeres (arranged in series)

2. Describe the characteristics of a sarcomere.

- In the middle of the sarcomere, the areas that appear dark are termed **anisotropic.** This portion of the sarcomere is known as the **A band.**
- Areas at the outer ends of each sarcomere appear light and are known as **I bands** because they are **isotropic** with respect to their birefringent properties.
- The **H band** is in the central region of the A band, where there is no myosin and actin filament overlap.
- The **H band** is bisected by the **M line,** which consists of proteins that keep the sarcomere in proper spatial orientation as it lengthens and shortens.
- At the ends of each sarcomere are the **Z disks.** The sarcomere length is the distance from one Z disk to the next.
- Optimal sarcomere length in mammalian muscle is 2.4 to 2.5 µm. The length of a sarcomere relative to its optimal length is of fundamental importance to the capacity for force generation.

3. What are the contractile and regulatory proteins?

The most prominent protein making up the myofibrillar fraction of skeletal muscle is **myosin,** which constitutes approximately one half of the total myofibrillar protein. The other contractile protein, **actin,** comprises about one fifth of the myofibrillar protein fraction. Other myofibrillar proteins include the regulatory proteins **tropomyosin** and **troponin complex.**

4. Name the structural proteins in skeletal muscle.

- C protein—part of the thick filament; involved in holding the tails of myosin in their correct spatial arrangement
- Titin—links the end of the thick filament to the Z disk
- M line protein—also known as myomesin; functions to keep the thick and thin filaments in their correct spatial arrangement
- α-Actinin—attaches actin filaments together at the Z disk
- Desmin—links Z disks of adjacent myofibrils together
- Spectrin and dystrophin—have structural and perhaps functional roles as sarcolemmal membrane proteins

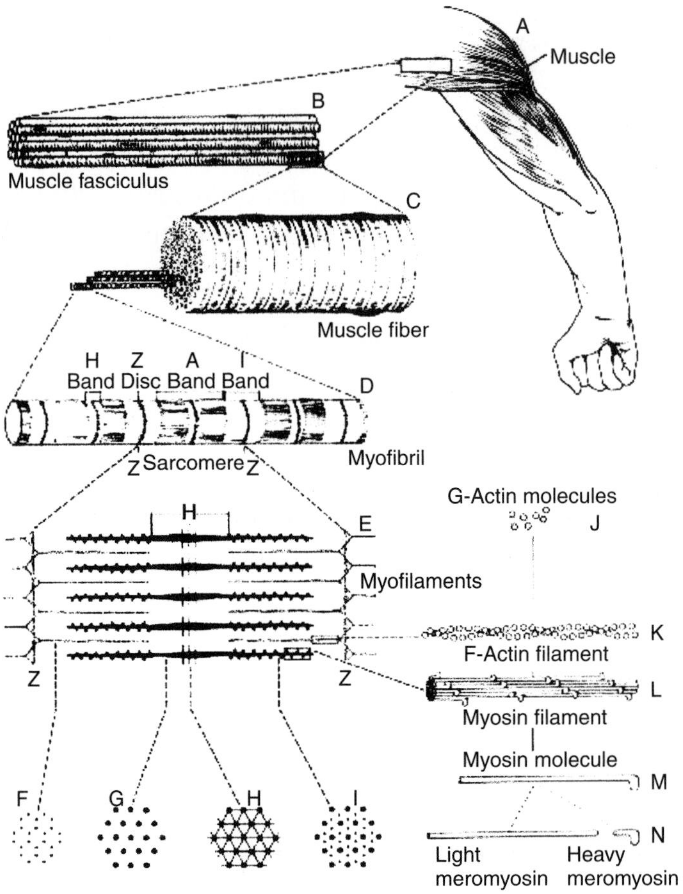

Organization of skeletal muscle, from the gross to the molecular level. F, G, H, and I are cross-sections at the levels indicated. (*Drawing by Sylvia Colard Keene. Modified from Bloom W, Fawcett DW:* A textbook of histology, *Philadelphia, 1986, WB Saunders.*)

5. What are the characteristics of myosin?

Myosin is of key importance for the development of muscular force and velocity of contraction. A myosin molecule is a relatively large protein (approximately 470 to 500 kD) composed of two identical myosin heavy chains (MHCs) (approximately 200 kD each) and four myosin light chains (MLCs) (16 to 20 kD each). In different muscle fibers, MHCs and MLCs are found in slightly different forms, called **isoforms.** The isoforms have small differences in some aspects of their structure that markedly influence the velocity of muscle contraction.

6. Describe the components of myosin.

Light-meromyosin (LMM) is the tail or backbone portion of the molecule, which intertwines with the tails of other myosin molecules to form a thick filament. Heavy-meromyosin (HMM) consists of two subfragments: S-1 and S-2. The S-2 portion of HMM projects out at an angle from LMM, and the S-1 portion is the globular head that can bind to actin. S-1 and S-2 together are also termed a **myosin cross-bridge.** There are approximately 300 molecules of myosin in 1 myofilament or thick filament. Approximately one half of the MHCs combine with their HMM at one end of the thick filament; the other half have their HMM toward the opposite end of the thick filament—a tail-to-tail arrangement. When molecules combine, they are rotated 60 degrees relative to the adjacent molecules and are offset slightly in the longitudinal plane. As a consequence of these three-dimensional structural factors, myosin has a characteristic bottlebrush appearance, with HMM projecting out along most of the filament.

7. Explain the role of the enzyme myosin adenosinetriphosphatase (ATPase).

A specialized portion of the MHC provides the primary molecular basis for the speed of muscular contraction. The **enzyme myosin ATPase** is located on the S-1 subfragment. In different fibers, the myosin ATPase can be one of several isoforms that range along a functional continuum from slow to fast. The predominant isoforms of MHC are the slow type I and the fast types IIa, IIx, and IIb.

8. What are the characteristics of actin?

Actin consists of approximately 350 monomers and 50 molecules of each of the regulatory proteins—tropomyosin and troponin. The actin monomers are termed **G-actin** because they are globular and have molecular weights of approximately 42 kD. G-actin normally is polymerized to **F-actin** (i.e., filamentous actin), which is arranged in a double helix. The polymerization from G-actin to F-actin involves the hydrolysis of ATP and the binding of adenosine diphosphate (ADP) to actin; 90% of ADP in skeletal muscle is bound to actin. The actin protein has a binding site that, when exposed, attaches to the myosin cross-bridge. The subsequent cycling of cross-bridges causes the development of muscular force. The actin filaments also join together to form the boundary between two sarcomeres in the area of the A band. **α-Actinin** is the protein that holds the actin filaments in the appropriate three-dimensional array.

9. Explain the sliding filament theory of muscle contraction.

A muscle shortens or lengthens because the myosin and actin myofilaments slide past each other without the filaments themselves changing length. The myosin cross-bridge projects out from the myosin tail and attaches to an actin monomer in the thin filament. The cross-bridges then move as **ratchets,** forcing the thin filaments toward the M line and causing a small amount of sarcomere shortening. The major structural rearrangement during contraction occurs in the region of the I band, which decreases markedly in size.

10. How is the hierarchical organization of skeletal muscle achieved?

The connective tissue that surrounds an entire muscle is called the **epimysium;** the membrane that binds fibers into fascicles is called the **perimysium.** Two separate membranes surround individual muscle fibers. The outer membrane of fibers has three names that are interchangeable: **basement membrane, endomysium,** or **basal lamina.** An additional, thin elastic membrane is found just beneath the basement membrane and is termed the **plasma membrane** or **sarcolemma.**

11. List the functions of myonuclei and satellite cells.

- Growth and development of muscle
- Adaptive capacity of skeletal muscle to various forms of training or disuse
- Recovery from exercise-induced or traumatic injury

12. What percentages of the nuclear material are myonuclei and satellite cells?

True myonuclei (located inside the plasma membrane) compose 85% to 95% of nuclear material with satellite cells (located between the basal lamina and plasma membrane) accounting for the remaining 5% to 15% of nuclear material.

13. How many nuclei are found in the skeletal muscle fiber?

There are approximately 200 to 3000 nuclei per millimeter of fiber length. This is in contrast to many other cells in the human body that have only a single nucleus.

14. What is the range of muscle fiber lengths?

Muscle fiber lengths range from a few millimeters in the intraocular muscles of the eye to >45 cm in the sartorius muscle.

15. Discuss the role of satellite cells in the formation of a new muscle fiber.

Satellite cells are normally dormant, but under conditions of stress or injury, they are essential for the regenerative growth of new fibers. Satellite cells have **chemotactic** properties, which means they migrate from one location to another area of higher need within a muscle fiber, and then undergo the normal process of developing a new muscle fiber. The process of new fiber formation begins with satellite cells entering a mitotic phase to produce additional satellite cells. These cells then migrate across the plasma membrane into the cytosol, where they recognize each other, align, and fuse into a **myotube,** an immature form of a muscle fiber. The multinucleated myotube then differentiates into a mature fiber.

16. Identify and define or describe muscle growth factors.

Muscle growth factors are proteins that either promote muscle growth and repair or inhibit muscle protein breakdown. Examples include insulin-like growth factors, fibroblast growth factor, hepatocyte growth factor, and transforming growth factors.

17. What are the characteristics of myofibrils?

Individual **myofibrils** are approximately 1 μm in diameter and comprise approximately 80% of the volume of a whole muscle. The number of myofibrils is a regulated variable during the hypertrophy of muscle fibers associated with growth; for example, the number of myofibrils ranges from 50 per muscle fiber in the muscles of a fetus to approximately 2000 per fiber in the muscles of an untrained adult. The hypertrophy and atrophy of adult skeletal muscle are associated with certain types of training and disuse and result from the regulation of the number of myofibrils per fiber. Training and disuse have negligible effects on the number of fibers in mammals.

18. Describe the characteristics of individual muscle fibers.

The cross-sectional area of an individual muscle **fiber** ranges from approximately 2000 to 7500 μm^2, with the mean and median in the 3000- to 4000-μm^2 range. Muscle fiber and muscle lengths vary considerably. For example, the length of the medial gastrocnemius muscle is approximately 250 mm, with fiber lengths of 35 mm, whereas the sartorius muscle is approximately 500 mm, with fiber lengths of 450 mm. The number of fibers ranges from several hundred in small muscles to >1 million in large muscles, such as those involved in hip flexion and knee extension.

19. Discuss the relationship between the size of the cell and diffusion of important nutrients.

The **radius** of muscle cells (typically 25 to 50 μm) is an important variable for sustained muscular performance because it affects the diffusion distance from the capillary network (which is exterior to the muscle cell) to the cell's interior. As the radius of muscle cells increases, the distance through which gases, such as oxygen, must travel to diffuse from the capillary blood to the center of the muscle cell increases. This can be a problem, limiting the muscle's ability to sustain endurance exercise, because **sufficient oxygen delivery** is needed for the mitochondria, where most energy for muscle contraction is produced.

20. What is a strap or fusiform muscle?

Muscles that have a **parallel-fiber** arrangement are strap or fusiform muscles. In a parallel-fiber muscle, the muscle fibers are arranged essentially in parallel with the longitudinal axis of the muscle itself. Muscles with a parallel-fiber arrangement generally produce a greater range of motion (ROM) and greater joint velocity than muscles with the same cross-sectional area but with a different fiber arrangement.

21. List examples of fusiform muscles.

- Sartorius
- Biceps brachii
- Sternohyoid

22. Explain the role of pennation in force production.

When muscles are designed with angles of pennation, which is the most common architecture, **more sarcomeres** can be packed in parallel between the origin and insertion of the muscle. By packing more sarcomeres in a muscle, **more force** can be developed. As the angle of pennation increases, an increasing portion of the force developed by sarcomeres is displaced away from the tendons. As long as the angle of pennation is <30 degrees, the force lost as a result of the angle of pennation is more than compensated for by the increased packing of sarcomeres in parallel, producing an overall benefit to the force-producing capacity of muscle.

23. Describe the differences among unipennate, bipennate, and multipennate muscles.

- In **unipennate** muscles, such as the flexor pollicis longus, the obliquely set fasciculi fan out on only one side of a central muscle tendon.
- In a **bipennate** muscle, such as the gastrocnemius, the fibers are obliquely set on both sides of a central tendon.
- In a **multipennate** muscle, such as the deltoid, the fibers converge on several tendons.

24. Define the force-velocity relationship.

The muscle shortens at different velocities depending on the load placed on the muscle. As the load is increased, the velocity decreases. When the load exceeds the maximal force capable of being developed by the muscle, a lengthening contraction ensues. The force developed during a shortening contraction is less than the isometric force. The force developed during a lengthening contraction exceeds the isometric force by 50% to 100% because of the increased extension of the attached cross-bridges.

25. Describe additional factors influencing muscle strength.

Myosin structural state, the ratio of strong binding and weak binding cross-bridges to actin, muscle innervation, motor unit recruitment, and synchronization are all factors influencing muscle strength.

26. What is active insufficiency at the sarcomere level?

Active insufficiency is the diminished ability of a muscle to produce or maintain active tension when a muscle is elongated to a point at which there is no overlap between myosin and actin or when the muscle is excessively shortened.

27. What is active insufficiency at the muscle level?

This type of insufficiency is most commonly encountered when the full ROM is attempted simultaneously at all joints crossed by a two-joint or multijoint muscle. During active shortening, a two-joint muscle becomes actively insufficient at a point before the end of a joint range, when full ROM at all joints occurs simultaneously. Active insufficiency also may occur in one-joint muscles but is not common.

28. Define excitation-contraction coupling.

Excitation-contraction coupling is the physiologic mechanism whereby an electric discharge at the muscle initiates the chemical events that lead to contraction.

29. Summarize how excitation-contraction coupling occurs in skeletal muscle.

1. Action potentials in the alpha motor neuron propagate down the axon to the axon terminals.
2. Acetylcholine, the neurotransmitter at the neuromuscular junction, is released from the axon terminals.
3. Acetylcholine diffuses across the neuromuscular junction and binds with acetylcholine receptors on the sarcolemma of the muscle.
4. A muscle action potential is generated at the motor end plate.
5. The muscle action potential travels along the sarcolemma and into the depths of the transverse tubules, which are continuous with the sarcolemma.
6. The action potential (voltage change) is sensed by the dihydropyridine receptors in the transverse tubules.
7. The dihydropyridine receptors communicate with the ryanodine receptors of the sarcoplasmic reticulum, a mechanism poorly understood.
8. Calcium is released from the sarcoplasmic reticulum through the ryanodine receptors.
9. Calcium binds to the regulatory protein troponin C, and the interaction between actin and myosin can occur.
10. Myosin cross-bridges, previously activated by the hydrolysis of ATP, attach to actin.
11. The myosin cross-bridges move into a strong binding state, and force production occurs.

30. What are the characteristics of the different skeletal muscle fiber types?

31. Define type IIx myosin heavy chain in human fibers.

The type IIx myosin heavy chain was first described in animals (rat, mouse). Type IIx myofibers have maximal shortening velocity and maximal isometric tension that are intermediate between types IIa and IIb. The fiber type IIb in animals is not found in humans. Rather, the type IIb that is described in humans has a myosin composition very similar to that of type IIx.

32. Define muscle spindles and their function in muscular dynamics and limb movement.

Muscle spindles provide sensory information concerning changes in the length and tension of the muscle fibers. Their main function is to respond to stretch of a muscle and, through reflex action, to produce a stronger contraction to reduce the stretch.

33. Describe the appearance of the muscle spindle.

The **spindle** is fusiform in shape and is attached in parallel to the regular or extrafusal fibers of the muscle. Consequently, when the muscle is stretched, so is the spindle. There are more spindles in muscles that perform complex movements. There are two specialized cells within the spindle, called **intrafusal fibers.** There are two sensory afferents and one motor efferent innervating the intrafusal fibers. The gamma efferent innervates the contractile portion—the striated ends of the spindle. These fibers, activated by higher cortex levels, provide the mechanism for maintaining the spindle at peak operation at all muscle lengths.

34. Discuss the function of the Golgi tendon organs.

Connected in series to 25 extrafusal fibers, these sensory receptors also are located in the ligaments of joints and are primarily responsible for detecting differences in muscle tension. The Golgi tendon organs respond as a feedback monitor to discharge impulses under one of two conditions: (1) in response to tension created in the muscle when it shortens and (2) in response to tension when the muscle is passively stretched. Excessive tension or stretch on a muscle activates the tendon's Golgi receptors. This causes a reflex inhibition of the muscles they supply. The Golgi tendon organ functions as a protective sensory mechanism to detect and inhibit subsequently undue strain within the muscle-tendon structure.

35. Describe the adaptations in muscle structure with progressive resistance exercises.

The major adaptation is an increase in the cross-sectional area of muscle, which is termed **hypertrophy.** The number of muscle fibers is minimally affected. Progressive resistive exercise involves 10 repetitions a day at 60% to 90% of maximal capacity; this results in an increase in strength by 0.5% to 1.0% per day over a period of several weeks. The fast-twitch type II fibers are more responsive to progressive resistance exercise than slow-twitch type I fibers. There are increases in the amounts of transverse tubular and sarcoplasmic reticulum membranes as well. There are neural adaptations, which result in an increased ability to recruit high-threshold motor units. The functional significance of the morphologic change is primarily a greater capacity for strength and power development.

Motor Unit Type and Muscle Fiber Types in the Motor Unit

Property	I (S) (SO)	IIa (FR) (FOG)	IIb (FF) (FG)
Contraction speed	Slow	Fast	Fast
Force production	Small	Intermediate	Large
Fatigue resistance	High	High (intermediate)	Low
Fiber diameter	Small	Intermediate	Large
Red color	Dark	Dark	Pale
Myoglobin	High	High	Low
Capillary supply	Rich	Rich	Poor
Respiration type	Aerobic	Aerobic	Anaerobic
Mitochondria	Many	Many	Few
Z line thickness	Intermediate (wide)	Wide (intermediate)	Narrow
Glycogen content	Low	High (intermediate)	High
Alkaline ATPase	Low	High	High
Acid ATPase	High	Low	Moderate
Oxidative capacity	High	Medium-high	Low
Glycolytic ability	Low	High	High

36. List the effects of progressive resistance exercise.

- Increased mass and strength
- Increased cross-sectional area of muscle (increased number of myofibrils, leading to hypertrophy)
- Increased type I and type II fiber area
- Decreased mitochondrial density per fiber and oxidative capacity
- Increased intracellular lipids and capacity to use lipids as fuel
- Increased intracellular glycogen and glycolytic capacity
- Increased intramuscular high-energy phosphate pool and improved phosphagen metabolism

37. Describe the adaptations in muscle structure with endurance exercises.

Endurance exercise has minimal impact on the cross-sectional area of muscle and muscle fibers. The smaller cross-sectional area allows better diffusion of metabolites and nutrients between the contractile filaments and the cytoplasm and between the cytoplasm and the interstitial fluid. There is a decrease in fatigability. The number of capillaries increases around each fiber, and there is an increase in mitochondria, especially in the type I fibers. The increased mitochondria can provide a good supply of ATP during exercise. The more extensive capillary bed improves the delivery of oxygen and circulating energy sources to the fibers, whereas the products of muscle activity are removed more efficiently. The functional significance of these changes is observed during sustained exercise, in which there is a delay in the onset of fatigue.

38. List the effects of endurance exercise.

- Improved ability to obtain ATP from oxidative phosphorylation
- Increased size and number of mitochondria
- Less lactic acid produced per given amount of exercise
- Increased myoglobin content
- Increased intramuscular triglyceride content
- Increased lipoprotein lipase (enzyme needed to use lipids from blood)
- Increased proportion of energy derived from fat; less from carbohydrates
- Lower rate of glycogen depletion during exercise
- Improved efficiency in extracting oxygen from blood
- Decreased number of type IIb fibers; increased number of type IIa fibers

39. What are the consequences of muscle disuse?

- The most striking consequence is **atrophy**—a reduction in muscle and muscle fiber cross-sectional area.
- The slow type I fibers show greater atrophy with disuse than the fast type II fibers.
- A few fibers undergo necrosis, and there is an increase in the endomysial and perimysial connective tissue.
- The muscles develop smaller twitch and tetanic tensions, beyond those expected on the basis of fiber atrophy.
- There is an increase in fatigability.
- There is a tendency for slow-twitch fibers to be transformed into fast-twitch fibers, with changes in the isoforms of the myofibrillar proteins.
- In the sarcolemma, there is a spread of acetylcholine receptors beyond the neuromuscular junction, and the resting membrane potential is diminished.
- The motor nerve terminals are abnormal in showing signs of degeneration in some places and evidence of sprouting in others.
- There is a loss of motor drive, such that the motor units cannot be recruited fully.

40. What physiologic adaptations occur if muscles are immobilized in a shortened position?

- Decrease in the number of sarcomeres
- Increase in the amount of perimysium
- Thickening of endomysium
- Increase in ratio of collagen concentration
- Increase in ratio of connective tissue to muscle fiber tissue
- Atrophy

41. List the changes that result from muscles being immobilized in a shortened position.

- Altered strength
- Increased stiffness to passive stretch
- Increased fatigability

42. What occurs as a result of lengthening the muscles?

Sarcomeres are added.

43. Does muscle splitting occur, or can there be an increase in the number of cells (hyperplasia)?

Hyperplasia, defined as an increase in fiber number, generally does not occur. Individual fiber splitting may occur in specific pathologic conditions, such as neuromuscular diseases.

44. Define disease-associated muscle atrophy, such as cachexia.

Disease-associated muscle atrophy is due to accelerated proteolysis. This form of skeletal muscle atrophy is systemic and associated with metabolic and/or inflammatory factors.

45. Differentiate apoptosis from necrosis as applied to skeletal muscle.

Apoptosis, or programmed cell death, is a regulated physiologic process critical to cellular homeostasis, which can become dysregulated, leading to disease states including muscle disease or dysfunction. Apoptosis results in cell shrinkage, DNA fragmentation, membrane blebbing, and disassembly into apoptotic bodies (membrane-bound cell fragments). Necrosis is a pathologic process caused by the progressive degradative action of enzymes that is generally associated with severe cellular trauma in muscles, leading to cell death.

46. Can changes in muscle temperature be beneficial?

Changes can be advantageous as well as deleterious to individuals. Before starting an exercise program, the **warming-up** period can have several beneficial effects. When a muscle warms up, it takes advantage of the local Q_{10} effect. $\mathbf{Q_{10}}$ is the ratio of the rate of a physiologic process at a particular temperature to the rate at a temperature 10° C lower, when the logarithm of the rate is an approximately linear function of temperature. Physiologically, the warming-up period can increase the speed of particular enzymatic processes in muscles through the Q_{10} effect.

Temperatures >40° C have been observed to decrease the efficiency of oxygen use in muscle.

Bibliography

Bagshaw CR: *Muscle contraction,* ed 2, London, 1993, Chapman & Hall.
Brooks S: Current topics for teaching skeletal muscle physiology, *Adv Physiol Educ* 27:171-182, 2003.
Enoka RM: *Neuromechanics of human movement,* ed 3, Champaign, Ill, 2002, Human Kinetics Publishers.

Franzini-Armstrong C, Engel A: *Myology*, ed 3, New York, 2004, McGraw-Hill.
Hawke TJ: Muscle stem cells and exercise training, *Exercise Sport Sci Rev* 33:63-68, 2005.
Jones DA, Round JM, deHaan A: *Skeletal muscle from molecules to movement,* Edinburgh, 2004, Churchill Livingstone.
Lieber RL: *Skeletal muscle structure, function, & plasticity: The physiological basis of rehabilitation,* ed 2, Baltimore, 2002, Lippincott Williams & Wilkins.
McArdle WD, Katch FI, Katch VL: *Exercise physiology: Energy, nutrition and human performance,* ed 5, Baltimore, 2001, Lippincott Williams & Wilkins.
Schiaffino S, Reggiani C: Molecular diversity of myofibrillar proteins: Gene regulation and functional significance, *Physiol Rev* 76:371-423, 1996.

Chapter 2

Biomechanics

Sean P. Flanagan, PhD, ATC, CSCS, and Kornelia Kulig, PT, PhD

1. Define the terms biomechanics and kinesiology.

Biomechanics is the study of the structure and function of biological systems by the methods of mechanics. Mechanics is a branch of physics that is concerned with the analysis of the action of forces on matter or material systems.

The term **kinesiology** combines two Greek words—**kinein,** which means to move, and **logos,** which means to discourse. Therefore kinesiology is the discourse of movement or the science of movement of the body. Because human movement is an expression of complex musculoskeletal, neural, and cardiovascular biological systems, kinesiology encompasses the sciences underlying the study of those systems.

2. Define the term kinematics.

Kinematics is the study of the geometry of motion without reference to the cause of motion. Kinematics is the analytical and mathematical description of motion (e.g., position, displacement, velocity, acceleration, and time). Displacement, velocity, and acceleration are vector quantities (they have magnitude and direction) and can be linear or angular in nature.

3. What is the difference between osteokinematics and arthrokinematics?

Osteokinematics describes the motion of bones around an axis. By convention, the motion is referenced relative to sagittal, frontal, and/or transverse planes. Terms such as flexion, extension, abduction, adduction, internal rotation, and external rotation are used to describe osteokinematics. Arthrokinematics describes the motion that occurs between the articular surfaces of the two bones of a joint. Terms such as spin, roll, and glide are used to describe arthrokinematics.

4. What are the various types of levers?

A **class 1 lever** has the axis of rotation between the resistance and effort (e.g., seesaw or scissors), and a **class 2 lever** has the resistance between the axis and effort (e.g., bottle opener or wheelbarrow). An example of a class 1 lever in the body is the head on the spinal column, and it is questionable whether there are any class 2 levers in the body (possibly the gastrocnemius/soleus attachment onto the calcaneus). A **class 3 lever** is one in which the effort is between the axis of rotation and the resistance to overcome (e.g., elbow [axis], biceps [effort], and weight [resistance] in a curl). This configuration provides us with the ability to move a resistance through a larger range of motion (moving through a greater range allows for greater speed of movement) but at the expense of using a greater force than the resistance we are overcoming.

5. What is the relation between the linear motion at the joint surface and the angular motion of a bone around the joint axis?

A theoretical construct, developed to describe this relation and advocated by Kaltenborn, is known as the **convex-concave rule.** In brief, if the convex surface of one bone is moving on the fixed concave surface of another bone, rotation and translation will occur in opposite directions. Additionally, if the concave surface of one bone is moving on the fixed convex surface of another bone, rotation and translation occur in the same direction. This rule should be appreciated when joint mobilizations are performed. It is proposed that in order to restore rotational motion at a joint, a linear mobilization is performed in relation to the treatment plane (in the concave joint surface) and in accordance with the convex-concave rule.

6. Has the convex-concave rule been experimentally verified?

No, at least not for all joints. For example, it has been demonstrated that the glenohumeral joint contradicts the convex-concave rule during external rotation when the humerus is abducted to 90 degrees, and there is no clear consensus that the femur translates anteriorly when the knee is flexing in a weight-bearing position. However, these findings may not violate the convex-concave rule if the amount of translation in the direction of rolling is less than what the curvature of the convex segment would predict. The amount of rolling in one direction may be greater than the sliding in the opposite direction. Furthermore, pathologic joints (e.g., ACL-deficient knees) have different arthrokinematics than normal joints. Further research is necessary, and the rationale for manual therapy techniques may have to be modified, for different joints, different motions of the same joint, and/or pathologic joints.

7. Where is the location of the joint axis of rotation?

The axis of rotation (AOR) must be determined experimentally, because the AOR may be located within the joint or outside the two bones composing a joint. In a nonpathologic joint, the AOR is generally within the convex joint member and may stay in the same location (fixed AOR). A degenerated joint may lose its integrity and the AOR may change its location throughout the range of motion. To reflect that change, the axis (or center) of rotation is called the instantaneous axis (or center) of rotation.

8. Why is it important to know the axis of rotation?

Knowing the location of the AOR is important for at least three reasons. First, motion will occur in a cardinal plane only if the AOR is perpendicular to that plane; otherwise, motion will occur in two or all three planes of motion. Second, a muscle's function is governed by the orientation of its line of pull with respect to the AOR of a joint. Third, when quantifying joint range of motion, the AOR of the goniometer should be aligned with the AOR of the joint.

9. What is the difference between an absolute and a relative joint angle?

An absolute angle is the angle that the distal point of a segment (e.g., foot, shank, thigh) makes with respect to some reference line (such as the horizontal for sagittal plane movements). A relative angle is the joint angle made by two segments (e.g., the knee angle is the angle between the shank and thigh). Relative angles can be stated as either internal (included) or external (anatomic) angles. An internal angle is the angle between the longitudinal axes of the two segments comprising a joint, while the external angle is the angular displacement from the anatomic position. For example, in the anatomic position, the internal knee angle is 180 degrees, while the external angle is 0 degrees. If this angle were decreased by 30 degrees, the internal angle would be 150 degrees while the external angle would be 30 degrees (see figure).

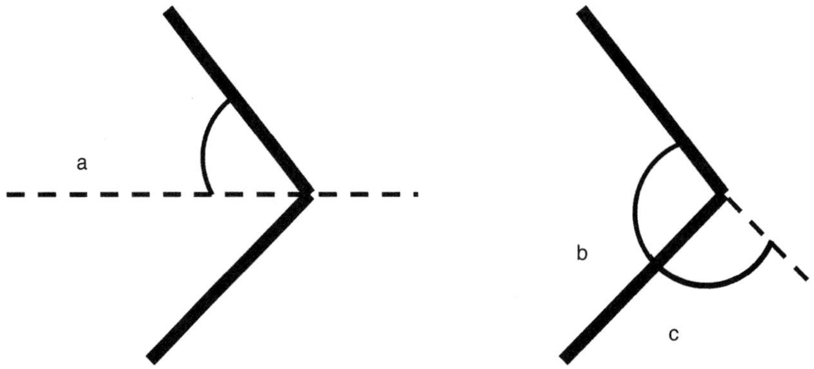

A graphic depiction of the three types of angles: **a**, absolute angle from the horizontal; **b**, relative, internal angle; **c**, relative, external angle.

It is important to understand the distinction between these three measures and to be consistent in their use. In observational gait analysis, for example, ankle and knee measures are usually external, relative angles while the thigh is usually an absolute angle with respect to the vertical; many motion capture systems, on the other hand, report internal angles for all three joints.

10. How are force and strength related? Define commonly used biomechanical terms and equations.

Force is a push or pull of one object on another. Force is a vector quantity, having both a magnitude and a direction. Strength may be thought of as the ability to produce or absorb force.

11. Does the amplitude of the electromyography (EMG) signal quantify a muscle's force-producing (absorbing) capability?

No. A muscle's force-producing (absorbing) capability is primarily determined by the:

- Type of muscle action (concentric, eccentric, isometric)
- Length of muscle (force-velocity relation)
- Physiologic cross-sectional area of the muscle
- Number of motor units within a muscle that are activated (intramuscular coordination)
- Rate of motor unit activation (rate-coding)
- Intrinsic force-generating capability of the muscle (specific tension)
- Contractile history of the muscle (e.g., prestretch)

Common Biomechanical Terms and Equations

Term (Linear; Angular)	Physical Meaning	Equation: Linear	Equation: Angular	Units: Linear (Metric, English)	Units: Angular (Metric, English)
Displacement (Δx; $\Delta\theta$)	A change in position	$x_2 - x_1$	$\theta_2 - \theta_1$	m ft	deg rad
Velocity (v; ω)	A change in displacement with respect to a change in time	$\Delta x/\Delta t$	$\Delta\theta/\Delta t$	m/sec ft/sec	deg/sec rad/sec
Acceleration (a; α)	A change in velocity with respect to a change in time	$\Delta v/\Delta t$	$\Delta\omega/\Delta t$	m/sec^2 ft/sec^2	deg/sec^2 rad/sec^2
Force; Moment (F; M)	A push or pull by one object on another object	$\sum F = ma$	$\sum M = I\alpha$	N lb	N-m lb-ft
Momentum (H; L)	Resistance to change in velocity	$H = mv$	$L = I\omega$	kg•m/sec	kg•m^2/sec
Impulse (I)	Effect of a force during the time the force acts	$\int F\,dt$	$\int M\,dt$	N-s lb-sec	N-m-sec lb-ft-sec
Work (W)	A change in energy	$\int F\,dx$	$\int M\,d\theta$	J ft-lb	
Gravitational potential energy	Energy caused by position	mgh		J	
Elastic potential energy	Energy caused by deformation	$\frac{1}{2}ks^2$		J	
Kinetic energy	Energy caused by motion	$\frac{1}{2}mv^2$	$\frac{1}{2}I\omega^2$	J	
Power (P)	Time rate of doing work	$\Delta W/\Delta t$		W hp	
Stress (Pressure) σ	Magnitude of force dispersed over an area	F/A		N/m^2 lb/in^2	
Strain	Amount of deformation	$\Delta L/L_0$		Unitless measure	

The EMG signal quantifies the number of motor units and their rate of activation within the electrode field. In addition, because electrode placement can affect the number of motor units within the field, it is important to compare relative values (usually normalized to a maximum voluntary isometric contraction) rather an absolute values when comparing differences in EMG signals.

12. Explain why it is useful to identify the components of a force.

Just as forces can be combined together to determine a resultant, they can also be broken into their **components.** The components are useful in identifying the different effects of a force on a joint. For example, a muscle force can be divided into the component that is perpendicular to the bone (causing it to rotate) and the component that is parallel to the bone (usually increasing the compressive force across a joint). Therefore in addition to causing movement at a joint, all muscle forces will affect the amount of compression at a joint. During rehabilitation of certain joint pathologies, it may be necessary to identify which therapeutic exercises will increase the force of a muscle (to strengthen it) without applying harmful compressive forces across the joint.

13. Explain how impulse can be manipulated in order to prevent injury.

Impulse is the area under the force-time curve, and accounts not only for the magnitude of the force but also for the duration over which the force is applied. Impulse determines the change in a body's **momentum,** which is the product of mass and velocity. Applying a smaller force over a longer period of time will have the same impulse (and effect on a body's momentum) as applying a larger force over a shorter period of time. Increasing the time of the impact, which can be accomplished by cushioned shoes and/or bending the knees when making contact with the ground, can attenuate the magnitude of an impact force, and may decrease the risk of injury.

14. What concept is analogous to force for angular motion?

The moment of a force (**"moment"** for short), or torque, is the turning effect of a force. A force will have a tendency to rotate a body according to its magnitude, its direction, and the perpendicular distance between its line of application and the axis of rotation. (This perpendicular distance is known as the **moment arm.**) As with a resultant force, it is the resultant moment that will ultimately determine the rotation of a body. Human movement occurs as a result of muscle forces producing a resultant moment about a joint axis of rotation. Even linear movement is a result of the coordinated rotation of two or more joints.

15. Provide examples of the concept of moment.

Knowing that the moment is the product of the force and the moment arm, the length of the moment arm can be manipulated to increase or decrease the force required to complete a task. For example, low back injury prevention strategies are based on the premise of decreasing the moment about the low back during lifting by keeping the load as close to the spine as possible, thus reducing the moment arm of the external resistance. Similarly, flexing the elbows during abduction will decrease the moment arm about the shoulder, thus making the movement easier to perform. On the other hand, during manual muscle testing, the therapist can increase the demand on a muscle by applying the resistance as far from the axis of rotation as possible.

16. When a study recommends a particular exercise because it produces a high net joint moment, what does that mean?

One of the greatest limitations in biomechanics is that we cannot, with current technology, measure muscle forces in a noninvasive way. However, we can measure the acceleration of the limbs, and forces between the body and the ground to calculate the net joint moment (NJM), which is the moment required to accelerate a limb in accordance with Newton's second law. Despite the fact that muscles and other soft tissue structures contribute to the NJM, and co-contractions of the antagonists can make the actual moment much greater than the NJM, we usually equate high NJMs with high muscle forces needed to produce that moment. So when a research study suggests that exercise A has a greater extensor NJM at the knee than exercise B, it assumes that there is no co-contraction of the hamstrings during both exercises, and exercise A has a higher demand on the quadriceps.

17. What are the benefits of having three different types of muscle actions?

Skeletal muscles are required to produce force, reduce (or absorb) force, or stabilize against a force. There is a different type of muscle action to fulfill each of these roles. A concentric muscle action produces force—the muscle moment is greater than the moment of an external force, and movement occurs in the direction of the muscle moment. An eccentric muscle action reduces force—the muscle moment is less than the moment of an external force, and movement occurs in the direction opposite of the muscle moment. The eccentric muscle action reduces the external force, and consequently decreases the acceleration caused by it. An isometric muscle action stabilizes against a force—the muscle moment is equal and opposite to the moment created by an external force, and no movement occurs.

18. What information can be obtained from studying the force-velocity curve?

Examining this relation reveals that greater force can be produced isometrically (when the velocity is zero) than can be produced concentrically, and greater force can be produced eccentrically than can be produced isometrically (see figure).

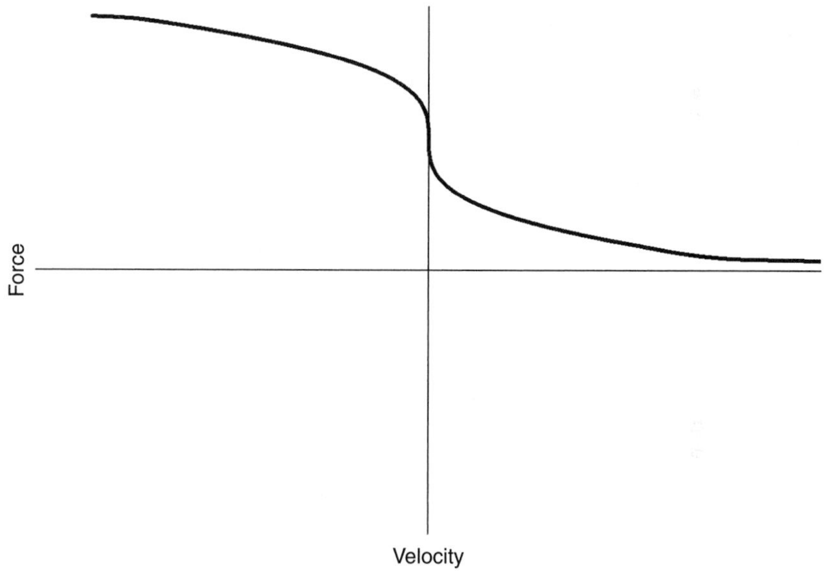

The force-velocity relation.

Peak eccentric force is estimated to be between 120% and 140% of peak concentric force. Additionally, there is a negative relation between force and velocity in the concentric range, while there is a positive relation between force and velocity in the eccentric range.

19. Is there a mechanical variable that can identify the type of muscle actions?

Yes; mechanical power is the product of the net joint moment and the angular velocity. If the NJM and the angular velocity are in the same direction, the power is positive and a concentric muscle action is controlling the velocity. If the NJM and angular velocity are in opposite directions, the work is negative and an eccentric muscle action is controlling the velocity. If there is an NJM but no angular velocity, the power is zero because there is no angular velocity, but the presence of an NJM indicates an isometric muscle action is preventing a velocity.

20. Why is eccentric strength important in the prevention of injury?

While energy can be absorbed by all of the tissues of the body (e.g., bone, ligament, muscle-tendon), the muscle-tendon complex has the greatest potential to safely absorb or distribute energy within the body. Eccentric muscle actions are the primary means by which energy is safely absorbed by the body. If the muscles are not strong enough, then other tissues must absorb this energy. Because the other tissues are not as capable of absorbing or distributing energy, energy levels can quickly exceed the tissues' limits, resulting in injury.

21. Is the definition of joint instability defined consistently throughout the clinical literature?

No, and that makes interpretation of different studies difficult. Investigators and clinicians have used at least three definitions: (1) excessive and occasionally uncontrolled range of motion resulting in frank joint dislocation; (2) small, abnormal movement in an otherwise normal range of motion that may result in pain because of "impingement" at the joint; and (3) a small amount of force necessary to move a joint through its range of motion (or low stiffness).

22. What factors determine if a force, or load, will cause an injury?

Several factors combine to determine the location, severity, and type of injury, including the:
- Magnitude
- Rate
- Duration
- Frequency
- Variability
- Location
- Direction

23. What is pressure, and how does it relate to pressure sores?

Pressure is force per unit area. The insensate and poorly vascularized foot, in association with connective tissue changes, is vulnerable to increases in pressure and consequently the development of pressure sores. If the body weight transmitted to the foot can be dispersed over a larger surface area of the foot, the magnitude of pressure is decreased as is the chance for ulceration. The same factors apply to a person confined to prolonged bed rest; pressure sores may develop on areas where bony prominences contact the bed.

24. Is patellofemoral pain related to pressure between the patella and femur?

Yes; this is likely the mechanical component of this symptom. However, a certain amount of pressure applied to cartilage is normal and desirable. The degree of pressure is governed by the amount of quadriceps contraction (producing stress or force) and the amount of contact between the patella and the femur. The smaller contact area seems to have a stronger relationship to symptoms than does the increased amount of force.

25. Do human tissues respond to all stresses the same way?

No. Depending on the tissue and its role, tissues respond quite differently, and this difference in response is called **anisotropic.** For example, tendon responds well to tension, not as well to shear, and not at all to compression. Cartilage, on the other hand, responds well to compression. Human bone can handle **compressive force** best (such as pushing both ends of the bone toward each other), followed by **tension** (such as pulling both ends of the bone away from each other) and then **shear** forces (such as pushing the top of the bone to the right and the bottom of the bone to the left). A **bending force** basically subjects one side of the bone to compression, while the other side experiences tension; therefore the side subjected to tension usually fails first (immature bone may fail in compression first). For **torsional loading** (such as twisting the top part of the bone, while holding the bottom of the bone fixed), fracture patterns typically show that the bone fails as a result of shear forces, and then tension.

26. Is stress the same as pressure?

It depends on whom you ask. Both determine the intensity of loading, and are quantified as force per unit area. Some scientists maintain that pressure represents the distribution of force external to a body and stress represents the distribution of force inside a body. Others maintain that pressure should be used in reference to fluids, while stress should be used in reference to solids. In orthopaedics, both are often used interchangeably.

27. What is the tissue response to a force (stress), and how is it measured?

The tissue response to a force (or load) is **deformation,** which is a change in the size or shape of the tissue. Deformation is usually expressed as the quotient of the change in tissue length divided by the tissue's original length, or **strain.** Laboratory experiments usually apply a given force (N) to a tissue of known cross-sectional area (mm^2) and specified length (mm), in which the resulting deformation (mm) is measured. Simple calculations will produce the applied stress and resulting strain.

28. Can tissue responses to stress be measured in vivo, and if so, how is that accomplished?

Yes; they can be measured in vivo but not in all tissues. For example, musculotendinous units are accessible to testing in vivo, but cartilage is not. The force, either exerted by subject (active) or caused by an apparatus (passive), is measured using a dynamometer and the deformation (here displacement) is measured using an imaging technique (i.e., ultrasound).

29. What information can be ascertained from studying stress-strain curves?

Plotting the stress (force per area) on the vertical axis and the corresponding strain (deformation) on the horizontal axis produces a stress-strain (force-deformation) curve, which graphically represents the relation between the two (see figure).

Several important qualities can be determined from this curve, including the tissue's:

- **Ultimate strength**—the point on the curve where the tissue fails
- **Yield point**—the point at which a permanent deformation occurs
- **Elastic region**—the portion of the curve preceding the yield point
- **Plastic region**—the portion of the curve following the yield point
- **Stiffness**—the slope of the curve in the elastic range, also known as Young's modulus
- **Energy**—the area under the curve

30. When the force is applied to the tissue externally, does the tissue return to its original state after the force is removed?

It depends on the amount of force applied. At lower levels of force the tissue returns to its original form, and therefore this stage is called the **elastic region.** It is in the elastic region that the characteristics of the tissue are stable and therefore are used to describe the tissues with a modulus. This **Young's modulus** is the change in stress over the change in strain during the elastic (or linear) range of the stress-strain testing.

If the force continues to increase, it reaches a transitional point—the **yield point.** The yield point is where the material changes from the elastic range to the **plastic range.** Beyond this yield point, permanent deformation will occur even after the load is removed.

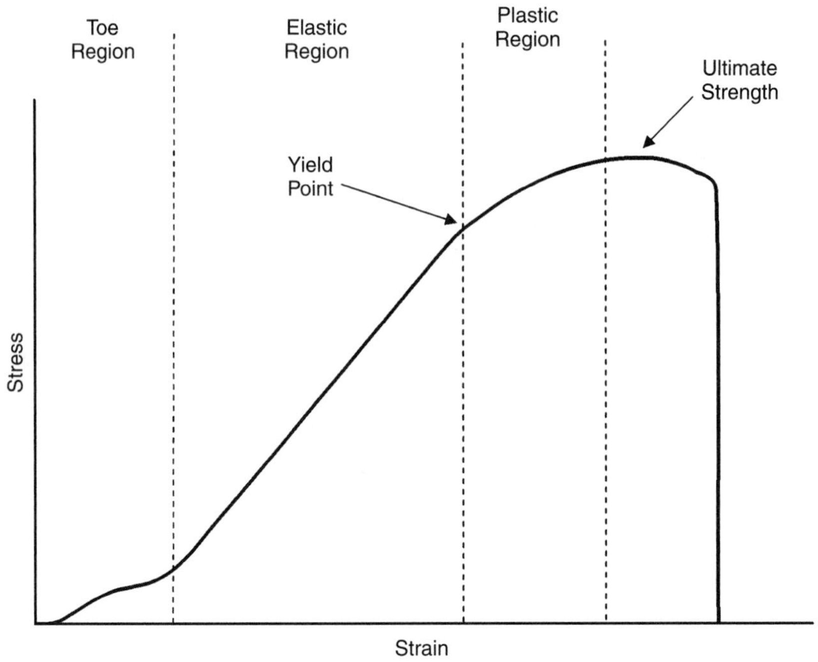

The stress-strain relation.

31. Give an example of the clinical implications of the stress-strain curve.

The stress-strain curve can be appreciated clinically most easily during ligamentous testing. If the injurious force did not exceed the yield point, the ligament would return to its original length with no detectable changes in joint laxity. This injury would be classified as a first-degree sprain. If the injurious force exceeded the yield point but did not reach the ultimate strength of the ligament, the ligament would experience a permanent deformation that would be manifested as an increase in joint laxity. This injury would be classified as a second-degree sprain. If the injurious force exceeded the ultimate strength of the ligament, the ligament would catastrophically fail and the subsequent force applied during ligamentous testing would be met with no resistance. This injury would be classified as a third-degree sprain.

32. Are tissue responses to a submaximal stress time dependent?

Yes; tissue responses do change with time of application. Even if the amount of load is in the elastic range, but it is applied for a longer time, it will continue to cause a deformation. This type of deformation is reversible and it is called **creep.** Creep is caused by the exudation of interstitial fluid. The fluid exits most rapidly at first and diminishes gradually over time. Human cartilage takes 4 to 16 hours to reach **creep equilibrium,** and this is why humans become slightly shorter as the day passes. Creep can also be associated with injury. Prolonged flexion of the lumbar spine results in a creep of the posterior ligaments, which decreases joint stiffness and may predispose the low back to injury. It is prudent to advise patients to allow this flexion-creep to reverse itself before performing activities that require lumbar stability.

33. What is hysteresis?

When viscoelastic tissue is loaded and then subsequently unloaded, the amount of stress is lower for a given amount of strain. This phenomenon is a consequence of the tissue's viscosity, and is called **hysteresis.** The area between the loading and unloading curves (shaded area, see figure) is a measure of hysteresis, and represents the energy absorbed by the tissue, which is usually lost in the form of heat (although it could cause tissue damage).

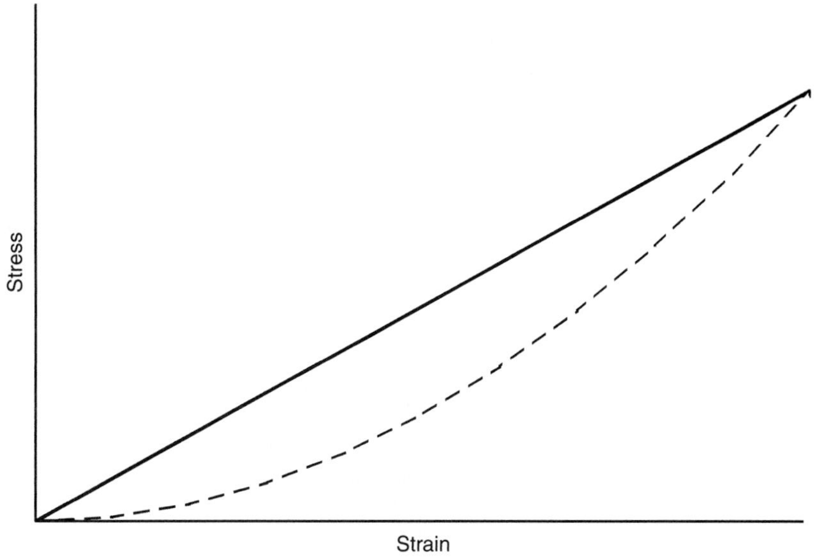

The hysteresis loop.

Repeated loadings, as well as acute and chronic stretching, increase a tendon's compliance and decrease the amount of hysteresis. These changes increase the energy returned during the stretch-shortening cycle (improving performance), and can decrease the risk of injury. These changes show that stretching has beneficial effects other than just improving the range of motion of a joint.

34. Explain the length-tension relationship of muscle.

The amount of force or **tension** that a muscle can produce varies with the **length** of the muscle at the time of contraction. Maximum force is produced when the muscle is approximately at its resting length. When the fibers shorten beyond resting length, the force production decreases slowly at first, and then rapidly. There is a progressive decline as the fibers are lengthened beyond resting length. This relationship can be used to help explain why surgically lengthened muscles are weak postoperatively (see figure).

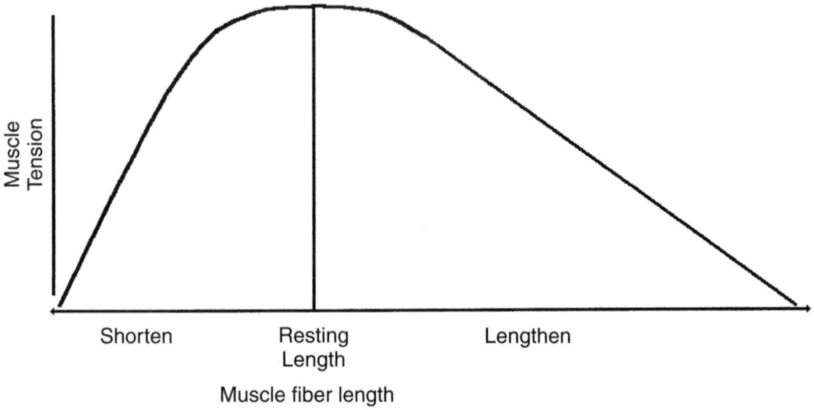

Length-tension curve.

35. Discuss some factors that affect the biomechanical properties of tendons and ligaments.

The most commonly cited factors affecting the biomechanical properties of tendons and ligaments are:

Factor	Physiologic Effect on Collagen	Mechanical Effect
Physical activity	↑ Glycosaminoglycan content ↓ Cross-linking ↑ Alignment of fibers	Strengthens
Disuse/immobilization	↑ Turnover ↑ Reducible cross-linking ↑ Nonuniform orientation ↓ Glycosaminoglycan and water content	Weakens
Aging	↓ In number and quality of cross-links ↓ In fibril diameter	Weakens
Corticosteroid use	↓ Collagen synthesis ↓ Stiffness ↓ Ultimate stress ↓ Energy to failure	Weakens
Pregnancy-induced hormones	↑ Collagen degradation	Increases laxity
NSAIDs	Variable, depending on specific drug	Inconclusive

36. Is cartilage the same in all joints?

No. There are morphological, biomechanical, metabolic, and histologic differences between types of cartilage in the joints of the lower extremities. Those differences, in part, are the reason why osteoarthritis is more prominent in the knee and hip joints than in the ankle joint.

37. What are the normal processes of joint lubrication?

There are two different types of joint lubrication processes. With **boundary lubrication,** a layer of fluid prevents direct contact between two surfaces, decreasing friction. With **fluid film lubrication,** the fluid between two surfaces separates the contact surfaces and distributes the loading between them. Fluid film lubrication works by:

- Increased fluid pressure creating a wedge, separating two surfaces (**hydrodynamic**)
- Increased fluid pressure deforming the articular surface, creating greater contact area (**elastohydrodynamic**)
- Increased pressure on the articular cartilage, forcing fluid out onto the surface (**weep**)

38. What is friction, and is it good or bad?

Friction is a force, parallel to the contact surface, that opposes motion between two objects. The interlocking of irregularities in the contact surfaces causes friction. The magnitude of the friction force will depend upon the material characteristics of the two contacting surfaces, and will be lower if there is relative motion between the two surfaces.

Friction may be good or bad, depending on the situation. A certain amount of friction between the ground and our shoes is necessary for efficient movement and to prevent slipping, but it also wears the soles of our shoes. High friction forces between the ground and the shoe increase the risk of ankle and knee injuries in sports where there is a lot of sudden turning or stopping, while repetitive friction forces to the skin can cause blisters.

39. Do all tissues adapt to change at the same rate?

No. An obvious example would be the difference in change in volume response to resistive exercise by a muscle and a tendon. A tendon adapts to change slower than muscle because it has fewer cells (in this case, tenocytes) that are capable of facilitating adaptation. Bone adapts more slowly than muscle. Evidence on the rate of adaptation of ligaments, cartilage, and intervertebral disks is scarce, but it is believed that they develop more slowly than muscle. It is important to realize, during rehabilitation, that a muscle will regain its strength before the other tissues of the musculoskeletal system, and therefore muscle strength alone is not a good indicator of the rehabilitation process.

40. Describe the difference in a spurt versus shunt muscle.

- A **spurt muscle** has the insertion close to the joint; there is a large change in distal bone motion for a short change in the muscle length (e.g., brachialis muscle at the elbow).
- A **shunt muscle** has its origin close to the joint; a short change in muscle length results in a small amount of distal bone motion (e.g., brachioradialis muscle at elbow).
- Spurt muscles are better at moving the joint rather than stabilizing it, and shunt muscles are better at stabilizing the joint rather than moving it.

41. List biomechanical factors that affect a joint implant.

- **Initial stability**—based mainly on the surgery technique used and the implant design
- **Late stability**—determined by the bone growth and remodeling of the bone around the implant
- **Stress shielding**—affects bone around the implant as the load typically goes through the stronger implant, not the bone surrounding the implant
- **Wear of the implant**—cobalt-chrome implants typically used to decrease wear
- **Wear debris**—polyethylene wear can cause osteolysis
- **Changing the anatomic alignments**—by the manner in which the implant is installed

42. List factors that affect the stability of an external fixator.

- Pin diameter—bending stiffness increasing by an order of the fourth power as the diameter increases

- Number of pins used
- Distance from the surface to the bone
- Stiffness of the frame
- Number of fixation planes

43. What happens to the strength of an intramedullary rod when its diameter is increased?

Strength increases as the rod size increases by an order of the third power.

44. What are the effects of increasing thickness and width of a fixation plate?

- Stability is determined by raising the thickness to the third power and the width to the first power.
- Strength is determined by raising the thickness to the second power and the width to the first power.

45. How do holes in bone (i.e., missing screw or following removal of plate) affect its strength?

- A hole decreases the cross-sectional area of the bone; there is less bone at the hole, and the strength is decreased.
- A hole decreases strength by causing a stress concentration point that is determined by the geometry of the hole and bone.
- A hole of 20% of the bone diameter decreases strength by 50%.

46. How long does it take for strength to return to normal levels after the removal of a screw?

It takes between 4 months and 1 year for strength to return to normal.

47. List the types of metals that are closest biomechanically to bone.

With Regard to Modulus:

- Aluminum
- Titanium (and titanium alloys)
- Stainless steel
- Cobalt-chromium

With Regard to Biocompatibility:

- Titanium (and titanium alloys)
- Cobalt-chromium
- Stainless steel
- Aluminum

48. How much strength does a well-placed lag screw add to fracture fixation?

One should be able to assume that the strength of the fixation is determined by the pull-out strength of the lag screw, or approximately a **40% increase** in strength over plating alone.

49. Why do we use the terms varus with talipes varus, varum with genu varum, and vara with coxa vara?

Varus and **valgus** are adjectives and should be used only in connection with the noun they describe. In Latin, the adjective takes the gender of the noun. **Talipes** is a form of the masculine noun **talus,** thus **talipes varus** (foot inverted and pointed, as in a clubfoot); **genu** is a neutral noun, thus **genu varum** or **valgus** (bowlegged or knock-kneed); and **coxa** is feminine, thus **coxa vara** (any decrease in the femoral neck shaft angle $<$120 to 135 degrees).

Bibliography

Adams MA et al: *The biomechanics of back pain,* Edinburgh, 2002, Churchill Livingstone.

Baeyens JP, van Roy P, Clarys JP: Intra-articular kinematics of the normal glenohumeral joint in the late preparatory phase of throwing: Kaltenborn's rule revisited, *Ergonomics* 43:1726-1737, 2000.

Cerny K: Kinesiology versus biomechanics: a perspective, *Phys Ther* 64:1809, 1984.
Hatze H: The meaning of the term "biomechanics," *J Biomech* 7:189-190, 1974.
Kubo K, Kanehisa H, Fukunaga T: Effects of resistance and stretching training programmes on the viscoelastic properties of human tendon structures in vivo, *J Physiol* 538:219-226, 2002.
Meriam JL, Kraige LG: *Engineering mechanics: dynamics,* New York, 1997, John Wiley and Sons.
McGill SM, Brown S: Creep response of the lumbar spine to prolonged full flexion, *Clin Biomech* 7:43-46, 1992.
Neumann DA: *Kinesiology of the musculoskeletal system: foundations for physical rehabilitation,* St Louis, 2002, Mosby.
Rasch PJ, Burke RK: *Kinesiology and applied anatomy: the science of human movement,* ed 4, Philadelphia, 1971, Lea & Febiger.
Smidt GL: Biomechanics and physical therapy: a perspective, *Phys Ther* 64:1807-1808, 1984.
Whiting WC, Zernicke RF: *Biomechanics of musculoskeletal injury,* Champaign, Ill, 1998, Human Kinetics.
Zatsiorsky VM: *Kinematics of human motion,* Champaign, Ill, 1998, Human Kinetics.
Zatsiorsky VM: *Kinetics of human motion,* Champaign, Ill, 2002, Human Kinetics.

Chapter 3

Soft Tissue Injury and Repair

Arthur J. Nitz, PT, PhD, ECS

1. What is the body's initial response to soft tissue injury? How is it identified?

The inflammatory response is characterized by a cascade of biochemical reactions and represents the body's initial reaction to injury, whether caused by trauma, surgery, or metabolic or infectious disease. The principal signs of the inflammatory response are erythema (rubor), swelling (tumor), elevated tissue temperature (calor), and pain (dolor). Local vasodilation, fluid leakage into the extracellular and extravascular spaces, and impaired lymphatic drainage are responsible for the erythema, swelling, and increased tissue temperature. The fourth cardinal sign of inflammation—pain—is the result of mechanical distention and pressure of the soft tissues and chemical irritation of pain-sensitive nerve receptors.

2. Describe the phases of soft tissue healing.

The acute **inflammatory phase** begins immediately after injury and lasts 24 to 48 hours, although some aspects may continue for up to 3 weeks. The **proliferative phase** may begin early in the inflammatory phase but is thought to be most extensive approximately 21 days after injury. The **matrix formation/remodeling phase** begins 3 weeks after injury and may last for up to 2 years, although in many cases the majority of remodeling has occurred by 2 months. Because the time frames for these three phases overlap considerably, the accepted delineations should be used as general guidelines only.

3. Describe the basic vascular and cellular activities associated with the inflammatory reaction and the primary function of each activity.

Blood vessels at the site of the injury initially undergo vasoconstriction, which is mediated by norepinephrine and usually lasts from a few seconds to a few minutes. If serotonin is released by mast cells in the area of injury, a secondary prolonged vasoconstriction occurs to slow blood loss in the affected region. Additional cellular activities after soft tissue injury include margination of leukocytes, which adhere to the vessel wall, and chemotaxis (movement of white blood cells through the extravascular space toward the site of injury), which begins the process of phagocytosis and removes the cellular debris caused by the injury.

4. Identify the key chemical mediators of the inflammatory response.

Both histamine and serotonin are released from granules of mast cells in the area of the injury. Histamine results in elevated vascular permeability, whereas serotonin is a potent vasoconstrictor. Kinins, notably bradykinin, also cause a marked increase in vascular permeability, much as histamine does. Pro-inflammatory prostaglandins are believed to sensitize pain receptors, attract leukocytes to the inflamed area, and increase vascular permeability by antagonizing vasoconstriction. The primary mode of action of aspirin, nonsteroidal antiinflammatory drugs (NSAIDs), and steroids is to inhibit prostaglandin synthesis by deactivation of a key enzyme (cyclooxygenase).

5. Which cell type is especially prominent in the proliferative and matrix formation phases of connective tissue healing?

The fibroblast is the most common connective tissue cell. It is responsible for synthesizing and secreting most of the fibers and ground substance of connective tissue. Soft tissue injury signals the fibroblast to multiply rapidly and mobilizes free connective tissue cells to the injured area.

6. Describe the elements that comprise the connective tissue matrix.

The connective tissue matrix is composed of fibrous elements (such as collagen, elastin, and reticulin) and ground substance, which consists principally of water, salts, and glycosaminoglycans (GAGs). The matrix provides the strength and support of the soft tissue and also serves as the means for diffusion of tissue fluid and nutrients between capillaries and cells.

7. What general factors affect connective tissue repair after tissue injury?

Healing after soft tissue injury is affected by the availability of a number of factors, including blood supply, proteins, minerals, and amino acids. Enzymes and hormones also play a role in tissue healing, as do mechanical stress and infection. Steroids suppress the mitotic activity of fibroblasts, which results in diminished deposition of collagen fibers and reduction in tensile strength. Antibiotic medicines inhibit protein synthesis and may adversely affect wound healing and scar formation. Disease processes such as diabetes mellitus significantly retard wound healing because small-vessel disease inhibits normal collagen synthesis.

8. What influence does nutrition play in the soft tissue repair process?

Collagen biosynthesis is especially sensitive to the availability of proper nutrients. Lack of vitamins C and A impedes the process of collagen synthesis. Glucosamine, found within collagen type II, is the critical compound in connective tissue repair and production. Glucosamine is the precursor for compounds important to connective tissue health, such as chondroitin sulfate and hyaluronic acid, and increases proteoglycan production. Whether dietary supplements such as glucosamine have a significant and lasting effect on joint disease has not been well established in controlled clinical trials, though mounting evidence suggests that such supplements are beneficial. Recent studies indicate that glucosamine may limit the advance of joint space narrowing associated with osteoarthritis, resulting in improved functional scores. Minerals such as zinc contribute to the normal rate of cell proliferation and ultimate wound strength.

9. What role does aging play in altering the soft tissue injury healing process?

Age-related effects on wound healing include attenuated metabolic activity, decreased vascular supply, diminished cellular biosynthesis, delayed collagen remodeling, and decreased wound strength. Despite these differences, many of which have been confirmed in animal studies, clinical experience indicates that older patients often undergo surgical treatment with no adverse healing responses related to aging.

10. How does tendinitis differ from tendinosis?

Tendinitis is a microscopic tear at the muscle-tendon junction, usually attended by localized swelling and tenderness. **Tendinosis** usually results from a degenerative process and manifests as chronic irritation or inflammation at the tendon-bone interface.

In most cases tendinitis and tendinosis can be differentiated on the basis of clinical examination findings. The paratenon, a double-layered sheath of loose areolar tissue, is attached to the outer connective tissue surface of tendons that do not have a synovial lining. Paratenonitis refers to inflammation and thickening of the paratenon sheath. In many cases it is difficult to differentiate between tendinitis and paratenonitis by clinical examination, although the distinction is evident with surgical exploration.

11. How does treatment for tendinitis differ from that for tendinosis?

The treatment for tendinitis is almost exclusively conservative, focusing on reducing the inflammatory process and underlying tissue stresses. Initial efforts to reduce the inflammation and tenderness include ice application, oral NSAID administration, iontophoresis, rest, and cortisone injection. Because tendinosis is a chronic condition, treatment using oral NSAIDs and cortisone injection does not appear to be as effective as with tendinitis. Tendinosis treatment focuses on a controlled eccentric training program, often is lengthy (10 to 12 weeks or more in some cases), and eventually may require surgical intervention to eliminate the diseased area of the bone-tendon interface.

12. What tissue changes occur in response to a period of immobilization after soft tissue injury?

Immobility after soft tissue injury alters the rate of the biological process of remodeling. Changes that result in this alteration include increased density of cells (usually fibroblasts), the presence of myofibroblasts, reduction in hyaluronic acid and chondroitin sulfate levels in the periarticular connective tissue, and a 4% to 6% reduction in water content of the same tissues after only 9 weeks of immobilization. Further changes include a shift in the balance between collagen synthesis and degradation, which results in a reduction in total collagen.

13. What is the effect of immobilization on stiffness and strength of injured soft tissue?

Experimental evidence in rabbits indicates that 9 weeks of immobilization results in a 50% reduction in the normal breaking strength of the medial collateral ligament. At the same time a significant increase in the intermolecular cross-links of collagen leads to contracture formation. Therefore the remodeled connective tissue after immobilization is both thicker (tendency toward contracture) and weaker, possibly because of the random alignment of collagen fibers.

14. How do stress and motion affect connective tissue repair after injury?

Stress and motion have a profound effect on the quality of soft tissue repair after injury or surgery. Many studies have documented that scar tissue forms earlier in mobilized tendon, is well-oriented, and is not attended by adhesions, in contrast to scar tissue that develops without physiologic stresses. Exposure of scar tissue to physiologic tensile forces during the healing process results in a more mature and stronger union of tendon and ligament. Healing of articular cartilage involves a greater amount of collagen and glycosaminoglycans, less cellularity, and fewer scar tissue adhesions when accompanied by modest joint movements. Some experimental evidence indicates that ultrasound application to tenotomized Achilles tendons improves tensile strength of the tissue if administered during postoperative days 2 to 4. This response appears to be time-dependent and may be related to limiting the inflammatory response and encouraging fibroplasia and fibrillogenesis. In a similar manner, high-voltage electrical stimulation appears to augment protein synthesis and the ultimate strength of the tendon if applied during the early stages of healing.

15. Define myositis ossificans. What is the histologic basis for its occurrence after soft tissue injury?

Myositis ossificans refers to the formation of heterotopic bone in soft tissue after contusion or trauma involving the muscle, connective tissue, blood vessels, and underlying periosteum. It occurs most often in males between the ages of 15 and 30 after contusions of the thigh or fractures/dislocations, especially of the elbow. Recent studies show the existence of an undifferentiated cell known as an **inducible osteogenic precursor cell**, which after stimulation by trauma can differentiate into an active osteoblast. Radiographic evidence of bone formation is usually seen 3 to 4 weeks after the initial injury. The precise mechanism by which trauma activates the stem cell remains elusive.

16. After ligament and tendon repair or reconstruction, when is the soft tissue the strongest and when is it the weakest?

Much of the information related to this question has been derived from studies using animal models (primates and others) and should be interpreted with caution. General data indicate that the strength of the patellar tendon autograft used in anterior cruciate ligament reconstruction cases is strongest on the day that it is surgically implanted. As the tissue heals in its new location, its strength diminishes to significantly <50% during the first 4 to 8 weeks postoperatively. In the ensuing 3 to 6 months, there is a slow transformation of collagen type and revascularization of the graft tissue. Stiffness and load to failure continue to increase for many months, and at 1 year the tissue is reported to have achieved 82% of its original strength. The clinical implications are fairly straightforward: protect the graft in the early stages of rehabilitation, encourage closed-chain axial loading activity to minimize shear forces (joint translation), and emphasize maximal motor unit activation throughout the rehabilitation process.

17. Does the location of a ligament or tendon repair (mid-substance versus insertion site) influence the rate of healing? Why?

Generally, insertion site repairs heal at a faster rate than mid-substance repairs. The primary reason is the availability of adequate blood supply to provide nutrients for the healing process. Other factors may include differences in the intra-articular and extra-articular environment, such as presence or absence of synovial lining and fluid, which usually encourage healing. Furthermore, the regional distribution and level of fibroblast activity may play a role in the healing rate.

18. What is the response of articular cartilage to chondroplasty (microfracture technique, abrasion, drilling) of the undersurface of the patella?

The microfracture technique is used to stimulate tissue repair of full-thickness articular cartilage defects. A drill is used to make multiple perforations in the subchondral bone in the area of the cartilage defect in an effort to produce a "super clot." Over a period of 8 weeks or more the super clot heals with a hybrid mixture of fibrocartilage and type II (hyaline-like) collagen. This hybrid repair tissue may be functionally better than fibrocartilage alone; early animal and human studies suggest that it is durable enough to function like articular cartilage.

19. Describe the scientific evidence supporting articular cartilage repair.

Reproduced chondrocyte cells harvested from the patient are injected under a periosteal flap covering the articular defect. Two-year follow-up studies of patients with femoral condyle transplants indicate excellent results; most patients developed hyaline-like cartilage in the defect site. Patellar lesions have not done as well, possibly because of shear forces or noncorrection of underlying malalignment abnormalities. Research is encouraging for focal chondral defects but not for generalized osteoarthritis of the joint. In addition, there is evidence that articular cartilage exposed to electric and electromagnetic fields can lead to a sustained upregulation of growth factors, enhancing its viability. The degradative enzymes in the synovial fluid of osteoarthritic joints are not conducive to cell transfer with cartilage transplant experimental procedures.

20. What growth factors are involved with soft tissue healing?

- Chemotactic factors—prostaglandins, complement, platelet-derived growth factor (PDGF), and angiokines
- Competence factors—activate quite cells, PDGF, and prostaglandins
- Progression factors—stimulate cell growth such as IL-1 and somatomedins
- Enhancing factors—fibronectin and osteonectin

21. What is the effect of NSAIDs on muscle recovery?

Short-term use (<1 week) of NSAIDs after muscular strain may improve recovery. However, long-term use (>1 month) may result in decreased recovery.

22. What factors affect allograft strength?

Freeze-drying reduces the immunogenic response but also decreases strength. Greater than 3-megarad irradiation will also decrease strength. Less radiation (2 megarad) in combination with ethylene oxide will decrease graft strength. Allografts have a slower, less predictable recovery than autografts.

23. What growth factors may aid in soft tissue repair?

Platelet-rich plasma (PRP) has been shown to improve soft tissue healing in horses with improved collagen abundance and organization. Macrophage-secreted myogenic factors may someday play a role in inducing muscle repair. Specific chondrocyte growth factors and bone morphogenetic proteins (BMP) have shown promise in improving cartilage repair.

Bibliography

Akeson WH et al: The connective tissue response to immobility: biochemical changes in periarticular connective tissue of the immobilized rabbit knee, *Clin Orthop* 93:356-361, 1973.

Alford JW, Cole BJ: Cartilage restoration, Part 1: Basic science, historical perspective, patient education, and treatment options, *Am J Sports Med* 33:295-306, 2005.

Carter CA et al: Platelet rich plasma promotes differentiation and regeneration during equine wound healing, *Exp Mol Pathol* 74:244-255, 2003.

Chen FS, Frenkel SR, DiCesare PE: Chondrocyte transplantation and experimental treatment options for articular cartilage defects, *Am J Orthop* 6:396-406, 1997.

Ciccone CD, Wolf SL: Non-steroidal anti-inflammatory drugs. In Ciccone CD, editor: *Pharmacology in rehabilitation,* Philadelphia, 1990, pp 160-172, FA Davis.

Curwin SL: The etiology and treatment of tendinitis. In Harris M, et al, editors: *Oxford textbook of sports medicine,* ed 2, Oxford, 1998, pp 610-627, Oxford University Press.

Devereux DF et al: The quantitative and qualitative impairment of wound healing by adriamycin, *Cancer* 43:932, 1979.
English T, Wheeler ME, Hettinga DL: Inflammatory response of synovial joint structure. In Malone TR, McPoil T, Nitz AJ, editors: *Orthopedic and sports physical therapy,* ed 3, St Louis, 1997, pp 81-113, Mosby.
Enwemeka CS: Inflammation, cellularity and fibrillogenesis in regenerating tendon: Implications for tendon rehabilitation, *Phys Ther* 69:816-825, 1989.
Frank C, Amiel D, Woo SL-Y: Normal ligament properties and ligament healing, *Clin Orthop* 196:15-25, 1985.
Goodson WH, Hung TK: Studies of wound healing in experimental diabetes mellitus, *J Surg Res* 22:211, 1977.
Goodson WH, Hunt TK: Wound healing and aging, *J Invest Dermatol* 73:88, 1979.
Gross MT: Chronic tendinitis: pathomechanics of injury, factors affecting the healing response and treatment, *J Orthop Sports Phys Ther* 16:248-261, 1992.
Kloth LC, McCulloch JM: The inflammatory response to wounding. In McCulloch JM, Kloth LC, Feedar JA, editors: *Wound healing alternatives in management,* ed 2, Philadelphia, 1995, pp 3-15, F.A. Davis.
Lieber RL, Bjorn-Ove L, Friden J: Sarcomere length in wrist extensor muscles, *Acta Orthop Scand* 68:249-254, 1997.
Lineaweaver W et al: Topical antimicrobial toxicity, *Arch Surg* 120:267, 1985.
Modolin M et al: Effects of protein depletion and repletion on experimental wound contraction, *Ann Plast Surg* 15:123, 1985.
Reginster JY et al: Long-term effects of glucosamine sulphate on osteoarthritis progression: a randomized, placebo-control clinical trial, *Lancet* 357:251-256, 2001.
Van Story-Lewis PE, Tennenbaum HC: Glucocorticoid inhibition of fibroblast contraction of collagen gels, *Biochem Pharmacol* 35:1283, 1986.
Videman T: Connective tissue and immobilization, *Clin Orthop* 221:26-32, 1987.
Weiss EL: Connective tissue in wound healing. In McCulloch JM, Kloth LC, Feedar JA, editors: *Wound healing alternatives in management,* ed 2, Philadelphia, 1995, pp 16-31, FA Davis.
Woo SL-Y et al: The importance of controlled passive mobilization on flexor tendon healing, *Acta Orthop Scand* 52:615-622, 1981.
Woo SL-Y et al: The response of ligaments to stress deprivation and stress enhancement. In Daniel D, Akeson W, O'Connor J, editors: *Knee ligaments: structure, function, injury and repair,* New York, 1990, pp 337-350, Raven Press.

Chapter 4

Bone Injury and Repair

Arthur J. Nitz, PT, PhD, ECS, and Patrick H. Kitzman, PT, PhD

1. What are the components that make up bone?

- Cells
- Ground substance
- Fibrous tissue network

The **cellular component** consists of **osteoblasts,** which produce and initiate mineralization of new bone and cartilage, and **osteoclasts,** which are essential for the removal of the callus for lamellar bone to be laid down. A third cell type found in mature adult bone is the **osteocyte.**

The **ground substance component** of bone contains mostly calcium phosphate, glycosaminoglycans, and hyaluronic acid. **Calcium phosphate** helps to add rigidity and hardness to the bone.

The **fibrous component** consists of **collagen** fibers, which help resist tensile stresses, and **elastin** fibers, which add a resilient aspect to the bone.

2. Describe the effects of aging on bone structure.

The most commonly known age-related change is a calcium-related loss of mass and density. This loss ultimately causes the pathologic condition of osteoporosis. **Osteoporosis** is a major bone mineral disorder in older adults that decreases the bone mineral content; as a result, bone mass and strength decline with age. In geriatric patients, the hormonal system regulating calcium metabolism is less efficient and responds poorly to the challenge of a calcium-incorporating process, such as callus formation. Aging influences tissues (i.e., kidneys, gastrointestinal tract, and endocrine system) of the body that affect calcium metabolism and bone physiology. Thus, the process of fracture healing in the geriatric patient is altered to some extent. **Calcitonin,** a hormone associated with decreasing serum calcium levels and possibly the remodeling of bone, has a decreased responsiveness to a calcium challenge with age. This decrease in calcitonin response may account, in part, for the slow bone healing in geriatric patients. Bones of older adults can withstand about half the strain of the bones of younger adults. Bones of older adults are less pliable and less able to store energy. Although there are physiologic changes that occur during the aging process that can affect bone health, the more sedentary lifestyle of many older individuals also may account for many of the age-associated changes in bone health.

3. List the different types of bone fractures.

- Compound (open)—fracture occurs when sharp ends of the broken bone protrude through the victim's skin or when some projectile penetrates the skin into the fracture site.
- Closed—skin remains intact.
- Perforating (e.g., gunshot-bullet penetration)—fracture may involve loss of bone from the effect of high-level energy at the fracture site.
- Depressed or fissured—fracture occurs when a sharply localized blow depresses a segment of cortical bone below the level of surrounding bone (e.g., a skull fracture).
- Greenstick—fracture is on one side of the bone but does not tear the periosteum of the opposite side (seen in children).
- Spiral—fracture is caused by opposite rotatory forces pulling on the bone (twisting).
- Oblique—fracture is oriented at an angle of ≥30 degrees to the axis of the bone.
- Transverse—fracture is oriented at a right angle to the axis of the bone.
- Avulsion—fracture may be produced by a sudden muscle contraction, with the muscle pulling off the portion of the bone to which it is attached; also may result from traction on a ligamentous or capsular attachment.
- Comminuted—fracture involves multiple fracture fragments.
- Stress—fracture results from stresses repeated with excessive frequency to a bone.
- Pathologic—fracture arises in abnormal or diseased bones; pathologic conditions that can lead to fractures include carcinomas, infection, and osteoporosis.

4. Discuss the stages of bone healing.

The **first stage** is referred to as the inflammatory phase, granulation stage, fracture stage, or clot stage. During this phase surviving cells are sensitized to chemical messengers that are involved with the healing process. This initial aspect of the first stage is probably completed within 7 days. A second feature of the initial stage is the development of a clot around the fracture site (not seen in stress fracture healing). After the formation of the clot, granulation tissue forms in the space between the fracture fragments. This granulation tissue activates macrophages, whose function is to remove the clot. This second aspect of the initial stage lasts about 2 weeks.

The **second stage** is known as the reparative phase or callous stage and can be divided further into soft callous and hard callous stages. Osteoblasts and chondrocytes within the granulation tissue begin to synthesize cartilage and woven bone matrices (soft callus). Approximately 1 week later, the newly formed soft callus begins to mineralize. This mineralization concludes several weeks later with the formation of a fracture (hard) callus. The hard callus is detectable on radiographs because of the calcium it contains. The creation and mineralization of the callus can require 4 to 16 weeks to complete.

The **third stage** is called the remodeling or consolidation phase and involves several processes. First the callus is replaced by woven bone, which, in turn, is replaced with packets of new lamellar bone. The callus plugging the marrow cavity is removed, restoring the cavity. It has been estimated that the complete replacement of the callus with functionally competent lamellar bone can take 1 to 4 years.

5. Name some conditions that have a negative effect on the bone healing process.

Technical Factors*	Biologic Failures†	Miscellaneous Conditions
Infection	Vascular injury	Poor nutrition
Poor reduction	Failure to make or mineralize callus (because of metabolic abnormalities)	Alcohol abuse
Distraction	Formation of scar and fat tissue instead of callus	Smoking
Repeated gross motion of fracture fragments	Inability to replace woven bone with lamellar bone (e.g., children with osteogenesis imperfecta)	
Loss of local blood supply because of injury and/or surgical procedure		

*In these situations, the potential for normal healing is present, but problems during the treatment have prevented the healing process from proceeding, resulting in delayed union or nonunion.

†Biologic failures refer to abnormalities in the biology of the healing process that delay or prevent union even with proper treatment.

6. Discuss the effect that smoking has on the bone healing process.

In studies in which animals were administered nicotine, a significant decrease in callous formation and an increase in the prevalence of nonunions were documented. Nicotine-exposed bones have been shown to be significantly weaker in a three-point bending test as compared with controls. Smoking and nicotine have been shown to delay the revascularization and incorporation of bone grafts and to increase the pseudarthrosis rate in spinal fusion patients. Nicotine has been shown to have a direct inhibitory effect on bone cellular proliferation and function. These changes, taken together with the vascular effects, result in a decrease in the quantity and maturity of the fracture callus. It has been estimated that the risk of fractures is 2 to 6 times higher in patients who smoke because of reduced bone density in these patients. Damaged soft tissue and impaired nerve function (neurogenic inflammation) can impede fracture healing by increasing the metabolic demand on the tissue repair system and limiting the benefit of supportive muscle function around the fracture site. Such failures usually require downward revisions of the rehabilitation timetable and ultimate recovery potential for the patient.

7. Discuss the effect nutrition has on bone healing.

Calcium plays an important role in helping attain peak bone mass during bone development and in preventing fractures in later life. The daily recommended allowance of calcium for nonpregnant, nonlactating women is 800 mg/day. This level increases to 1500 mg/day in postmenopausal, estrogen-depleted women. It is estimated that 75% of all women ingest less than the recommended daily allowance. Men tend to meet their calcium needs more successfully by consuming twice as much calcium at the same age. Multiple factors can affect the bioactivity of calcium. High-fat or high-fiber diets can interfere with or decrease the activity of calcium. Large doses of zinc supplementation or megadoses of vitamin A can lower calcium bioactivity. High-protein diets can decrease calcium reserves by increasing urinary excretion of calcium.

8. What other factors affect calcium absorption?

Alcohol consumption can decrease the absorption of calcium by a direct cytotoxic effect on intestinal mucosa. Various **medications,** such as glucocorticoids, heparin, and anticonvulsants, can affect calcium activity.

Vitamin D increases serum calcium levels by enhancing intestinal absorption of calcium and enhancing parathyroid hormone–stimulating reabsorption of bone. A low level of vitamin D impairs the ability of the body to adapt to low levels of calcium intake and may contribute to the pathogenesis of osteoporosis. Intake of vitamin D alone has never been shown to improve fracture healing.

9. How does Wolff's law apply to bone healing?

The ability of bone to adapt by changing size, shape, and structure depends on the mechanical stresses on the bone. When optimal stress is placed on bone, there is greater bone deposition than bone reabsorption. This results in hypertrophy of periosteal bone and increased bone density. When bone is subjected to less than optimal stresses, reabsorption of periosteal bone can occur, resulting in a decrease in strength and stiffness. Optimal stress within an appropriate range is essential for bone strength.

10. Define closed reduction, open reduction, and rigid external fixation in fracture treatment.

- **Closed reduction**—use of casting or traction
- **Open reduction**—surgical intervention using plates, screws, or other internal fixation devices
- **Rigid external fixation**—combination of closed and open reduction using percutaneous pins and external stabilizing bars

11. What are the advantages of closed reduction?

Avoidance of surgery, reduction of the fracture, and usually (except in the case of traction) a shorter hospital stay are all advantages of closed reduction. Usually the patient can safely begin gentle range of motion exercises several weeks before the fractured limb is strong enough to return to normal weight-bearing function or to withstand resistance at the fracture site. In later stages of fracture healing, splints can be worn to protect the fractured limb, to be removed at intervals to permit joint mobilization or bathing.

12. List advantages and disadvantages of open reduction.

ADVANTAGES

- Precise bone reduction
- Early mobilization of joints
- Immediate stability, allowing earlier return to full function

DISADVANTAGES

- Increased possibility of infection
- Increased hospital stays
- Metal devices may require subsequent removal

13. How does rigid fixation affect bone healing?

When rigid fixation is used, there is no stimulus for the production of the external callus from the periosteum or the internal callus from the endosteum (**secondary bone healing**). Instead the fracture healing occurs directly between the cortex of one fracture fragment and the cortex of the other fracture fragment (**primary bone healing**). Primary bone healing involves a direct repair of the bone lesion by new bridging osteons that become oriented through haversian remodeling to the long axis of the bone.

14. What effects can internal fixation have on bone healing?

- Improper placement or tightening of plates, screws, nut, or bolts in bone surgery may cause **bone reabsorption** because of local stress concentration or decreased vascular perfusion.
- Plates that are too rigid may cause **bone atrophy** secondary to preventing the bone from perceiving intermittent compressive stresses.
- If the hardware needs to be removed, a secondary inflammatory response occurs that leads to **weakening of the bone.** The bone needs to be protected until it regains strength.
- If the plates are left in place, problems with **stress** along the plate-bone interface can occur.

15. List some advantages of weight-bearing activities after sustaining a fracture.

- Enhanced rehabilitation (e.g., improved range of motion)
- Shorter hospital stays
- Less overall postfracture morbidity

16. How do Salter-Harris fractures influence the pediatric population?

The growth plate appears on a radiograph as a lucent line near the joint, and a fracture through that line can be missed easily unless there is some disturbance in the alignment of the bone. When there is an injury to the growth plate, growth disturbances may occur in that bone. The younger the patient, the greater the growth potential remaining; however, there is also the danger of significant growth disturbance.

17. Describe a radiologic sign of a fracture of the radial head/neck.

Fat-pad signs constitute radiologic evidence of an effusion in the elbow joint and appear as areas of translucency on the lateral radiograph of the elbow flexed to a right angle. The fat-pad sign has an overall high negative predictive value (87%). The absence of the fat-pad sign can exclude a fracture and is a reliable indicator of the absence of a fracture. The presence of a fat-pad sign should only raise the suspicion of a fracture being present, however, because there may be a positive fat-pad sign with no fracture.

18. What is the most commonly overlooked fracture in adults at the time of injury?

Carpal scaphoid fractures are easily overlooked. Because fractures of the scaphoid may result in loss of blood supply to the bone and consequent avascular necrosis, most physicians elect to treat wrist injuries as a fracture (immobilization) until properly interpreted radiographs indicate otherwise.

19. Discuss the role of ultrasound in the treatment of acute fractures.

Ultrasound stimulation can accelerate the normal repair process in a fresh fracture. Ultrasound may help stimulate the healing process of nonunions. In animal models low-intensity pulsed ultrasound at 0.1 to 0.5 W/cm^2 accelerated fracture healing. Pulsed ultrasound at higher doses (1.0 to 2.0 W/cm^2) significantly inhibited the synthesis of collagen and noncollagenous protein, however. In clinical double-blind studies, ultrasound has been shown to decrease significantly the time for overall healing of grade I open tibial fractures and distal radial fractures. Ultrasound has been shown to reduce significantly the prevalence of delayed union in nonsmokers and smokers. In animal studies ultrasound increased bone mineral content and density, increased peak torque, and accelerated the overall endochondral ossification process. Ultrasound stimulation may increase the mechanical properties of the healing fracture callus by stimulating earlier synthesis of extracellular matrix proteins in cartilage.

20. What effect does bioelectric stimulation have on fracture healing?

Implantable electric stimulation and pulsed electromagnetic field (surface application) have been used for healing nonunion tibial fractures with some success. Electric stimulation generally is thought to convert fibrous connective tissue to bone, possibly by simulating mechanical stress in the bone. The best results with implantable electrodes in animal studies have been associated with the cathode located in the fracture gap and the anode in adjacent bone or in the soft tissue. Ionic migration in response to external direct current is believed to be one probable explanation for the apparent efficacy of electric stimulation on bone healing.

21. What is the effect of NSAIDs on bone healing?

While there is still no well-defined answer, prostaglandins are known to participate in the inflammatory response and to stimulate osteoclasts as well as increase osteoblastic activity and subsequent new bone formation. Long-term excessive use of these medications may reduce normal bone healing.

22. What are stress fractures, and how do they occur?

Fatigue or stress fractures occur in otherwise healthy individuals usually in response to a sudden increase in physical activity of several weeks duration. First described in military training as "march fractures," they are now fairly common in young individuals engaged in athletic activities and almost always represent a form of training error. In weight-bearing bones the overactivity causes microscopic fractures (debonding of osteons) that do not totally heal from day to day, eventually resulting in macroscopic bone failure and severe pain during ambulation or running. Though more common in the lower extremities, they can also occur in the medial epicondyle of the elbow with excessive throwing. Standard treatment involves early identification and rest of the involved extremity with avoidance of high-impact activities until healing has occurred. Signs of healing include resolution of bone tenderness with palpation and radiographic indication of healing—bone sclerosis.

23. What is the best imaging method for detecting stress fractures?

In spite of severe pain experienced by the patient, initial plain film radiographs of individuals suspected of a stress fracture are usually normal (up to 3 to 4 weeks following the initial onset of symptoms). Consequently, MRI and technetium bone scans are considered the best imaging studies for identifying stress fractures. Bone scans, in particular, may show signs of bone uptake as early as 72 hours after the onset of symptoms. However, radionucleotide (bone) scans have the disadvantage, as compared to the MRI, of exposing the patient to ionizing radiation.

24. Describe how the bone marrow signal with magnetic resonance imaging is assisting clinicians in establishing bone injury and patterns of soft tissue lesion.

Bone marrow contusions are often seen by MR imaging after a musculoskeletal injury and may result from a direct blow to the bone, from compressive forces of adjacent bones impacting on one another, or from traction forces experienced by the bone during avulsion injuries. The distribution of bone marrow edema has been likened to a footprint left behind by the musculoskeletal injury. Since MR imaging is able to identify bone marrow edema, patterns of soft tissue injury about the knee have been established for various complex ligamentous injuries and for traumatic injuries to the knee (e.g., dashboard injury from a motor vehicle accident). This method of investigation allows the clinician to predict with accuracy the specific soft tissue abnormalities likely to attend the presentation of bone marrow edema.

25. What is bone transplantation (replacement), and why is it used?

Bone transplantation (replacement) is an aggressive surgical technique whereby an entire diseased bone is excised and a cadaveric allograft replacement is transplanted in its place. This is usually necessitated by malignant bone tumors—primary or metastatic—and most of the descriptions in the current literature are of cases of femur transplantation. The alternative is typically an above-knee amputation or a hip disarticulation. Allograft replacement of the femur is prone to a number of complications, such as refracture, infection, nonunion, and resorption of the graft.

26. What treatments are available for nonunions?

- Autogenous bone grafting and appropriate stable fixation
- Vascularized bone grafting
- Use of allografts or autografts with the addition of platelet-rich plasma (contains high levels of PDGF and TGF-β1)
- Use of bone morphogenic proteins such as BMP-2

27. What are the roles of various growth factors on bone healing?

- BMP—bone morphogenic protein induces metaplasia of undifferentiated perivascular mesenchymal cells into osteoblasts.
- PDGF—platelet-derived growth factor is chemotactic for inflammatory cells at the fracture site.
- TGF-β—transforming growth factor–β stimulates the production of type II collagen and proteoglycans at the fracture callus.
- IGF-II—insulin-like growth factor II stimulates type I collagen production and cellular proliferation.

Bibliography

Ahl T, Dalen N, Selvik G: Mobilization after operation of ankle fractures: good results of early motion and weight bearing, *Acta Orthop Scand* 59:302-306, 1988.

Cimino W, Ichtertz D, Slabaugh P: Early mobilization of ankle fractures after open reduction and internal fixation, *Clin Orthop* 267:152-156, 1991.

Colson DJ et al: Treatment of delayed and nonunion of fractures using pulsed electromagnetic fields, *J Biomed Eng* 10:301-304, 1988.

Cook et al: Acceleration of tibia and distal radius fracture healing in patients who smoke, *Clin Orthop* 337:198-207, 1997.

Eckardt H et al: Recombinant human bone morphogenetic protein 2 enhances bone healing in an experimental model of fractures at risk of nonunion, *Injury* 36:489-494, 2005.

Einhorn TA, Levine B, Michel P: Nutrition and bone, *Orthop Clin North Am* 21:43-50, 1990.

Frost HM: The biology of fracture healing: an overview for clinicians: Part I, *Clin Orthop* 248:283-293, 1989.

Frost HM: The biology of fracture healing: an overview for clinicians: Part II, *Clin Orthop* 248:294-309, 1989.

Hadjiargyrou M et al: Enhancement of fracture healing by low intensity ultrasound, *Clin Orthop* 355(suppl): S216-S229, 1998.

Harder AT, An YH: The mechanism of the inhibitory effects of nonsteroidal anti-inflammatory drugs on bone healing: a concise review, *J Clin Pharmacol* 43:807-815, 2003.

Hayes CW et al: Mechanism-based pattern approach to classification of complex injuries of the knee depicted at MR imaging, *Radiographics* 20:S121-134, 2000.

Hulth A: Current concepts of fracture healing, *Clin Orthop* 249:265-284, 1989.
Khasigian HA: The results of treatment of nonunions with electrical stimulation, *Orthopedics* 31:32, 1980.
Kristiansen TK et al: Accelerated healing of distal radial fractures with the use of specific, low intensity ultrasound, *J Bone Joint Surg* 75A:961-973, 1997.
Levangie PK, Norkin CC: *Joint structure and function: a comprehensive analysis,* ed 4, Philadelphia, 2005, F.A. Davis.
Levine JD et al: Reflex neurogenic inflammation: I. Contribution of the peripheral nervous system to spatially remote inflammatory responses that follow injury, *J Neurosci* 5:1380-1386, 1985.
Malone TR, McPoil T, Nitz AJ, editors: *Orthopedic and sports physical therapy,* ed 3, St Louis, 1997, Mosby.
McRae R, editor: *Practical fracture treatment,* ed 3, New York, 1994, Churchill Livingstone.
Meller Y et al: Parathormone, calcitonin, and vitamin D metabolites during normal fracture healing in geriatric patients, *Clin Orthop* 199:272-279, 1985.
Mooney V: A randomized double-blind prospective study of efficacy of pulsed electromagnetic fields for interbody lumbar fusion, *Spine* 15:708-712, 1990.
Raikin SM et al: Effect of nicotine on the rate and strength of long bone fracture healing, *Clin Orthop* 353:231-237, 1998.
Sanders TG et al: Bone contusion patterns of the knee at MR imaging: footprint of the mechanism of injury, *Radiographics* 20:S135-151, 2000.
Skaggs DL, Vmirzayan R: The posterior fat pad sign in association with occult fracture of the elbow in children, *J Bone Joint Surg* 81A:1429-1433, 1999.

Chapter 5

Exercise Physiology

Victoria L. Veigl, PT, PhD

1. What measurement is considered the best indicator of an individual's level of aerobic fitness?

Maximal oxygen uptake ($\dot{V}O_2max$) is the best indicator of aerobic fitness.

2. Why is $\dot{V}O_2max$ considered the best indicator of aerobic fitness?

It is dependent on several factors:

- Cardiac output
- Ventilatory capacity
- Circulation
- Ability of the tissues to remove oxygen from the blood

3. What are limiting factors in determining $\dot{V}O_2max$?

- In healthy individuals, **maximal cardiac output**
- In individuals with asthma, chronic bronchitis, or emphysema, **ventilatory compromise**
- In individuals with emphysema, **abnormalities in the ventilation-perfusion ratio of the lungs**
- In individuals with peripheral vascular disease, **decreased tissue perfusion**

4. Define other common indicators of physical fitness.

- **Blood lactate threshold**—the intensity of exercise when there is a sudden increase in the amount of lactate in the blood
- **Ventilatory threshold**—the intensity of exercise when there is an increase in ventilation corresponding to the development of metabolic acidosis during exercise

5. Are the $\dot{V}O_2max$ values the same in an individual performing various exercises (e.g., treadmill, cycling, arm ergometry)?

No; the $\dot{V}O_2max$ value is different for each exercise. Differences are thought to be a result of the amount of muscle mass involved in the exercise. If similar muscle mass is involved, the $\dot{V}O_2max$ value is highest when the individual is performing the specific exercise for which he or she has trained.

6. What is oxygen deficit?

Oxygen deficit is the difference between the amount of oxygen that is consumed and the amount of oxygen that is required to perform an exercise.

7. What effect does warming up have on the oxygen deficit?

It decreases it. Warming up increases blood flow, muscle temperature, and mitochondrial respiration, and these factors enable oxygen to be delivered to and used by the tissues more rapidly. There is less time for a deficit to develop, and this results in a smaller deficit.

8. How do the resting stroke volume, heart rate, and cardiac output of a well-trained athlete compare with those of a sedentary individual?

The resting **stroke volume** of an athlete is greater than that of a sedentary individual because of hypertrophy of the cardiac muscle in the athlete, which results in an increase in contractility and an increase in venous tone that lead to more blood being returned to the heart. Both the increased contractility and increased venous tone cause an increase in the strength of contraction of cardiac muscle and in the stroke volume.

The resting **heart rate** of an athlete is lower than that of a sedentary individual (athlete, 40 to 60 beats/min; sedentary individual, 70 to 75 beats/min).

The higher stroke volume of an athlete is canceled out by the lower heart rate, resulting in the resting **cardiac output** of an athlete being similar to that of a sedentary individual.

9. How does the stroke volume response to exercise in the upright position differ between individuals who are physically fit and those who are not?

In a trained individual, stroke volume continues to increase until Vo_2max is reached; in an untrained individual, stroke volume increases as exercise intensity increases up to about 50% of $\dot{V}O_2max$, and then remains steady. Maximal stroke volume is higher in fit individuals, and the stroke volume for any submaximal exercise intensity is higher in a fit individual.

10. How do heart rate, stroke volume, mean total peripheral resistance, mean arterial blood pressure, and respiratory rate change when exercise is performed with the upper extremities compared with a similar amount of exercise using the lower extremities?

These changes occur mainly because vasodilation occurs in exercising muscles, and vasoconstriction occurs in nonexercising muscles. Upper extremity exercise involves smaller muscles than lower extremity exercise. During upper extremity exercise, more vasoconstriction is occurring than vasodilation. This causes an increase in total peripheral resistance, and changes in the other variables occur as a result of this.

Higher	Slightly Lower	Much Lower
Heart rate	Cardiac output	Stroke volume
Mean arterial blood pressure		
Respiratory rate		
Total peripheral resistance		

11. Describe the normal interaction of inotropes and chronotropes during exercise.

During exercise the initial chronotropes and inotropes are the sympathetic nerves that directly innervate the heart. A slightly delayed chronotrope and inotrope come from the adrenal medulla. When sympathetic nerves innervating the adrenal medulla are stimulated, epinephrine and norepinephrine are released into the blood. These hormones travel to the heart and perpetuate the response that was initiated by the sympathetic nerves.

12. What happens to systolic, diastolic, and mean arterial pressures during exercise?

- Systolic and mean arterial pressures increase because of a higher stroke volume.
- Diastolic pressure remains constant or drops slightly because of a decrease in total peripheral resistance.

13. What effect does a low partial pressure of oxygen (Po_2) have on blood vessel diameter in the lung and in the systemic circulation?

Vessels in the lung constrict when exposed to a low Po_2, whereas vessels in the systemic circulation dilate. The constriction of vessels in the lung shunts blood to the areas of the lung that are better ventilated. This results in better ventilation-perfusion matching, which causes more effective oxygenation of blood. Dilation of systemic vessels enables more blood to be delivered to the area. This results in better oxygenation of the localized tissues.

14. Why is the arteriovenous oxygen difference ($A - Vo_2$) larger in endurance athletes?

- Regular exercise results in an increase in the size of mitochondria and in the mitochondrial enzyme activity. This allows each mitochondrion to extract more oxygen from the blood in a given time period.
- Exercise results in an increase in the density of mitochondria, which leads to more oxygen extraction.

- Exercise results in an increase in capillary density of skeletal muscle. This allows the velocity of blood flow through each vessel to decrease, and the amount of time for oxygen extraction by the mitochondria increases.

15. Discuss the effect long-term endurance training has on the heart and on blood volume.

Increases in plasma volume occur shortly after the initiation of intense endurance training. This appears to be caused by an increase in plasma albumin levels, which osmotically draws fluid into the vasculature. Higher plasma volumes cause an increase in venous return, left ventricular end-diastolic volume, and stroke volume. These changes can occur within 1 week of the initiation of endurance training. Hypertrophy of myocardial muscle also occurs with endurance training, but this is a slower process.

16. Describe the contributions of stored adenosine triphosphate (ATP), creatine phosphate, glycolysis, and aerobic metabolism toward providing ATP during intense exercise over time.

- Stored ATP is used primarily for maximal intensity exercise causing fatigue after about 4 seconds.
- If the intensity of exercise is such that fatigue occurs after about 10 seconds, **creatine phosphate** is used to supply the energy to replenish the ATP stores during the last 6 seconds of the exercise.
- Intense exercise lasting between 10 seconds and 2 minutes depends on **anaerobic glycolysis** for ATP production. The maximal intensity of exercise is not as great as it was when creatine phosphate was being used.
- For intense exercise lasting longer than 2 minutes, **aerobic metabolism** provides most of the ATP, and the maximal intensity of the exercise that can be sustained is only about half of what it was during anaerobic glycolysis.

17. What can be done to improve the systems for providing ATP during intense exercise?

To improve the ability of **creatine phosphate** to provide energy, several bouts of intense exercise should be performed for 5 to 10 seconds with a 30- to 60-second rest between bouts. To improve **anaerobic capacity**, several bouts of intense exercise should be performed for at most 1 minute in duration with 3 to 5 minutes of recovery between bouts.

18. Compare differences in size, velocity of contraction, fatigability, and metabolism among type 1, type 2a, and type 2b muscle fibers.

	Fiber Type		
	Type 1	**Type 2a**	**Type 2b**
Fiber name	Slow twitch	Intermediate twitch	Fast twitch
Velocity of shortening	Low	Intermediate	High
Resistance to fatigue	Good	Average	Poor
Diameter	Small	Intermediate	Large
Type of metabolism	Aerobic	Aerobic and anaerobic	Anaerobic

19. Which type of muscle fiber is activated during moderate-intensity, long-duration exercise, such as jogging?

Slow-twitch type 1 fibers are activated.

20. Which type of muscle fiber is activated during high-intensity, short-term exercise, such as sprinting?

Slow-twitch type 1 and fast-twitch type 2 fibers are activated.

21. Why are specific muscle fiber types activated during different kinds of exercise?

The activation of a particular motor unit depends on the size of the α-motor neuron that innervates it. Type 1 fibers are innervated by small α-motor neurons, which have a lower threshold of stimulation than type 2 fibers; type 1 fibers always are stimulated first. Type 2 fibers are stimulated only if the intensity of the exercise requires it.

22. Explain why movements become less precise and refined as low-intensity exercise is continued for a prolonged period of time.

Initially, low-intensity exercise uses motor units consisting of slow-twitch muscle fibers. These motor units have fewer muscle fibers than motor units with fast-twitch fibers, and this accounts for better control during low-intensity exercises compared with high-intensity exercises. If low-intensity exercise is prolonged to the point that glycogen is depleted, the fast-twitch motor units are recruited. These motor units have more muscle fibers and result in less control of movements.

23. Can the three muscle fiber types be changed as a result of exercise?

Type 1 fibers cannot be converted to type 2 fibers, but type 1 fibers can improve their ability to use anaerobic metabolism, and type 2 fibers can improve their ability to use aerobic metabolism. Type 2b fibers can be converted to type 2a fibers with endurance training, or strength training.

24. What changes occur in muscle with endurance training?

Endurance training results in improvements in oxygen delivery and use. This is caused by an increase in capillary and mitochondria content and aerobic oxidative enzyme activity. Type 2b muscle fibers are converted to type 2a. The cross-sectional area of the muscle decreases, resulting in shorter diffusion distances for oxygen and carbon dioxide.

25. What changes occur in muscle with resistance training, and how long does it take for those changes to occur?

Resistance training causes synthesis of proteins in thick and thin filaments, resulting in an increase in cross-sectional area. The ratio of mitochondrial volume to contractile protein volume decreases. The aerobic capacity of the muscle decreases, which hinders performance in endurance activities. Type 2b muscle fibers are converted to type 2a. It takes about 6 to 8 weeks for the addition of protein filaments, but conversion of type 2b to type 2a fibers begins after about 2 weeks.

26. What causes improvements in strength with resistance training?

In the first 2 weeks, 90% of the improvements are attributed to neural changes, including improvements in recruitment pattern of motor units, increases in CNS activation, more synchronization of motor units, and less neural inhibition. After about 6 weeks of training, 80% of the improvements are from an increase in contractile proteins.

27. How does the $\dot{V}O_2max$ of a well-trained man compare with the $\dot{V}O_2max$ of a well-trained woman?

When $\dot{V}O_2max$ is expressed per kilogram of body weight, the $\dot{V}O_2max$ of a well-trained man is approximately 20% higher than that of a well-trained woman. If $\dot{V}O_2max$ is expressed relative to lean body mass, it is only about 9% higher in men. The cause of the difference is not known, but it may be due to a greater oxygen-carrying capacity in men caused by a higher hemoglobin content and larger blood volume as well as a higher cardiac output.

28. What is the cause of athletic amenorrhea?

Women who train heavily have higher levels of catecholamines, cortisol, and β-endorphins. These hormones inhibit the release of luteinizing hormone and follicle-stimulating hormone, which results in decreased levels of estradiol. This contributes to the cause of athletic amenorrhea. Studies have shown that physical and emotional stress, diet, and the presence of menstrual irregularity before training also contribute. The exact mechanism is not known.

29. Is it true that pregnant women who are physically fit deliver more easily?

No. The duration and intensity of labor are not affected by the level of fitness of the mother, although the perception of pain may be less in physically fit women.

30. Summarize some physiologic changes that occur during pregnancy that affect exercise.

The American College of Obstetrics and Gynecology (ACOG) recognizes the following:

A. After the first trimester, the supine position results in relative obstruction of venous return by the enlarging uterus and a significant decrease in cardiac output.
B. Stroke volume and cardiac output during steady-state exercise are increased significantly.
C. Exercise during pregnancy induces a greater degree of hemoconcentration than does exercise in the nonpregnant state.
D. There is a 10% to 20% increase in baseline oxygen consumption during pregnancy.
E. Because of the increased resting oxygen requirements and the increased work of breathing brought about by physical effects of the enlarged uterus on the diaphragm, decreased oxygen is available for the performance of aerobic exercise during pregnancy.
F. There is a shift in the physical center of gravity that may affect balance.
G. Basal metabolic rate and heat production increase during pregnancy.
H. Approximately 300 extra kilocalories per day are required to meet the metabolic needs of pregnancy; this caloric requirement is increased further in pregnant women who exercise regularly.
I. Pregnant women use carbohydrates during exercise at a greater rate than do nonpregnant women; adequate carbohydrate intake for exercising pregnant patients is essential.

31. List general guidelines for an exercise program to increase aerobic fitness.

The American College of Sports Medicine (ACSM) recommends:

A. Exercise should be performed 3 to 5 days per week.
B. The intensity of exercise should be such to maintain the heart rate at 65% to 90% of the maximal heart rate except for individuals who are quite unfit; 55% to 64% of maximal heart rate should be used for these individuals.
C. The duration of training should be 20 to 60 minutes of continuous or intermittent (minimum of 10-minute bouts accumulated throughout the day) aerobic activity.
D. The mode of activity should be any activity that uses large muscle groups, which can be maintained continuously and is rhythmic and aerobic in nature, such as walking, jogging, or bicycling. Higher intensity exercise does not need to be performed as long as lower intensity exercises. The total amount of work done seems to be the most important variable.

E. Proper warm-up and cool-down periods of exercise should be performed: these are increasingly important as the intensity of exercise increases.

32. List the general ACSM guidelines for an exercise program to increase muscular strength.

A. Resistance training should be progressive, should be individualized, and should provide a stimulus to all major muscle groups.
B. One set of 8 to 10 exercises that conditions the major muscle groups 2 to 3 days per week is recommended. Multiple sets may provide greater benefits.
C. A range of 8 to 12 repetitions of each exercise should be performed; older or more frail individuals should do 10 to 15 repetitions of a lower intensity.
D. Strength is developed best by using heavier weights that require near-maximal tension, with few repetitions. Muscular endurance is developed by using lighter weight with more repetitions. Use of 8 to 12 repetitions seems to cause improvements in both areas.
E. For upper body strengthening, 65% to 70% of the maximal amount of weight that can be moved through the full range of motion one time (1-RM) frequently is recommended for the amount of weight to use. For lower body strengthening, 75% to 80% of 1-RM should be used. These amounts need to be individualized.

33. List the general ACSM guidelines for an exercise program to decrease body weight.

A. The most successful program to decrease body weight is one that combines exercise with dieting. Such a program decreases weight, decreases fat mass, and maintains or increases fat-free mass. If one diets without exercising, one may lose more weight than by combining diet and exercise, but fat-free mass is lost in addition to fat mass.
B. An aerobic exercise program is most effective.
C. Exercise should be performed at least 3 days per week at an intensity and duration to expend 250 to 300 kilocalories per exercise session for a 75-kg person. This usually requires a duration of at least 30 to 45 minutes for a person in average physical condition.

34. List the general ACSM guidelines for an exercise program to preserve bone health.

A. Type of exercise should include weight-bearing endurance activities such as tennis, stair climbing, and jogging intermittently during walking; jumping activities such as volleyball and basketball; and resistance exercise that involves all major muscle groups, such as weight lifting.
B. Intensity should be moderate to high, in terms of bone-loading forces.
C. The frequency of weight-bearing endurance activities should be 3 to 5 times per week, resistance exercise 2 to 3 times per week.
D. Duration should be 30 to 60 minutes per day.
E. The older adult should also perform activities to improve balance for the prevention of falls.

35. How do exercise and training affect the endocrine system and the resting levels of hormones?

Most hormone levels increase during submaximal, short-term exercise with the exception of insulin, which decreases, and thyroid hormones, which do not change. Resting levels of ACTH, cortisol, catecholamines, insulin, and glucagons decrease with training. This may be related to greater energy stores or a decreased perception of stress.

36. Discuss prolonged, moderate-intensity exercise training and blood glucose levels in individuals with type I and type II diabetes.

Blood glucose levels do not seem to change with a prolonged exercise program in individuals with type I diabetes, but they decrease in individuals with type II diabetes. Exercise causes the cells of type II diabetic patients to be less resistant to insulin. This seems to be most effective if exercise is performed at an intensity of 60% to 75% of $\dot{V}O_2max$. Most type II diabetic patients are overweight. Exercise causes a decrease in weight, which results in an increase in the number of insulin receptors, an increase in their sensitivity, or both. It is not certain which mechanism is occurring, but the end result is lower blood glucose levels. Exercise reduces the cholesterol level of type II diabetic patients. This along with the accompanying weight loss decreases the cardiovascular risk factors of these individuals, which is the most significant benefit of performing exercise.

Although exercise has not been shown to improve blood glucose levels in individuals with type I diabetes, it is still recommended for the same reasons that exercise is recommended for individuals without diabetes.

37. Does exercise affect the prevalence of upper respiratory tract infections (URTI)?

Few studies have addressed the effect of moderate-intensity exercise on URTI. Preliminary results indicate a decrease in URTI with moderate exercise. More evidence indicates an increased prevalence of URTI during heavy endurance training and 1 to 2 weeks following a marathon-type event.

38. Does exercise lower resting blood pressure (BP) in normal and hypertensive individuals?

Yes; exercise, especially aerobic exercise, lowers both resting systolic pressure (SP) and resting diastolic pressure (DP); however, authors disagree on the amount respective BPs are decreased. The decrease is more pronounced in hypertensive individuals. Estimates range between 2 and 10 mm Hg for both SP and DP in these subjects. Exercise is particularly effective in reducing blood pressure if it is combined with weight reduction and a decrease in salt intake.

39. Should patients with chronic obstructive pulmonary disease (COPD) be encouraged to exercise?

Ambulation distance and feeling of well-being can increase significantly with an exercise program in individuals with mild or moderate COPD. There is controversy regarding the benefits of exercise for individuals with severe COPD. Some studies have shown improvements in endurance, whereas others have found no change. Only patients with stable COPD should be allowed to participate in an exercise program in a nonmedical setting.

40. How does the heart rate response to exercise differ between normal individuals and individuals who have had heart transplants?

In normal individuals, heart rate increases rapidly with moderate exercise as a result of a decrease in parasympathetic nerve activity and an increase in sympathetic nerve activity. Transplanted hearts are denervated. Any change in heart rate must be caused by changes in circulating levels of catecholamines, which takes more time than altering nerve activity. It takes longer for the heart rate to increase when exercise is initiated, and it takes longer for it to return to resting levels after exercise.

41. How does resting heart rate differ between normal individuals and individuals who have had heart transplants?

Resting heart rate is higher in individuals who have had a heart transplant because they no longer have the normal parasympathetic tone to slow the intrinsic rate of depolarization of the sinoatrial node.

42. Why are individuals with thoracic level spinal cord injuries at risk for fainting after exercising in the upright position with the upper extremities?

There is no sympathetic innervation to the lower limb vasculature, and there may not be any innervation to the adrenal glands (depending on how high the injury is). This results in a lack of vasoconstriction of the vessels of the lower extremities, venous pooling occurs, and syncope follows.

43. What is the most common problem associated with exercising in cold environments?

When people know they are going to be exercising in cold environments, they usually overdress, resulting in **hyperthermia.**

44. List strategies to avoid hypothermia and hyperthermia when exercising in a cold environment.

- Dress in layers that can be removed as the exercise progresses.
- Stay dry; heat is lost much more rapidly when you are wet than when you are dry.

45. Describe the physiologic changes that occur when exercising in a cold environment.

Vasoconstriction of cutaneous and nonexercising skeletal muscle blood vessels occurs. This provides a thicker layer of insulation between the body core and the environment, which minimizes heat loss. Vasoconstriction does not occur in the cerebral circulation, and 25% of the total heat loss from the body can occur through the head if a hat is not worn. **Shivering** occurs; these involuntary skeletal muscle contractions increase heat production, which warms the body. Shivering also causes blood flow to skeletal muscle to increase, which decreases the insulation layer; therefore shivering is not an effective means of conserving heat. $\dot{V}O_2max$ decreases, and maximal muscle strength and power decrease with hypothermia.

46. List possible causes for decreased maximal muscle strength and power with hypothermia.

- Increased viscosity of skeletal muscle
- Increased resistance to blood flow
- Decreased maximal nerve conduction velocity

47. What are the two most common problems associated with exercising in hot environments?

Dehydration and hyperthermia are the two most common problems in this situation.

48. How can dehydration and hyperthermia be avoided?

These problems cannot be avoided totally, but they can be limited by ingesting fluid while exercising. There appears to be a similar benefit between ingestion of pure water compared with carbohydrate and electrolyte drinks as far as controlling core temperature and cardiovascular changes.

49. Describe the physiologic changes that occur when exercising in a hot environment.

Sweat production can increase to 2 to 3 L/hr. This fluid comes from interstitial fluid, intracellular fluid, and plasma. **Dehydration** occurs quickly if fluid intake does not increase. If dehydration occurs, the sweat rate decreases to conserve water, but this causes the core temperature to increase. **Cardiovascular changes** include a decrease in venous return caused by dehydration. This results in an increase in heart rate and a decrease in stroke volume and cardiac output. **Blood flow to the skin** increases, especially in the forearms in an attempt to increase heat loss from the body, but if dehydration is severe, vasoconstriction of cutaneous vessels occurs to maintain central blood volume. This also causes the core temperature to increase. Skeletal muscles respond by producing more lactate; this may be related to an increase in the recruitment of fast-twitch motor units as well as decreased removal of blood lactate.

50. Does living at high altitude improve exercise tolerance at high altitude?

Yes. The exercise response at high altitude of subjects who live at moderate altitudes compared with subjects who live at sea level shows that individuals who live at moderate altitude have less of a decrease in $\dot{V}O_2$max and blood lactate accumulation. They also have a larger maximal ventilation during maximal exercise. Hematocrit levels increase after about 25 days of exposure to high altitude, which should increase performance. Some studies indicate that pulmonary function, cardiac output, muscle enzyme capacity, and lean body mass decrease at high altitudes. World-class athletes performing endurance exercise consistently seem to perform better if they train at moderate altitude.

Bibliography

American College of Obstetricians and Gynecologists: *Exercise during pregnancy,* Washington, DC, 1994, ACOG (technical bulletin 189).

American College of Sports Medicine: Position stand: the recommended quantity and quality of exercise for developing and maintaining cardiorespiratory and muscular fitness, and flexibility in healthy adults, *Med Sci Sports Exerc* 30:975-991, 1998.

American College of Sports Medicine: Position stand: progression models in resistance training for healthy adults, *Med Sci Sports Exerc* 34:364-375, 2002.

American College of Sports Medicine: Position stand: exercise and hypertension, *Med Sci Sports Exerc* 36:533-546, 2004.

American College of Sports Medicine: Position stand: physical activity and bone health, *Med Sci Sports Exerc* 36:1985-1993, 2004.

Artal Mittelmark R et al: Exercise guide for pregnancy. In Artal Mittelmark R, Wiswell RA, Drinkwater BL, editors: *Exercise in pregnancy,* ed 2, Baltimore, 1991, pp 299-319, Williams & Wilkins.

Bacon SL et al: Effects of exercise, diet and weight loss on high blood pressure, *Sports Med* 34:307-314, 2004.

Fahay TD: Endurance training. In Shangold M, Mirkin G, editors: *Women and exercise: Physiology and sports medicine,* ed 2, Philadelphia, 1994, pp 73-86, FA Davis.

Hasson SM, editor: *Clinical exercise physiology,* St Louis, 1994, Mosby.

Katch FI, McArdle WD: *Introduction to nutrition, exercise, and health,* ed 4, Philadelphia, 1993, Lea & Febiger.

McArdle WD, Katch FI, Katch VL: *Exercise physiology,* ed 5, Philadelphia, 2001, Lippincott Williams & Wilkins.

McMurray RG, Hackney AC: Endocrine responses to exercise and training. In Garrett WE, Kirkendall DT, editors: *Exercise and sport science,* Philadelphia, 2000, pp 135-161, Lippincott Williams & Wilkins.

Nieman DC: Exercise, the immune system, and infectious disease. In Garrett WE, Kirkendall DT, editors: *Exercise and sport science,* Philadelphia, 2000, pp 177-190, Lippincott Williams & Wilkins.

Robergs RA, Roberts SO: *Exercise physiology: exercise, performance, and clinical applications,* St Louis, 1997, Mosby.

Roberts SO: Principles of prescribing exercise. In Roberts SO, Robergs RA, Hanson P, editors: *Clinical exercise testing and prescription theory and application,* Boca Raton, Fla, 1997, pp 235-259, CRC Press.

Shephard RJ, Astrand PO, editors: *The encyclopedia of sports medicine endurance in sport,* London, 1992, Blackwell Scientific.

Staron SS, Hikida RS: Muscular responses to exercise and training. In Garrett WE, Kirkendall DT, editors: *Exercise and sport science,* Philadelphia, 2000, pp 163-176, Lippincott Williams & Wilkins.

Tipton CM: Exercise and hypertension. In Shephard RJ, Miller HS, editors: *Exercise and the heart in health and disease,* ed 2, New York, 1999, pp 463-484, Marcel Dekker.

Viru A, Viru M: Nature of training effects. In Garrett WE, Kirkendall DT, editors: *Exercise and sport science,* Philadelphia, 2000, pp 67-95, Lippincott Williams & Wilkins.

Zernicke RF, Salem GF, Alejo RK: Endurance training. In Reider B, editor: *Sports medicine: the school age athlete,* Philadelphia, 1996, pp 3-16, WB Saunders.

Section II

Disease Processes

Chapter 6

Arthritis

Judith L. Bateman, MD

1. List uses, mechanisms of action, and potential side effects of medications commonly used to treat types of arthritis.

Medication Name or Class	Use	Mechanism of Action	Side Effects
NSAIDs	OA, RA, sprains, inhibition of heterotopic ossification	Inhibits COX	GI upset, peptic ulcers, renal function, excessive bleeding
COX-2 inhibitors	As above	Inhibits COX-2 specifically	Renal and possibly cardiac function
Glucocorticoids	RA, SLE, gout, other inflammatory diseases	Inhibits many inflammatory mediators	Weight gain, bone/muscle loss, hyperglycemia
Methotrexate	RA, seronegative arthritis	Inhibits adenosine metabolism	Pneumonitis, leukopenia, liver disease, infection
Sulfasalazine	RA, seronegative arthritis	Inhibits B cell activity	Bone marrow suppression, rash, hepatitis
Anti-TNF therapy	RA, psoriatic arthritis, AS	Inhibits TNF activity	Infection (especially TB), heart failure, possibly lymphoma
Antimalarials	RA, SLE	Inhibits enzyme activity	Eye changes, vision loss
Gold	RA	Inhibits WBC activity	Anemia, low WBC count, lung disease, proteinuria
Minocycline	RA, Reiter syndrome	Inhibits metalloproteinase activity	Hepatitis, lupus-like reactions
Colchicine	Gout, pseudogout	Inhibits microtubule movement	Diarrhea, bone marrow suppression
Leflunomide	RA, psoriatic arthritis	Inhibits IMP	Diarrhea, liver toxicity, hypertension

AS, Ankylosing spondylitis; *COX,* cyclooxygenase; *NSAIDs,* nonsteroidal antiinflammatory drugs; *OA,* osteoarthritis; *RA,* rheumatoid arthritis; *SLE,* systemic lupus erythematosus; *TB,* tuberculosis; *TNF,* tumor necrosis factor; *WBC,* white blood cell.

2. Describe characteristic signs and symptoms of rheumatoid arthritis.

Symmetric arthritis of small joints of the hands (sparing distal interphalangeals [DIPs]), wrists, feet, and knees that is associated with morning stiffness is present. Rheumatoid nodules as well as serum rheumatoid factor may be evident, and radiographic changes may also be seen. Symptoms and signs should be present for 6 weeks before the diagnosis is made.

3. What x-ray changes are typical of rheumatoid arthritis?

- Periarticular osteopenia occurs first.
- Erosions may develop at joint margins.
- Loss of joint space, malalignment, and progressive osteopenia may be seen.

4. Who may be affected by rheumatoid arthritis (RA)?

RA affects approximately 1% of the population worldwide. It may begin at any age, but there is a peak in onset in women of childbearing years and a second peak in elderly men and women. Genetic influences are important, and HLA-DR4 subtypes are associated with more severe forms of the disease.

5. Describe joint pathology in RA.

Chronic changes include thickening and edema of the synovial lining of the affected joints. The underlying connective tissue cells become activated and invade and destroy cartilage and bone at the margins of joints. This is called pannus formation.

6. List the most common hand and wrist deformities associated with rheumatoid arthritis.

- Swan neck deformity (flexion at DIP, extension at proximal interphalangeal [PIP])
- Boutonnière deformity (extension at DIP, flexion at PIP)
- Ulnar deviation at metacarpophalangeals (MCPs)
- Flexion, radial deviation, and subluxation at wrist
- Extensor tendon rupture at wrist

7. Name the types of juvenile RA.

- Pauciarticular, involving ≤4 joints, the most common presentation
- Polyarticular, similar in nature to adult RA
- Systemic onset, with fever, arthritis, rash, and other organ involvement

8. What is the prognosis for patients with RA?

The course is variable, with some individuals never seeking treatment. Half of RA patients may be disabled at work within 10 years, and two thirds may have significant trouble with activities of daily living after 15 years. Patients with severe disease may die 10 to 15 years sooner than expected.

9. Define rheumatoid factor (RF).

RF is an antibody, most often an IgM antibody directed against IgG antibodies, that precipitates immune complex formation. It is found in approximately 80% of patients with RA. RF is associated with nodule formation, extra-articular disease, and more severe joint disease. RF is not diagnostic of RA, because it is present in many chronic diseases (low specificity).

Higher specificity for RA (approximately 98%) is found by testing for anticyclic citrullinated peptide antibodies (anti-CCP Ab)—antibodies directed against specifically modified proteins found in the rheumatoid synovium.

10. Does RA affect the spine?

The synovium of the odontoid process of C2 and the transverse ligament that holds C2 to C1 may become involved and cause erosion, leading to instability at C1-C2. Patients may have pain and may develop myelopathy. The thoracic and lumbar spines are not affected by RA.

11. List physical therapy treatments that are helpful for RA.

Acutely Inflamed Joint	Decreased Inflammation
• Heat	• Isometric exercise
• Rest	• Range of motion exercise
• Splinting, to avoid contracture	• Strengthening exercise
	• Paraffin baths
	• Transcutaneous electric nerve stimulation

12. List the types of orthopaedic procedures that most often are used for RA involving the hand and wrist.

- Synovectomy
- Arthrodesis (joint fusion)
- Soft tissue reconstruction
- Arthroplasty

13. What is the Darrach procedure?

This is a common procedure that involves excision of the distal ulna, often accompanied by synovectomy and extensor tendon repair when needed.

14. What is systemic lupus erythematosus?

Systemic lupus erythematosus (SLE) is a multisystem inflammatory disease that may cause fever, fatigue, rash, cytopenia, renal disease, serositis, lung disease, nervous system changes, joint pain, and other problems.

15. Is lupus diagnosed by the presence of antinuclear antibodies (ANA)?

ANA are present in 99% of patients with SLE, but false positive results are very common (up to 30% to 40% false positives, especially with low-titer ANA). Lupus is a clinical diagnosis.

16. List musculoskeletal problems that patients with systemic lupus erythematosus can develop.

- Arthralgia and arthritis
- Osteonecrosis
- Tendinitis and tendon rupture
- Fibromyalgia
- Steroid myopathy
- Polymyositis

17. Describe typical lupus arthritis.

- Arthralgias are most common, without visible joint swelling.
- When inflammation is present, it often involves the small joints of the hands, similar to the pattern in RA.
- The arthritis is not erosive, although joint deformities may be seen (e.g., Jaccoud's arthropathy, with swan neck deformities).

18. Name the seronegative arthropathies.

- Ankylosing spondylitis
- Reiter syndrome (reactive arthritis)
- Psoriatic arthritis
- Arthritis associated with inflammatory bowel disease

19. List the clinical features that the seronegative arthropathies share.

- Enthesitis (inflammation at sites of insertion of tendons or ligaments into bone)
- Sacroiliitis and other axial skeletal involvement
- Asymmetric, peripheral pauciarticular inflammatory arthritis
- Extra-articular disease involving the gastrointestinal or genitourinary systems, skin, and eye
- Association with HLA-B27 (in patients with spondylitis)

20. List clinical features of psoriatic arthritis.

- Psoriatic skin lesions (nail changes are common)
- Asymmetric peripheral arthritis with DIP involvement
- Sausage digits and other tendinitis
- Occasional spondylitis and sacroiliitis
- Occasional arthritis deformans with telescoping of digits

21. What is Reiter syndrome?

Reiter syndrome is a seronegative arthritis that is triggered by infection, typically by *Chlamydia, Shigella,* or *Yersinia.*

The classic triad of arthritis, conjunctivitis, and urethritis is seen in a minority of cases.

22. How does the back pain of ankylosing spondylitis differ from mechanical back pain clinically?

	Ankylosing Spondylitis	Mechanical Back Pain
Age of onset	Late teens to 20s	Any age
Timing of onset	Insidious, nontraumatic	Often sudden, traumatic
Pain with rest	Increased	Decreased
Pain with activity	Decreased	Increased
Stiffness	+++	±, usually <15 min

23. What treatments are available for ankylosing spondylitis?

- Education and exercise are most important.
- Extension exercises 3 times daily (swimming recommended), attention to erect posture, and sleeping without a pillow to prevent kyphosis are recommended.
- Nonsteroidal antiinflammatory drugs (NSAIDs) can help relieve pain and stiffness, and methotrexate and sulfasalazine improve inflammation in peripheral joints.
- Tumor necrosis factor (TNF) inhibitors have been shown to cause clinical improvement in the axial skeleton.

24. Describe x-ray changes in ankylosing spondylitis.

- Erosion, sclerosis, pseudowidening, and ultimately fusion of sacroiliac joints
- Squaring of vertebrae with shiny corners

- Syndesmophyte formation (ossification of the outer layer of the intervertebral disk), leading to bamboo spine
- Fusion of apophyseal joints

25. What causes gout?

Gout is caused by the accumulation of uric acid crystals in synovial joints. Polymorphonuclear leukocytes are attracted to the joint, try to engulf the crystals, and release digestive enzymes and proinflammatory mediators.

26. What causes pseudogout?

Calcium pyrophosphate crystals initiate inflammation.

27. How can the crystal types in gout and pseudogout be distinguished?

Examination of synovial fluid under a polarizing microscope helps differentiate gout from pseudogout: uric acid crystals are needle-like and negatively birefringent whereas pseudogout crystals are rod-shaped and positively birefringent.

28. Name the phases of gout.

- Asymptomatic hyperuricemia (elevated serum uric acid level predisposes people to develop gout)
- Acute gouty arthritis
- Intercritical gout (asymptomatic between episodes of acute gout)
- Chronic gout (tophi, deposits of uric acid, are often seen)

29. Describe a typical episode of acute gout.

Acute gout episodes typically begin with the sudden onset of severe burning pain, often in the middle of the night, usually involving the first metatarsophalangeal (MTP) joint. The pain may be so severe that even the weight of the bed sheets may be unbearable. The joint appears red, swollen, and hot to touch. Episodes usually resolve within 7 to 10 days. They may be precipitated by alcohol consumption, trauma, surgery, or immobilization.

30. What joints other than the first MTP may be affected in gout?

Any joint in the body can be affected, but the knee, ankle, midfoot, wrist, and hand are commonly affected. Tophi are seen as painless lumps in chronic gout, often at the olecranon, fingers, toes, or outer ear.

31. How is acute gout treated?

Cold packs may be helpful, but no other modalities or exercise is recommended. NSAIDs are the mainstay of treatment; however, local injection or oral administration of corticosteroids is another form of treatment. Colchicine often causes severe diarrhea and nausea with oral use and may be associated with severe bone marrow toxicity or skin damage with intravenous use, so it generally is not recommended.

32. Can gout be diagnosed by an elevated serum uric acid level?

No. Of patients with elevated serum uric acid levels, <20% develop gout; 30% of patients do not have elevated uric acid levels at the time of a joint flare-up. The diagnosis must be made by examining joint fluid.

33. How does pseudogout differ from gout?

Calcium pyrophosphate deposition disease can present similarly to gout (pseudogout) but also may present similarly to RA (pseudo-RA) or as aggressive osteoarthritis (OA). Calcium pyrophosphate deposits (chondrocalcinosis) often can be seen on radiographs as opacities in the knee joint space or in the triangular fibrocartilage of the wrist.

Definitive diagnosis requires examination of joint fluid. Aspiration of fluid often is adequate to relieve symptoms. Local steroid injection or NSAIDs are used.

34. What is the differential diagnosis of a single red, hot joint?

Infection is the most dangerous condition associated with this diagnosis and must immediately be ruled out by testing a sample of synovial fluid. Other diagnoses include acute gout, hemarthrosis with or without trauma, pseudogout, RA, seronegative arthropathy, and other less common etiologies (e.g., tumor or pigmented villondular synovitis).

35. Describe clinical signs of infected total joint prostheses.

With acute infection, wound dehiscence or drainage may be seen along with classic signs of inflammation (pain, redness, swelling, heat). Later, pain and loosening of the joint may be the only signs. If acute infection is suspected, patients should be referred back to their orthopaedist for immediate evaluation.

36. How are infected total joint arthroplasties treated?

If detected early, infected joint arthroplasties may be salvaged with aggressive lavage and intravenous antibiotics. If not caught early or if gram-negative bacteria are present, the joint must be removed and often cannot be replaced until after extensive antibiotic treatment.

37. How common is OA?

OA is the most common type of arthritis. Prevalence increases with age, and it has been estimated to affect >80% of individuals >75 years of age.

38. List the pathologic changes in OA.

- Thinning and damage to articular cartilage
- Subchondral bone sclerosis
- Marginal bone and cartilage growth as osteophytes
- Periarticular muscle wasting

39. Which joints are commonly involved in OA?

- DIPs (Heberden's nodes) and PIPs (Bouchard's nodes)
- Hips
- Lumbar spine
- Knees
- Feet (especially first MTP)

40. Have treatments been found to stop the progression of OA?

No, but a few studies have suggested that minocycline may slow the progression of OA, presumably by inhibiting metalloproteinases, which cause cartilage damage. In one study glucosamine sulfate was shown to increase the joint space in osteoarthritic knees.

Bibliography

Cush JJ: Safety overview of new disease-modifying antirheumatic drugs, *Rheum Dis Clin North Am* 30:237-255, 2004.

D'Ambrosia RD: *Musculoskeletal disorders: regional examination and differential diagnosis,* Philadelphia, 1977, JB Lippincott.

Deyle GD et al: Effectiveness of manual physical therapy and exercise in osteoarthritis of the knee: a randomized, controlled trial, *Ann Intern Med* 132:173-181, 2000.

Ekblom B et al: Effects of short-term physical training on patients with rheumatoid arthritis, *Scand J Rheumatol* 4:80-86, 1975.

Kelley WN, editor: *Textbook of rheumatology,* Philadelphia, 2005, WB Saunders.

Klippel JH, editor: *Rheumatology,* ed 2, Philadelphia, 1998, Mosby.

Nordemar R et al: Physical training in rheumatoid arthritis: a controlled long-term study: I, *Scand J Rheumatol* 10:17-23, 1981.

Schumacher HR, editor: *Primer on the rheumatic diseases,* Atlanta, 1997, Arthritis Foundation.

Solomon D et al: Evidence-based guidelines for the use of immunologic tests: antinuclear antibody testing, *Arthritis Rheum* 47:434-444, 2002.

Vallbracht I et al: Diagnostic and clinical value of anti-cyclic citrullinated peptide antibodies compared with rheumatoid factor isotypes in rheumatoid arthritis, *Ann Rheum Dis* 63:1079-1084, 2004.

van Baar ME et al: Effectiveness of exercise therapy in patients with osteoarthritis of the hip or knee: a systematic review of randomized clinical trials, *Arthritis Rheum* 42:1361-1369, 1999.

Chapter 7

Deep Venous Thrombosis

Michael Quinn, MD

1. Define Virchow's triad.

This is the classic triad for the pathogenesis of venous thrombosis:

1. Endothelial injury—change to the vascular wall that serves as a potent thrombogenic influence. It may be caused directly by surgical trauma or indirectly by hematoma formation or thermal injury from electrocautery or cement polymerization.
2. Alteration in blood flow—arterial turbulence or venous stasis that contributes to the development of thrombi. Stasis occurs while on the operating table and postoperatively because of immobilization or impaired ambulation.
3. Hypercoagulability—alteration in the blood coagulation mechanism that predisposes to thrombosis. A transient hypercoagulable state may exist as part of the normal host response to surgery.

2. List states that are associated with hypercoagulability.

GENETIC

- Antithrombin C deficiency
- Protein C deficiency
- Protein S deficiency
- Factor V Leiden deficiency

ACQUIRED

- Postoperative
- Postpartum
- Prolonged bed rest or immobilization
- Severe trauma
- Cancer
- Oral contraceptives
- Malignancy
- Congestive heart failure
- Advanced age
- Nephrotic syndrome
- Obesity
- Prior thromboembolism

3. How common are genetic factors in association with hypercoagulability?

Approximately 20% to 30% of patients with deep venous thrombosis (DVT) have a predisposing genetic factor.

4. Where do venous thrombi occur?

They occur mostly in the lower extremities, in the superficial or deep veins.

5. When do venous thrombi develop?

- DVT may begin during the surgical procedure.
- Patients may present with signs and symptoms of DVT 24 to 48 hours postoperatively.
- The risk of late postoperative DVT is recognized to continue for 3 months.

6. Describe the incidence of DVT after total joint arthroplasty.

Patients who undergo total hip arthroplasty or total knee arthroplasty are at high risk for DVT. If no prophylaxis is used, DVT occurs in 40% to 80% of these patients, and a proximal DVT occurs in 15% to 50%. Thromboembolic prophylaxis, early mobilization, and modern surgical techniques have reduced the incidence of fatal pulmonary embolism to ≤0.18%. Despite prophylaxis, venous thromboembolism remains the most common reason for emergency department readmission after a total joint arthroplasty.

7. Does the type of anesthetic used during surgery affect the incidence of DVT?

Regional epidural anesthesia has been associated with a reduction in overall, proximal, and distal DVT. Epidural anesthesia may reduce the overall incidence of DVT by 40% to 50%. Hypotensive anesthesia may also be beneficial.

8. List the clinical signs and symptoms of DVT.

- Calf pain
- Swelling
- Calf cramping
- Warmth
- Erythema
- Pain along the course of the involved vein
- Engorged veins
- Edema
- Low-grade fever
- Palpable cord along the course of the involved vein

9. Is DVT easily clinically diagnosed?

No. DVT may be difficult to diagnose on the basis of physical examination. In one study, the diagnosis was confirmed with diagnostic studies in less than half of those suspected of having a DVT. Most venous thrombi are clinically silent. A clinician may not rely on physical examination findings alone to diagnose a DVT.

10. What is Homans' sign?

Homans' sign is calf pain with forced passive foot dorsiflexion; it is a physical examination finding suggestive of DVT.

11. List differential diagnoses of DVT.

- Muscle strain
- Cellulitis
- Superficial thrombophlebitis
- Chronic venous insufficiency
- Nerve compression syndromes
- Lymphedema
- Arterial occlusion
- Baker cyst

12. Name the most dreaded complication from a DVT.

Pulmonary embolism is the most feared complication.

13. Describe the signs and symptoms of pulmonary embolism.

Pulmonary embolism (PE) may be the first clinical sign of a DVT. The clinical signs of PE are nonspecific, and, as with DVT, diagnostic studies are needed to confirm the diagnosis. A classic presentation of pulmonary embolism consists of pleuritic chest pain and dyspnea (40%). Patients also may present with cough, diaphoresis, apprehension, altered mental status, hemoptysis, tachypnea, tachycardia (most common finding, 85%), rales, fever, bulging neck veins (30%), and a pleural friction rub. In one study, nearly 40% of patients who had a DVT but no symptoms of pulmonary embolism had evidence of pulmonary embolism on diagnostic studies. Massive pulmonary embolism may present as syncope or sudden death. Two thirds of patients who suffer a fatal pulmonary embolus do so within 30 minutes of becoming symptomatic.

14. What are the electrocardiogram findings of pulmonary embolism?

Typical ECG findings include ST segment depression or T wave inversion, right axis deviation, or right bundle branch block. The classic electrocardiogram pattern $S_1Q_3T_3$ is rare.

15. What long-term complications are associated with DVT?

Chronic venous insufficiency secondary to venous dilation and valvular incompetence is a typical long-term DVT complication. At 5 years post-DVT, symptoms may include:

- Night pain (45%)
- Pigmentation changes (50%)
- Pain with prolonged standing (39%)
- Venous ulceration (7%)
- Edema (52%)

16. Discuss the modalities that are available to prevent the formation of a DVT.

- Heparin—may be given subcutaneously in the perioperative period. It may be given as a fixed dosage (5000 units every 8 to 12 hours) or as an adjusted low dosage (3500 units every 8 hours; then adjust the dose to desired anticoagulation).

- Low-molecular-weight heparin—typically given at a fixed dosage without the need for outpatient monitoring. However, it may be associated with a slightly increased incidence of postoperative bleeding and wound problems.
- Fondaparinux (Arixtra)—a selective factor Xa inhibitor. This medication was recently approved for prevention of venous thromboembolism after hip and knee arthroplasty.
- Warfarin—the most commonly used single agent for DVT prophylaxis for patients who have undergone total hip arthroplasty. Warfarin may take several days to reach therapeutic levels, and patients often are placed on heparin until the warfarin is therapeutic.
- Aspirin—the benefit for patients after joint arthroplasty is not conclusively proven. Aspirin has been proven to be a safe drug, but more study is needed to prove its efficacy for prevention of thromboembolism. Aspirin has been found to be effective in decreasing DVT when combined with exercise and graded stockings or leg pumps.
- Dextran—should be used cautiously. The additional fluid volume may result in heart failure in patients with low cardiac reserve. A decrease in renal function also may occur from excessive diuresis after administration of dextran.
- Mechanical—a variety of mechanical modalities exist. External pneumatic compression devices decrease the risk of DVT without bleeding risk by decreasing venous stasis and stimulating fibrinolytic activity. Calf and thigh sleeves exist as well as pneumatic foot pumps. The devices should not be used on patients who have an acute DVT or lower extremity fracture. Compression stockings also may help prevent venous thrombosis.

17. What actions should a therapist take if a DVT is suspected to be present?

The therapist should hold the therapeutic interventions and inform the physician. The patient should be non–weight-bearing on the affected lower extremity until they are evaluated by the physician. Diagnostic tests may be ordered by the physician to confirm the suspicion. A period of bed rest may be prescribed to prevent the clot from dislodging and developing into a pulmonary embolus.

18. Discuss the sensitivity and specificity of diagnostic tests for DVT.

- Duplex ultrasound—the screening test of choice for initial evaluation of patients with suspected DVT. Color flow Doppler imaging improves the ability to detect a clot. In patients with asymptomatic DVT, the sensitivity and specificity have been found to be 89% and 100%, respectively. When used as a screening tool in asymptomatic patients, the sensitivity and specificity are 62% and 97%, respectively. Duplex ultrasound imaging is highly operator dependent, and these values vary widely among institutions. It is less sensitive for detecting calf vein thrombi than those located more proximally.
- Venography—the gold standard for the diagnosis of DVT in the calf and thigh, with sensitivity and specificity almost 100%. The procedure is not an ideal screening test because of cost and potential morbidity related to the test. The detection of pelvic thrombi is poor, unless direct femoral vein puncture is performed.
- Impedance plethysmography—poor sensitivity (30%) for large thigh thrombi. Plethysmography is even less sensitive for small thigh and calf thrombi.
- ^{125}I-Fibrinogen scanning—90% accurate in detecting calf vein DVT. It may be falsely positive in the thigh after total hip arthroplasty in which there is fibrin present at the surgical site.
- Magnetic resonance imaging—also may be used to image DVT, particularly in the pelvis (100% sensitivity, 95% specificity), where it is more sensitive than venography. Magnetic resonance imaging is equally sensitive for detection of DVT in the thigh but inferior in the calf (87% sensitivity and 97% specificity).
- D-dimer—a blood assay that can significantly reduce the need for emergent venous Doppler examinations. It has a sensitivity of 100%, specificity of 49%, positive predictive value of 22%, and negative predictive value of 100%.

19. If the presence of a DVT is confirmed, what treatments are available?

- Heparin is initiated to prevent propagation and promote stabilization of the clot.
- Warfarin (Coumadin) therapy may be delayed for 1 day because warfarin may cause an initial thrombogenic effect before acting as an anticoagulant.
- Fondaparinux (Arixtra) is a selective factor Xa inhibitor.
- Low-molecular-weight heparin—enoxaparin (Lovenox) or dalteparin (Fragmin)—is another treatment option.

20. What are the mechanisms of action of heparin and warfarin?

- Heparin acts by binding to antithrombin III, increasing its inhibitory effects on thrombin and activated factors II, VII, IX, X, XI, and XII.
- Warfarin acts by inhibiting vitamin K–dependent factors II, VII, IX, and X.

21. Define PTT, PT, and INR.

- PTT is partial thromboplastin time—used to monitor anticoagulation while on heparin.
- PT is prothrombin time—used to monitor anticoagulation while on warfarin.
- INR is the abbreviation for international normalized ratio—represents measured PT adjusted by reference thromboplastin so that all laboratories have a universal result of patient PT; usually kept between 2 and 3 for treatment or prevention of DVT.

Bibliography

Buller HR et al: Fondaparinux or enoxaparin for the initial treatment of symptomatic deep venous thrombosis: a randomized trial, *Ann Intern Med* 140:867-873, 2004.

Della Valle CJ, Steiger DJ, Di Cesare PE: Thromboembolism after hip and knee arthroplasty: diagnosis and treatment, *J Am Acad Orthop Surg* 6:327-336, 1998.

Diamond S, Goldbweber R, Katz S: Use of D-dimer to aid in excluding deep venous thrombosis in ambulatory patients, *Am J Surg* 189:23-26, 2005.

Haas S: Deep vein thrombosis: beyond the operating table, *Orthopedics* 6:629-632, 2000.

Simon SR: *Orthopaedic basic science,* Rosemont, Ill, 1994, American Academy of Orthopaedic Surgeons.

Chapter 8

Complex Regional Pain Syndromes

Susan W. Stralka, PT, MS

1. What is complex regional pain syndrome (CRPS)?

CRPS is a syndrome in which pain is out of proportion to the injury and the symptoms are characterized by autonomic dysregulation, such as swelling, vasomotor instability, abnormal sweating, trophic changes, and abnormal motor activity. CRPS I was formerly called reflex sympathetic dystrophy, and CRPS II was formerly called causalgia.

2. Before being named CRPS, what other terms were used to describe this dysfunction?

- Algodystrophy
- Sudeck's atrophy
- Bone loss dysfunction
- Reflex sympathetic dystrophy
- Causalgia
- Reflex neurovascular dystrophy
- Sympathalgia
- Neurodystrophy
- Traumatic arthritis
- Minor causalgia
- Posttraumatic osteoporosis
- Posttraumatic pain syndrome
- Posttraumatic edema
- Posttraumatic angiospasms
- Shoulder-hand syndrome

3. What is the difference between CRPS I and CRPS II?

CRPS I does not have a history of nerve involvement, whereas CRPS II has nerve involvement, which starts as a peripheral nerve injury that may spread to regional involvement. Clinical findings are the same for CRPS I and II with the exception of nerve involvement in CRPS II.

4. Describe the cardinal signs seen in patients with CRPS.

- Pain—Classically the pain is a burning type of pain. It generally is felt in the distal part of the extremity in a nonsegmented distribution. As the symptoms continue, the pain becomes more diffuse and may spread gradually proximal to the involved limb and can spread to other parts of the body.
- Trophic change—Edema often is the first notable change in the skin, with gradual thickening and coarsening of the skin and wrinkle distribution changes, or the skin may become thin, smooth, and tight. The hair becomes coarse, and nails often are thickened, ridged, and brittle. As the process of CRPS continues, muscle shortening, atrophy, and weakness may occur.
- Autonomic instability (vasomotor/sudomotor)—Vasomotor instability indicates that the sympathetic nervous system (SNS) is involved in the pathophysiology. Initially the dystrophic limb is cool, pale, and cyanotic with sweating changes that indicate sympathetic hyperactivity. This state may occur any time throughout the disorder. The onset is after the initiating event or onset of problems. At times, the limb may be warm, red, and dry. Skin dryness may predominate for a while; then there may be increased sweating.

- Sensory abnormalities—Dysesthesia and allodynia often occur. Sensory abnormalities are not always dermatomal in distribution and can spread from distal to proximal or to the uninvolved limb.
- Bony changes—Initially, radiographs may reveal patchy osteoporosis that appears in the juxta-articular bone of the affected limb. Osteopenia begins in the metacarpal or metatarsal joint but can spread more proximally. A more generalized osteoporosis of subchondral bone of the involved joints may be observed. On three-phase bone scans, changes usually result in increased periarticular uptake and blood flow on the affected side.

5. Describe the pain terms that are associated with a patient having symptoms of CRPS I and II.

- Allodynia is pain caused by a stimulus that does not normally provoke pain. Example: Patients with CRPS cannot tolerate clothes or bed clothing on their injury because the fabric hurts their skin.
- Hyperalgesia refers to a stimulus that is normally more painful than usual or an exaggerated response to a normally painful stimulus.
- Hyperesthesia refers to an unusual sensitivity to repetitive stimuli. Example: Initial tapping on the skin is not painful, but with repetition it becomes more painful.

6. Summarize the different staging and time courses for CRPS.

	Acute	Dystrophic	Atrophic
Pain	Burning/neuralgia, +++	Burning/throbbing, +++	Burning/throbbing, ++
Dysesthesia	++	+++	+
Function	Minimal impairment	Restricted	Severely restricted
Autonomic dysfunction	Increased blood flow	Decreased flow	Decreased blood flow
Temperature	Increased	Decreased	Decreased
Discoloration	Erythematous	Mottled, dusky	Cyanotic
Sudomotor dysfunction	Minimal	++	+++
Edema	++	+++	+
Trophic changes	0	++	++++
Three-phase bone scan	Increased activity, all images	Normal uptake, all phases except increased static phase	Decreased activity
Osteoporosis	–	+	+++

7. List some of the precipitating events that cause reflex sympathetic dystrophy (CRPS I).

- Fractures
- Soft tissue trauma
- Frostbite
- Burns
- Multiple sclerosis and other central nervous system diseases
- Wearing of a tight cast
- Cerebral vascular accidents
- Myocardial infarction
- Crushing injuries
- Amputations
- Surgical procedures

8. How common are CRPS I and CRPS II?

The exact figures and the exact number of individuals with CRPS are unknown because there is relatively little information available regarding the overall incidence. Carron and Weller documented 123 patients who met criteria for CRPS. These 123 patients were of a general population of 1156 patients seen at a pain clinic and represented 10.7% of overall patients treated in a 2-year period. The Reflex Sympathetic Dystrophy Syndrome Association estimates that 6 million adults and children suffer from the condition in the United States. Women seem to be more likely to suffer from this disorder than men (ratio, 2:1 to 3:1). All ages can develop this syndrome, but more commonly the distribution seems to be in women between the ages of 30 and 55.

9. Discuss treatment of CRPS.

The most helpful guideline is early recognition and early treatment intervention, in which a multidisciplinary approach is used. Initial treatment should focus on locating and eliminating the initiating cause of pain. The treatment primarily is aimed toward interruption of the abnormal sympathetic response as well as interruption of the vicious cycle of dysfunction, including pain, swelling, immobility, and decreased weight-bearing. Interruption of the abnormal sympathetic reflex is by means of surgical decompression, nerve blocks, ganglion blocks, and axillary blocks in conjunction with physical, occupational, and psychological therapies.

10. What is triple-phase scintigraphy?

It is an imaging approach that is helpful in confirming the diagnosis of CRPS and eliminating other conditions that may be causing these symptoms. The skin pattern most commonly associated with CRPS is increased flow in the involved extremity with delayed static images showing diffuse increased activity in a periarticular distribution. Delayed imaging shows that diffuse increased tracer uptake is diagnostic for CRPS with 96% sensitivity and 98% specificity. Studies show the specificity for bone scans in diagnosing CRPS varies from 75% to 98%, whereas sensitivity is greatly variable (50% to ≤96%).

11. What should be seen in a three-phase bone scan for the scan to be considered diagnostic of CRPS?

The delayed phase (3 to 4 hours after injection) must show diffusely increased activity in the involved joints with periarticular accentuation.

12. How is radiography useful in diagnosing CRPS?

Radiographic evidence of sympathetic hyperdysfunction includes patchy demineralization of the epiphyses and metacarpal and metatarsal bones of the hands and feet. Tunneling of the cortex may occur with subperiosteal reabsorption and striation formation. Endosteal bone resorption and surface erosions in subchondral bone may be seen. Patchy osteopenia usually is not seen on radiographs until the late stages of the disease.

13. Do children develop CRPS?

The earliest reported age of an individual with CRPS was a 3-year-old child who received immunization in the buttocks and developed lower extremity CRPS. Most pediatric patients who develop CRPS are adolescent girls.

14. List drugs that are effective in treating CRPS.

Drug*	Type of Pain	Action
Anticonvulsants (Topamax, Neurontin, Keppra, Trileptal)	Neuropathic pain	Change rate of nerve firing
Antidepressants (Prozac, Pomelor, Paxil, Zoloft, Wellbutrin)	Multiple pain syndromes; associated sleep problems	Block reuptake of serotonin and norepinephrine in descending pathway modulation
Second-generation antidepressants (Seroquel, Cymbalta)	Multiple pain syndromes, including nerve pain	Block selective serotonin reuptake
NSAIDs (nonsteroidal antiinflammatory drugs)	Inflammatory pain	Decrease production of prostaglandins to reduce inflammatory mediators
Systemic corticosteroids (Medrol dose pack)	Painful and edematous pain syndromes such as CRPS I and II	Act as antiinflammatory drugs; reduce nerve firing
Calcitonin spray	Bone pain	Unknown, but modulates actions in SNS
Opioids (hydrocodone, Vicodin, Duragesic, Kadian, Avinza)	Extreme pain or intractable pain	Directly interact with opioid receptor
Antipsychotics (Zyprexa)	Pain caused by anxiety	Act on serotonin and dopamine receptors to reduce anxiety

*Drugs listed are just a few examples.

15. How are capsaicin and clonidine patches helpful in treating pain associated with CRPS?

Capsaicin decreases primary afferent neurons involved in pain transmission. It has been shown to decrease the peptide substance P, which mediates pain transmission in the dorsal horn of the spinal cord. Some patients with neuropathic pain respond to topical application. Clonidine stimulates α-adrenoreceptors, leading to decreased sympathetic outflow. Both of these medications should be prescribed by the physician, and the patient's blood work should be monitored.

16. Discuss outcomes that are associated with CRPS.

In a prospective follow-up study at the University of Washington of 103 children with CRPS (87 girls; mean age, 13 years), 49 subjects were followed for 2 years. They received an intensive exercise program of hydrotherapy, desensitization, aerobics, and functionally directed exercise. No medications or modalities were used. All had psychological evaluations, and 79% were referred for psychological counseling. A total of 95 (92%) subjects initially became symptom-free. Of the subjects followed for >2 years, 43 (88%) were symptom-free (15, or 31%, of these patients had a recurrence), 5 (10%) were fully functional but had some continued pain, and 1 (2%) had functional limitations. Case studies by Menke et al. show that therapy and mobilization were successful in treating CRPS in a patient with wrist tendon lacerations and carpal fracture. Exercise programs emphasizing compression and distraction have been shown to improve function in patients with CRPS.

17. Is the timing of the initiation of treatment important in CRPS?

Yes. Of patients treated within 1 year of onset, 80% show significant improvement. If treatment is begun after 1 year, 50% improve significantly. Powlaski reviewed 126 cases of CRPS and found that the most important factor in predicting response to treatment was an interval of less than 6 months before treatment and therapy.

18. What role does smoking play in aggravating the symptoms of CRPS?

It is believed that the sympathetic nervous system can be stimulated by the products in cigarettes, causing an increase in the plasma levels of epinephrine and norepinephrine.

It is also known that smoking decreases blood flow to the extremities, especially the distal portions, which leads to ischemia.

19. Can the development of CRPS be prevented?

The following principles play a major role in CRPS prevention and further deterioration:
- Early recognition of symptoms
- Use of appropriate medications
- Early referral to PT and OT
- Avoidance of unnecessary immobilization
- Avoidance of narcotics in the early stages
- Avoidance of smoking and drinking alcohol
- Avoidance of unnecessary surgery, especially reentry into areas of scars, amputation, and sympathectomy. Regional anesthesia instead of general anesthesia is preferred if surgery is warranted.

20. What should nonaggressive PT and OT programs use immediately after a nerve block?

Exercises are best performed during the analgesic periods following sympathetic blocks. Exercise (nonaggressive) increases proprioception into the spinal cord. This may result in inhibition of the overactive sympathetic nervous system. Exercise also increases blood flow to the extremity and may cause central inhibition of the sympathetic nervous system.

21. It is not uncommon for the involved limb with CRPS to lack volitional motor control. What terms are commonly used to describe these motor abnormalities?

- Hypokinesia—delay of movement
- Akinesia—reduced spontaneous movement
- Bradykinesia—slowness of movement
- Hypometria—small amplitude of movement
- Asomatognosia—lack of awareness of a body part

22. What are common types of neuropathic pain?

PERIPHERAL NEUROPATHIC PAIN

- Painful diabetic neuropathy
- Postherpetic neuralgia
- Complex regional pain syndrome
- Entrapment neuropathies
- Radiculopathy
- Phantom limb pain

CENTRAL NEUROPATHIC PAIN
- Compressive myelopathy
- Poststroke pain
- Spinal cord injury pain
- Multiple sclerosis
- Parkinson's disease

23. In a CRPS II patient, when is surgical intervention appropriate?

Traditionally, surgical treatment for a CRPS patient has been discouraged. Recent research has show that when a patient with CRPS II has positive electrophysiological testing (e.g., median nerve or ulnar nerve compression) that does not respond to conservative treatment, then it is appropriate for decompression to be performed. Research has shown that patients with CRPS II that have a positive EMG have done well after surgery. In this study, the patient had immediate or near-complete resolution of symptoms.

Bibliography

Baron R, Blumberg H, Janig W: Clinical characteristics of patients with CRPS in Germany with special emphasis on vasomotor function. In Janig WS, Stanton-Hicks M, editors: *RSD: a reappraisal,* Vol 6, Seattle, 1996, pp 25-28, IASP Press.

Boas RA: Complex regional pain syndromes: Symptoms, signs and differential diagnosis. In Janig WS, Stanton-Hicks M, editors: *RSD: a reappraisal,* Seattle, 1996, pp 79-92, IASP Press.

Bonica JJ: Causalgia and other reflex sympathetic dystrophies. In Bonica JJ, editor: *The management of pain,* ed 2, Philadelphia, 1990, pp 220-243, Lea & Febiger.

Colton AM, Fallat LM: Complex regional pain, *J Foot Joint Surg* 35:284-295, 1996.

Galer BS, Butler S, Jensen MP: Case reports and hypothesis: a neglect-like syndrome may be responsible for the motor disturbance in reflex sympathetic dystrophy (complex regional pain syndrome-1), *J Pain Symptom Management* 10:385-391, 1995.

Hollister L: Tricyclic antidepressants, *N Engl J Med* 99:1044-1048, 1988.

IASP Subcommittee on Pain Taxonomy: Reflex sympathetic dystrophy, 1-5, *Pain* (suppl 3):29-30, 1986.

Kozin F, et al: Bone scintigraphy in RSDS, *Radiology* 138:437-443, 1981.

Livinston WK: *Pain mechanisms: a physiologic interpretation of causalgia and its related states,* New York, 1944, MacMillan.

Menke J, Mais S, Kulig K: Mobilization of the thoracic spine: management of a patient with CRPS in upper extremity: a case report. Poster presentation at the American Physical Therapy Association, Combined Sections Meeting, Seattle, 1999.

Placzek JD et al: Nerve decompression for complex regional pain syndrome type II following upper extremity surgery, *J Hand Surg* 30:69-74, 2005.

Poplawski ZJ, Wiley AM, Murray JF: Post-traumatic dystrophy of the extremities: a clinical review and trial of treatment, *J Bone Joint Surg* 65A:642-655, 1983.

Price DD, Mao J, Mayer DJ: Neural mechanisms of normal and abnormal pain states. In Raj PP, editor: *Current review of pain,* Philadelphia, 1994, Current Medicine.

Ruggeri SB et al: Reflex sympathetic dystrophy in children, *Clin Orthop* 163:670-673, 1982.

Stralka SW, Akin K: Reflex sympathetic dystrophy syndrome. In *Orthopaedic home study course: the elbow, forearm, and wrist,* Fairfax, Va, 1997, American Physical Therapy Association Orthopedic Section.

Watson HK, Carlson L: Treatment of reflex sympathetic dystrophy of the hand with an active "stress loading" program, *J Hand Surg* 12A:779-785, 1987.

Section III

Electrotherapy and Modalities

Chapter 9

Cryotherapy and Moist Heat

Kathleen Galloway, PT, MPT, DSc

1. At what depth have tissue temperature changes been recorded after treatment with superficial ice?

Ice application is reported to lower tissue temperature in the skin, subcutaneous tissue, and muscle, depending on the amount of subcutaneous tissue (adipose), type of cold application, and length of time treated. Measurements of decreased temperature have been recorded at a 4-cm depth. Patients with little subcutaneous tissue showed more significant cooling with a much shorter treatment time.

2. Which method is more effective in lowering tissue temperature: ice massage or ice pack?

Both are effective. A 5-minute ice massage treatment in the lower extremity decreased skin temperature by 20° C, subcutaneous tissue by 15° C, and muscle temperature at a depth of 2 cm by 5° C and a depth of 4 cm by 4° C. Zemke et al., measuring at an average depth of 1.7 cm, found that a 15-minute ice massage treatment of a 4-cm^2 area created an intramuscular temperature drop of >4° C, reaching its lowest temperature at 17.9 minutes after the initiation of treatment. Zemke et al. also found that an ice pack treatment produced an intramuscular temperature drop of >2° C and had its maximum effect at 28.2 minutes. The ice pack and ice massage resulted in the same minimum skin temperature of 29.67° C. The extent of the temperature change seems to relate more to the length of application and the amount of subcutaneous adipose tissue. Clinical considerations include the size and location of the affected area, time allotted for ice application, and patient preference. Ice massage may produce its maximum effect sooner than an ice pack; however, if a large area is to be treated, an ice pack may be more efficient.

3. What is the effect of ice application on metabolic rate?

Lower tissue temperatures produce a decrease in metabolic rate and subsequently a decrease in demand for oxygen. This decreased need for oxygen serves to limit further injury, particularly in the case of acute tissue damage, when the blood supply and oxygen delivery are impaired, resulting in hypoxia.

4. What is the physiologic effect of cold application on the muscle spindle?

Cold-induced lower tissue temperature raises the threshold of activation of the muscle spindle, rendering it less excitable.

5. How may the physiologic effect of cold application be successful in reducing muscle spasm or cramp?

A decrease in muscle tension is produced by the less-excitable muscle spindle that is not altered by active or passive stretching exercises, which means that an ice pack can be employed successfully during a passive or active stretch of a muscle that is in spasm.

6. Describe the effect of therapeutic ice on local blood flow.

Maximum vasoconstriction occurs at tissue temperatures of 15° C (59° F). Normal skin temperature is 31° to 33° C. The superficial vasculature has a sympathetic innervation that produces vasoconstriction when stimulated. The neurotransmitters for this system are norepinephrine and epinephrine. Norepinephrine secretion and epinephrine secretion are stimulated by exposure to ice and are secreted into the blood vessels, resulting in vasoconstriction. If the tissue temperature drops to below 15° C, vasodilation occurs as a result of a paralysis of the musculature, which provides the vasoconstriction or a conduction block of the sympathetic nervous system. Vasoconstriction can lead to vasodilation if ice application is such that a tissue temperature <15° C is reached. If vasodilation results, there is no definite consensus regarding the overall effect on the blood flow. A decrease in the amount of blood lost was reported in patients who showed lower joint temperatures; this would seem to indicate that the overall blood flow remains decreased. Intramuscular temperature recordings have shown a range of 1.5° C drop in the calf to a 17.9° C drop in the biceps. Neither of these temperature ranges should bring the muscle tissue temperature to <15° C and should not produce vasodilation within the deeper or target tissues.

7. At what temperature does local tissue damage occur with ice application?

Although the core body temperature is 98.6° F, the shell temperature (temperature in the extremities) can vary depending on exposure to the environment. Frostbite occurs when the extremities or face has been exposed to cold such that there is a drop in shell temperature, resulting in freezing of the tissue. Tissue freezing occurs as ice crystals form in the extracellular areas, causing fluids to be drawn out of the cells. The earliest or precursor stage of frostbite begins with tissue temperatures of 37° to 50° F (3° to 10° C). Zemke et al. indicated that tissue temperatures of 19° to 25° C after ice treatment had no adverse effect and that consistent tissue damage does not occur until tissue temperature declines to –10° C. Cold-induced vasodilation occurs at temperatures <15° C, reaching a maximum at tissue temperatures of 0° C (32° F).

8. What is the ideal tissue temperature to achieve the optimal physiologic effects of cryotherapy?

Optimal physiologic effects from cryotherapy are achieved at tissue temperatures of 15° to 25° C.

9. How long do tissue blood flow and tissue temperature remain decreased after application of an ice pack?

Forearm blood flow has been shown to return to normal gradually over a 35-minute period after a 20-minute ice pack treatment. A 15-minute ice pack treatment has been shown to produce a maximum intramuscular cooling effect at 28.2 ± 12.5 minutes, and a 15-minute ice massage has been reported to produce a maximum intramuscular cooling effect at 17.9 ± 2.4 minutes from the start of treatment. Zemke et al. indicate that, for a 15-minute treatment, the maximum cooling effect does not occur until the ice treatment is completed. Myrer et al. report that tissue rewarming begins at 5 minutes after ice pack or cold whirlpool (10° C) treatment; however, the intramuscular temperature remains decreased relative to pretreatment temperatures for up to 50 minutes posttreatment.

10. Which form of cold treatment is the most effective at relieving postoperative pain and swelling?

There does not seem to be a consensus in the literature. Dervin et al. found no difference in pain level or total wound drainage between post–acromioclavicular ligament reconstruction patients treated with a cryotherapy cuff device (Cryocuff) using cold water and those treated with room temperature water. Previous researchers reported a greater decrease in pain in those treated with a Cryocuff than in those treated with an ice pack. It is possible that, because of the postoperative dressing, the tissue temperature is not decreased to an effective level to produce analgesia or to decrease swelling in some cases.

Crushed ice was compared to continuous flow cold therapy in patellar tendon graft anterior cruciate ligament (ACL) reconstructions. Patients receiving continuous flow cold therapy demonstrated statistically significant decreases in pain, decreased pain medication usage, and increases in range of motion 1 week after surgery when compared with the patients receiving crushed ice.

11. Explain the impact of cold application on the diabetic patient.

Caution should be exercised when using modalities in the diabetic patient. Non–insulin-dependent diabetes mellitus (NIDDM) patients exposed to cold-water immersion have been found to have a significantly reduced capacity to recover skin temperature when compared with healthy controls. There did not appear to be a correlation between the severity of the disease process and the length of recovery time required. Underlying pathology to explain the slow recovery is probably related to sympathetic nervous system involvement and associated peripheral vascular disease. This needs to be considered in addition to the possibility of peripheral polyneuropathy resulting in impaired touch and hot/cold temperature sensation.

12. Should ice be used in the treatment of a subacute or chronic injury?

Ice may be used for pain relief or decreases in muscle guarding or spasm, which may allow the therapist to achieve other objectives such as joint mobilization, stretching, or strengthening exercises.

13. What is the hunting response?

The hunting response is proposed to occur as a mechanism by which the body responds to extreme cold by a vasodilation that occurs secondary to the extreme cold temperature. This vasodilation is proposed to last for 4 to 6 minutes and to be followed by a vasoconstriction lasting 15 to 30 minutes. Recent studies have not been able to demonstrate this cycle. Cold-induced vasodilation has been shown at tissue temperatures <15° C, and some researchers recommend treatment duration of no greater than 20 minutes to avoid the peripheral vasodilation effect. The maximum temperature effect may not be achieved because recent studies indicate that ice pack treatment may not reach its maximum effect until nearly 39 minutes.

14. Why does skin appear red after ice application?

It is red because of the lack of blood in the capillary bed, secondary to the body's attempt to conserve heat by trying to pool the blood in the area.

15. At what depth have tissue temperature changes been recorded after treatment with superficial heat?

Tissue temperature changes have been recorded at 1- to 2-cm depth. This may reach all desired tissues in the hand; however, in other areas of the body, subcutaneous tissue may prevent adequate heating of the desired structures. Superficial heat is proposed to affect deeper structures by conduction heating.

16. What is the desired therapeutic tissue temperature produced by heat?

Therapeutic heating effects are achieved when a tissue temperature of 41° to 45° C is reached. When tissue temperatures are >45° C, tissue damage can occur. Much greater temperatures than can be achieved with superficial heat (60° to 65° C) have been proposed to provide a breakdown and structural change in the collagen fiber, resulting in tissue shrinkage. This tissue shrinkage may be useful in the treatment of capsular laxity or instability of the shoulder.

17. What is the oxygen-hemoglobin dissociation curve?

At rest, tissues require approximately 5 ml of oxygen from each 100 ml of blood traveling through the area. At the level of the lung where oxygen is transferred into the bloodstream, the Po_2 is normally 104 mm Hg. This Po_2 facilitates the association of oxygen to hemoglobin. At the level of the tissues, oxygen needs to be dissociated from the hemoglobin to allow it to be delivered. The Po_2 at the level of the tissues needs to be <40 mm Hg to allow this dissociation to occur.

18. What does a shift in the oxygen-hemoglobin dissociation curve to either the right or the left signify?

- A shift to the right is called the Bohr effect, producing an enhanced dissociation of oxygen from hemoglobin and improving delivery of oxygen to the tissues from the bloodstream.
- A shift to the left produces an enhanced association of oxygen to hemoglobin, enhancing the delivery of oxygen from the alveolus to the blood and improving the oxygen saturation level.

19. Explain the mechanism by which heat reduces muscle spasm or cramp.

Either type of heating modality—superficial or deep—has been reported to decrease muscle tone. The physiologic mechanism for this effect may be caused by the decrease in firing rates of the efferent fibers in the muscle spindle when heat is applied. Heat also lowers the threshold for activation of the muscle spindle afferent fibers. This makes the spindle more excitable when movement is applied to the body part and results in increased muscle tension if the heat is applied during a passive or active stretching treatment. For example, application of a hot pack to a muscle in spasm during a passive stretch technique may result in increased muscle tension. Superficial heat can help to decrease spasm but works better if the muscle is heated while at rest.

20. Describe the effect of heat on a tight or shortened muscle, capsule, or tendon during stretching.

Application of a heating modality before or during stretching may yield a benefit resulting from increased extensibility of collagen fibers in the associated supporting structures and tendons as well as decreased firing rates of the efferent muscle spindle fibers. In an environment of connective tissue healing, the immature collagen bonds can be degraded by heat. This allows the tissue to be stretched more effectively. A 25% increase in potential elongation of mature connective tissue is noted if the temperature of the collagen tissue reaches 40° C. The therapist needs also to consider the possibility of increased excitability of the muscle spindle during passive and active stretching.

21. What is the effect of heat application on local blood flow?

The application of heat to the skin results in increased local blood flow as a consequence of vasodilation. This increase in blood flow increases the delivery of oxygen, nutrients, and metabolites to the area.

22. Describe the physiologic effect of heat on muscle performance during exercise.

- During strenuous exercise, there is an increase in blood flow to the muscle of up to 25 times that which occurs at rest, which is important to provide adequate oxygen to the area. Much of the increase in blood flow is because of vasodilation instigated by increases in muscle metabolism.
- Although during the actual contraction there is a decrease in blood flow, resulting from a wringing effect of contraction providing compression on the blood vessels, muscle heating also occurs during contraction because much of the energy that makes muscle function is directed into production of heat within the muscle.
- Treatment of an area with superficial heat can affect tissues directly to 1 to 2 cm in depth and is suggested to heat deeper than 1 to 2 cm by compression and conduction.

- If a relatively superficial muscle is heated, such as in the forearm or hand, the result is increases in muscle metabolism and blood flow secondary to vasodilation. This, in turn, allows an increased supply of oxygen, which may be beneficial as a warm-up before initiating exercise with a patient. Heating the area has a similar, but less dramatic, effect on muscle metabolism and blood flow as activity does, and together there is an additive effect.
- Heat has been reported to produce a decrease in muscle strength for the first 30 minutes after treatment. Heat treatment after exercise may prove to be even more beneficial because it can have the effect of continued elevation in muscle metabolism and blood flow, providing greater levels of oxygen to the tissue during the period of recovery from activity.

23. What is the effect of heat and ice on nerve conduction velocity?

Heat results in increases in local nerve conduction, whereas the lower tissue temperatures resulting from ice treatment produce a relative slowing of nerve conduction. Skin temperature values need to be monitored when performing nerve conduction studies because a cool extremity may produce nerve conduction values that appear to be pathologic but are the result of lower skin temperatures.

24. How do the superficial heat and ice modalities act to reduce pain?

Heat and ice serve to stimulate the thermoreceptors, which transmit the message proximally to the dorsal horn and may act to inhibit transmission of the painful stimulus by the gate control theory. Sluka et al. report that arthritic rats treated with ice had a delayed pain response, which indicated some effect of ice application on pain response. They also treated the arthritic rats with heat and found no change in the pain response but did notice a decrease in muscle guarding with heat application.

25. Are home heat wraps effective in treating low back pain?

A group of researchers examined this topic using prospective, randomized, single blinded placebo controlled clinical trials. The first study involved 219 subjects between 18 and 55 years of age with acute, nonspecific low back pain. Treatment was for 3 consecutive nights while outcome measures were taken for an additional 2 days. There was a significant difference in pain relief and decreases in muscle stiffness and disability as well as increases in flexibility when compared with the placebo over all 5 days of outcome measurement.

26. Do heat wraps provide an increase in muscle temperature or is the heating more superficial?

A group of researchers studied three different types of heat wraps in a double blinded randomized crossover design. They inserted a thermometer at a 2-cm depth at the L3 level, and placed thermometers on the skin before applying the heat wraps. There was a significant increase in muscle temperature only with the use of the ThermaCare heat wrap. All tested heat wraps produced an increase in skin interface temperature and increases in subjective reports of superficial warming.

27. Is heat wrap therapy a cost-effective method of delivering superficial heat?

A group of researchers in the United Kingdom examined the cost effectiveness of different treatments for low back pain. They compared outcome measures of pain and disability reduction between patients being treated with low-level heat wrap therapy and those being treated with medications. The cost per application was greater for heat wrap therapy; however, the cost per patient was lower with heat wrap therapy. They also identified heat wrap therapy as providing significantly greater reductions in pain and disability than did treatment with medication.

Bibliography

Barber FA: A comparison of crushed ice and continuous flow cold therapy, *Am J Knee Surg* 13:97-101, 2000.

Belitsky RW, Odam SJ, Hubley-Kozey C: Evaluation of the effectiveness of wet ice, dry ice, and cryogen packs in reducing skin temperature, *Phys Ther* 67:1080-1084, 1987.

Bell GW, Prentice WE: Infrared modalities. In Prentice WE, editor: *Therapeutic modalities for allied health professionals,* New York, 1998, pp 201-239, McGraw-Hill.

Bullough PG: *Orthopedic pathology,* ed 3, London, 1997, Mosby-Wolfe.

Dervin GF, Taylor DE, Keene GC: Effects of cold and compression dressings on early postoperative outcomes for the arthroscopic anterior cruciate ligament reconstruction patient, *J Orthop Sports Phys Ther* 27:403-406, 1998.

Fedorczyk J: The role of physical agents in modulating pain, *J Hand Ther* 10:110-121, 1997.

Fujiwara Y et al: Thermographic measurement of skin temperature recovery time of extremities in patients with type 2 diabetes mellitus, *Exp Clin Endocrinol Diabetes* 108:463-469, 2000.

Greenberg RS: The effects of hot packs and exercise on local blood flow, *Phys Ther* 52:273-278, 1972.

Hardy M, Woodall W: Therapeutic effects of heat, cold and stretch on connective tissue, *J Hand Ther* 11:148-156, 1998.

Hayes KW: *Manual for physical agents,* ed 5, Upper Saddle River, NJ, 2000, Prentice Hall Health.

Karunakara RG, Lephart SM, Pincivero DM: Changes in forearm blood flow during single and intermittent cold application, *J Orthop Sports Phys Ther* 29:177-180, 1999.

Lloyd A et al: Cost effectiveness of low level heatwrap therapy for low back pain, *Value health* 7:413-422, 2004.

Michlovitz SL: *Thermal agents in rehabilitation,* ed 2, Philadelphia, 1990, FA Davis.

Minor M, Sanford M: The role of physical therapy and physical modalities in pain management, *Rheum Dis Clin North Am* 25:233-248, 1999.

Myrer JW, Measom G, Fellingham GW: Temperature changes in the human leg during and after two methods of cryotherapy, *J Athletic Training* 33:25-29, 1998.

Nadler SF et al: Continuous low-level heatwrap therapy for treating acute nonspecific low back pain, *Arch Phys Med Rehabil* 84:329-334, 2003.

Okoshi Y, Ohkoshi MN, Shinya Ono A: The effect of cryotherapy on intraarticular temperature and postoperative care after anterior cruciate ligament reconstruction, *Am J Sports Med* 27:357-362, 1999.

O'Toole G, Rayatt S: Frostbite at the gym: a case report of an ice pack burn, *Br J Sports Med* 33:278-279, 1999.

Prentice WE: An electromyographic analysis of the effectiveness of heat or cold and stretching for inducing relaxation in injured muscle, *J Orthop Sports Phys Ther* 3:133-146, 1982.

Sallis R, Chassay CM: Recognizing and treating common cold-induced injury in outdoor sports, *Med Sci Sports Exercise* 31:1367-1373, 1999.

Sluka KA et al: Reduction of pain-related behaviors with either cold or heat treatment in an animal model of acute arthritis, *Arch Phys Med Rehabil* 80:313-317, 1999.

Trowbridge CA et al: Paraspinal musculature and skin temperature changes: comparing the Theracare HeatWrap, the Johnson & Johnson Back Plaster and the ABC Warme-Pflaster, *J Orthop Sports Phys Ther* 34:549-558, 2004.

Wall MS et al: Thermal modification of collagen, *J Shoulder Elbow Surg* 8:339-344, 1999.

Waylonis GW: The physiologic effects of ice massage, *Arch Phys Med Rehabil* 48:37-42, 1967.

Zemke JE et al: Intramuscular temperature responses in the human leg to two forms of cryotherapy: ice massage and ice bag, *J Orthop Sports Phys Ther* 27:301-307, 1998

Chapter 10

Electrotherapy

Fredrick D. Pociask, PT, PhD, OCS, and
Tracey M. Fleck, PT, MPT

MUSCLE AND NERVE ANATOMY AND PHYSIOLOGY

1. Define cellular membrane potentials.

All living cells are electrically charged or polarized, the inside of the cell being relatively negative in charge when compared with the outside of the cell. The polarization is a result of the unequal distribution of ions on either side of the cell membrane. This polarity can be measured as a difference in electrical potential between the inside and the outside of the cell and is referred to as the membrane potential. A change in the membrane potential is referred to as an action potential and is the basis for the transmission of a nerve impulse. Nerve cells are specialized in detecting changes in their surroundings. If a change in their surroundings reaches a certain intensity or threshold, it can disturb the membrane's resting state and trigger a nerve impulse.

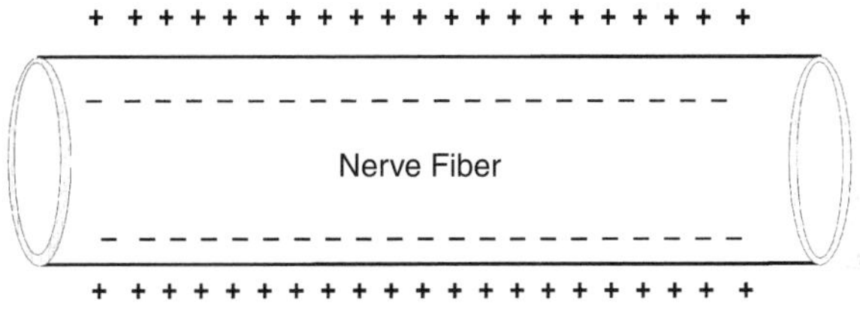

2. Define refractory period.

Immediately after a nerve impulse is triggered, an ordinary stimulus is not able to generate another impulse. This brief period is termed the refractory period. The refractory period consists of two phases—the absolute refractory period and the relative refractory period. The absolute refractory period lasts about 1/2500 of a second and is followed by the relative refractory period. During the relative refractory period, a higher intensity stimulus can trigger an impulse.

3. What is saltatory, or jumping, conduction?

Saltatory (jumping) conduction of a nerve impulse occurs in myelinated nerve axons because myelin is an excellent insulator with a high resistance to current flow. Because myelin does not cover the nodes of Ranvier, current flows from one node of Ranvier to the next. The action potentials do not travel along the entire length of the axon; consequently, the nerve impulses can travel much faster in myelinated axons when compared with unmyelinated axons. This jumping of nerve impulses also is much more efficient from a metabolic and physiologic standpoint. Fewer sodium and potassium ions are necessary to cross the cell membrane during the nerve impulse, and as a result, resting potentials are reestablished at a much faster rate while conserving metabolic energy.

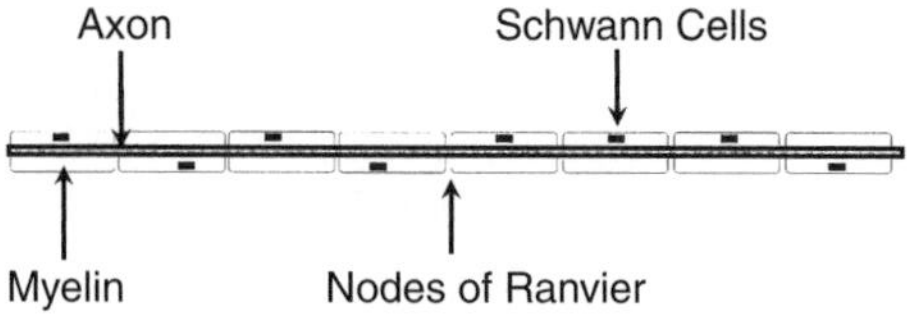

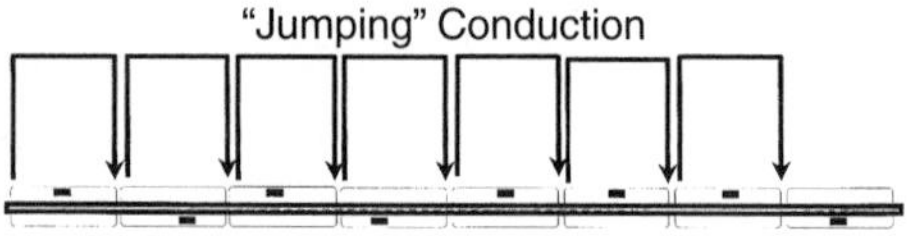

4. What are the average conduction velocities for myelinated and unmyelinated nerve fibers?

- Myelinated: ≈130 m/sec
- Unmyelinated: ≈0.5 m/sec

PHYSICS OF ELECTRICAL FORCES

5. What is an ion?

An ion is an atom or a group of atoms that has acquired a net electrical charge by gaining or losing one or more electrons. Ions are present in electrolytic solutions, such as acids, bases, and salts. Bases, alkaloids, and metals form positive ions, whereas acid radicals form negative ions.

6. What is ionization?

Ionization is the process of changing the electrically neutral state of an atom. A positive ion is an atom that has lost one or more electrons, whereas a negative ion is an atom that has gained one or more electrons.

7. What is an electrical current?

Current—the natural drifting of ions that occurs within all matter—is defined as the directed flow of free electrons from one place to another. The unit of current is the ampere (A), which is the amount of electrical charge flowing past a specified circuit point per unit of time. The drifting is somewhat random and involves free electrons, positive ions, and negative ions.

8. How does the number of electrons in the valence shell of an atom relate to the conductivity of a material?

The tendency for an atom to give or receive electrons depends on the structure of the atom's orbital shells.

- Atoms with valence shells that are almost full tend to be stable and are called insulators.
- Atoms possessing only one or two valence electrons tend to relinquish their electrons willingly and are called conductors.
- In general, conductors, such as metal, readily permit electron movement, whereas resistors, such as adipose tissue, tend to impede electron movement.

9. Clinically, therapeutic intensities should not exceed what amperage?

Therapeutic intensities should not exceed 80 to 100 mA.

10. What is electromotive force?

The rate of current flow depends on a source of free electrons, positive ions, materials that allow the electrons to flow, and on the electromotive force that concentrates electrons in one place. The volt is the International System unit of electrical potential and electromotive force, whereas voltage is the driving force of the electrons. One volt (V) is the electromotive force required to move 1 ampere (A) of current through a resistance of 1 ohm (Ω).

11. What role does voltage play in nerve cell membrane depolarization?

For a nerve cell membrane to depolarize, an adequate number of electrons must be forced to move through conductive tissues. Given that likes repel and opposites attract, a high concentration of electrons flows to an area of low concentration. The greater the difference in concentrations, the greater the potential for electron flow.

12. How does Ohm's law express the relationship between current (I), voltage (V), and resistance (R)?

$$V = IR$$
$$I = V/R$$
$$R = V/I$$

Therefore:
- When resistance decreases, current increases.
- When resistance increases, current decreases.
- When voltage decreases, current decreases.
- When voltage increases, current increases.
- When voltage is zero, current is zero.

13. What properties of a material tend to make it resist electrical currents?

Conductors have low resistance, whereas insulators have high resistance. The actual resistance of a material is determined by the formula:

R = P ∞ length of the material/cross section

where R = resistance and P = resistivity. Therefore:
- Greater cross-sectional area = decreased resistance
- Greater temperature = decreased resistance = increased conductivity
- Longer resistor = increased resistance

14. What factors typically alter skin impedance?

Increases Skin Impedance	Decreases Skin Impedance
• Cooler skin temperature	• Increasing electrode surface
• Electrode type/surface factors	• Removing excess hair
• Hair and oil present	• Warming skin
• Increased skin dryness	• Washing skin
• Increased skin thickness	

PRINCIPLES OF ALTERNATING AND DIRECT CURRENT

15. What criteria are used to describe direct current (DC)?

DC is the flow of electrons in one direction for >1 second. A current is considered DC if it meets the following criteria:

- The flow of electrons is unidirectional.
- The polarity is constant.
- The current produces a twitch response only at the time of make (when the circuit is closed).
- The membrane is hyperpolarized as long as the current is on.
- The duration of current flow is >1 second.

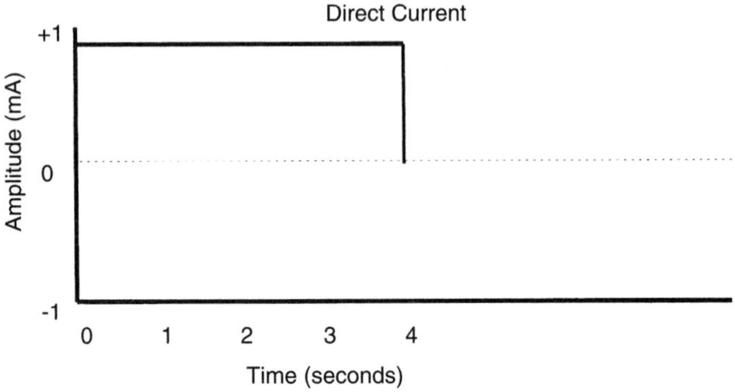

16. Direct currents produce polar effects. What polar effects are produced by the anode and the cathode?

Positive (Anode)	Negative (Cathode)
Hyperpolarizes nerve fibers	Depolarizes nerve fibers
Repels bases	Attracts bases
Hardens tissues	Softens tissues
Stops hemorrhage	Increases hemorrhage
Sedates, calms	Stimulates
Reduces pain in acute situations	Reduces pain in chronic situations

17. What are the criteria used to describe alternating current (AC)?

AC is characterized by sine wave modulation and has a constantly fluctuating voltage and a symmetric pattern. A current is termed AC if it meets the following criteria:

- The magnitude of flow of electrons changes.
- The direction of flow reverses.
- There are no polar effects.

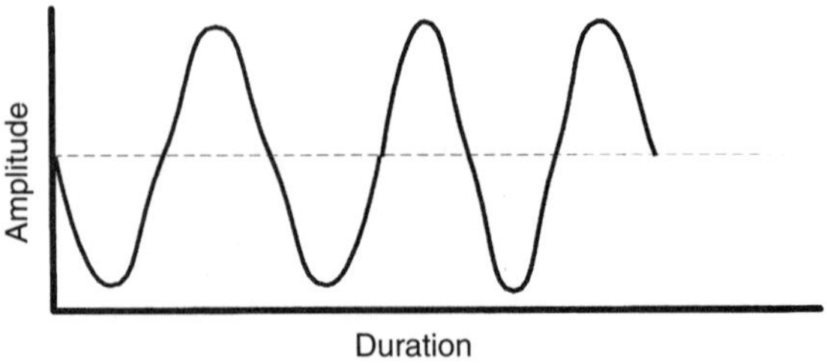

18. List the typical frequencies (ranges of currents, if applicable) used in therapeutic applications.

Frequency (Hz)	Classification
0	Direct current
0-1000	Low frequency
1000-100,000	Medium frequency
>100,000	High frequency

19. Does medium-frequency stimulation (MFS) differ from low-frequency stimulation in terms of skin resistance (capacitive impedance)?

Yes. When electrical current passes through cutaneous tissues, by surface electrodes, an opposition to the flow of current is encountered. When electrical currents are introduced into the body, ions accumulate at tissue interfaces, and cell membranes create a charge that opposes the applied voltage. This opposing voltage is referred to as reactance or capacitive impedance. The capacitive impedance can be calculated using the following formula:

$$Z = C(F) \bullet 2\pi f(Hz)$$

where Z = capacitance impedance, C = polarization capacitance of tissues in farads (constant), and F = frequency of current.

This formula shows that capacitance impedance decreases as the frequency increases.

20. Describe the key attributes of interferential currents.

With an interferential current (IFC), two separate current generators produce electrical currents that vary in relation to one another in amplitude or frequency, or both. Where these two distinct currents meet in the tissue, an electrical interference pattern is created based on the summation or the subtraction of the respective amplitudes or frequencies. With a sinusoidal wave pattern, when oscillations from two unlike frequencies or amplitudes are out of phase and blend (heterodyne), they produce the interference effect for which this modality was given its name. The typical depiction of the interference pattern is that which may be produced in homogeneous tissues, which would differ in human tissues. With IFC, the patient perceives the resulting signal or beat signal produced by the heterodyned alternating current as amplitude-modulated electrical pulses.

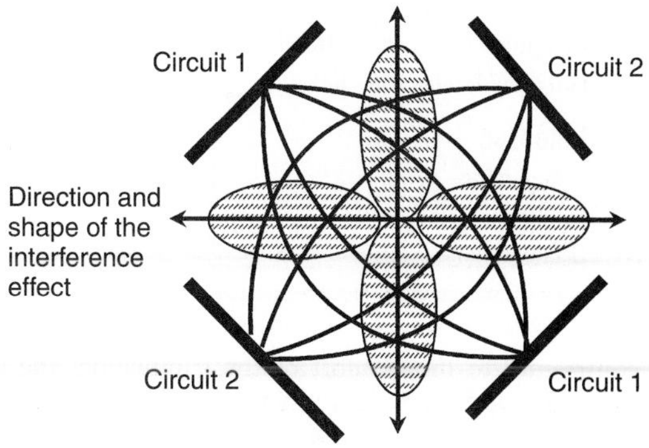

The beat signal often is described as being comparable to low-frequency pulse rates. For example, a 4100-Hz frequency and a 4200-Hz frequency could produce a constant beat frequency of 100 Hz.

The phase duration of the delivered current can be easily calculated as follows:

Frequency = 1
2 ∞ phase duration

WAVEFORM CHARACTERISTICS

21. Draw and label the following waveform characteristics: (1) pulse duration, (2) phase duration, and (3) amplitude.

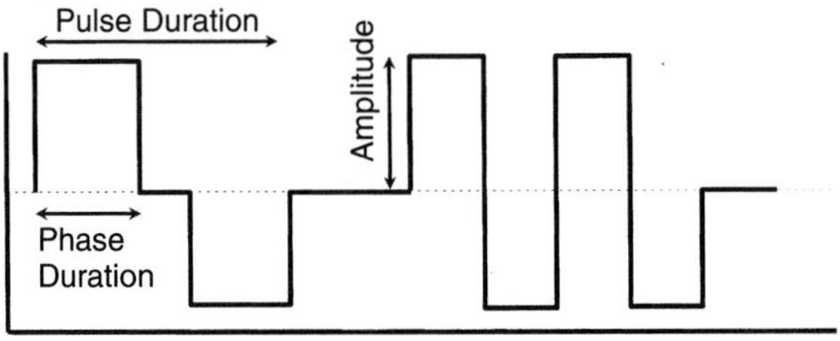

22. What is the typical nomenclature and the appropriate units of measurement used to describe waveform characteristics?

- Amplitude = intensity (mA)
- Frequency = pulse rate or pulses per second (Hz)
- Phase duration = pulse width (μsec)

23. Discuss the practical and clinical implications for frequency, phase duration, and amplitude.

Frequency contributes to the type of contraction as well as theorized opiate-mediated effects:

Frequency (Hz)	Type of Contraction	
1-10	Twitch contraction	
>30	Tetanic contraction	
30-70	Nonfatiguing tetanic contraction	
100-1000	Fatiguing tetanic contraction	
Pulse Rate (Hz)	**Released**	**Carryover**
40-150 (110-120)	Enkephalins	Short
15-100 (40-60)	Serotonin	Longer
1-4	β-Endorphins	Longest

Phase duration contributes to the comfort of the stimulation, the amount of chemical change that occurs in the tissues, and nerve discrimination. A duration of 50 to 100 μsec typically is used for sensory stimulation, and 200 to 300 μsec is typically used for motor stimulation.

Amplitude is best described by the following characteristics:

- Is less discriminatory than phase duration and pulse rate
- Greater intensity yields greater depths of penetration (generally speaking)
- Low intensities used for sensory stimulation
- High intensities used for motor stimulation

24. What is the clinical relevance of the pulse characteristics that are labeled in the diagram?

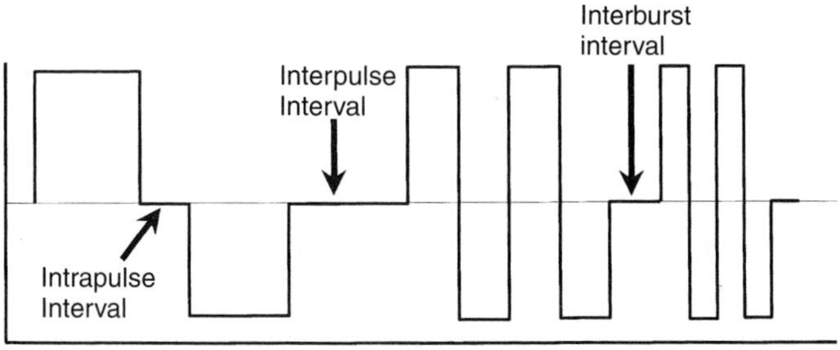

- Intrapulse interval—used to increase patient comfort
- Interpulse interval—needed to ensure the absolute refractory period
- Interburst interval—used with some protocols as a form of modulation

25. Define rise time, fall time, and duty cycle.

- Rise time is the time that it takes the wave to travel from zero to its peak amplitude.
- Fall time is the time that it takes the wave to travel from its peak amplitude to zero.
- Duty cycle is the relative proportion of time between the stimulation period and the rest period.

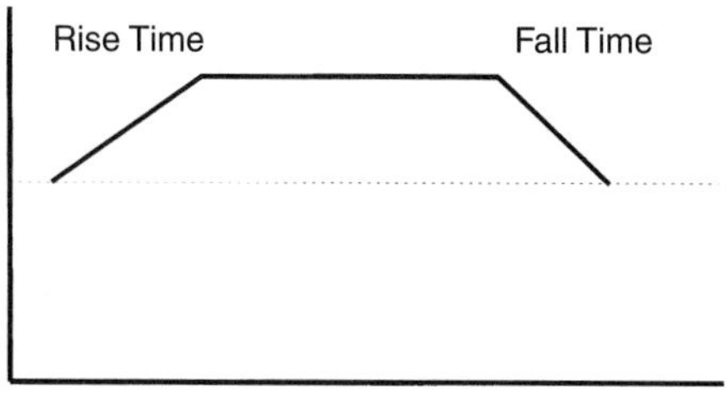

26. Describe the key attributes of high-volt current and the unique characteristics of high-volt units.

High-volt galvanic currents are unique because they are not grouped with alternating or direct currents. The typical high-volt current stimulator produces a twin-peak monophasic waveform. Because the waveform is fixed and small in duration, two peaks are required to depolarize nerve cells. High-volt current stimulators are constant voltage units capable of delivering amplitudes >100 V. They also have a high peak current; however, the average current is only 50% of the peak current.

High-volt units typically have two electrode leads—one active and one dispersive—with the active electrode being much smaller than the dispersive electrode. A variety of hand applicators and probes are available for the high-volt unit. A polarity switch typically is present and can be used to set the polarity of the active electrode.

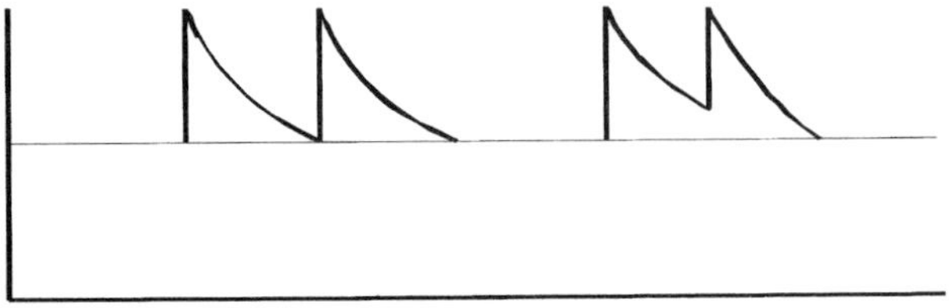

27. High-volt current therapy often is referred to as high-voltage galvanic therapy or high-voltage pulsed galvanic therapy. Discuss how high-volt currents differ from direct currents.

High Voltage	Direct Current
Used to excite peripheral nerves	Useless in exciting peripheral nerves
Useless in exciting denervated tissues	Used to excite denervated tissues
Creates no measurable thermal reaction under electrodes	Creates thermal and chemical reactions under electrodes
Ineffective current for iontophoresis	Effective current for iontophoresis
Affects superficial and deep tissues	Affects only superficial tissues
Useful in discriminating between sensory, motor, and painful stimulation	Discrimination is almost impossible and stimulation usually is painful
Used to resolve many clinical pathologies	Restricted benefit to limited number of clinical pathologies

ELECTRODES AND ELECTRODE PLACEMENT

28. What is the relationship between interelectrode distance and depth of penetration?

Current travels through areas of least resistance; electrodes placed at greater distances from each other result in deeper penetration, provided that all other parameters and variables remain constant.

29. List the potential sites for electrode placement used in the treatment of pain.

- At the location of the pain
- Over acupuncture points
- Over trigger points
- Over motor points related to the origin of the pain
- Along peripheral nerve roots

- Paravertebral, even if the pain is only on one side
- Contralateral to the pain
- Distal or proximal

30. Name the two electrode placement strategies for neuromuscular electrical stimulation (NMES).

1. Unipolar method: The active electrode is placed on the motor point, and the dispersive electrode is placed on some other point such as the nerve trunk.
2. Bipolar method: Two electrodes of equal size are placed along the length of the muscle belly. Usually the active electrode is placed over the motor point.

STIMULATION OF HEALTHY AND DENERVATED TISSUES

31. List electrically excitable and nonexcitable tissues.

Excitable Tissues	Nonexcitable Tissues
Abdominal organ cells	Bone
Autonomic motor fibers	Blood cells
Cardiac muscle fibers	Cartilage
Cells that produce glandular secretion	Collagen
Nerve axons of all types	Extracellular fluid
Nerve cells of all types	Ligaments
Voluntary motor fibers	Tendon

32. Discuss Pflüger's law and its implications in the stimulation of human tissues.

According to Pflüger's law, healthy muscle contracts with less current if stimulated by the cathode compared with stimulation by the anode. When stimulating a muscle with a direct current, the cathode should be the active electrode because the amount of current required to acquire a muscle contraction is less with the active cathode than with the anode:

$$\text{CCC} > \text{ACC} > \text{AOC} > \text{COC}$$

where CCC = cathode closing current, ACC = anode closing current, AOC = anode opening current, COC = cathode opening current, closing = starting the current, and opening = stopping the current.

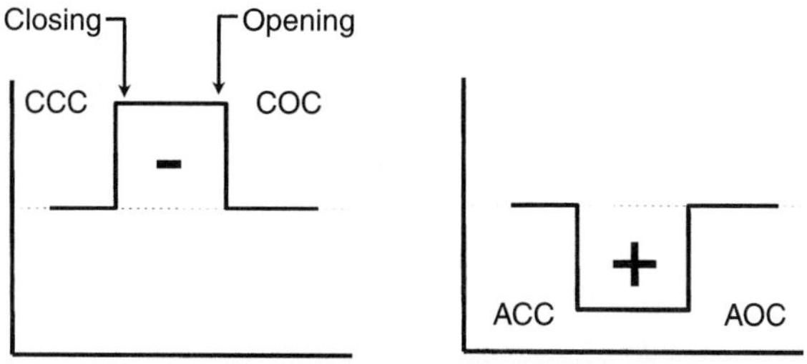

33. What is accommodation?

Accommodation is the increased threshold of excitable tissue when a slowly rising stimulus is used. Both nerve and muscle tissues are capable of accommodating to an electrical stimulus; nerve tissue accommodates more rapidly than muscle tissue. Understanding the process of accommodation is important when stimulating healthy muscle by the motor axon because the electrical stimulus must be applied somewhat rapidly to avoid accommodation.

34. What is the strength-duration curve?

The strength-duration curve describes the relationship between the strength of the stimulus (intensity) and the duration of the stimulus (on time) required to reach a specified level of activation. By varying the intensity and duration of an electrical stimulus, it is possible to plot a strength-duration curve. The strength-duration curve gives a graphic representation of the excitability of nerve and muscle tissues. Although the strength-duration curves are comparable for healthy nerve and muscle tissues, they are different from denervated nerve and muscle tissues. As a result, we are clinically able to stimulate healthy, innervated muscles with a stimulus of adequate amplitude and of short duration. It also is shown by this curve that greater amplitudes of stimulus and longer durations are necessary to stimulate denervated muscles effectively.

TEST	NORMAL	DENERVATING	DENERVATED	REINNERVATING	REINNERVATED
Chronaxie	< 1 msec	begins to rise	30 to 50 msec	begins to decrease	approaches normal
Strength Duration Curve	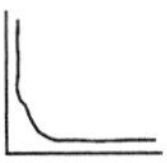	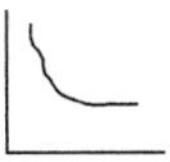	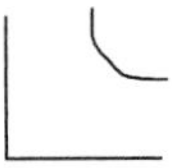	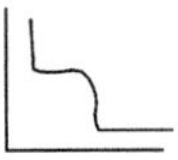	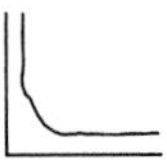
Reaction of de-generation	AC = DC	DC > AC	DC only	AC begins	AC = DC
Nerve Conduction	40 to 60 m/sec	No conduction after 3 days	No conduction	Conduction increses	WNL

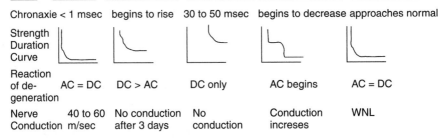

35. What are identified contraindications and precautions for electrotherapy application?

CONTRAINDICATIONS (ABSOLUTE AND RELATIVE)

- Cardiac pacemaker of synchronous or demand type
- Patients prone to seizures
- Placement of electrodes across or around the heart
- Placement of electrodes over a pregnant uterus, especially during the first trimester (this is controversial, and delivery itself presents with relative precautions)
- Placement of electrodes over an area suspected of arterial or venous thrombosis or thrombophlebitis
- Placement of electrodes over the pharyngeal area
- Placement of electrodes over protruding metal
- Placement of electrodes over the carotid sinus

PRECAUTIONS

- Allergies to tapes and gels
- Areas of absent or decreased sensation
- Electrically sensitive patients
- Patients with advanced cardiac disease
- Patients with severe hypotension or hypertension
- Placement of the electrode over area with significant adipose tissue
- Placement of the electrode over damaged skin (with the exception of tissue healing protocols)
- Placement of the electrode over or near the stellate ganglion
- Placement of the electrode over the temporal and orbital region
- Patients who are unable to communicate clearly

APPLICATION

36. Electrical stimulation has been reported in the literature to be useful in what conditions?

- Edema management
- Endurance training
- Improvement of muscle contractures
- Maintaining and improving range of motion
- Management of spasticity and spasm
- Muscle strengthening
- Neuromuscular facilitation and reeducation
- Orthotic substitution

37. Is there a difference between use of NMES or voluntary exercise or use of combined NMES and voluntary exercise in terms of muscle strength?

Yes. Recent evidence suggests that NMES combined with voluntary exercise may accelerate gains in quadriceps muscle strength and activation greater than voluntary exercise alone following total knee arthroplasty. For example, Stevens and colleagues showed that the addition of ten 10-second NMES-elicited quadriceps contractions to treatment sessions significantly improved quadriceps strength, with the most dramatic improvement noted in the first 3 weeks of treatment.

38. Outline an appropriate protocol for neuromuscular facilitation and reeducation including purpose, rationale, indications, parameters, and special considerations.

1. Purpose—To barrage the central nervous system (CNS) with appropriate sensory information
2. Rationale—By supplying the proper sensory input of what a muscle contraction or limb movement feels like and visual information about the appearance of the action, electrical stimulation can enhance a motor response. It also may prevent decreases in muscle oxidative capacity and provide an artificial drive to inactive synapses in some circumstances.
3. Indications—Any patient for whom a motor- and sensory-augmented muscle response would assist in better performance of his or her own voluntary actions
4. Parameters—Pulse duration, 100 to 200 msec; pulse rate, 35 to 50 Hz; intensity, to a tolerable motor level up to $3^{+}/5$; ramp, 1 to 3 sec up/down; on/off, 1:1 ratio set or hand-held switch; treatment time, 5 to 30 min, 1 to 3 times/day, 3 to 7 days/week, 1 to 2 weeks; polarity, not applicable
5. Special considerations—Facilitation and reeducation require active participation by the patient and may be limited by patient tolerance, cooperation, and attention span.

39. When is NMES indicated after knee surgery and immobilization?

- Prevention of muscle atrophy associated with prolonged immobilization
- Prevention of decreases in muscle strength
- Prevention of decreases in muscle mass
- Prevention of decreases in muscle oxidative capacity

40. Is there a difference between the use of high-intensity electrical stimulators and low-intensity or battery-powered stimulators with regard to quadriceps femoris muscle force production in the early phases of anterior cruciate ligament (ACL) rehabilitation?

Yes. Studies support the use of high-intensity electrical stimulation but do not consistently support the use of low-intensity or battery-powered stimulators when the desired objective is the recovery of quadriceps femoris muscle force production. A study by Snyder-Mackler and colleagues indicates that training contraction intensity is positively correlated with quadriceps femoris muscle recovery, with an apparent threshold training contraction intensity of 10% of the maximal voluntary contraction of the uninvolved quadriceps femoris muscle.

41. Outline an appropriate protocol for muscle strengthening in terms of purpose, rationale, indications, parameters, and special considerations.

1. Purpose—To increase muscle strength, encourage muscle hypertrophy, and facilitate normal motor response
2. Rationale—Electrical stimulation can be used to help patients achieve a volitional contraction sufficient to increase strength and prevent disuse atrophy if they are unable to do so on their own.
3. Indications—Any patient in need of increasing girth and strength of an atrophied muscle
4. Parameters—Pulse duration, 200 to 300 msec; pulse rate, 35 to 80 Hz; intensity, motor, 60% ± maximal voluntary contraction (MVC); ramp, 1 to 5 sec up/down, as tolerated; on/off, 1:5 ratio; treatment time, activity specific, 10 to 20 repetitions, 3 to 5 days/week, 2 to 3 weeks; polarity, not applicable
5. Special considerations—This program should be used with patients with sufficient innervation to make muscle strengthening practical. It is important to avoid muscle fatigue with this type of stimulation.

42. Can NMES be used to augment ROM and strength of the shoulder musculature?

Yes. Strengthening and muscle girth improve in orthopaedic patients, and shoulder subluxation, in particular, can be prevented or corrected in neurologically involved patients.

43. What are the benefits of NMES after ACL reconstruction?

Reduced postsurgical muscle atrophy, increased muscle torque values, improved quadriceps femoris muscle strength, and improved functional recovery are some of the benefits. For example, in a study by Fitzgerald and colleagues, subjects receiving NMES (2500-Hz alternating current, time modulated to deliver 75 bursts per second, with a 2-second ramp-up and ramp-down time, a 10-second stimulation period at the maximum amplitude, followed by a 50-second rest period) twice a week in treatment sessions of 11 to 12 minutes showed significantly greater maximum voluntary isometric torque of the quadriceps femoris muscle and significantly improved functional status (per patient self-report) at 12 weeks following initiation of treatment than subjects not receiving NMES.

44. Is NMES more effective for strength training after ACL reconstruction when performed against isometric resistance?

Yes. Recent evidence suggests that the strength training effect is decreased when NMES is applied without isometric resistance. However, use of NMES without resistance is considered to be an acceptable alternative when clinicians do not have access to a dynamometer or for patients who do not tolerate NMES-induced contractions against isometric resistance.

45. Should the presence or absence of a knee extensor lag be a criterion for using or not using NMES after ACL reconstruction?

No. No relationship has been found between knee extensor lag and treatment outcomes following use of NMES. Data indicate that NMES is beneficial regardless of whether or not an extensor lag is present.

46. Is there a relationship between the number of NMES training sessions per week and strength outcomes?

Yes. Three training sessions per week for 4 weeks have been shown to be effective for strength gains versus two training sessions per week for 4 weeks.

47. Can electrical stimulation protocols developed for a certain muscle group be used for training muscles with a different fiber-type composition?

Yes. Research suggests that variable frequency stimulation can augment the force of skeletal muscle irrespective of fiber type.

48. Is there a relationship between muscle contraction strength or fatigue and type of waveform used with electrical stimulation?

Yes. Recent evidence suggests that monophasic and biphasic waveforms generate greater torque and are less fatiguing than polyphasic waveforms.

49. What are the appropriate parameters and rationale for conventional, low-rate, and brief intense transcutaneous electrical nerve stimulation (TENS)?

	Conventional	Low Rate	Brief Intense
Phase duration	60-100 μsec	200-400 μsec	250 μsec
Pulse rate	80-125 Hz	2-4 Hz	125 Hz
Intensity	Sensory just below motor	Muscle fasciculation	Sensory just below muscle
Treatment duration	As needed	30-45 min	10-15 min
Onset of relief	10-20 min	25-30 min	1-5 min
Carryover	30 min to 2 hr	Hours to days	Short
Indications	Acute, superficial pain, first time application	Acute to chronic pain	Wound debridement and deep fiber massage
Theory	Gate theory Opiate mediated Placebo	Gate theory Opiate mediated Placebo Other	Gate theory Opiate mediated Placebo Other

50. Does TENS aid in the management of chronic low back pain when administered in isolation or when combined with an exercise program?

In general, there is no strong support that TENS is any more effective than a placebo in the management of chronic low back pain. TENS offers no apparent benefit to the patient as compared with exercise alone. Follow-through with exercise programs or TENS often is poor in this specific patient population.

51. Discuss appropriate considerations for maintaining range of motion.

Protocols should begin with simple one-plane joint movements, use antigravity starting positions with a rest between movements, and progress to antigravity positions without a rest between movements (i.e., flexion-rest-extension-rest > flexion-extension-flexion) as tolerated. Reasonable parameters are the following: intensity, to a tolerable motor level up to $3^+/5$; frequency, 35 to 50 Hz; phase duration, 100 to 200 msec; ramp, 4 to 5 sec progressing to 3 sec; on/off, as required to achieve desired range of motion; treatment time, 30 min/day, 50 to 100 repetitions, as needed.

52. Discuss appropriate considerations for edema control.

Muscular activity is an important aspect of lymphatic and venous flow. The contraction of skeletal muscles by electrical stimulation can produce a muscle contraction capable of aiding lymphatic and venous flow. The intervention can be enhanced further by combining it with other forms of management, such as elevation, rest, and compression. Muscle pumping protocols are valuable for pain modulation. Reasonable stimulation parameters should focus on producing a nonfatiguing muscle contraction: pulse rate, 4 to 10 Hz; phase duration, ±300 μsec; waveform, biphasic or high volt; polarity, not applicable with this protocol; intensity, visible contraction of muscles in the area where edema is noted, 1/5 to 3/5; time of treatment, 30 min, 2 to 3 times/day, 1 to 2 weeks; electrode placement, muscle bulk of an involved muscle or an involved joint.

This protocol should be used in conjunction with ice application and elevation of the affected area.

53. Can electromyographic biofeedback aid in the recovery of quadriceps femoris muscle function following ACL reconstruction?

Yes. Findings from studies by Draper and by Draper and Ballard suggest (1) biofeedback is more effective than electrical stimulation in promoting recovery of peak torque, (2) biofeedback and electrical stimulation are comparable in terms of recovery of active knee extension, and (3) biofeedback combined with muscle strengthening exercises facilitates a more rapid recovery of quadriceps femoris peak torque following ACL reconstruction as compared to electrical stimulation alone.

Bibliography

Baker LL, Parker K: Neuromuscular electrical stimulation of the muscles surrounding the shoulder, *Phys Ther* 66:1930-1937, 1986.

Baker LL et al: *Neuromuscular electrical stimulation: a practical guide,* ed 4, Downey, Calif, 2000, Rancho.

Bickel CS et al: Fatigability and variable-frequency train stimulation of human skeletal muscles, *Phys Ther* 83:366-373, 2003.

Currier DP, Mann R: Muscular strength development by electrical stimulation in healthy individuals, *Phys Ther* 63:915-921, 1983.

Delitto A, Snyder-Mackler L: Two theories of muscle strength augmentation using percutaneous electrical stimulation, *Phys Ther* 70:158-164, 1990.

Delitto A et al: Electrical stimulation versus voluntary exercise in strengthening thigh musculature after anterior cruciate ligament surgery, *Phys Ther* 68:660-663, 1988.

Deyo RA et al: A controlled trial of transcutaneous electrical nerve stimulation (TENS) and exercise for chronic low back pain, *N Engl J Med* 322:1627-1634, 1990.

Draper V: Electromyographic biofeedback and recovery of quadriceps femoris muscle function following anterior cruciate ligament reconstruction, *Phys Ther* 70:11-17, 1990.

Draper V, Ballard L: Electrical stimulation versus electromyographic biofeedback in the recovery of quadriceps femoris muscle function following anterior cruciate ligament surgery, *Phys Ther* 71:455-461, 1991.

Faghri PD et al: The effects of functional electrical stimulation on shoulder subluxation, arm function recovery, and shoulder pain in hemiplegic stroke patients, *Arch Phys Med Rehabil* 75:73-79, 1994.

Fitzgerald GK, Piva SR, Irrgang JJ: A modified neuromuscular electrical stimulation protocol for quadriceps strength training following anterior cruciate ligament reconstruction, *J Orthop Sports Phys Ther* 33:492-501, 2003.

Gersh MR: *Electrotherapy in rehabilitation,* Philadelphia, 1992, FA Davis.

Lake DA: Neuromuscular electrical stimulation. An overview and its application in the treatment of sports injuries, *Sports Med* 13:320-336, 1992.

Laufer Y et al: Quadriceps femoris muscle torques and fatigue generated by neuromuscular electrical stimulation with three different waveforms, *Phys Ther* 81:1307-1316, 2001.
McArdle WD, Katch FI, Katch VL: *Exercise physiology: Energy, nutrition, and human performance,* ed 5, Philadelphia, 2001, Lippincott Williams & Wilkins.
Nelson RM, Karen HW, Currier DP: *Clinical electrotherapy,* ed 3, Norwalk, Conn, 1999, Appleton & Lange.
Parker MG et al: Strength response in human femoris muscle during 2 neuromuscular electrical stimulation programs, *J Orthop Sports Phys Ther* 33:719-726, 2003.
Robinson AJ, Snyder-Mackler L: *Clinical electrophysiology: Electrotherapy and electrophysiologic testing,* ed 2, Baltimore, 1995, Williams & Wilkins.
Snyder-Mackler L et al: Use of electrical stimulation to enhance recovery of quadriceps femoris muscle force production in patients following anterior cruciate ligament reconstruction, *Phys Ther* 74:901-907, 1994.
Snyder-Mackler L et al: Strength of the quadriceps femoris muscle and functional recovery after reconstruction of the anterior cruciate ligament. A prospective, randomized clinical trial of electrical stimulation, *J Bone Joint Surg Am* 77:1166-1173, 1995.
Stevens JE, Mizner RL, Snyder-Mackler L: Neuromuscular electrical stimulation for quadriceps muscle strengthening after bilateral total knee arthroplasty: a case series, *J Orthop Sports Phys Ther* 34:21-29, 2004.

Chapter 11

Iontophoresis, Ultrasound, Phonophoresis, and Laser Therapy

Fredrick D. Pociask, PT, PhD, OCS, Kathleen Galloway, PT, MPT, DSc, and Tracey M. Fleck, PT, MPT

IONTOPHORESIS

1. Are iontophoresis and phonophoresis interchangeable clinically?

No. Ions are introduced with iontophoresis, whereas molecules are introduced by the ultrasound waves. Furthermore, because sound waves are not electrical in nature, no ionization takes place.

2. Describe Leduc's classic experiment.

In 1908 Leduc showed that ionic medication could penetrate intact skin and produce local and systemic effects in animals. Two rabbits were placed in series in the same direct current circuit so that the current had to pass through both rabbits to complete the circuit. The electrical current entered into the first rabbit by a positive electrode soaked in strychnine sulfate and exited the rabbit by a negative electrode soaked in water. The current then entered the second rabbit by an anode soaked in water and exited by a cathode soaked in potassium cyanide. When a current of 40 to 50 mA was used, the first rabbit exhibited tetanic convulsions secondary to the introduction of the strychnine ion, and the second rabbit died quickly secondary to cyanide poisoning. When the animals were replaced and the flow of current was reversed, the animals were not harmed because the strychnine ion was not repelled by the positive pole, and the cyanide was not repelled by the negative pole.

3. Describe the potato experiment.

Two electrodes were implanted at opposite ends of a potato, and a potassium iodine solution was placed in a depression that was made in the central-top portion of the potato. Direct current (DC) attracted the iodine anion toward the positive pole, and the free iodine formed blue starch iodine.

4. Define direct current.

Direct current is the flow of electrons in one direction for >1 second. A current is termed a direct current if:
- The flow of electrons is unidirectional.
- The polarity is constant.
- The current produces a twitch response only at the time of make.
- The membrane is hyperpolarized as long as the current is on.
- The duration of current flow is >1 second.

With iontophoresis, the current is on for the duration of the treatment.

5. List some commonly used ionic solutions and their proposed indications.

Ionic Solution	Indications	Polarity	% Solution
Acetic acid	Calcium deposits	Negative	2-5%
Dexamethasone sodium phosphate	Inflammatory conditions	Negative	4 mg/ml
Lidocaine hydrochloride	Skin anesthesia	Positive	4-5%
Potassium iodide	Scar tissue	Negative	5-10%
Water	Hyperhidrosis	Alternate	100%
Zinc oxide	Ulcers, antiseptic	Positive	20%

6. Why are the effects of iontophoresis often longer lasting than those of phonophoresis?

Ions are introduced into the superficial tissues, where circulation is limited, giving the ions time to be absorbed and used. Phonophoretically introduced molecules are delivered to deeper layers, where vascularization is more abundant, leading to early transport out of the area before effective breakdown and reuse are possible.

7. Does increasing the concentration of the drug increase the amount delivered to the target tissue?

No. While concentrations vary based on the applied ion (e.g., dexamethasone sodium phosphate [$DexNa_2PO_3$] at 0.04% and sodium salicylate [NASal] at 2%), higher concentrations have not been shown to be more effective.

8. Are there concerns with using direct current?

Yes. Intact skin cannot tolerate current density >1 mA/cm^2.

9. Ion transfer depends on what factors?

1. The concentration of the ions in solution
2. The current density of the active electrode
3. The duration of the current flow

10. List the polar effect on treated tissues produced by the anode and the cathode.

Positive (Anode)	Negative (Cathode)
Hyperpolarizes nerve fibers	Depolarizes nerve fibers
Repels bases	Attracts bases (more damaging to skin)
Hardens tissues	Softens tissues
Stops hemorrhage	Increases hemorrhage
Sedates, calms	Stimulates
Reduces pain in acute situations	Reduces pain in chronic situations

11. Why do burns occur with iontophoresis?

Most burns are caused by poor technique, which can be greatly negated by the use of quality, commercial products. Some conditions that can produce burns are the following:

- Poor skin-electrode interfaces
- Intensity too high
- Velcro straps too tight
- Electrodes too small, too dry, with not enough of a size differential between anode and cathode
- Wrong polarity
- Use of current other than continuous DC

12. Where should iontophoretic electrodes be placed?

The active electrode containing the ion that is to be repelled is placed over the treatment tissues, and the depressive electrode is placed about 18 inches away to encourage a greater depth of penetration. Because electrodes and units typically come with specific instructions, it is wise to read both sets of instructions before attempting the procedure.

13. What are advantages of iontophoresis as compared to injection?

- No carrier fluids required
- Reduced risk of infections secondary to noninvasive application
- Relatively painless for most patients
- Able to deliver antiinflammatory medication locally without the gastrointestinal side effects associated with oral ingestion or the systemic effects noted with injection

14. What are the disadvantages of iontophoresis?

- Numerous treatments may be required to obtain results.
- Depth of penetration is limited to approximately 8 to 10 mm (depth of penetration has been reported at up to 2 cm).
- Electrodes are costly.
- There are risks of polar effects and skin damage.
- Setup and application are time consuming.

15. How many serial iontophoretic treatments are safe?

One to six treatments of dexamethasone are considered safe when administered alone.

16. Does the magnitude of iontophoretic current determine the depth of penetration?

No. Recent evidence suggests that diffusion, rather than magnitude of current, determines depth of drug penetration. Comparable doses delivered at low magnitude currents over several hours may be more effective than those delivered by higher magnitude currents for 10 to 30 minutes.

17. Do buffered electrodes stabilize skin pH under the cathode?

The literature suggests that when iontophoresis is properly delivered at 20 to 40 mA/min, pH changes with or without a buffer are not significantly different. In contrast, when iontophoresis is delivered at 80 mA/min, significant changes in pH are stabilized by the addition of buffers.

ULTRASOUND

18. How is ultrasound generated and what is a piezoelectric effect?

The natural quartz or synthetic crystal housed within the sound head, classified as a piezoelectric material, will mechanically respond or deform when subjected to alternating current (AC) by expanding and contracting at the same frequency at which the current changes polarity. When the crystal expands, it compresses the material in front of it, and when it contracts, it rarefies the material in front of it. This process is described as a piezoelectric effect.

19. What is the beam nonuniformity ratio (BNR)?

BNR is the measure of the variability of the ultrasound wave intensity produced by the machine. If the machine is set at 1.5 W, BNR is the range of possible intensities actually delivered by the machine. The lower the ratio, the more uniform the machine output, resulting in a more uniform treatment. A higher ratio, 8 W, for example, means that when the machine is set at 1 W, it could deliver in the range of 1 to 8 W.

20. What is the effective radiating area (ERA) of a transducer?

ERA is the effective radiating area that corresponds to the part of the sound head that produces the sound wave. The ERA should be close to the size of the sound head or transducer. If it is smaller than the sound head, it may be misleading when treating the patient. The recommended treatment area is only 2 to 3 times the ERA.

21. What are nonthermal and thermal ranges of therapeutic ultrasound?

Intensities between 0.1 and 0.3 W/cm^2 are considered nonthermal, and intensities above approximately 0.3 W/cm^2 are considered thermal.

22. What are the reported nonthermal effects of ultrasound?

- Increases cell membrane permeability
- Increases vascular permeability
- Increases blood flow in chronically ischemic tissue
- Stimulates collagen synthesis
- Stimulates phagocytosis
- Promotes tissue regeneration
- Breaks down scar tissue in acute injuries
- Kills bacteria and viruses in chronic situations

23. What are the reported thermal effects of ultrasound?

- Preferentially heats collagen-rich tissues
- Increases tissue elasticity of collagen-rich tissue
- Increases blood flow
- Increases pain threshold
- Decreases muscle spasm
- Decreases pain and joint stiffness
- Causes a mild inflammatory response

24. How does ultrasound frequency relate to depth of penetration?

Increasing the frequency of ultrasound causes a decrease in its depth of penetration and concentration of the ultrasound energy in the superficial tissues. For example, the approximate depth of penetration at 1 MHz is 2 to 5 cm and the approximate depth of penetration at 3 MHz is 1 to 2 cm.

25. Will tissue temperature increases in human muscle vary between pulsed and continuous ultrasound application when administered at equivalent temporal average intensities?

The literature suggests that equivalent temporal average intensities will produce similar increases in intramuscular tissue temperature. For example, 3 MHz at a 50% duty cycle and an intensity of 1.0 W/cm^2 over a 10-minute period produced similar heating as compared to 3 MHz at a 100% duty cycle and an intensity of 0.5 W/cm^2 over a 10-minute treatment.

26. Is a metal implant an absolute contraindication for the use of ultrasound?

No. However, caution should be exercised because ultrasound is contraindicated over plastic implants and joint cement, which are often components of a total joint replacement.

27. Is ultrasound effective in treating calcific tendonitis of the shoulder?

Yes. It has been suggested that ultrasound treatment helps resolve calcifications and is associated with short-term improvements in pain and quality of life. In a study by Ebenbichler and colleagues, patients received 24 15-minute sessions of 25% pulsed ultrasound (0.89 MHz at 2.5 W/cm^2) over a 6-week period. After 6 weeks of treatment, calcifications resolved in 19% of patients and decreased by at least 50% in 28% of patients (compared to zero and 10% in those receiving sham ultrasound). At the 9-month follow-up, calcifications resolved in 42% of patients and improved in 23% of patients receiving ultrasound (compared to 8% and 12% in those receiving sham ultrasound).

28. Is ultrasound effective in treating carpal tunnel syndrome?

A study by Ebenbichler and colleagues suggests that ultrasound may be effective in reducing pain and improving electroneurographic variables (motor distal latency and nerve conduction velocity) in patients with carpal tunnel syndrome. In this study, 20 sessions of ultrasound treatment were performed over a 6-week period (1 MHz, 1.0 W/cm^2, pulsed mode 1:4, 15 minutes per session).

Controversy

29. Is there sufficient support for the use of ultrasound in a physical therapy treatment program?

Based on a review of randomized controlled trials (RCTs) published between 1975 and 1999 in which ultrasound was used for patient treatment (Robertson and Baker, 2001), it was suggested that there is little evidence to support the use of active therapeutic ultrasound versus placebo ultrasound. It was also noted that 25 out of the 35 studies reviewed were methodologically inaccurate, and the 10 remaining studies had significant variability in dosages used and patient problems treated. A more recent RCT (Gursel, 2004) drew the conclusion that "there is insufficient evidence to support the use of 1-MHz ultrasound in combination with other interventions in the management of painful shoulder conditions." However, the validity of these conclusions may be questioned when the parameters of the interventions are analyzed against current evidence-based recommendations; further research is required to answer this question.

ULTRASOUND AND PHONOPHORESIS

30. How does phonophoresis work?

It was once thought that ultrasound exerted pressure on the drug, driving it through the skin. However, ultrasound exerts only minimal pressure. Another explanation is that ultrasound changes the permeability of the stratum corneum (the most superficial skin layer) through thermal and nonthermal effects. Ultrasound performed before the application of a drug to the skin has been found to increase drug penetration, supporting this theory.

31. When performing phonophoresis, what dosage is preferred?

In several animal studies Griffin and colleagues demonstrated that ultrasound allowed cortisone to penetrate paravertebral muscles and nerves under a variety of treatment dosages (e.g., 1.0 W/cm^2 for 5 minutes, 3.0 W/cm^2 for 5 minutes, 0.3 W/cm^2 for 17 minutes, and 0.1 W/cm^2 for 51 minutes; with frequencies that ranged from 0.09 to 3.6 MHz). Griffin's work demonstrated the greatest penetration with higher intensities at shorter durations and with lower intensities at longer durations. Results favored lower intensities at longer durations in terms of greatest delivery of cortisone to muscles and nerves. Clinically, modest intensities at longer durations using a nonstationary sound mode of application within carefully constrained areas of treatment are recommended for patient comfort and to prevent tissue damage.

32. When performing phonophoresis, what concentrations of hydrocortisone are most effective?

A study by Kleinkort and Wood suggests that treatments using 10% hydrocortisone are more effective than those using 1% hydrocortisone for relieving pain associated with tendonitis or bursitis.

33. How many serial phonophoretic treatments are safe?

Once a drug passes through the skin, it is circulated through the body and can become systemic; this is also true in the case of phonophoresis. It is recommended that a drug administered in any fashion should not be administered again by phonophoresis without the consent of a physician to rule out the possibility of elevating the therapeutic dose of the drug beyond desired levels.

34. What are examples of drugs that can be administered by phonophoresis?

The following drugs have been identified as phonophoretic agents: dexamethasone (0.4% ointment), hydrocortisone (0.5 to 1.0% ointment), iodine (10% ointment), lidocaine (5% ointment), magnesium sulfate (2% ointment), salicylates (10% trolamine salicylate or 3% sodium salicylate ointment), zinc oxide (20% ointment).

35. Provide an example of a topical nonsteroidal antiinflammatory drug (NSAID) that may be administered by phonophoresis.

Fastum gel (ketoprofen 2.5%) has been shown to be an effective phonophoretic agent. Phonophoretic application of this drug appears to be superior to topical application. In a study by

Cagnie and colleagues, the concentration of ketoprofen in synovial tissue was significantly greater in the groups receiving phonophoresis with either continuous (1 MHz at 1.5 W/cm^2) or pulsed (20%) ultrasound than in the group receiving only topical application.

36. What is the most efficiently transmitted topical antiinflammatory media used in phonophoresis?

Fluocinonide 0.05% (Lidex) gel and methyl salicylate 15% (Thera-Gesic) cream transmit ultrasound the best—97% relative to water.

37. Is phonophoresis effective in treating lateral epicondylitis?

A study by Baskurt and colleagues suggests that phonophoresis of naproxen (10%) may be equally as effective as iontophoresis of naproxen (10%) in reducing pain and improving grip strength in patients with lateral epicondylitis.

LASER THERAPY

38. Is laser treatment effective for relieving symptoms of arthritis?

A meta-analysis of the randomized controlled trials of low level laser therapy (LLT) was conducted. Short-term pain relief and a decrease in morning stiffness were noted with LLT interventions in patients with rheumatoid arthritis (RA). The results for osteoarthritis (OA) were more inconsistent. The Ottawa Panel formed a board of experts to review the use of modalities for intervention in rheumatoid arthritis using the Cochrane data collection method. They recommended the use of thermotherapy and low level laser therapy as well as the use of electrical stimulation and therapeutic ultrasound for patients with rheumatoid arthritis.

39. Has low level laser therapy been found to be effective for any other conditions?

A placebo-controlled clinical trial of low level laser therapy in addition to rest, ice, compression, and elevation was conducted with soccer players following lateral ankle sprains. Researchers used an 820-nm gallium/aluminum/arsenide (GaAlAs) wave with a frequency of 16 Hz and an output of 40 mW over a 0.16-cm^2 area. Volumetric measurements found a significant decrease in edema in the ankles receiving laser therapy when compared with controls.

The effectiveness of low level laser therapy in treating Raynaud's disease was studied in another randomized placebo controlled double blind crossover study. The frequency and intensity of Raynaud attacks were significantly decreased during laser treatment when compared with the sham treatment.

40. Is low level laser therapy effective for the treatment of carpal tunnel syndrome?

Irvine et al compared the use of an 860-nm gallium/aluminum/arsenide laser at 6 J/cm^2 with a sham laser treatment over the carpal tunnel. There was no difference between treatment and sham groups in outcome measurements that included the Levine carpal tunnel syndrome questionnaire, electrophysiological measurements, and the Purdue pegboard test.

Bibliography

Anderson CR et al: Effects of iontophoresis current magnitude and duration on dexamethasone deposition and localized drug retention, *Phys Ther* 83:161-170, 2003.

Apostolos S: Low-level laser treatment can reduce edema in second degree ankle sprains, *J Clin Laser Med Surg* 22:125-128, 2004.

Apostolos S: Low level laser therapy in primary Raynaud's phenomenon—Results of placebo controlled, double blind intervention study, *J Rheumatol* 31:2408-2412, 2004.

Banga AK, Bose S, Ghosh TK: Iontophoresis and electroporation: comparisons and contrasts, *Int J Pharm* 179:1-19, 1999.

Baskurt F, Ozcan A, Algun C: Comparison of effects of phonophoresis and iontophoresis of naproxen in the treatment of lateral epicondylitis, *Clin Rehabil* 17:96-100, 2003.

Berliner MN: Skin microcirculation during tapwater iontophoresis in humans: cathode stimulates more than anode, *Microvasc Res* 54:74-80, 1997.

Brosseau L et al: Low level laser therapy for osteoarthritis and rheumatoid arthritis: a meta-analysis, *J Rheumatol* 27:1961-1969, 2000.

Cagnie B et al: Phonophoresis versus topical application of ketoprofen: comparison between tissue and plasma levels, *Phys Ther* 83:707-712, 2003.

Cameron MH, Cameron R, Kuhn S: *Physical agents in rehabilitation: from research to practice,* ed 2, St Louis, 2003, Elsevier.

Ciccone CD: *Pharmacology in rehabilitation,* Philadelphia, 1990, FA Davis.

Costello CT, Jeske AH: Iontophoresis: applications in transdermal medication delivery, *Phys Ther* 75:554-563, 1995.

Demirtas RN, Oner C: The treatment of lateral epicondylitis by iontophoresis of sodium salicylate and sodium diclofenac, *Clin Rehabil* 12:23-29, 1998.

Ebenbichler GR et al: Ultrasound treatment for treating the carpal tunnel syndrome: randomised "sham" controlled trial, *BMJ* 316:731-735, 1998.

Ebenbichler GR et al: Ultrasound therapy for calcific tendonitis of the shoulder, *N Engl J Med* 340:1533-1538, 1999.

Gallo JA et al: A comparison of human muscle temperature increases during 3-MHz continuous and pulsed ultrasound with equivalent temporal average intensities, *J Orthop Sports Phys Ther* 34:395-401, 2004.

Glass JM, Stephen RL, Jacobson SC: The quantity and distribution of radiolabeled dexamethasone delivered to tissue by iontophoresis, *Int J Dermatol* 19:519-525, 1980.

Griffin JE, Touchstone JC: Ultrasonic movement of cortisol into pig tissues. I. Movement into skeletal muscle, *Am J Phys Med* 42:77-85, 1963.

Griffin JE, Touchstone JC: Low-intensity phonophoresis of cortisol in swine, *Phys Ther* 48:1336-1344, 1968.

Griffin JE, Touchstone JC, Liu AC: Ultrasonic movement of cortisol into pig tissue. II. Movement into paravertebral nerve, *Am J Phys Med* 44:20-25, 1965.

Griffin JE et al: Patients treated with ultrasonic driven hydrocortisone and with ultrasound alone, *Phys Ther* 47:594-601, 1967.

Guffey JS et al: Skin pH changes associated with iontophoresis, *J Orthop Sports Phys Ther* 29:656-660, 1999.

Hasson SM et al: Dexamethasone iontophoresis: effect on delayed muscle soreness and muscle function, *Can J Sport Sci* 17:8-13, 1992.

Irvine J et al: Double-blind randomized controlled trial of low level laser therapy in carpal tunnel syndrome, *Muscle Nerve* 30:182-187, 2004.

Kahn J: *Principles and practice of electrotherapy,* ed 3, New York, 1994, Churchill Livingstone.

Kassan DG, Lynch AM, Stiller MJ: Physical enhancement of dermatologic drug delivery: iontophoresis and phonophoresis, *J Am Acad Dermatol* 34:657-666, 1996.

Kleinkort JA, Wood F: Phonophoresis with 1 percent versus 10 percent hydrocortisone, *Phys Ther* 55:1320-1324, 1975.

Lark MR, Gangarosa LP Sr: Iontophoresis: an effective modality for the treatment of inflammatory disorders of the temporomandibular joint and myofascial pain, *Cranio* 8:108-119, 1990.

Lewis C: Ultrasound efficacy, *Phys Ther* 84:984, 2004 (author reply 984-985, discussion 985-987).

Morrisette DC, Brown D, Saladin ME: Temperature change in lumbar periarticular tissue with continuous ultrasound, *J Orthop Sports Phys Ther* 34:754-760, 2004.

Nelson RM, Karen HW, Currier DP: *Clinical electrotherapy,* ed 3, Norwalk, Conn, 1999, Appleton & Lange.

Ottawa Panel: Evidence based clinical practice guidelines for electrotherapy and thermotherapy interventions in the management of rheumatoid arthritis in adults, *Phys Ther* 84:1016-1043, 2004.

Robertson VJ, Baker KG: A review of therapeutic ultrasound: Effectiveness studies, *Phys Ther* 81:1339-1350, 2001.

Romani WA et al: Identification of tibial stress fractures using therapeutic continuous ultrasound, *J Orthop Sports Phys Ther* 30:444-452, 2000.

Singh S, Singh J: Transdermal drug delivery by passive diffusion and iontophoresis: a review, *Med Res Rev* 13:569-621, 1993.

Wieder DL: Treatment of traumatic myositis ossificans with acetic acid iontophoresis, *Phys Ther* 72:133-137, 1992.

Section IV

Special Topics

Chapter 12

Stretching

David A. Boyce, PT, EdD, OCS

1. What is stress relaxation?

It is a physical property of viscoelastic structures, such as a muscle tendon unit (MTU). If an MTU is elongated to a specific length and held in that position, the internal tension within the MTU decreases with the passage of time. Clinically, this is what occurs during a static stretch of an MTU.

2. Define creep.

Creep occurs when an MTU is elongated to a specific length, and then allowed to continue to elongate as stress relaxation occurs. Clinically, this is what occurs when a therapist performs a stretch in which joint range is increased during the stretch repetition. Creep is partially responsible for the immediate increase in joint range of motion (ROM) during a stretch repetition.

3. When stretching a muscle joint complex, what structures are influenced?

- Joint capsule
- Ligaments
- Nerves
- Vessels
- Skin
- MTU

4. What is ballistic stretching?

Ballistic stretching places the muscle joint complex at or near its limit of available motion, and then cyclically loads the muscle joint complex (bouncing motion at the end ROM). The rate and amplitude of the stretch are variable. Ballistic muscle stretching is indicated for preconditioning a muscle joint complex for activities such as sprinting, high jump, or other events that depend on the elastic energy in an MTU to enhance the performance of a particular movement pattern.

5. Define static stretching.

Static stretching is a technique that places a muscle joint complex in a specific ROM until a stretch is perceived. The position is held for a specific period of time and repeated as necessary to increase joint ROM.

6. Describe some commonly used proprioceptive neuromuscular facilitation (or active inhibition) stretching techniques.

- Hold-relax—the muscle to be stretched is placed in a lengthened but comfortable starting position. The patient is instructed to contract the target muscle for approximately 5 to 10 seconds. After the 10-second contraction, the patient is instructed to relax the target muscle completely as the therapist passively increases joint ROM. This is repeated for a specific number of repetitions. Intensity of the stretch is limited by the patient.

- Hold-relax-antagonist contraction—the muscle to be stretched is placed in a lengthened but comfortable starting position. The patient is instructed to contract the target muscle for approximately 5 to 10 seconds. After the 10-second contraction, the patient is instructed to relax, and then contract the muscle opposite (reciprocally inhibiting the target muscle) the target muscle, actively increasing joint ROM. Intensity of the stretch is limited by the patient.
- Antagonist contraction—the muscle to be stretched is placed in a lengthened but comfortable starting position. The patient is instructed to contract the muscle opposite (reciprocally inhibiting the target muscle) the target muscle, actively increasing joint ROM. Intensity of the stretch is limited by the patient.

7. What is the optimal number of stretch repetitions?

The optimal number of stretch repetitions is 1 to 4.

8. How is the optimal number of stretch repetitions determined?

According to Taylor, 80% of an MTU's length is obtained by the fourth repetition of a static stretch. The first stretch repetition results in the greatest increase in MTU length. Application of this information suggests that only 1 to 4 stretch repetitions may be necessary during a clinical or self-stretching session. Other studies have suggested 5 to 6 stretch repetitions, however.

9. What is the optimal amount of time that a stretch should be held?

Recent literature suggests that optimal stretch times are between 15 and 60 seconds. Most of the literature advocates stretch times between 15 and 30 seconds.

10. How often must stretching be performed to maintain gains experienced during a stretch session?

Bohannon found that stretch gains lasted 24 hours after a stretching session of the hamstrings. Zito reported no lasting effect of two 15-second passive stretches of the ankle plantar flexors after a 24-hour period. Clinically, this suggests that stretching should be performed at least every 24 hours.

11. If an individual stretches on a regular basis, how long will the gains realized during the stretching regimen be retained?

According to Zebas, after a 6-week regimen of stretching, gains realized during that period were retained for a minimum of 2 weeks and in some subjects a maximum of 4 weeks.

12. Does muscle stretching increase performance?

It depends on the activity. Athletes that perform ballistic events depend on stored elastic energy within tight muscle joint complexes to generate force beyond standard contractile force production. Stretching has been found to decrease performance in elite runners and sprinters. Research has shown, however, that stretching can increase performance, especially as it relates to the economy of gait.

13. Does stretching decrease the chance of injury?

Yes, usually. Flexibility imbalances can predispose an individual to injury. Some research has suggested that stretching was associated with increased injury rates in female athletes. The athletes created a flexibility imbalance from stretching, which ultimately resulted in injury. The key to injury prevention is to eliminate or prevent flexibility imbalances.

14. Does stretching decrease pain?

Yes. Personal testimony abounds that stretching decreases soreness. Research suggests that stretching is successful in decreasing delayed-onset muscle soreness.

15. Should a muscle joint complex be warmed up to optimize the effects of a stretch?

Not necessarily. Logically, it seems that increasing tissue temperature before stretching would increase viscoelastic properties of the soft tissues surrounding a muscle joint complex; however, research has shown that stretching with or without a warm-up yields the same results.

16. Should joint mobilization precede stretching?

Yes. Joints exhibiting decreased joint play should be mobilized before stretching to decrease the effects of abnormal joint compression and distraction.

17. What stretching technique results in the greatest flexibility gains?

According to a recent systematic review, static stretching of the hamstrings seems superior to other forms of stretching (e.g., proprioceptive neuromuscular facilitation techniques). However, based on the literature, it is difficult to state this with certainty.

18. What effect does stretching position have on hamstring flexibility gains?

Range of motion improvements when stretching the hamstring muscles are not dependent upon the position that the stretch is performed. Thus whether stretching in the standing, seated, or supine position, range of motion gains appear to be the same.

19. Does age influence the extensibility of muscle and tendon?

It does appear that with increasing age the extensibility of the muscle tendon unit decreases (related directly to the calf muscle tendon unit). This is important with regard to normal ambulation, balance, and fall prevention in the older adult. A flexibility program directed toward the calf musculature appears to be a logical prevention program for the older adult.

20. Does stretching the gastrocnemius muscle in subtalar supination result in greater ankle dorsiflexion range of motion?

It is often theorized that stretching the gastrocnemius muscle in subtalar neutral position will result in increased gastrocnemius muscle length because the totality of the stretch will be directed more specifically towards the target muscle (gastrocnemius) rather than the stretch force being dissipated across the midtarsal and subtalar joints. The literature suggests that there is no significant difference in the dorsiflexion ROM gains between individuals that stretched while maintaining the subtalar joint in supination versus pronation.

21. Does stretching alter joint position sense?

A brief stretching regimen of 3 stretches held for 30 seconds had no effect on knee joint position sense.

Bibliography

Bohannon R: Effect of repeated eight-minute muscle loading on the angle of straight leg raising, *Phys Ther* 64:491-497, 1984.

Gajdosik R, Vander Linden D, Williams A: Influence of age on length and passive elastic stiffness characteristics of the calf musle-tendon unit of women, *Phys Ther* 79:827-838, 1999.

Godges J: The effects of two stretching procedures on gait economy, *J Orthop Sports Phys Ther* 10:350-357, 1989.

Kisner C, Colby L: Stretching. In *Therapeutic exercise: foundations and techniques,* ed 3, Philadelphia, 1996, FA Davis.

Larsen R et al: Effect of static stretching of quadriceps and hamstring muscles on knee joint position sense, *Br J Sports Med* 39:43-46, 2005.
Smith CA: The warm up procedure: to stretch or not to stretch, *J Orthop Sports Phys Ther* 19:12-16, 1994.
Taylor DC: Viscoelastic properties of muscle tendon units: the biomechanical effects of stretching, *Am J Sports Med* 18:24-32, 1990.
Zito M: Lasting effects of one bout of two 15-second passive stretches on ankle dorsiflexion range of motion, *J Orthop Sports Phys Ther* 26:214-220, 1997.

Chapter 13

Manual Therapy

Richard Erhard, PT, DC, and Sara R. Piva, PT, MS, OCS

1. What is manual therapy?

Manual therapy is the use of skilled hand movements performed by physical therapists, chiropractors, or other health professionals to improve tissue extensibility, increase range of motion, induce relaxation, mobilize or manipulate soft tissue and joints, modulate pain, and reduce soft tissue swelling, inflammation, or restriction. Manual therapy uses joint or soft tissue techniques. Joint technique intends primarily to increase joint mobility, whereas soft tissue technique intends to increase soft tissue mobility. Hands-on procedures such as mobilization, manipulation, massage, stretching, and deep pressure are all components of manual therapy.

2. When is manual therapy treatment indicated?

This therapy is used to treat detected motion impairment that causes pain, loss of range of motion, and disability. Joint techniques are indicated when the motion impairment is caused by loss of the normal joint play and the assessment reveals a reversible joint hypomobility. When motion impairment is caused by excessive joint mobility, manual therapy techniques that involve the thrust component are generally contraindicated. Motion impairment caused by weakened or shortened muscles is an indication to use soft tissue techniques. Once pain has been reduced and joint mobility improved by using manual therapy, it is much easier for a patient to regain more efficient movement patterns and restore maximal function by combining manual therapy with therapeutic exercise and other rehabilitative activities. Therefore manual therapy is not a technique to be used in isolation during the overall episode of care.

3. What is joint play?

The normal movement that occurs between two articular surfaces is termed joint play. Because there is no perfect congruency between joint surfaces, joint play has to exist for full movement to occur. Mennell defined joint play movement as "a movement that cannot be produced by the action of voluntary muscles." Joint play movements include distractions, compressions, slides, rolls, or spins at a joint. Loss of joint play movement may impair range of motion. Manual therapy techniques use joint play movements for treating joint impairments.

4. Is manual therapy always passive?

Most of the time the movements used in manual therapy are not under the patient's voluntary control. Some manual therapy techniques, however, use the patient's muscle contraction or self-corrections during treatment. In these cases, the patient's participation is an expected extra force that helps the technique. Manual therapy occurs in response to existing extrinsic forces (therapist or gravity force) or intrinsic forces (patient's muscle contraction or breathing) acting on the patient's body.

5. Describe the basic types of manual therapy.

Manual Therapy Technique	Description	Comments
Joint manipulation (thrust)	Is passive movement that uses high-velocity, low-amplitude movement. Brings joint beyond its physiologic barrier and creates distraction or translation of joint surfaces. Does not exceed anatomic barrier.	Is direct or indirect technique. May present occasional hazards in untrained hands.
Joint mobilization	Is passive movement that uses slower motions than thrust. Moves joint within physiologic ROM. Uses three types of motion application: graded oscillation, progressive loading, sustained loading.	Is direct technique. Is controlled technique that uses patient feedback about effect during application, thus providing patients a sense of security and increased safety.
Muscle energy	Uses patient active muscle contraction after joint is passively taken to restrictive motion. Indicated when limiting factor to motion is neuromuscular system. Uses post-isometric relaxation principles.	Is direct technique. Demands fair degree of palpatory skill. Is contraindicated for patients with severe heart disease.
Soft tissue	Aims at enhancing status of muscle activity and/or extensibility in tissues. May produce effects on muscular, nervous, lymph, and circulatory systems.	Is indirect technique. Demands high degree of palpatory skill.

6. What are physiologic barrier and anatomic barrier?

- Physiologic barrier—the point at which voluntary range of motion in an articulation is limited by soft tissue tension. When the joint reaches the physiologic barrier, further motion toward the anatomic barrier can be induced.
- Anatomic barrier—the point at which passive range of motion is limited by bone contour or soft tissues (especially ligaments), or both. The anatomic barrier serves as the final limit to motion in an articulation. Movement beyond the anatomic barrier causes tissue damage.

7. What are direct and indirect manual therapy techniques?

- Direct technique—movement and force are in the direction of the motion restriction. Direct technique allows maximal restoration of movement; however, it may be painful when pain and muscle guarding are present.
- Indirect technique—movement and force are not both in the direction of the motion restriction. This technique is indicated in acute stages.

8. What is the difference between general and specific manual therapy techniques?

- General technique—the force is transmitted to a number of joints that have been determined to be hypomobile. General technique can increase motion in an unstable joint not previously detected.
- Specific technique—the force is localized to one joint; therefore force transmission is minimized through the uninvolved joints.

9. Is there evidence that specific manipulation techniques are delivered accurately to the targeted segment?

No. Only one study compared the target location of the technique with the location of the joints that actually produced an audible pop in response to manipulation therapy. They reported that spinal manipulation was accurate about half of the time. However, part of this accuracy was due to most procedures being associated with multiple pops, and in most cases, at least one pop emanated from the target joints. Therefore it seems that the clinical success of spinal manipulation is not dependent on the accurate delivery of that therapy to the target spinal joints.

10. What is the pop?

Popping of the joint frequently accompanies a manipulative thrust. The crack noise or joint cavitation is the result of generation or collapse of a gaseous bubble in the synovial fluid. Cineradiographic studies reported increased joint space and carbon dioxide gas production/breakdown after thrust manipulation. Because carbon dioxide is the gas with the higher miscibility within the synovial fluid, this increase in carbon dioxide levels has been suggested as the mechanism to increase range of motion in the joint after manipulation. It has also been hypothesized that the cavitation would initiate certain reflex relaxation of the periarticular musculature. After the manipulation, the joint takes approximately 15 minutes to rearrange the gas particles and allow another cavitation sound. Some people believe that if there is no noise, nothing has happened; this belief is incorrect. Recent studies suggest there is no relationship between the occurrence of an audible pop during joint manipulation and improvement in pain, ROM, and disability in patients with nonradicular low back pain.

11. Describe the grading systems for joint mobilization.

Different grading systems exist for joint mobilization: (1) grading for traction mobilization technique; (2) grading for sustained joint-play technique; (3) grading for oscillatory technique. The most widespread system used is the grading system for oscillatory technique proposed by Maitland, which has five grades of movement:

- Grade 1—slow, small-amplitude movements performed at the beginning of the range
- Grade 2—slow, large-amplitude movements that do not reach the resistance or limit of the range
- Grade 3—slow, large-amplitude movements performed to the limit of the range
- Grade 4—slow, small-amplitude movements performed at the limit of the range
- Grade 5—fast, small-amplitude, high-velocity movements (thrust) performed beyond the pathologic limitation of the range

Grades 1 through 4 are used for mobilization techniques and generally use oscillatory movements. Grades 1 and 2 are used mainly to reduce pain. Grades 3 and 4 are used primarily to increase mobility. Grade 5 is used for the thrust technique and is indicated when resistance limits movement, in the absence of pain in that direction.

12. Is there evidence that manual therapy is effective in the treatment of spinal conditions?

Yes. In fact there is a growing body of evidence of the effectiveness of manual therapy for several spinal conditions.

LOW BACK PAIN

- A systematic review of randomized trials reported that spinal manipulation and/or mobilization provides either similar or better pain outcomes in the short term and long term when compared with placebo and with other treatments, such as McKenzie therapy, medical care, management by physical therapists, soft tissue treatment, and "back school" for people with both acute and chronic low back pain. Therefore, to date it seems that joint techniques are more effective than muscle or soft tissue techniques. Among the joint techniques for individuals with acute low back pain, there is moderate evidence that manipulation provides more short-term pain relief than mobilization.
- A recent high-quality randomized trial investigated the effect of adding exercise classes, spinal manipulation, or manipulation followed by exercise to "best care" in general practice for patients complaining of back pain. This study reported that although all groups improved over time, manipulation followed by exercise achieved the most significant benefits, followed by the spinal manipulation group and lastly by the exercise group. Other more recent studies have validated the idea that a high probability of success from spinal manipulation depends on the importance of matching individual patients with the correct intervention. These studies developed a clinical prediction rule that demonstrated that clinicians can accurately identify patients with low back pain who are likely to benefit (achieve at least 50% improvement in disability) from spinal manipulation. The five predictors of success were short symptom duration, low treatment apprehension levels, lumbar hypomobility, adequate hip internal rotation range of motion, and no symptoms distal to the knee. The probability of a successful outcome among patients who met at least four of the five criteria in the rule increased from 45% to 95%. In essence, the combination of both manual therapy with exercises and the appropriate patient intervention selection to apply the techniques seems to increase the beneficial effects of manual therapy techniques.

THORACIC PAIN

- Limited evidence indicates that an intensive rehabilitation program decreased pain intensity in young patients with Scheuermann's disease.

NECK PAIN

- Evidence suggests manual therapy directed to the neck, particularly when combined with exercise, is an effective intervention for patients with mechanical neck pain with no radicular symptoms. A recent systematic review reported that spinal manipulation and/or mobilization is superior to general practitioner management for short-term pain reduction in patients with chronic neck pain. There is moderate evidence that mobilization is superior to physical therapy and family physician care. There is no evidence to support the use of manipulation versus mobilization for patients with neck pain.
- Manual therapy interventions directed to the thoracic region, instead of the cervical spine, have been shown to cause an immediate decrease in pain and increase in neck range of motion. It is theorized that biomechanical relationships between the cervical spine and thoracic spine make it possible that disturbances in joint mobility in the thoracic spine may

contribute to movement restrictions and pain in the cervical region. There is also limited evidence that the combination of thoracic spine manipulation and intermittent cervical traction for patients with cervical compressive myelopathy attributes to herniated disk and that patients with cervical radiculopathy show decreased pain and improved function.

13. Is there evidence that manual therapy is effective in treating cervicogenic headache?

Systematic reviews suggest that mobilization/manipulation is effective for patients with cervicogenic headache. A more recent trial of patients with cervicogenic headaches compared a control group to groups receiving cervical manipulation/mobilization, strengthening of the deep neck flexor and scapular muscles, and a combined manual therapy and exercise group. The results showed significant reductions in headache symptoms in all treatment groups versus the control group. At 7- and 12-week follow-up visits, the combined exercise and manual therapy group showed some advantages over the other groups.

14. Is there evidence that manual therapy is effective to treat conditions of the extremities?

HIP JOINT

A recent randomized trial compared manual therapy (manipulations and mobilization of the hip joint) with an exercise therapy program in patients with osteoarthritis of the hip. Success rates after 5 weeks were 81% in the manual therapy group and 50% in the exercise group. Furthermore, patients in the manual therapy group had significantly better outcomes on pain, stiffness, hip function, and range of motion.

KNEE JOINT

One study compared a group who received manual therapy combined with exercise to a placebo group. Subjects in the manual therapy group received joint mobilization techniques to the lumbopelvic region, hip, knee, and/or ankle, depending on whether they exhibited pain or reduced mobility. The manual therapy plus exercise group showed improvements in pain, stiffness, and function. The control group did not change. Yet again, the combination of manual therapy and exercise results in positive effects.

SHOULDER JOINT

Manual therapy used alone or combined with exercise has shown to be effective in the treatment of patients with shoulder problems. One trial studied the effectiveness of manipulative therapy for the shoulder girdle in addition to usual medical care. At 12 and 52 weeks after treatment, the manipulation group reported better rates of full recovery. A consistent between-group difference in severity of the shoulder pain and disability, and in general health favored manipulative therapy. Another randomized clinical trial compared a group of patients with shoulder impingement syndrome who performed supervised flexibility and strengthening exercises with a group who performed that same exercise program plus received manual physical therapy treatment. They reported significantly more improvement in pain and function in the exercise plus manual therapy group.

ELBOW JOINT

Limited evidence indicates that mobilization with movement may help reduce painful movements and improve grip strength in patients with lateral epicondylalgia.

15. Is there evidence that manual therapy is effective for other conditions?

Less rigorous studies indicate that the use of manual therapy techniques may help in decreasing pain in patients with temporomandibular joint osteoarthrosis and in patients with fibromyalgia.

There is also some indication that manual therapy may have positive effects on cervical radiculopathy, cervicogenic dizziness, carpal tunnel syndrome, and thoracic outlet syndrome. Few studies that have dealt with manipulation effectiveness used muscle energy or soft tissue techniques.

16. What are the side effects expected with spinal manipulation?

Reactions after spinal manipulation are very common in clinical practice. A recent study reported that approximately 61% of patients complain of at least one postmanipulative reaction. The most common side effects are stiffness (20%), local discomfort (15%), headache (12%), radiating discomfort (12%), fatigue (12%), muscle spasms (6%), dizziness (4%), and nausea (3%). Most reactions begin within 4 hours and generally disappear within 24 hours after treatment. Women are more likely to report side effects than men.

17. Is there any evidence to support the use of craniosacral therapy?

Although research exists reporting the presence of cranial bone motion, there is no single study to support craniosacral therapy as an effective therapeutic intervention.

18. Does manual therapy affect the visceral organs?

Some patients report improvement in their gastrointestinal discomfort or in constipation after thoracic or lumbar manipulation. Joint dysfunction facilitates the corresponding spinal cord segment, which can excite any of the neural elements arising from that segment, causing adverse visceral symptoms. There is a belief that when joint lesion is addressed, it may suppress or attenuate visceral complaints. To date, however, little evidence exists to validate the use of manual therapy for visceral problems.

19. Can manual therapy straighten a spinal deformity?

When there are structural spinal deformities such as scoliosis and hyperkyphosis, manipulation cannot straighten the curves.

20. Can manual therapy restore spinal curvatures?

When there is a temporary loss of spinal curvature, such as in a lateral lumbopelvic list or in a straightened cervical spine because of muscle spasm, nonaggressive manipulative techniques can be used to decrease spasm and increase movement.

21. How does manual therapy help to increase range of motion and decrease pain and disability?

The specific in vivo effects of manual therapy are not known. Suggested theories include:

- Manual therapy moves or frees the mechanical impediment (loose body, disk material, synovial fringe, or meniscoid entrapment) to joint movement, permitting movement and halting nociceptive input and associated reflex muscle spasm.
- Improvement in range of motion helps to relieve pain that is the direct result of such hypomobility.
- Manual therapy stretches or ruptures periarticular scar tissues.
- Manual therapy may improve nerve conductivity and circulation by means of increasing the space where nerves and blood vessels exit or cross.
- Manual therapy improves muscle function and decreases stress on bones and ligaments by improving the distribution of joint forces and levers.
- Manual therapy may affect neural activity as a result of afferent stimulation.

22. Should joint hypomobility be treated in the absence of symptoms?

No. Despite the fact that some clinicians advocate a prophylactic treatment for joint hypomobility, there is no evidence that this approach prevents dysfunction.

23. When is manual therapy contraindicated?

Manual therapy is a safe approach in well-trained hands. Contraindications are specific to each technique. General contraindications are:

- Fracture
- Infectious arthritis
- Tumors
- Joint ankylosis
- Acute inflammatory disorders
- Lack of diagnosed joint lesion
- Presence of pathologic end-feel

24. What is end-feel and how is it classified?

End-feel is the type of resistance felt by an examiner at the end range of a passive range of motion test. Its assessment is used to guide diagnosis and treatment. End-feels can be normal or pathologic, depending on the movement they accompany at a particular joint and where in the range of movement they are felt. When a hard end-feel is felt in a joint where one would expect a soft one, or vice versa, it is considered a pathologic end-feel. Other pathologic end-feels are muscle spasm, sensation of mushy end-feel, springy rebound, and severe pain without any motion restriction (empty end-feel).

CYRIAX END-FEEL CLASSIFICATION

- Bone to bone—abrupt stop to the movement that is felt when two hard surfaces meet, e.g., passive extension of the elbow
- Capsular—feeling of immediate stop of movement with some give, e.g., end range of shoulder flexion
- Tissue approximation—limb segment cannot be moved farther because the soft tissues surrounding the joint cannot be further compressed, e.g., end range of knee flexion
- Empty—patient complains of severe pain from the movement without the examiner perceiving increase in resistance to the movement; indicates acute inflammation or extra-articular lesions
- Springy block—rebound is felt at the end of the range; results from displacement of an intra-articular structure
- Spasm—feeling of a muscle coming actively into play during the passive movement; indicates the presence of acute or subacute condition

KALTENBORN END-FEEL CLASSIFICATION

- Hard—occurs when bone meets bone (e.g., resistance felt at the passive extension of the elbow)
- Firm—results from capsular or ligamentous stretching (e.g., resistance felt at the end range of external rotation of the glenohumeral joint)
- Soft—results from soft tissue approximation or soft tissue stretching (e.g., resistance felt at the end range of knee flexion)

25. List contraindications for thrust techniques.

- Cranial nerve signs or symptoms and dizziness of unknown origin (specific for cervical spine)
- Sacroperineal numbness or loss of bowel and bladder control (specific for lumbar spine)
- Painful movements in all joint directions or just one degree of movement free of pain and restriction

- Bilateral or multisegmental neurologic signs or symptoms
- Paralysis in nonperipheral nerve distribution
- Hyperreflexia or positive pathologic reflexes
- Presence of emotional disorders
- Patient taking anticoagulant medication or steroidal medication for a long time period
- Clinician not proficient in the indicated technique

26. Describe the convex-concave rule and explain how it influences manual therapy.

When a convex joint surface moves on a concave joint surface, joint rolling and gliding occur in opposite directions. Conversely, when a concave joint surface is moved on a convex joint surface, rolling and gliding occur in the same direction. This rule helps clinicians to decide the direction to apply joint manipulation therapy. When performing mobilization, the therapist moves a bone with a convex joint surface in the direction opposite to the restriction, whereas mobilization of a concave joint surface is performed in the same direction as the restriction.

27. Describe loose-packed and close-packed positions.

- Loose-packed position—resting position in which the joint capsule is most relaxed, the articular surfaces are least congruent, and the greatest amount of joint play is possible. This resting position does not take into account extra-articular structures, such as muscles and fascia.
- Close-packed position—the joint capsule and ligaments are tight or at maximal tension. In this position there is maximal contact between the concave and convex articular surfaces, and separation between the articular surfaces by traction forces is difficult.

28. How do the loose-packed and close-packed positions influence manual therapy treatment?

Knowledge of these positions allows clinicians to determine which movement compresses and tightens the joint and which movement distracts and loosens the joint. The loose-packed position is the position used for testing joint play and to start treatment of restricted joint movement. The close-packed position is used to avoid joint movement. As an example, in order to isolate the mobilizing force to a particular level of the spine, the adjacent vertebral joints are *locked* in the close-packed position.

29. Define capsular pattern.

Capsular pattern is a limitation of joint movement or a pattern of pain that occurs in a predictable fashion. Cyriax suggested that these patterns are a result of lesions in the joint capsule or the synovial membrane. It indicates loss of mobility of the entire joint capsule from fibrosis, effusion, or inflammation, which may occur in arthrosis, arthritis, prolonged immobilization, or acute trauma. Joints not controlled by muscles, such as the sacroiliac or tibiofibular joints, do not exhibit a capsular pattern.

30. Compare loose-packed position, close-packed position and capsular pattern for all joints.

Joint	Loose-Packed	Close-Packed	Capsular Pattern
Temporomandibular	Mouth slightly open	Teeth clenched	Limited mouth opening
Cervical spine	Midway between flexion and extension	Maximal extension	Limitation in all motion, except flexion

Continued

Continued

Joint	Loose-Packed	Close-Packed	Capsular Pattern
Sternoclavicular	Arm resting by side	Maximal shoulder elevation	Limited full elevation; pain at end ranges
Acromioclavicular	Arm resting by side	Arm abducted 90°	Limited full elevation; pain at end ranges
Glenohumeral	55° shoulder abduction, 30° horizontal adduction	Maximal abduction and external rotation	Loss in external rotation > loss in abduction > loss in internal rotation
Humeroulnar	70° flexion, 10° supination	Full extension and supination	Loss of flexion > loss in extension
Humeroradial	Extension and supination	90° flexion, 5° supination	Loss of flexion > loss in extension
Radioulnar: proximal	70° flexion, 35° supination	5° supination, full extension	Limited pronation = limited supination
Radioulnar: distal	10° supination	5° supination	Limited pronation = limited supination
Radiocarpal	Neutral, slight ulnar deviation	Full extension, radial deviation	Limited flexion = limited extension
Midcarpal	Neutral, slight flexion and ulnar deviation	Full extension	Equal limitation in all directions
Trapeziometacarpal	Neutral	Full opposition	Limited abduction > extension
Carpometacarpal	Neutral	Full opposition	Equal limitation in all directions
Metacarpophalangeal	Slight flexion, ulnar deviation	Full flexion	
Interphalangeal	Slight flexion	Full extension	Limited flexion > extension
Thoracic spine	Midway between flexion and extension	Maximal extension	Side-bending and rotation > extension > flexion
Lumbar spine	Midway between flexion and extension	Maximal extension	Equal limitation of side-bending and rotation; extension > flexion
Hip	30° flexion, 30° abduction, slight external rotation	Full extension, abduction, internal rotation	Flexion and internal rotation > abduction > adduction > external rotation
Tibiofemoral	25° flexion	Full extension and external rotation	Limited flexion > extension
Talocrural	10° plantar flexion, neutral inversion/eversion	Full dorsiflexion	Plantar flexion > dorsiflexion
Subtarsal	10° plantar flexion, neutral inversion/eversion	Full inversion	Limitation in varus
Midtarsal	10° plantar flexion, neutral inversion/eversion	Full supination	Supination > pronation

Continued

Joint	Loose-Packed	Close-Packed	Capsular Pattern
Tarsometatarsal	Neutral supination and pronation	Full supination	
Metatarsophalangeal	Neutral	Full extension	Extension > flexion
Interphalangeal	Slight flexion	Full extension	Limited extension

Bibliography

Abbott JH, Patla CE, Jensen RH: The initial effects of an elbow mobilization with movement technique on grip strength in subjects with lateral epicondylalgia, *Manual Ther* 6:163-169, 2001.

Bang MD, Deyle GD: Comparison of supervised exercise with and without manual physical therapy for patients with shoulder impingement syndrome, *J Orthop Sports Phys Ther* 30:126-137, 2000.

Bergman GJ et al: Manipulative therapy in addition to usual medical care for patients with shoulder dysfunction and pain: a randomized, controlled trial, *Ann Intern Med* 141:432-439, 2004.

Bronfort G et al: Efficacy of spinal manipulation for chronic headache: a systematic review, *J Manipulative Physiol Ther* 24:457-466, 2001.

Bronfort G et al: Efficacy of spinal manipulation and mobilization for low back pain and neck pain: a systematic review and best evidence synthesis, *Spine* 4:335-356, 2004.

Browder DA, Erhard RE, Piva SR: Intermittent cervical traction and thoracic manipulation for management of mild cervical compressive myelopathy attributed to cervical herniated disc: a case series, *J Orthop Sports Phys Ther* 34:701-712, 2004.

Cagnie B et al: How common are side effects of spinal manipulation and can these side effects be predicted?, *Manual Ther* 9:151-156, 2004.

Childs JD: A clinical prediction rule to identify patients with low back pain most likely to benefit from spinal manipulation: a validation study, *Ann Intern Med* 141:920-928, 2004.

Cleland JA et al: Immediate effects of thoracic manipulation in patients with neck pain: a randomized clinical trial, *Man Ther* 10:127-135, 2005.

Deyle GD et al: Effectiveness of manual physical therapy and exercise in osteoarthritis of the knee: a randomized, controlled trial, *Ann Intern Med* 132:173-181, 2000.

Flynn T et al: A clinical prediction rule for classifying patients with low back pain who demonstrate short-term improvement with spinal manipulation, *Spine* 27:2835-2843, 2002.

Flynn T et al: The audible pop is not necessary for successful spinal high-velocity thrust manipulation in individuals with low back pain, *Arch Phys Med Rehabil* 84:1057-1060, 2003.

Hoeksma HL et al: Comparison of manual therapy and exercise therapy in osteoarthritis of the hip: a randomized clinical trial, *Arthr Rheum* 51:722-729, 2004.

Jull G et al: A randomized controlled trial of exercise and manipulative therapy for cervicogenic headache, *Spine* 27:1835-1843, 2002.

Ross JK, Bereznick DE, McGill SM: Determining cavitation location during lumbar and thoracic spinal manipulation: is spinal manipulation accurate and specific?, *Spine* 29:1452-1457, 2004.

UK BEAM Trial Team: United Kingdom back pain exercise and manipulation (UK BEAM) randomised trial: effectiveness of physical treatments for back pain in primary care, *BMJ* 329:1377, 2004.

Vernon H, McDermaid CS, Hagino C: Systematic review of randomized clinical trials of complementary/alternative therapies in the treatment of tension-type and cervicogenic headache, *Complement Ther Med* 7:142-155, 1999.

Weiss HR, Dieckmann J, Gerner HJ: Effect of intensive rehabilitation on pain in patients with Scheuermann's disease, *Studies Health Technol Informatics* 88:254-257, 2002.

Chapter 14

Massage and Soft Tissue Mobilization

John R. Krauss, PT, PhD, OCS

1. Discuss briefly the common approaches to massage.

Massage techniques differ in origin and basic premise behind their effectiveness. Classic Western massage was developed in Europe and the United States over the past 2 centuries. Western massage is based on the Western medical model of disease, with mechanical and neurologic rationales supporting its use as therapy. Contemporary massage and bodywork and Asian bodywork are widely diverse in their rationale, which includes energy balancing, myofascial softening and lengthening, and traditional Chinese medicine and meridian theories.

2. Does massage boost the immune system?

Many advocates of massage suggest that it has the potential to produce a number of physical, mental, and emotional effects. Birk et al. studied the effects of massage therapy on immune system measures and concluded there was no significant effect.

3. Does massage improve lymphatic drainage?

Bass et al. investigated the effect of massage on the sensitivity of lymphatic mapping in breast cancer. Following the injection of a blue dye and radiocolloid, the patient received a 5-minute massage. They concluded that massage significantly improved the uptake of blue dye by sentinel lymph nodes.

4. Does massage increase tissue temperature?

Drust et al. examined the effects of massage on intramuscular temperature in the vastus lateralis in humans. They concluded that when comparing massage with ultrasound, changes in muscle temperature were significantly higher for massage at 1.5 to 2.5 cm below the skin. They also determined that thigh skin temperatures were significantly higher in massage-treated patients.

5. Does massage decrease depression?

Field et al. studied massage therapy effects on depressed pregnant women. The massage therapy group participants received two 20-minute massage therapy sessions by their significant others for 16 weeks of pregnancy starting during the second trimester. By the end of the study, the massage group had higher dopamine and serotonin levels and lower levels of cortisol and norepinephrine.

6. How does massage generate pain relief?

Several mechanisms have been proposed and researched as possible sources of pain relief following massage. One of the oldest theories is that light to moderate mechanical stimulation of cutaneous and subcutaneous tissues results in increased activity in somatosensory neurons, which may inhibit activity in pain-mediating neurons in the spinal cord. This is based on the gate control theory of pain developed by Melzack and Wall in 1965. Another proposed theory is that increased stimulation activation of the descending pain inhibitory system, starting in the periaqueductal gray matter (PAG) and continuing to the dorsal horn of the spinal cord, may reduce pain. In conjunction with this theory is the belief that opioid receptors in the PAG are activated as a result of massage. Lastly, Lund et al. investigated the mechanisms behind the effects of massage on animals. They concluded that long-term pain relief effects of massage may be attributed, at least in part, to the oxytocinergic system and its interaction with the opioid system. While this mechanism is not well understood, it is theorized that increased endogenous oxytocin may result in greater synthesis of endogenous opioids.

7. Does massage aid in sports performance?

Hemmings et al. examined the effects of massage on physiologic restoration, perceived recovery, and repeated sports performance on eight amateur boxers. They concluded that while there were significantly increased perceptions of recovery following massage there were no significant differences in blood lactate or glucose levels. Another study by Hilbert et al. examined the effects of massage on delayed-onset muscle soreness. They determined that massage administered 2 hours after exercise-induced muscle injury to the hamstrings did not improve function but did reduce the intensity of soreness 48-hours postinjury. Another study examined the effects of leg massage on recovery from high-intensity cycling exercise. They concluded that massage had no effect on blood lactate concentration, heart rate, and maximum and mean power. They did find that the massage group had a significantly lower fatigue index.

8. Does massage increase blood flow?

Hinds et al. examined the effects of massage on limb and skin blood flow after quadriceps exercise. A total of 13 participants performed three 2-minute bouts of concentric quadriceps exercise followed either by two 6-minute bouts of deep effleurage and pétrissage massage or by a rest period of similar duration. Measures of femoral artery blood flow, skin blood flow, skin temperature, muscle temperature, blood lactate concentration, heart rate, and blood flow were compared. They concluded that skin temperature and skin blood flow were significantly elevated following the application of massage. There were no significant differences between the massage and control groups for the remaining measurements.

9. Does massage decrease the frequency of chronic tension headaches?

Quinn et al. investigated the effect of massage therapy on chronic nonmigraine headaches. Chronic tension headache sufferers received structured massage therapy treatment to the neck and shoulder muscles. They concluded that headache frequency was significantly reduced within the first week of treatment and continued throughout the study. The duration of headaches also tended to decrease during the massage treatment period. Headache intensity was unaffected by massage.

10. What is the purpose of Cyriax transverse friction massage?

It provides movement to the muscle or tendon while inducing traumatic hyperemia in order to stimulate healing.

11. What are the basic principles of transverse friction massage?

- The soft tissue lesion must be properly treated.
- Friction is given across the grain of the soft tissue.
- The therapist's fingers must move together with the patient's skin.
- Friction must have sufficient depth and sweep.
- The patient must be comfortable.
- Tendon is put on stretch, whereas muscle is massaged in a relaxed position.

12. Does transverse friction massage induce healing?

No well-performed studies have shown histologic support for the promotion of healing of soft tissue with transverse friction massage. Walker examined the use of transverse friction massage on medial collateral ligaments of rabbits and found no difference between massaged and control rabbits. However, the experimentally induced sprain may have been insufficient to promote an inflammatory response.

13. How long should transverse friction massage be performed?

The dosing of transverse friction massage is based on the intended or expected outcomes of the massage. If the intention is to decrease pain, then the massage may be performed until the patient reports decreased pain. If the intention is to improve tissue pliability, then the massage may be performed until a palpable change in pliability is noted by the therapist. If the intention is to stimulate a mild inflammation in a tendon that is degenerative but nonpainful, then the massage may be performed until a mild sensation of discomfort is perceived by the patient. Because of the diverse intentions of transverse friction massage, individual treatment doses may vary from a few minutes up to 15 to 20 minutes. The total number of treatment sessions is also dependent on the intended outcomes of the treatment. Changes from friction massage are often noted within one treatment session and at the very least should be noted within two treatment sessions. Failure to achieve results should lead to a careful consideration of the specific treatment parameters (rate, depth, direction, and duration, for example) and of the treatment choice itself. Typically, friction massage is used for up to four to six treatment sessions, with a great deal of variability in the total number of treatment sessions depending on the nature of the specific condition/impairment undergoing treatment.

Bibliography

Bass SS et al: The effects of postinjection massage on the sensitivity of lymphatic mapping in breast cancer, *J Am Coll Surg* 192:9-16, 2001.

Birk TJ et al: The effects of massage therapy alone and in combination with other complementary therapies on immune system measures and quality of life in human immunodeficiency virus, *J Altern Complement Med* 6:405-414, 2000.

Drust B et al: The effects of massage on intramuscular temperature in the vastus lateralis in humans, *Int J Sports Med* 24:395-399, 2003.

Field T et al: Massage therapy effects on depressed pregnant women, *J Psychosomatic Obstet Gynaecol* 25:115-221, 2004.

Fields HL, Basbaum AI: Central nervous system mechanisms of pain modulation. In *Textbook of pain,* Edinburgh, 1994, pp 243-257, Churchill Livingstone.

Hammer WI: *Functional soft tissue examination and treatment by manual methods,* ed 2, Gaithersburg, Md, 1999, Aspen Publishers.

Harris JA: Descending antinociceptive mechanisms in the brainstem: their role in the animal's defensive system, *J Physiol Paris* 90:15-25, 1996.

Hemmings B et al: Effects of massage on physiological restoration, perceived recovery, and repeated sports performance, *Br J Sports Med* 34:109-114, 2000 (discussion 115).

Hilbert JE, Sforzo GA, Swensen T: The effects of massage on delayed onset muscle soreness, *Br J Sports Med* 37:72-75, 2003.

Hinds T et al: Effects of massage on limb and skin blood flow after quadriceps exercise, *Med Sci Sports Exercise* 36:1308-1313, 2004.

Holey E, Cook E: *Therapeutic massage,* Philadelphia, 1998, WB Saunders.

Lederman E: *Fundamentals of manual therapy, physiology, neurology, and psychology,* New York, 1997, Churchill Livingstone.

Lund I et al: Repeated massage-like stimulation induces long-term effects on nociception: contribution of oxytocinergic mechanisms, *Eur J Neurosci* 16:330-338, 2002.

Salvo SG: *Massage therapy principles and practice,* Philadelphia, 1999, WB Saunders.

Tappan FM, Benjamin PJ: *Tappan's handbook of healing massage techniques: classic, holistic, and emerging methods,* Norwalk, Conn, 1998, Appleton & Lange.

Quinn C, Chandler C, Moraska A: Massage therapy and frequency of chronic tension headaches, *Am J Public Health* 92:1657-1661, 2002.

Walker JM: Deep transverse frictions in ligament healing, *J Orthop Sci Phys Ther* 6:89-94, 1984.

Chapter 15

Spinal Traction

H. Duane Saunders, PT, MS, and
Robin Saunders Ryan, PT, MS

1. What are the theoretical effects of spinal traction?

Spinal traction is theorized to have several effects. Among these are distraction or separation of the vertebral bodies, a combination of distraction and gliding of the facet joints, tensing of the ligamentous structures of the spinal segment, widening of the intervertebral foramen, straightening of spinal curves, and stretching of the spinal musculature. There is evidence that a disk protrusion can be reduced and spinal nerve root compression symptoms relieved with the application of relatively high-force spinal traction (approximately 50% of the body weight). Epidurography studies demonstrate temporary reductions of the disk protrusions, along with clinical improvement. Onel et al. used computed tomography to demonstrate lumbar disk reduction in 21 of 30 patients (70%), and theorized that the reduction was due to a suction effect caused by decreased intradiskal pressure. The change in intradiskal pressure caused by traction also has been theorized to positively affect the disk's nutrition.

2. What are the indications for spinal traction?

Given the above theoretical effects, the significant indications are (A) herniated disk or radiculopathy, (B) any condition in which mobilization and stretching of soft tissue are desired, and (C) any condition in which opening the neural foramen is desired.

3. What are the contraindications for spinal traction?

Traction is contraindicated in patients with structural disease secondary to tumor or infection, rheumatoid arthritis, severe vascular compromise, and any condition for which movement is contraindicated. Relative contraindications include acute strains and sprains and inflammatory conditions that may be aggravated by traction. Strong traction applied to patients with spinal joint instability may cause further strain. Traction should be avoided if the patient has had recent spinal fusion. Because spinal fusion techniques and healing rates vary from patient to patient, the surgeon should be consulted before applying traction if the fusion is less than 1 year old. Other relative contraindications may include pregnancy, osteoporosis, hiatal hernia, and claustrophobia.

4. How much force is optimal for cervical traction?

In the cervical spine, Judovich found that 25- to 45-lb forces were necessary to demonstrate a measurable change in the posterior cervical spine structures. Colachis and Strohm demonstrated that a traction force of 30 lb produced separation of the cervical spine, and that a 50-lb force produced more separation than a 30-lb force. There is no evidence that midcervical and lower cervical spine separation occurs at forces less than 20 lb.

5. Is cervical traction effective for treatment of cervical radiculopathy?

One MRI study showed either complete or partial reduction of herniated disk in 21 of 29 patients who received 30-lb seated traction with an inflatable traction device. Honet and Puri provided a progressively more intense cervical traction treatment, depending on severity of symptoms and neurological findings. Subjects received traction treatment at home, in an outpatient facility, or in the hospital. The percentage of patients with excellent or good outcomes was 92% in the home treatment category, 77% in the outpatient treatment category, and 65% in the hospital treatment category.

6. Is cervical traction effective for treatment of cervicogenic headache?

No clinical trials have been performed using cervical traction to treat cervicogenic headache, but two case studies suggest that cervicogenic headache can be treated successfully with traction. Using 25- to 30-lb home traction and cervical exercise, Olson reported success with two difficult cases of headache caused by chronic whiplash. The cervical exercise consisted of postural correction and stabilization exercises.

7. What are the important treatment variables for cervical traction?

- Chin halter versus occipital wedges—When traction is provided with a standard head halter with a chin strap, force is transmitted through the chin strap to the teeth, and the temporomandibular joints become weight-bearing structures. A common problem from administering cervical traction is aggravation of the temporomandibular joints because of the force applied at the chin. It is generally advisable to use a cervical traction system that pulls from the occiput, rather than placing pressure on the chin. If the patient has known temporomandibular dysfunction, a chin halter should never be used.
- Force—To effectively treat cervical radiculopathy, herniated disk, or other conditions requiring a separation of the intervertebral space, the traction force should be great enough to cause movement at the spinal segment. Based on our experience and the evidence available in the literature, we typically use a force of 25 to 40 lb for the midcervical and lower cervical spine. Less force is necessary when treatment is directed to the upper cervical area.
- Patient position—We recommend the supine position to facilitate patient relaxation, proper force application, and optimal cervical angle. The supine position is favored in the literature. Cervical traction studies show that *narrowing* of the intervertebral spaces can actually occur during the traction treatment in patients who are unable to relax.
- Cervical angle—Cervical traction is performed with the head and neck in some degree of flexion. Some clinicians believe that the greater the angle of flexion, the greater the intervertebral separation in the lower cervical spine. While it is true that posterior separation does increase with more flexion, anterior separation *decreases* with flexion. In most cases, clinicians should try to achieve a combination of a posterior and anterior stretch. Thus the ideal traction device will flex the head and neck somewhat, but pull at a relatively flat angle. We recommend a 15-degree angle to accomplish this goal.
- Mode (static or intermittent)—The traction mode selected will depend on the disorder being treated and the comfort of the patient. Herniated disk is usually treated more effectively in static mode or with longer hold-rest periods (3- to 5-minute hold, 1-minute rest) in intermittent mode. Joint dysfunction and degenerative disk disease usually respond to shorter hold-rest periods (1- to 2-minute hold, 30-second rest) in intermittent mode.
- Time—When treating herniated disk, the treatment time should be relatively short. As the disk space widens, the intradiskal pressure decreases, causing the herniated disk material to be retracted into the disk space. The decrease in pressure is temporary, however, because eventually the decreased intradiskal pressure will cause fluid to be imbibed into the disk. When pressure equalization occurs, the suction effect on the disk protrusion is lost, and it is possible for patients to experience a sudden increase in pain when traction is released. If the traction time is 8 to 10 minutes, this effect is minimized. For other conditions, a treatment time of up to 20 minutes is often used. As a general rule, the higher the force, the shorter the treatment time. Often the first treatment is only 3 to 5 minutes long. This gives the clinician a chance to determine the patient's reaction to treatment and plan treatment progression accordingly.

8. How much force is optimal for lumbar traction?

There is consensus in the literature that a force of 40% to 50% of the patient's body weight is necessary to cause vertebral separation. In one of the earliest lumbar traction studies, Cyriax reported a visible separation between lumbar vertebrae with static traction of 120 lb for 15 minutes. Other studies have reported measurable separation in the lumbar spine at forces ranging from 80 to 200 lb. Judovich advocated a force equal to one half the patient's body weight on a friction-free surface as the minimum force necessary to cause therapeutic effects in the lumbar spine.

9. Is lumbar traction effective for lumbar radiculopathy?

Epidurography and CT investigations have shown that high-force traction can reduce disk protrusions and relieve spinal nerve root compression symptoms. Despite these findings, lumbar traction is currently out of favor in the literature. Four reviews summarizing lumbar traction studies have concluded that there is no significant benefit for patients treated with lumbar traction compared to a control group. However, wide variations of methods and techniques were described in the studies cited. Some of the studies that showed lumbar traction was ineffective were performed with low forces. In many of the studies, patient selection criteria were poorly defined. Most studies tended to group all patients with low back pain together and did not distinguish between subgroups or by diagnosis. The only two studies that looked specifically at traction for herniated disk did not use forces generally considered sufficient to separate the intervertebral spaces.

10. What are the most important treatment variables for lumbar traction?

- Force—To effectively treat lumbar radiculopathy, herniated disk, or other conditions requiring a separation of the intervertebral space, the traction force should be great enough to cause movement at the spinal segment. Based on our experience and the evidence available in the literature, we typically use a force of 40% to 50% of the patient's ideal body weight. Often the first treatment is a little less to ensure patient tolerance.
- Spinal position—The position of the spine during traction is an important treatment variable. In our experience, disk herniation is most effectively treated with the patient lying prone with a normal lordosis. However, this position is not always possible because the patient with acute herniated disk may not tolerate any position of normal lordosis. If this is the case, the treatment must be given in flexion initially with the goal of gradually working toward neutral lumbar lordosis. Foraminal (lateral) stenosis is usually more effectively treated with the lumbar spine in a flexed (flattened) position initially, with the goal of achieving a neutral lordosis when possible. Soft tissue stiffness/hypomobility and degenerative disk or joint disease may be treated in neutral position or some degree of flexion or extension, depending on the goals of treatment. Patient comfort and the patient's ability to remain relaxed during the treatment are important considerations when choosing the most beneficial position, and no absolute rule applies. Variations of flexion, extension, and lateral bending should be tried to find the most beneficial position for each patient.
- Mode (static or intermittent) and time—See question 7.

11. Does spinal traction change somatosensory evoked potentials (SSEPs)?

SSEP latencies were decreased after cervical traction in patients with radiculopathy and cervical sprain. In patients with severe myelopathy, latencies may increase. Traction may improve conduction by improving blood flow to cervical nerve roots.

Bibiolography

Beurskens A et al: Efficacy of traction for nonspecific low back pain: 12-week and 6-month results of a randomized clinical trial, *Spine* 22:2756-2762, 1997.

Chung TS et al: Reducibility of cervical disk herniation: evaluation at MR imaging during cervical traction with a nonmagnetic traction device, *Radiology* 225:895-898, 2002.
Colachis S, Strohm M: Cervical traction: relationship of traction time to varied tractive force with constant angle of pull, *Arch Phys Med* 46:815-819, 1965.
Colachis S, Strohm M: A study of tractive forces and angle of pull on vertebral interspaces in cervical spine, *Arch Phys Med* 46:820-830, 1965.
Constantoyannis C et al: Intermittent cervical traction for cervical radiculopathy caused by large-volume herniated disks, *J Manipulative Physiol Ther* 25:188-192, 2002.
Cyriax J: The treatment of lumbar disk lesions, *BMJ* 2:14-34, 1950.
Franks A: Temporomandibular joint dysfunction associated with cervical traction, *Ann Phys Med* 8:38-40, 1967.
Harris P: Cervical traction: review of literature and treatment guidelines, *Phys Ther* 57:910, 1977.
Hattori M, Shirai Y, Aoki T: Research on the effectiveness of intermittent cervical traction therapy using short-latency somatosensory evoked potentials, *J Orthop Sci* 7:208-216, 2002.
Honet JC, Puri K: Cervical radiculitis: treatment and results in 82 patients, *Arch Phys Med Rehabil* 57:12-16, 1976.
Komori H et al: The natural history of herniated nucleus pulposus with radiculopathy, *Spine* 21:225-229, 1996.
Mathews J: The effects of spinal traction, *Physiotherapy* 58:64-66, 1972.
Moetti P, Marchetti G: Clinical outcome from mechanical intermittent cervical traction for the treatment of cervical radiculopathy: a case series, *J Orthop Sports Phys Ther* 31:207-213, 2001.
Olivero WC, Dulebohn SC: Results of halter cervical traction for the treatment of cervical radiculopathy: rRetrospective review of 81 patients, *Neurosurg Focus* 12:1-3, 2002.
Olson V: Case report: chronic whiplash associated disorder treated with home cervical traction, *J Back Musculoskel Rehabil* 9:181-190, 1997.
Olson V: Whiplash-associated chronic headache treated with home cervical traction, *Phys Ther* 77:417-423, 1997.
Onel D et al: Computed tomographic investigation of the effect of traction on lumbar disc herniations, *Spine* 14:82-90, 1989.
Philadelphia Panel Evidence-Based Clinical Practice Guidelines on Selected Rehabilitation Interventions for Low Back Pain, *Phys Ther* 81:1641-1674, 2001.
Saal J et al: Nonoperative management of herniated cervical intervertebral disc with radiculopathy, *Spine* 21:1877-1883, 1996.
van der Heijden G et al: The efficacy of traction for back and neck pain: a systematic, blinded review of randomized clinical trial method, *Phys Ther* 75:93-104, 1995.
Yates D: Indications and contraindications for spinal traction, *Physiotherapy* 58:55, 1972.

Chapter 16

Normal and Pathologic Gait

Judith M. Burnfield, PT, PhD, and
Christopher M. Powers, PT, PhD

1. What is the average adult walking velocity?

- On level surfaces, approximately 80 m/min
- In men, 82 m/min
- In women, 79 m/min

2. Does walking velocity decline with age?

Yes. Declines of 3% to 11% in healthy adults >60 years old have been reported.

3. Name contributors to an individual's walking velocity.

- Step (or stride) length
- Cadence

4. What is considered normal stride and step length?

- Stride length is the distance from ipsilateral heel contact to the next ipsilateral heel contact during gait (i.e., right-to-right or left-to-left heel contact). Normal adult stride length averages approximately 1.39 m, with the mean stride length of men (1.48 m) being slightly longer than that of women (1.32 m).
- Step length is the distance between ipsilateral and contralateral heel contact (e.g., right-to-left heel contact) and is on average equal to half of stride length.

5. What is normal cadence?

Cadence is the number of steps per minute.

- In adults without pathology, average 116 steps/min
- In women, 121 steps/min
- In men, 111 steps/min

6. Define gait cycle.

Gait cycle is a repetitive pattern that extends from heel contact to the next episode of heel contact of the same foot. The gait cycle can be further subdivided into a period of stance, when the limb is in contact with the ground (approximately 60% of the gait cycle), and a period of swing, when the limb is not in contact with the ground (approximately 40% of the gait cycle).

7. Describe the functional tasks associated with normal gait.

Functionally, each gait cycle can be divided into three tasks:

1. Weight acceptance
2. Single limb support
3. Swing limb advancement

During weight acceptance, body weight is accepted onto the limb that has just completed swinging forward. The limb must absorb shock arising from the abrupt transfer of body weight, while remaining stable and allowing continued forward progression of the body.

During single limb support, only the stance limb is in contact with the ground, and the limb must remain stable while allowing continued forward progression of the body over the foot.

Swing limb advancement includes the phase when weight is being transferred from the reference limb to the opposite limb as well as the entire reference limb swing period. During swing limb advancement, the foot must clear the ground to ensure forward progression.

8. Describe the key motions and muscular activity patterns at the ankle, knee, and hip during weight acceptance.

At the beginning of weight acceptance, the ankle is positioned in neutral, the knee observationally appears to be fully extended (it is actually in 5 degrees of flexion), and the hip is flexed approximately 20 degrees (relative to vertical) in the sagittal plane. These combined joint positions allow the heel to be the first part of the foot to contact the ground. During weight acceptance, as the foot positions itself flat on the ground, the ankle moves into 5 degrees of plantar flexion, controlled by eccentric activity of the dorsiflexors. The knee moves into 15 degrees of flexion, controlled by eccentric activity of the quadriceps. The hip remains in 20 degrees of flexion, primarily owing to isometric activity of the single joint hip extensors.

9. Describe the key motions and muscular activity patterns at the ankle, knee, and hip during single limb support.

Movement of the ankle from 5 degrees of plantar flexion to 10 degrees of dorsiflexion is controlled by eccentric activity of the calf. The knee moves from 15 degrees of flexion to what observationally appears to be full extension (actually 5 degrees of flexion by motion analysis), in part as a result of concentric activity of the quadriceps (early single limb support) in combination with passive stability achieved when the ground reaction force vector moves anterior to the knee joint (late single limb support). The hip moves from 20 degrees of flexion to 20 degrees of apparent hyperextension (a combination of full hip extension, anterior pelvic tilt, and backward pelvic rotation), in part as a result of concentric activity of the single joint hip extensors (early single limb support) in combination with passive stability achieved when the ground reaction force vector moves posterior to the hip joint.

10. Describe the key motions and muscular activity patterns at the ankle, knee, and hip during swing limb advancement.

Initially, as the more proximal joints begin to flex, the foot remains in contact with the ground and the ankle moves passively into a position of 15 degrees of plantar flexion. Once the foot lifts from the ground, the ankle moves to neutral dorsiflexion owing to concentric activity of the pretibial muscles. The knee initially moves into 40 degrees of flexion (while the foot is still on the ground) primarily as a result of passive forces. As the foot is lifted from the ground, the knee moves into 60 degrees of flexion, owing to concentric activity of knee flexors (biceps femoris short head, gracilis, and sartorius). During late swing limb advancement, the knee fully extends, in part as a result of momentum and quadriceps activity. The hip moves from 20 degrees of apparent hyperextension to 25 degrees of flexion by the middle of swing because of a combination of hip flexor muscle activity and momentum. In late swing, hip flexion decreases to 20 degrees as the hamstrings decelerate further progression of the leg.

11. What factors contribute to shock absorption during weight acceptance?

- Eccentrically controlled knee flexion to 15 degrees allows for dissipation of forces generated by the abrupt transfer of body weight onto the limb.

- Movement of the foot into 5 degrees of eversion functions to unlock the midtarsal joints (talonavicular and calcaneocuboid), creating a more flexible foot that is able to adapt to uneven surfaces. The rate of this motion is controlled by eccentric activity of the tibialis anterior and posterior.

12. What allows for stance stability during single limb support?

- Stability arises primarily from the action of the calf muscles that restrain excess forward collapse of the tibia. As a result, the knee and hip are able to achieve a fully extended position with only minimal muscle activity requirements.
- In late single limb support, a reduction in the amount of subtalar joint eversion functions to lock the midtarsal joints and creates a rigid forefoot over which body weight can progress.

13. What allows for foot clearance during swing limb advancement?

- Early in swing limb advancement, knee flexion to 60 degrees (owing to passive and active factors) assists in clearing the limb.
- As swing limb advancement progresses, hip flexion to 25 degrees, in combination with ankle dorsiflexion to neutral, becomes critical to achieve foot clearance.

14. Name key factors that are essential to ensure forward progression during the gait cycle.

- Forward progression during weight acceptance results primarily from eccentric activity of the dorsiflexors, which not only lower the foot to the ground but also draw the tibia forward.
- During single limb support, controlled tibial progression resulting from eccentric calf activity allows forward progression without tibial collapse.
- The 20 degrees of apparent hyperextension achieved at the hip contributes to a trailing limb posture that increases step length and forward progression.
- During swing limb advancement, knee extension and hip flexion to 20 degrees in late swing contribute to forward progression and step length.

15. Describe the role of the heel, ankle, and forefoot "rockers" during gait.

Collectively, the three rockers reflect a combination of joint motions and muscle actions that contribute to the smooth transition of body weight from the heel to the forefoot during stance. The heel rocker occurs during weight acceptance. Eccentric activity of the pretibial muscles lowers the forefoot to the ground and draws the tibia forward, allowing body weight to roll across the heel. Next is the ankle rocker, occurring during the first half of single limb support. The ankle moves from 5 degrees of plantar flexion to slight dorsiflexion. A gradual increase in eccentric calf muscle activity allows the tibia to remain stable as body weight progresses in front of the ankle. The forefoot rocker occurs during the last half of single limb support. A modulated increase in eccentric calf muscle activity permits the ankle to move into 10 degrees of dorsiflexion (without collapsing) and the heel to rise. Body weight smoothly transitions across the forefoot.

16. What is the functional significance of normal subtalar joint eversion/inversion during the stance phase of gait?

During weight acceptance, subtalar eversion is important for unlocking the midtarsal joints (calcaneocuboid and talonavicular) and creating a more flexible foot that is able to adapt to uneven surfaces. During single limb support, a reduction in the amount of subtalar eversion (motion toward inversion) functions to lock the midtarsal joints, creating a rigid forefoot lever over which the body weight can progress.

17. What effects would a weak tibialis anterior have on gait?

- Foot slap immediately after initial contact (lack of eccentric control)
- Footdrop during swing
- Excessive hip and knee flexion (steppage gait) to clear the toes during swing

18. Describe gait deviations that likely would be evident in a patient with plantar fasciitis or a heel spur.

Patients typically exhibit a forefoot initial contact, avoiding the pressure associated with heel impact during weight acceptance. As the plantar fascia becomes tight with the combination of heel rise and metatarsal-phalangeal joint dorsiflexion during late stance, patients may avoid this posture by prematurely unweighting the limb.

19. What are the consequences of a triple arthrodesis on gait function?

- Loss of subtalar joint motion results in reduced shock absorption during weight acceptance.
- The inability to supinate in terminal stance diminishes the forefoot rocker effect.
- The ability to progress beyond the supporting foot is compromised.
- Stride length is diminished.

20. Describe the effect of calf weakness on ankle function during gait.

Calf weakness results in the inability to control forward advancement of the tibia, causing excessive dorsiflexion during single limb support and a lack of heel rise during late stance. As a result of the inability to control the tibia through eccentric action, the tibia advances faster than the femur, causing knee flexion during stance. The flexed knee posture necessitates activity of the quadriceps, which normally are quiescent during single limb support.

21. Describe the effect of a plantar flexion contracture on ankle function during gait.

A plantar flexion contracture (>15 degrees) results in either a flat-foot or a forefoot-initial contact. This disrupts normal advancement of the tibia and may limit the knee from flexing to dissipate the forces associated with weight acceptance. During single limb support, the primary limitation is the inability to progress over the foot. Because 10 to 15 degrees of ankle dorsiflexion is necessary for normal stance phase function, compensatory mechanisms are necessary. Progression may be augmented through a premature heel rise, forward trunk lean, knee hyperextension, or a combination thereof. The inability to achieve a neutral ankle position during swing also necessitates compensatory movements to ensure foot clearance.

22. What are the characteristics of quadriceps avoidance?

Quandriceps avoidance manifests as reduced knee flexion during weight acceptance. This compensatory strategy results in decreased quadriceps demand and diminished muscular forces acting across the knee.

23. With what orthopaedic conditions could quadriceps avoidance be associated?

- Patellofemoral pain
- Anterior cruciate ligament deficiency
- Quadriceps weakness
- Quadriceps inhibition (owing to pain or effusion)

24. Discuss the penalty associated with a knee flexion contracture.

A knee flexion contracture (>15 degrees) results in excessive knee flexion during weight acceptance, during single limb support, and at the end of swing limb advancement. The penalties include altered shock absorption during weight acceptance and instability during single limb support. Excessive knee flexion during stance requires greater amounts of quadriceps activity to support the flexed knee posture, increasing the energy cost of gait. Excess knee flexion at the end of swing limb advancement shortens step length.

25. Name typical compensatory strategies associated with reduced knee flexion range of motion.

Hip hiking or circumduction on the affected side is necessary to clear the foot during swing.

26. What is the penalty associated with reduced knee flexion range of motion?

The muscle activity associated with compensatory strategies increases the energy cost of gait.

27. What is a Trendelenburg gait pattern?

It is a contralateral pelvic drop during single limb support, usually caused by weakness of the ipsilateral gluteus medius.

28. Describe a typical compensation associated with Trendelenburg gait.

A lateral trunk lean to the same side as the weakness functionally serves to move the body center of mass over the involved hip, reducing the demand on the ipsilateral hip abductors.

29. Discuss the penalty associated with a hip flexion contracture.

A hip flexion contracture results in inadequate hip extension during late stance. Failure to obtain a trailing limb posture during late stance limits forward progression and stride length. To compensate for the lack of hip extension, an anterior pelvic tilt may be employed.

30. Explain the effect of hip extensor weakness on gait function.

Because adequate hip extensor strength is necessary to support the flexed hip posture during weight acceptance, substantial weakness necessitates less hip flexion at initial contact, resulting in a reduced stride length.

31. How does decreased proprioception influence gait?

Individuals with proprioceptive deficits (secondary to peripheral nerve injury, partial spinal cord injury, or brain lesions) require additional sensory input regarding joint position; typically this can be achieved through a forward trunk lean (to augment visual feedback) or through a more abrupt transfer of weight during the loading response (to augment sensory feedback).

32. How does an ankle fusion alter gait and energy consumption?

Persons who have sustained an ankle fusion often substitute for losses in talocrural joint motion (i.e., dorsiflexion) by increasing midfoot and forefoot motion. This permits forward progression over the supporting foot in late stance. Stride length is often reduced, resulting in a slower walking velocity. Gait compensations resulting from an ankle fusion cause individuals to expend a slightly greater amount of energy during walking.

33. What are the energy costs of using various assistive devices (e.g., crutches, standard walker, wheeled walker, cane) when compared with using no equipment?

Energy Cost Associated with Walking Using Assistive Devices

Assistive Device	Energy Cost
Crutches	Energy demand increased 30-80%, in part because of increased demands placed on arms and shoulder girdle muscles
Standard walker	Oxygen consumption increased >200%
Front-wheeled walker	Less impact compared with standard walker
Cane	No significant contribution

34. How are energy costs of assistive devices affected by the presence of significant gait pathology?

When significant gait pathology is present (e.g., excess ankle dorsiflexion and knee flexion secondary to a weak calf), use of an assistive device may **lessen** the energy demands of ambulation by reducing the demands on lower extremity muscles, allowing achievement of a more normal, energy-efficient gait pattern.

35. How does osteoarthritis of the knee influence gait?

- Patients walk with a slower velocity, owing to reductions in stride length and cadence.
- Many patients are not able to tolerate the demands of loading onto a flexed knee and may purposefully reduce loading response knee flexion.
- Many patients decrease knee flexion during early swing in an effort to limit painful joint movement.

36. How does the energy cost of walking with a total hip fusion compare with that of walking with a total hip arthroplasty?

HIP FUSION

The average rate of oxygen consumption increases 32% when compared with normal values at the same walking speed. Increased energy cost likely results from the compensations required for forward progression during gait (e.g., excess lumbar lordosis and an anterior pelvic tilt to enable the fused hip to achieve a trailing limb posture in late stance).

TOTAL HIP ARTHROPLASTY

Energy expenditure (1 year postoperatively) is approximately 17% less compared with walking with a fused hip.

37. What influences do various levels of amputation have on walking velocity and energy cost?

- In persons with unilateral amputations, the more proximal the level of amputation (e.g., transfemoral versus transtibial) the slower the customary walking speed and the greater the energy cost (milliliters of oxygen per kilogram of body weight per meter of walking) of walking.
- Energy expenditure, heart rate, and oxygen consumption are typically lower during ambulation with a prosthesis as compared with ambulation with crutches.

38. What are common gait deviations in a person with a transtibial amputation?

- Limited dorsiflexion during single limb support
- Diminished plantar flexion in preswing
- Forward trunk lean
- Reduced knee flexion during weight acceptance

39. List the pros and cons of using an ankle-foot orthosis (AFO) for the treatment of footdrop.

Advantages and Disadvantages of Using an Ankle-Foot Orthosis (AFO) to Manage Footdrop

Pros	Cons
Assists with foot clearance during swing Reduces need for compensatory maneuvers	If AFO is too rigid, then during weight acceptance: • normal movement of ankle into plantar flexion is disrupted • heel rocker effect is accentuated, resulting in increased knee flexion and greater quadriceps demand

40. What are typical above-normal energy expenditures for level walking with various amputation levels?

- Transtibial = 25% increase
- Bilateral below-knee amputation (BKA) = 41% increase
- Above-knee amputation (AKA) = 65% increase

Bibliography

Foley MP et al: Effects of assistive devices on cardiorespiratory demands in older adults, *Phys Ther* 76:1313-1319, 1996.

Györy AN, Chao EYS, Stauffer RN: Functional evaluation of normal and pathologic knees during gait, *Arch Phys Med Rehabil* 57:571-577, 1976.

Perry J: *Gait analysis: normal and pathological function,* Thorofare, NJ, 1992, Slack.

Reischl SF et al: The relationship between foot pronation and rotation of the tibia and femur during walking, *Foot Ankle Int* 20:513-520, 1999.

Rose J, Gamble JG: *Human walking,* Baltimore, 1994, Williams & Wilkins.

The Pathokinesiology Service and the Physical Therapy Department, Rancho Los Amigos National Rehabilitation Center: *Observational gait analysis,* Downey, Calif, 2001, Los Amigos Research and Education Institute, Inc.

Waters RL, Mulroy S: The energy expenditure of normal and pathologic gait, *Gait Posture* 9:207-231, 1999.

Waters RL et al: Energy cost of walking of amputees: the influence of level of amputation, *J Bone Joint Surg* 58A:42-46, 1976.

Waters RL et al: Comparable energy expenditure after arthrodesis of the hip and ankle, *J Bone Joint Surg* 70A:1032-1037, 1988.

Chapter 17

Pharmacology in Orthopaedic Physical Therapy

Charles D. Ciccone, PT, PhD

1. Discuss the two primary categories of analgesic medications.

- **Opioids**—Opioids, also known as **narcotic analgesics,** are powerful pain medications that typically are administered to treat moderate-to-severe pain. These drugs are similar in structure and function to morphine, although individual agents vary in terms of potency and duration of analgesic effects.
- **Nonopioids**—Nonopioid analgesics consist primarily of **nonsteroidal antiinflammatory drugs (NSAIDs)** and **acetaminophen.** NSAIDs consist of about 20 medications, including aspirin, ibuprofen, and similar agents. These drugs are not usually as powerful as opioid analgesics, but NSAIDs can be helpful in treating mild-to-moderate pain. Acetaminophen is technically not a member of the NSAID category because acetaminophen does not decrease inflammation. Acetaminophen does have analgesic properties similar to the NSAIDs, but it does not cause the gastric side effects typically associated with NSAIDs.

2. Summarize properties of common opioid analgesics.

Common Opioid Analgesics

Generic Name	Trade Name	Administration Routes	Onset of Analgesic Action (min)	Peak Analgesic Effect (min)	Duration of Analgesic Action (hr)
Butorphanol	Stadol	IM	10-30	30-60	3-4
		IV	2-3	30	2-4
Codeine		Oral	30-45	60-120	4
		IM	10-30	30-60	4
		Sub-Q	10-30		4
Hydrocodone	Hycodan	Oral	10-30	30-60	4-6
Hydromorphone	Dilaudid, Hydrostat	Oral	30	90-120	4
		IM	15	30-60	4-5
		IV	10-15	15-30	2-3
		Sub-Q	15	30-90	4
Levorphanol	Levo-Dromoran	Oral	10-60	90-120	4-5
		IM		60	4-5
		IV		Within 20	4-5
		Sub-Q		60-90	4-5

Common Opioid Analgesics ***continued***

Generic Name	Trade Name	Administration Routes	Onset of Analgesic Action (min)	Peak Analgesic Effect (min)	Duration of Analgesic Action (hr)
Meperidine	Demerol	Oral	15	60-90	2-4
		IM	10-15	30-50	2-4
		IV	1	5-7	2-4
		Sub-Q	10-15	30-50	2-4
Methadone	Dolophine	Oral	30-60	90-120	4-6
		IM	10-20	60-120	4-5
		IV		15-30	3-4
Morphine	Kadian, MS Contin, many others	Oral	Slower than IM	60-120	4-5
		IM	10-30	30-60	4-5
		IV	10-30	20	4-5
		Sub-Q	15-60	50-90	4-5
		Epidural	15-60		Up to 24
		Intrathecal	15-60		Up to 24
Nalbuphine	Nubain	IM	Within 15	60	3-6
		IV	2-3	30	3-4
		Sub-Q	Within 15		3-6
Oxycodone	OxyContin, Roxicodone	Oral		60	3-4
Oxymorphone	Numorphan	IM	10-15	30-90	3-6
		IV	5-10	15-30	3-4
		Sub-Q	10-20		3-6
Pentazocine	Talwin	Oral	15-30	60-90	3
		IM	15-20	30-60	2-3
		IV	2-3	15-30	2-3
		Sub-Q	15-20	30-60	2-3
Propoxyphene	Darvon	Oral	15-60	120	4-6

IM, Intramuscular; *IV,* intravenous; *Sub-Q,* subcutaneous.
(Information adapted with permission from Klasco RK, editor: *USP DI drug information for the health care professional,* vol 1, ed 24, Greenwood Village, Colo, 2004, Thompson Healthcare.)

3. List the common NSAIDs and compare them.

Common Nonsteroidal Antiinflammatory Drugs

Generic Name	Trade Name	Specific Comments—Comparison with Other NSAIDs
Aspirin	Many trade names	Most widely used NSAID for analgesic and antiinflammatory effects; also used frequently for antipyretic and anticoagulant effects
Diclofenac	Voltaren	Substantially more potent than naproxen and several other NSAIDs; adverse side effects occur in 20% of patients
Diflunisal	Dolobid	Has potency 3-4 times greater than aspirin in terms of analgesic and antiinflammatory effects but lacks antipyretic activity
Etodolac	Lodine	Effective as analgesic/antiinflammatory agent with fewer side effects than most NSAIDs; may have gastric-sparing properties
Fenoprofen	Nalfon	GI side effects fairly common but usually less intense than those occurring with similar doses of aspirin
Flurbiprofen	Ansaid	Similar to aspirin's benefits and side effects; also available as topical ophthalmic preparation (Ocufen)
Ibuprofen	Motrin, many others	First nonaspirin NSAID also available in nonprescription form; fewer GI side effects than aspirin, but GI effects still occur in 5-15% of patients
Indomethacin	Indocin	Relatively high incidence of dose-related side effects; problems occur in 25-50% of patients
Ketoprofen	Orudis, Oruvail, others	Similar to aspirin's benefits and side effects but has relatively short half-life (1-2 hr)
Ketorolac	Toradol	Can be administered orally or by intramuscular injection; parenteral doses provide postoperative analgesia equivalent to opioids
Meclofenamate	Meclomen	No apparent advantages or disadvantages compared with aspirin and other NSAIDs
Mefenamic acid	Ponstel	No advantages; often less effective and more toxic than aspirin and other NSAIDs
Nabumetone	Relafen	Effective as analgesic/antiinflammatory agent with fewer side effects than most NSAIDs
Naproxen	Anaprox, Naprosyn, others	Similar to ibuprofen in terms of benefits and adverse effects
Oxaprozin	Daypro	Analgesic and antiinflammatory effects similar to aspirin; may produce fewer side effects than other NSAIDs
Phenylbutazone	Cotylbutazone	Potent antiinflammatory effects but long-term use limited by high incidence of side effects (10-45% of patients)
Piroxicam	Feldene	Long half-life (45 hr) allows once daily dosing; may be somewhat better tolerated than aspirin
Sulindac	Clinoril	Relatively little effect on kidneys (renal-sparing) but may produce more GI side effects than aspirin

Common Nonsteroidal Antiinflammatory Drugs *continued*

Generic Name	Trade Name	Specific Comments—Comparison with Other NSAIDs
Tolmetin	Tolectin	Similar to aspirin's benefits and side effects but must be given frequently (4 times daily) because of short half-life (1 hr)

GI, Gastrointestinal.
(From Ciccone CD: *Pharmacology in rehabilitation,* ed 3, Philadelphia, 2002, FA Davis.)

4. How do opioid analgesics decrease pain?

Opioids bind to specific neuronal receptors located at synapses in the brain and spinal cord. These synapses are responsible for transmitting painful sensations from the periphery to the brain. Opioid drugs bind to protein receptors on the presynaptic terminal of these synapses and inhibit the release of pain-mediating chemicals, such as substance P. Opioids also bind to receptors on the postsynaptic neuron and cause hyperpolarization, which decreases the excitability of the postsynaptic neuron. These drugs limit the ability of these central nervous system synapses to transmit painful sensations to the brain.

Opioid drugs also may affect neurons outside the central nervous system. Opioid receptors have been identified on the distal ends of peripheral sensory neurons that transmit pain. Opioid drugs can bind to these peripheral receptors and decrease pain sensation by decreasing the sensitivity of nociceptive nerve endings.

5. Discuss side effects of opioids that can be especially troublesome in patients receiving physical therapy.

Sedation and **mood changes** (e.g., confusion, euphoria, dysphoria) can be bothersome because patients receiving physical therapy may be less able to understand instructions and participate in therapy sessions. Opioid drugs cause **respiratory depression** because they decrease the sensitivity of the respiratory control center in the brain stem. Although respiratory depression is not especially troublesome at therapeutic doses, this side effect can be serious or fatal if patients overdose on opioid medications. **Orthostatic hypotension** (a decrease in blood pressure when the patient becomes more upright) may occur during opioid use, and therapists should look for signs of dizziness and syncope, especially during the first 2 to 3 days after a patient begins taking opioid analgesics. Opioids are associated with several **gastrointestinal side effects,** including nausea, cramps, and vomiting. **Constipation** may also occur, and this side effect can be a serious problem if these drugs are used for extended periods in people who are susceptible to fecal impaction (e.g., people with spinal cord injuries).

6. Does long-term opioid use always result in addiction?

No. Addiction is characterized by **tolerance** (the need to increase drug dosage progressively to achieve therapeutic effects) and **physical dependence** (onset of withdrawal when the drug is discontinued suddenly). Although indiscriminate or excessive use of opioids can lead to addiction, tolerance and physical dependence do not necessarily occur when these agents are used appropriately for the treatment of pain. Appropriate use entails that the drug dosage match the patient's pain as closely as possible. If the dosage is adjusted carefully to meet each patient's needs, these drugs can be used for extended periods (several weeks to several months) without the patient developing tolerance and physical dependence.

7. List advantages of using a patient-activated electronic drug delivery system, known commonly as patient-controlled analgesia (PCA), to administer opioids.

- Increases patient satisfaction because the patient feels more in control of his or her ability to manage pain.
- Provides more consistent pain control while avoiding many of the side effects associated with excessive amounts of opioids.

8. Describe the disadvantages of using PCA to administer opioids.

One disadvantage is the inability of some patients to understand fully how to use the PCA device. For example, patients with cognitive problems or unreasonable fear of addiction may not understand that they must activate the PCA device when they feel pain. Other disadvantages include human error in programming the PCA device (the PCA pump can be programmed incorrectly and overdose or underdose the patient) and various technical problems (pump failure, displacement, or blockage of intravenous catheters).

9. List the primary effects of NSAIDs.

- Decreased pain (analgesia)
- Decreased inflammation (antiinflammatory)
- Decreased fever (antipyresis)
- Decreased blood clotting (anticoagulation)

10. How do NSAIDs exert their primary beneficial effects?

NSAIDs work by inhibiting the synthesis of prostaglandins. **Prostaglandins** are lipid-like compounds that are synthesized by cells throughout the body. These compounds help regulate normal cell activity, and they are synthesized as part of the cellular response to injury. Prostaglandins can increase sensitivity to pain, help promote inflammation, raise body temperature during fever, and increase platelet aggregation and platelet-induced clotting. Prostaglandin biosynthesis is catalyzed within the cell by the **cyclooxygenase (COX) enzyme.** This enzyme transforms a 20-carbon precursor (arachidonic acid) into the first prostaglandin (PGG_2). Cells then use PGG_2 to form various other prostaglandins depending on their physiologic status and whether or not they are injured. By acting as a potent inhibitor of the COX enzyme, NSAIDs block the production of all prostaglandins in the cell.

11. How do prescription NSAIDs differ from nonprescription (over-the-counter) NSAIDs?

When used to treat pain and inflammation, prescription NSAIDs do not differ appreciably from an equivalent dose of a nonprescription product. Dosage of nonprescription NSAIDs may be relatively lower than prescription NSAIDs. The major difference between prescription and over-the-counter NSAIDs is their cost; prescription products may be substantially more expensive than their nonprescription counterparts.

12. Discuss potential problems associated with the long-term use of NSAIDs.

NSAIDs are relatively safe when taken at recommended doses for long periods (e.g., several weeks or months). The most common side effect associated with these drugs is gastric irritation. Most NSAIDs inhibit the production of prostaglandins that help protect the gastric mucosa, and loss of these beneficial prostaglandins renders the mucosa vulnerable to damage from gastric acids. This problem can be minimized by taking each dose with food or by administering NSAIDs with other medications (antacids, proton pump inhibitors, histamine type-2 receptor blockers) that reduce the effects or secretion of gastric acid. Other potential problems during long-term use include hepatic and renal toxicity. These problems are especially prevalent if other risk factors are present, including preexisting liver and kidney dysfunction, excessive alcohol consumption, and excessive or unnecessary use of other prescription drugs. NSAIDs probably should not be used for extended periods in people who have one or more of these risk factors.

13. Can NSAIDs inhibit healing of bone and soft tissues?

As indicated in question 10, NSAIDs inhibit prostaglandin biosynthesis. Certain prostaglandins, however, appear to be important during bone healing because these prostaglandins increase the activity of osteoblasts and osteoclasts that promote new bone formation. It follows that NSAIDs could impair bone healing by depriving bone of these important prostaglandins. As indicated in a review by Harder and An, much of the evidence for this detrimental effect has been derived from studies using laboratory animals and in vitro cellular models. Retrospective studies have found a significant relationship between NSAID use and nonunion of the femoral diaphysis; a relationship was also observed in patients who used NSAIDs postoperatively after spinal fusion surgery compared with patients who did not use these drugs. Consequently, many clinicians feel it is prudent to avoid use of NSAIDs immediately following fracture and bone surgery.

The effects of NSAIDs on soft tissue healing (cartilage, tendons, ligaments, skin) remain unclear. For example, a study using rat tissues suggested that certain NSAIDs (aspirin, indomethacin, phenylbutazone) may increase collagen synthesis and subsequent strength in cartilage, tendons, and skin. While Moorman et al. indicated that ibuprofen did not have a positive or negative effect on ligament healing in rabbits, Elder et al. found a 32% decrease in load to failure in rabbit medial collateral ligaments (MCLs) when treated with celecoxib. The effects of NSAIDs on the growth and healing of soft tissues in humans are difficult to determine and likely differ between drugs. Because of their effective antiinflammatory and analgesic effects, NSAIDs remain an important and popular treatment for soft tissue injuries.

14. What are the COX-2 inhibitors?

These are drugs that inhibit a specific subtype of the COX enzyme. There are two major subtypes of this enzyme known as COX-1 and COX-2. The COX-2 subtype is produced within various cells that are injured or damaged, and the COX-2 enzyme synthesizes prostaglandins associated with pain and inflammation. Drugs that are more selective for the COX-2 enzyme can help control production of prostaglandins that cause pain and inflammation, while sparing the production of beneficial prostaglandins, including the prostaglandins that help protect the stomach lining.

15. Give examples of COX-2 inhibitors and their benefits.

Celecoxib (Celebrex) may decrease pain and inflammation similar to the traditional NSAIDs, with less chance of causing gastric irritation in some patients. An additional benefit is that this drug does not inhibit platelet function, and therefore does not need to be stopped before surgery to prevent bleeding complications.

16. Are COX-2 inhibitors safe?

COX-2 inhibitors can produce side effects such as headache, abdominal pain, and diarrhea. Moreover, there is concern that these drugs may increase the risk of serious cardiovascular problems, including heart attack and stroke. For this reason, two of the original COX-2 drugs, rofecoxib (Vioxx) and valdecoxib (Bextra), were withdrawn from the market. Research continues to determine if the COX-2 drugs that are currently being developed have an acceptable risk-benefit ratio in certain patients. It seems reasonable that people who are at risk for cardiovascular disease should use these drugs cautiously, or perhaps avoid them altogether.

17. How is acetaminophen different from the NSAIDs?

Acetaminophen versus NSAIDs

Similarities	Differences
Analgesic effects	Does not decrease inflammation
Antipyretic effects	Does not have anticoagulant effects
	Does not irritate gastric mucosa

18. Does acetaminophen have any side effects?

Yes. Liver toxicity is the major side effect, especially if high doses are taken or the patient already has some degree of liver failure.

19. Can analgesics be applied topically or transdermally to decrease pain?

Certain analgesics can be applied to the skin to treat pain in fairly superficial structures. Trolamine salicylate (an aspirin-like drug) is available in several over-the-counter creams; this drug penetrates the skin and decreases pain in underlying tissues, such as muscle and tendon. Penetration of trolamine and certain other NSAIDs (ketoprofen) can be enhanced by ultrasound (phonophoresis) or by electric current (iontophoresis).

Certain opioids, including morphine and fentanyl, can also be administered transdermally. The goal of this administration is typically to achieve systemic levels that ultimately reach the central nervous system rather than to treat a specific subcutaneous structure or tissue. The use of opioid patches or other transdermal techniques (including iontophoresis) may offer a noninvasive way to provide fairly sustained administration and pain relief with opioid medications.

20. Are medications from other drug categories effective in treating chronic pain?

Yes. Traditional antidepressants such as nortriptyline (Aventyl, Pamelor) and amitriptyline (Elavil, Endep) and some of the newer antidepressants such as paroxetine (Paxil) and venlafaxine (Effexor) are often incorporated in the analgesic regimen for people with various types of chronic pain (such as fibromyalgia and chronic back and neck pain). In some patients depression may be present along with chronic pain, so it seems reasonable that managing the depression will help provide better outcomes when also trying to manage pain. There is evidence, however, that antidepressants can help improve pain even when a patient is not clinically depressed. Antidepressants prolong the activity of neurotransmitters in the brain such as norepinephrine, dopamine, and serotonin. It follows that their analgesic effects are probably related to their ability to affect these same neurotransmitters, but the exact reason they are effective in treating pain remains to be determined.

Certain antiseizure drugs such as gabapentin (Neurontin) are also helpful in treating chronic pain, especially neuropathic pain. Again, the reason for this drug's analgesic effects is not clear, but seems to be related to the ability of gabapentin to enhance the inhibitory effects of γ-aminobutyric acid (GABA) throughout the brain. That is, gabapentin and other antiseizure drugs might decrease neuronal excitability in central pain pathways, thereby reducing the sensitivity of neurons involved in pain perception.

21. What are the two primary categories of antiinflammatory medications?

NSAIDs and antiinflammatory steroids (glucocorticoids) are the two major types of antiinflammatory medications.

22. List the common glucocorticoids and their antiinflammatory activity.

Common Glucocorticoids

Generic Name	Trade Name	Antiinflammatory Dose (mg)*	Relative Antiinflammatory Activity†
Short-Acting‡			
Cortisone	Cortone acetate	25-300	0.8
Hydrocortisone	Cortef, Hydrocortone	20-240	1
Intermediate-Acting			
Methylprednisolone	Medrol, others	4-48	5
Prednisolone	Prelone, Delta-Cortef, others	5-60	4
Prednisone	Deltasone, Orasone, others	5-60	4
Triamcinolone	Aristocort, Kenacort	8-16	5
Long-Acting			
Betamethasone	Celestone	0.6-7.2	20-30
Dexamethasone	Decadron, Dexone, others	0.75-9.0	20-30

*Typical daily adult and adolescent dose, administered orally in single or divided doses.
†Antiinflammatory potency relative to hydrocortisone (e.g., prednisone is 4 times more potent than hydrocortisone).
‡Duration of activity related to tissue half-life (i.e., short-acting, tissue half-life 8-12 hr; intermediate-acting, tissue half-life 18-36 hr; long-acting, tissue half-life 36-54 hr).
(Data from Klasco RK, editor: *USP DI drug information for the health care professional,* vol 1, ed 24, Greenwood Village, Colo, 2004, Thompson Healthcare.)

23. How do glucocorticoids decrease inflammation?

Glucocorticoids enter the cell, bind to a specific receptor in the cytoplasm, and form a glucocorticoid-receptor complex that moves to the cell's nucleus. At the nucleus, the drug-receptor complex increases the transcription of genes that code for antiinflammatory proteins (e.g., certain interleukins, neutral endopeptidase) while inhibiting genes that code for inflammatory proteins (e.g., cytokines, inflammatory enzymes). Glucocorticoids also inhibit directly the function of various cells involved in the inflammatory response, including macrophages, lymphocytes, and eosinophils.

24. How do glucocorticoids compare with NSAIDs in terms of efficacy and safety?

Glucocorticoids are generally much more effective in reducing inflammation compared with NSAIDs, but glucocorticoids are not as safe as NSAIDs, and glucocorticoid use can produce several serious side effects when these drugs are administered systemically for periods of ≥3 weeks.

25. Discuss the serious side effects of glucocorticoids.

Glucocorticoids can cause hypertension, muscle wasting, glucose intolerance, gastric ulcers, and glaucoma. Patients may be more prone to infections because these drugs suppress the immune system. Prolonged glucocorticoid administration causes adrenocortical suppression, in which the adrenal gland stops synthesizing endogenous glucocorticoids (cortisol) because of the negative feedback effect of the drugs on the endocrine system. Because it takes the adrenal gland several days to regain normal function and begin synthesizing cortisol, adrenocortical suppression can be life-threatening if the glucocorticoid drug is suddenly discontinued. Consequently, patients who receive systemic doses of glucocorticoids for extended periods should not discontinue these medications suddenly but should gradually taper off the dosage under medical supervision.

26. Can delivery of antiinflammatory steroids via iontophoresis or phonophoresis cause adrenocortical suppression?

Iontophoresis or phonophoresis, when applied to a single joint or tissue and used at a reasonable frequency (i.e., 3 or 4 times each week), does not pose a serious threat for causing adrenocortical suppression.

27. Which side effect of glucocorticoids can be especially troublesome in patients receiving physical therapy?

One of the most troublesome side effects of glucocorticoids is the tendency of these drugs to cause breakdown (catabolism) of muscle, tendon, bone, and other supporting tissues.

28. How can the catabolic side effects of glucocorticoids be overcome?

Catabolic side effects can be overcome by subjecting muscle and other tissues to resistance exercise. For example, renal transplant patients receiving glucocorticoids to prevent organ rejection were trained using an isokinetic cycle ergometer, and these patients experienced an increase in thigh girth and thigh muscle area of 9% to 44% compared with healthy control subjects. This relative protection against muscle atrophy is variable and depends on the type and intensity of the exercise, the dosage of the glucocorticoid, and the amount of catabolism that may already be present because of high glucocorticoid dosage and prolonged administration. Nonetheless, judicious use of progressive resistance training and other strengthening techniques (e.g., walking, aquatic exercise) can be invaluable in minimizing the catabolic side effects.

29. Is there a critical dosage or frequency of administration that contraindicates further intra-articular injections of glucocorticoids?

A given joint should receive no more than four injections within a 12-month period.

30. What are the fluoroquinolones?

They are a group of antibacterial drugs that includes ciprofloxacin (Cipro) and ofloxacin (Floxin). These drugs have a fairly broad antibacterial spectrum, and are used frequently to treat urinary tract infections, respiratory tract infections, and other infections caused by gram-negative bacteria.

31. Why are the fluoroquinolones potentially harmful to patients with orthopaedic conditions?

Some patients experience tendinopathy (pain, tenderness), especially in the Achilles tendon and other large tendons that are subjected to high amounts of stress. The exact reasons for this effect are unclear, but fluoroquinolone-induced tendinopathy can be severe and lead to tendon rupture. Risk factors include advanced age, renal failure, use of glucocorticoids, and a history of tendinopathy caused by these drugs. Therapists should be especially cognizant of tendinitis in patients who are taking these drugs, and any increase in tendon problems should be brought to the attention of the medical staff. Exercise involving the affected tendon should be discontinued until the source of the pain and tenderness can be evaluated.

32. What medications are available to treat skeletal muscle spasms associated with orthopaedic impairments (e.g., nerve root impingement or direct injury to the muscle)?

Diazepam (Valium) and a diverse group of drugs such as carisoprodol and other so-called polysynaptic inhibitors are available to treat these conditions. The drugs commonly used to control muscle spasms act on the central nervous system and attempt to reduce excitatory input onto the α-motor neuron. Valium increases the inhibitory effects of γ-aminobutyric acid (GABA) in the spinal cord. GABA, an inhibitory neurotransmitter in the central nervous system, tends to decrease neuronal activity, including the activity of the α-motor neuron that activates skeletal muscle. Valium increases GABA-mediated inhibition of the α-motor neuron, which, in turn, causes decreased muscle activation, with subsequent relaxation of muscles that are in spasm. The actions of the polysynaptic inhibitors are poorly understood. The term polysynaptic inhibitor refers to the idea that these drugs decrease α-motor neuron activity by inhibiting polysynaptic reflex pathways in the spinal cord. There is little evidence that these drugs act selectively on the spinal cord, and it seems likely that any muscle relaxant properties of these drugs are caused by their sedative effects.

33. Discuss the efficacy of the drugs commonly used to treat skeletal muscle spasm.

Antispasm drugs typically have been shown to be more effective than placebo in reducing the pain associated with skeletal muscle spasms. These drugs may not be any more effective than simple analgesic medications (e.g., NSAIDs, acetaminophen), however, when treating orthopaedic conditions that include spasms. All of the commonly prescribed antispasm drugs cause sedation, and the ability of these drugs to relax skeletal muscle is probably related more to their sedative properties than to a direct effect on muscle spasms. Many practitioners are foregoing use of these muscle relaxants in lieu of pain medications and other nonpharmacologic interventions, including physical therapy.

34. How do antispasm medications differ from drugs used to treat spasticity?

Antispasm medications consist primarily of diazepam (Valium) and other drugs that act in the central nervous system and attempt to decrease excitation of the α-motor neuron. Diazepam also can be used to treat spasticity (i.e., increased stretch reflex activity secondary to central nervous system lesions). The other traditional antispasm drugs (e.g., carisoprodol) typically are used only for spasms.

Antispasticity drugs, including baclofen (Lioresal), tizanidine (Zanaflex), gabapentin (Neurontin), dantrolene (Dantrium), and botulinum toxin (Botox), act at various sites to decrease the hyperexcitability of skeletal muscle. Baclofen, tizanidine, and gabapentin act within the spinal cord to increase inhibition and decrease excitation of the α-motor neuron. Dantrolene acts directly on the skeletal muscle cell and causes relaxation by inhibiting the release of calcium from the sarcoplasmic reticulum. Botulinum toxin can be injected directly into spastic muscles and causes relaxation by inhibiting the release of acetylcholine at the neuromuscular junction. Botulinum toxin can be used to treat severe, chronic muscle spasms in conditions such as torticollis.

35. What are the primary medications used to treat osteoarthritis?

Acetaminophen and NSAIDs are the primary medications used in the treatment of osteoarthritis. NSAIDs can be used as an alternative or as a supplement to acetaminophen, especially in more advanced stages of osteoarthritis where some inflammation (synovitis) may occur secondary to other degenerative changes in the joints. Other drugs can be used to help restore joint function and prevent further degeneration. Viscosupplementation involves injection of hyaluronan directly into the joint in an attempt to restore viscosity of the synovial fluid. Another strategy uses over-the-counter dietary supplements, such as glucosamine and chondroitin sulfate, to provide substrates for the formation of healthy articular cartilage and synovial fluid.

36. Is there evidence that dietary supplements (e.g., glucosamine, chondroitin) can improve joint function in people with osteoarthritis?

A recent systematic review by Towheed et al. analyzed 20 randomized controlled trials (RCTs) of varying quality, and suggested that glucosamine may decrease pain and improve function in people with osteoarthritis. When only high-quality studies were analyzed, however, the benefits to pain and function were not apparent. On the other hand, some studies suggested that glucosamine may have beneficial effects on structural changes in knee osteoarthritis, but this effect seems limited to a certain type of glucosamine product (i.e., the Rotta preparation), and beneficial structural effects such as decreased joint space narrowing have not been documented in other joints.

Some older studies suggest that these supplements may decrease pain and improve function, but many of these studies have design or methodological flaws that limit their interpretation. More recent, high-quality studies cast doubt on the effects of these supplements in the general population. Given the relative safety of these interventions, these nutritional supplements might be worth a trial in certain people with osteoarthritis.

37. Discuss the primary pharmacologic strategies available for treating rheumatoid arthritis.

- NSAIDs typically are the first drugs used to control pain and inflammation, and these agents often are the cornerstone of treatment throughout the course of the disease.
- Glucocorticoids are especially effective in controlling inflammation, but these drugs must be used cautiously because of their catabolic properties and other side effects. Glucocorticoids often are used for short periods to help control flare-ups or acute exacerbations of rheumatoid arthritis.
- Disease-modifying antirheumatic drugs (DMARDs) include methotrexate (Mexate, Rheumatrex), azathioprine (Imuran), penicillamine (Cuprimine), etanercept (Enbrel), and several other agents. These drugs are grouped together because they can slow or reverse the joint destruction that typifies rheumatoid arthritis. DMARDs seem to work by suppressing the immune response that causes the degenerative changes associated with rheumatoid arthritis. DMARDs tend to be fairly toxic, and their use is limited to patients who are able to tolerate long-term administration.

38. How can physical therapists help patients deal with the residual effects of general anesthesia?

Residual effects such as confusion, drowsiness, and lethargy can be resolved to some extent by increasing the patient's respiration and activity level. Therapists should instruct patients in deep-breathing exercises to help eliminate any remaining anesthesia and to help prevent any respiratory complications from extensive or prolonged surgeries. Therapists can institute active range of motion exercises of the upper and lower extremities to help increase metabolism and excretion of the anesthetic. Progressive ambulation, as tolerated by the patient, should help eliminate any lasting anesthetic effects.

39. Why are local anesthetics used to treat acute and chronic pain?

Local anesthetics (e.g., lidocaine, bupivacaine) block transmission of action potentials in nerve axons. This effect occurs because these drugs inhibit sodium channels from opening in the nerve membrane, rendering the membrane inexcitable for a short period. By blocking transmission in sensory axons, local anesthetics prevent painful sensations from reaching the brain. These drugs can be administered in conditions such as reflex sympathetic dystrophy (also known as complex regional pain syndrome) to try to interrupt painful afferent sensations and to decrease efferent sympathetic discharge to the affected extremity. By using a PCA pump and delivery system, local anesthetics can be administered epidurally to the area surrounding the spinal cord. This type of anesthesia can be especially helpful in decreasing severe pain and improving quality of life in conditions such as cancer.

40. How can medications decrease the risk of thromboembolic disease in patients recovering from hip arthroplasty and other surgeries?

Anticoagulant drugs such as heparin and warfarin (Coumadin) are invaluable in maintaining normal hemostasis after surgery. Heparin is a sugarlike molecule that delays blood clotting by decreasing the activity of thrombin, a key component of the clotting mechanism. Heparin acts rapidly but typically must be administered parenterally by intravenous or subcutaneous routes. Warfarin and similar oral anticoagulants are administered by mouth, and these drugs work by decreasing the production of certain clotting factors in the liver. Oral anticoagulants take several days to affect blood clotting because they have a delayed effect on clotting factor biosynthesis. Heparin and oral anticoagulants often are used sequentially to control excessive clotting; drug therapy begins with parenteral administration of heparin but is switched after a few days to oral anticoagulants (warfarin), which can be administered for several weeks or months to maintain normal coagulation after surgery.

41. Is aspirin effective in preventing deep venous thrombosis?

Yes. Aspirin exerts anticoagulant effects by inhibiting the production of prostaglandins that cause platelets to aggregate and participate in clot formation. Aspirin can be administered alone or with other anticoagulants (heparin, warfarin), especially in patients who are at high risk for developing deep venous thrombosis.

42. Is ambulation safe for a patient newly diagnosed with deep vein thrombosis (DVT)?

There is no evidence that ambulation increases the risk of pulmonary embolism after an uncomplicated DVT. That is, immediate ambulation seems to be safe provided that the patient does not have a current or recent pulmonary embolism (symptomatic or asymptomatic) or other risk factors that would increase the likelihood of an embolism (e.g., malignant cancer, prolonged immobilization, advanced age). An adequate level of anticoagulant therapy using heparin and warfarin should also be achieved before starting ambulation. Graduated compression stockings should also be considered because there is evidence that proper use of these garments can prevent complications related to DVT.

43. What drugs are contraindications to upper cervical manipulation?

Anticoagulant drugs such as heparin, warfarin, and traditional NSAIDs (i.e., aspirin and other antiplatelet drugs) can increase the risk of vertebral artery damage and bleeding in patients receiving upper cervical manipulation. In patients taking anticoagulant drugs, therapists should avoid using upper cervical manipulation until laboratory tests indicate that the patient's clotting time is being maintained within normal limits. If these tests indicate relatively normal hemostasis, upper cervical manipulation still must be used cautiously, and the velocity and force of the manipulation must be reduced to decrease the risk of bleeding caused by vertebral artery damage.

44. Discuss medications that are currently available to treat osteoporosis.

- Calcitonin, a hormone normally produced within the body, can be administered to help increase the storage of calcium and phosphate in bone.
- Estrogen is likewise important in the hormonal control of bone mineral content in women, and estrogen replacement (using patches or oral supplements) can be especially valuable in women after menopause.
- Bisphosphonates, including etidronate (Didronel) and pamidronate (Aredia), may help stabilize bone mineral content by binding directly to calcium in the bone and preventing excessive calcium turnover.

- Calcium supplements can help provide a dietary source of this essential mineral, and vitamin D supplements can increase absorption of calcium and phosphate from the gastrointestinal tract.

45. What is heterotopic ossification?

It is the abnormal formation of bone in muscle and other periarticular tissues. This condition is one of the most common complications that occurs in patients recovering from hip arthroplasty and similar surgical procedures.

46. Discuss drugs that are effective in treating heterotopic ossification.

NSAIDs can reduce significantly the prevalence of heterotopic ossification associated with orthopaedic surgeries and other conditions (e.g., fracture, rheumatoid arthritis). Treatment with NSAIDs has been successful in reducing the prevalence and severity of heterotopic ossification after total hip arthroplasty. These drugs inhibit prostaglandin biosynthesis, and their ability to limit heterotopic ossification undoubtedly is related to a reduction of proinflammatory prostaglandins in periarticular soft tissues. These drugs seem to work best when used prophylactically, and they often are administered a day or so before surgery and continued for 1 to 6 weeks after surgery.

47. Discuss how cardiovascular medications affect exercise responses.

Certain cardiovascular medications blunt the cardiac response to an exercise bout. β-Blockers typically decrease heart rate and myocardial contractility, resulting in a decrease in blood pressure and heart rate at submaximal and maximal workloads. Digitalis increases myocardial contraction force and can increase left ventricular ejection fraction in patients with heart failure. Other cardiovascular drugs, such as diuretics, vasodilators, antiarrhythmics, angiotensin-converting enzyme inhibitors, and calcium channel blockers, can have variable effects on exercise responses, depending on the drug and dosage used, the type of cardiac disease, and the presence of comorbidity.

48. List specific concerns for physical therapists regarding cardiac medications and exercise.

1. Exercise tolerance may improve when the drug is in effect. This is true even for drugs that blunt cardiac function (e.g., β-blockers) because the drug may control symptoms of angina and arrhythmias, allowing the patient to exercise longer and at a relatively higher level.
2. Exercise prescriptions must take into account the medication effects. The prescription should be based on exercise testing that was performed while the drug was acting on the patient. Formulas that estimate exercise intensity based on age, resting heart rate, and other variables may not be accurate because these formulas fail to account for the effect of each medication on these variables.
3. Therapists should look carefully for medication-related side effects and adverse effects while the patient is exercising. These effects may be latent when the patient is inactive, but exercise may unmask certain side effects, such as arrhythmias and abnormal blood pressure responses.

49. Can lipid-lowering medications cause skeletal muscle damage?

Lipid-lowering drugs such as the statins (e.g., simvastatin [Zocor], atorvastatin [Lipitor]) are generally well tolerated. In rare cases, however, they can cause myopathy that is characterized by skeletal muscle pain, weakness, and inflammation (myositis). In severe cases, myopathy can lead to severe muscle damage (rhabdomyolysis) with disintegration of the muscle membrane and release of myoglobin and other muscle proteins into the bloodstream. This situation can lead to renal damage because the kidneys must try to filter and excrete large quantities of muscle protein. Hence, any patient who is taking lipid-lowering drugs and spontaneously develops muscle pain and weakness should be referred to his or her physician immediately to rule out the possibility of drug-induced myopathy.

50. Can physical agents affect drug absorption, distribution, and metabolism?

Physical agents (e.g., heat, cold, and electricity) can have dramatic effects on drug disposition in the body; this is especially true for drugs that are injected into a specific area. Insulin typically is administered through subcutaneous injection into adipose tissue in the trunk or extremities. Insulin is absorbed into the bloodstream more rapidly if heat and other physical interventions (e.g., electric stimulation, massage, exercise) are applied to the injection site. Application of cold agents delays insulin absorption.

Use of physical agents or manual interventions at the site of the injection should be avoided when the rate of absorption must remain constant or the goal is to keep a drug localized in a specific area. Conversely, heat, massage, and exercise could be applied to a certain area of the body with the idea that a systemically administered drug (i.e., a drug that is in the bloodstream) might reach the area more easily because of an increase in local blood flow and tissue metabolism. This idea has not been proved conclusively.

Bibliography

Aldrich D, Hunt DP: When can the patient with deep venous thrombosis begin to ambulate?, *Phys Ther* 84:268-273, 2004.

Bjordal JM et al: Non-steroidal anti-inflammatory drugs, including cyclo-oxygenase-2 inhibitors, in osteoarthritic knee pain: meta-analysis of randomised placebo controlled trials, *BMJ* 329:1317, 2004.

Ciccone CD: Basic pharmacokinetics and the potential effect of physical therapy interventions on pharmacokinetic variables, *Phys Ther* 75:343-351, 1995.

Ciccone CD: *Pharmacology in rehabilitation,* ed 3, Philadelphia, 2002, FA Davis.

Colwell CW Jr: The use of the pain pump and patient-controlled analgesia in joint reconstruction, *Am J Orthop* 33(suppl):10-12, 2004.

Cush JJ: Safety overview of new disease-modifying antirheumatic drugs, *Rheum Dis Clin North Am* 30:237-255, 2004.

Dahners LE, Mullis BH: Effects of nonsteroidal anti-inflammatory drugs on bone formation and soft-tissue healing, *J Am Acad Orthop Surg* 12:139-143, 2004.

Dews TE, Mekhail N: Safe use of opioids in chronic noncancer pain, *Cleveland Clin J Med* 71:897-904, 2004.

Doggrell SA: Present and future pharmacotherapy for osteoporosis, *Drugs Today* 39:633-657, 2003.

Elder CL, Dahners LE, Weinhold PS: Cyclooxygenase-2 inibitor impairs ligament healing in the rat, *Am J Sports Med* 29:801-805, 2001.

Harder AT, An YH: The mechanisms of the inhibitory effects of nonsteroidal anti inflammatory drugs on bone healing: A concise review, *J Clin Pharmacol* 43:807-815, 2003.

Hinz B, Brune K: Pain and osteoarthritis: New drugs and mechanisms, *Curr Opin Rheumatol* 16:628-633, 2004.

Moorman CT et al: The early effect of ibuprofen on the mechanical properties of healing medial collateral ligament, *Am J Sports Med* 27:738-741, 1999.

Olsen NJ, Stein CM: New drugs for rheumatoid arthritis, *N Engl J Med* 350:2167-2179, 2004.

Peel C, Mossberg KA: Effects of cardiovascular medications on exercise responses, *Phys Ther* 75:387-396, 1995.

Richy F et al: Structural and symptomatic efficacy of glucosamine and chondroitin in knee osteoarthritis: a comprehensive meta-analysis, *Arch Intern Med* 163:1514-1522, 2003.

Rosenson RS: Current overview of statin-induced myopathy, *Am J Med* 116:408-416, 2004.

Stichtenoth DO: The second generation of COX-2 inhibitors: clinical pharmacological point of view, *Mini Rev Med Chem* 4:617-624, 2004.

Toth PP, Urtis J: Commonly used muscle relaxant therapies for acute low back pain: a review of carisoprodol, cyclobenzaprine hydrochloride, and metaxalone, *Clin Ther* 26:1355-1367, 2004.

Towheed TE et al: Glucosamine therapy for treating osteoarthritis, *Cochrane Database Syst Rev* CD002946, 2005.

Townsend HB, Saag KG: Glucocorticoid use in rheumatoid arthritis: benefits, mechanisms, and risks, *Clin Exp Rheumatol* 22(suppl 35):S77-S82, 2004.

Chapter 18

Evaluation of Medical Laboratory Tests

Douglas Boyce, MD, RPh

1. List various nondisease states that can result in an abnormal laboratory test result.

- Pregnancy
- Exercise
- Posture
- Food intake and nutritional state
- Drugs, alcohol, vitamin and dietary supplements
- Specimen complications (hemolysis, stasis, sampling error, storage, exposure)
- Circadian rhythms, diurnal variation
- Technician error
- Reference range variations between different laboratories
- Normal variations based on patient age, gender, race, body weight

2. What two characteristics are important for diagnostic laboratory testing?

Sensitivity and specificity. Sensitivity is the percentage of persons with the disease that are correctly identified by the test. Specificity is the percentage of persons without the disease that are correctly excluded by the test. Clinically, these concepts are important for confirming or excluding disease during screening. Ideally, a test should provide a high sensitivity and specificity. Sensitivity = TP/(TP + FN). Specificity = TN/(TN + FP). Abbreviations: TP, true positive; TN, true negative; FP, false positive; FN, false negative.

3. Explain the concepts of positive predictive value (PPV) and negative predictive value (NPV).

PPV is defined as the percentage of persons with a positive test result who actually have the disease. NPV is the percentage of persons with a negative test result who do not have the disease. Predictive value therefore is the probability a person's test result (positive or negative) is correct. PPV = TP/(TP + FP). NPV = TN/(TN + FN).

4. Where is albumin produced and what are its functions?

Albumin is synthesized in the liver. Albumin functions to maintain osmotic pressure in the vasculature and also serves as a transport protein. Hypoalbuminemia leads to abnormal distribution of body water. This occurs because of decreased osmotic pressures within the vasculature and resultant tissue edema. Albumin serves to transport various drugs, ions, pigments, bilirubin, and hormones.

5. What is the normal range for serum albumin levels?

Normal levels are 3.5 to 5.5 g/dl.

6. What conditions result in decreased albumin levels (hypoalbuminemia)?

- Poor absorption of albumin (malabsorption, malnutrition)
- Decreased synthesis of albumin (chronic liver disease)
- Catabolic states (infection, burns, malignancy, chronic inflammation)
- Increased losses of albumin (hemorrhage, renal disease, protein-losing enteropathies)
- Albumin dilution

7. Where does alkaline phosphatase originate?

Liver (cells of the biliary tract), intestine (mucosal cells of the small intestine), placenta (pregnancy), and bone (osteoblasts) are sources of alkaline phosphatase. Biliary obstruction and Paget's disease (liver and bone) can result in a marked increase in alkaline phosphatase levels compared to intestinal or placental sources.

8. Explain alkaline phosphatase elevation as it relates to bone.

Any bone lesions (such as sarcoma or metastatic lesions) that produce increased osteoblastic activity will result in elevated alkaline phosphatase levels. Normal bone growth in children and adolescents will also result in alkaline phosphatase elevations.

9. What are the two hepatic conditions that result in elevation of alkaline phosphatase concentration?

- Extrahepatic obstruction—Obstruction of the large, extrahepatic bile ducts occurs with bile duct stones, strictures, or tumors. This obstructive process of the biliary system can result in significant enzyme elevation.
- Intrahepatic obstruction—Processes within the liver parenchyma can also lead to alkaline phosphatase elevation because of interference with bile flow or transport. Examples include leukemia, sarcoidosis, amyloid, malignancy, primary biliary cirrhosis (PBC), and primary sclerosing cholangitis (PSC).

10. How can liver- versus bone-related elevations in alkaline phosphatase levels be differentiated?

Measure 5′-nucleotidase, gammaglutamyl transpeptidase (GGTP), or fractionation of alkaline phosphatase. If nucleotidase or GGTP is elevated, alkaline phosphatase elevations are caused by a liver, not bone, source. Nucleotidase is present in the bile canaliculi of the liver. GGTP is not present in bone or placental tissue; therefore elevations are because of an underlying liver condition.

11. What is the normal range for alkaline phosphatase?

The normal range is 25 to 100 units/L.

12. What are aminotransferases?

They are enzymes involved in liver synthetic function and/or liver injury. Elevations in both aspartate transaminase (AST) and alanine transaminase (ALT) levels occur with liver inflammation, necrosis, or biliary obstruction. These enzymes are found in many other tissues beside the liver. Together with alkaline phosphatase and bilirubin, aminotransferase evaluation can help the clinician determine the pattern or cause of underlying liver disease.

13. What are nonhepatic sources of AST and causes for its elevation?

In addition to liver, AST is found in the heart, kidney, and skeletal muscle. When AST is elevated without elevation of ALT, a nonhepatic source (i.e., muscle, heart) should be considered. Examples include (1) skeletal muscle injury from intramuscular injection, muscle trauma with severe/prolonged exercise, polymyositis, and seizure disorder or (2) myocardial damage as seen in acute myocardial infarction. Both of these nonhepatic conditions can result in isolated AST elevation.

14. List the common pancreatic causes for elevated amylase and lipase levels.

- Acute or chronic pancreatitis
- Pancreatic pseudocyst
- Pancreatic trauma

Amylase is the most sensitive test for pancreatitis; lipase is the most specific indicator of pancreatitis. Often the degree of enzyme elevation does not correlate with the severity of disease.

Alcohol and gallstones are the most common causes of acute pancreatitis. Chronic pancreatitis is a result of chronic alcohol abuse, hypercalcemia, hyperlipidemia, trauma, or hereditary causes. Any of these conditions can result in elevated amylase/lipase values.

15. List some of the nonpancreatic causes for elevated amylase and lipase levels.

- Salivary gland disorders (amylase)
- Intestinal perforation or ischemia (amylase and lipase)
- Perforated peptic ulcer (amylase and lipase)

16. What are antinuclear antibodies (ANAs)?

ANAs are used to detect the presence of antinucleoprotein factors associated with certain autoimmune diseases. ANAs are γ-globulins that react with the nuclei of various tissues. The ANA test is reported as a pattern and a titer. The presence of a positive result (1) can occur in normal individuals, (2) may not indicate disease, or (3) may indicate persons destined to develop disease. ANA positivity usually requires confirmatory testing with other disease-specific tests, e.g., anti–double-stranded DNA (anti-dsDNA), anti-Smith antibody (anti-Sm antibody), or antiscleroderma antibody, depending on the suspected disease.

17. List diseases associated with a positive ANA (conditions associated with the disease or specific lab abnormality in parentheses).

- Systemic lupus erythematosus (SLE) (anti-dsDNA, anti-Sm antibody)
- Rheumatoid arthritis (rheumatoid factor [RF], erythrocyte sedimentation rate [ESR])
- Scleroderma/CREST [calcinosis, Raynaud's, esophageal, sclerodactyly, telangiectasia)] (Scl-70 [anti-topoisomerase antibodies]/anti-centromere)
- Polymyositis
- Drugs (antideoxyribonucleoprotein [anti-DNP])
- Mixed connective tissue disease (antiribonucleoprotein [anti-RNP])
- Sjögren's syndrome (anti-SSA, anti-SSB [antinuclear antibodies detected in patients with Sjögren's Syndrome])
- Chronic hepatitis
- Tuberculosis

18. What is bilirubin and what are its two forms?

Bilirubin is a by-product of hemolysis (red blood cell destruction). It is taken up by the liver, conjugated, and secreted into bile. It is eliminated in the stool and urine. Bilirubin exists as a conjugated and an unconjugated form.

19. Why does jaundice occur with hyperbilirubinemia?

Jaundice is yellow discoloration of the skin because of bile deposition in the skin and sclerae. Jaundice can result from abnormal processing of bilirubin, excess bilirubin production, biliary obstruction, or liver damage. Jaundice is clinically evident when the total bilirubin level is >2.5 mg/dl.

20. What conditions are associated with hyperbilirubinemia?

- Liver disease (hepatitis, cirrhosis, biliary obstruction)
- Hereditary disorders (Gilbert syndrome, Dubin-Johnson syndrome, Crigler-Najjar disease)
- Drugs
- Hemolysis

21. What is blood urea nitrogen (BUN)?

BUN is the end product of protein catabolism. BUN is formed in the liver and excreted by the kidneys. Impairment in kidney function, protein intake, and protein catabolism will affect BUN levels. It is used clinically as an estimate of renal function along with serum creatinine levels.

22. What are causes for elevated BUN levels?

- Inadequate excretion because of kidney disease/impairment
- Urinary obstruction
- Dehydration
- Drugs (aminoglycosides, diuretics)
- Gastrointestinal bleeding
- Decreased renal blood flow (shock, congestive heart failure [CHF], myocardial infarction [MI])

23. What is the normal range for BUN levels?

Typical BUN levels range from 8 to 18 mg/dl.

24. Where is the majority of calcium stored in the body?

Almost 98% to 99% is found in bone; 1% is found in the intracellular/extracellular space.

25. What factors affect serum calcium levels?

- Parathyroid hormone
- Calcitonin
- Vitamin D
- Estrogens and androgens
- Carbohydrates and lactose

These factors have a wide range of effects on calcium homeostasis (i.e., GI tract absorption, renal excretion and reabsorption, and also bone calcium mobilization).

26. What conditions are associated with hypercalcemia?

Hyperparathyroidism, malignancy, sarcoidosis, Paget's disease, vitamin D intoxication, and thiazide diuretics are all causes of hypercalcemia. The two most common causes are hyperparathyroidism and malignancy.

27. What are signs and symptoms of hypercalcemia?

The phrase "bones, stones, and psychiatric overtones" is often used to remember signs and symptoms of hypercalcemia. Here, bones refer to bone pain, stones to nephrolithiasis, and psychiatric overtones to confusion and altered concentration. Hypercalcemia is defined as a serum calcium concentration >10.5 mg/dl.

28. What are signs and symptoms of hypocalcemia?

- Neuromuscular irritability: Chvostek's sign (facial twitch after tapping facial nerve), Trousseau's sign (carpopedal spasm after inflation of blood pressure cuff), tetany, paresthesias
- Psychiatric disturbances
- Cardiovascular abnormalities (arrhythmias, CHF)

29. What causes the neuromuscular irritability (tetany) seen with hypocalcemia?

This is a result of the decrease in the excitation threshold of neural tissue, with a resultant increase in excitability, repetitive response to a stimulus, and continued activity of the affected tissue.

30. What is the prothrombin time (PT) and what does its value signify?

Prothrombin time is a measurement of the clotting ability of five plasma coagulation factors (prothrombin, fibrinogen, factor V, factor VII, and factor X). The PT is commonly used for monitoring warfarin therapy (an anticoagulant) and evaluating liver function (liver normally produces clotting factors).

31. How does warfarin function as an anticoagulant?

It interferes with vitamin K dependent clotting factors (II, V, VII, X). As a result, the PT will increase (or prolong), and coagulation will be delayed.

32. What conditions can lead to an increased PT?

- Anticoagulant use (warfarin)
- Vitamin K deficiency
- Liver disease (with decreased clotting factor production)
- Factor deficiency (II, V, VII, X)

33. What medical therapy requires monitoring of the PTT (partial thromboplastin time)?

Heparin use requires monitoring of the PTT because heparin is involved in the intrinsic clotting pathway. Heparin acts as a cofactor for antithrombin III, and down-regulates coagulation. Heparin is used for treatment of pulmonary embolism, prophylaxis of deep vein thrombosis, and treatment of various coronary conditions such as acute MI.

34. What is the INR (international normalized ratio)?

INR = patient PT divided by the mean PT for the laboratory reference range. INR provides a universal result indicative of what the patient's PT result would have been if measured using the primary World Health Organization International Reference reagent.

35. What components constitute the CBC (complete blood count)?

- Red blood cell (RBC) count
- White blood cell (WBC) count
- Differential white cell count (Diff)
- Platelet (Plt) count
- Hemoglobin (Hgb) level
- Hematocrit (Hct) level
- Red cell indices (MCV, MCH, MCHC)

36. What are causes of leukocytosis (elevated WBC count)?

Acute infections, hemorrhage, trauma, malignant disease, toxins, drugs, tissue necrosis/inflammation, and leukemia can all contribute to elevated WBC count.

37. Within the differential white cell count (Diff), name the five white blood cell types, their percentages, and what they protect against.

- Neutrophils (58%)—bacterial infections
- Eosinophils (3%)—allergic disorders and parasitic infections
- Basophils (1%)—parasitic infections
- Monocytes (5%)—severe infections
- Lymphocytes (30%)—viral infections

38. List causes of neutrophilia.

Acute bacterial infections, acute MI, stress, malignancy, and leukemias can all cause neutrophilia.

39. List causes of neutropenia.

Neutropenia can be caused by viral infections, aplastic anemias, drugs, radiation, and leukemias.

40. List causes of eosinophilia.

The acronym NAACP is used to remember causes of eosinophilia, where N= neoplasms, A = allergies, A = Addison's disease, C = collagen vascular disorders, and P = parasitic infection.

41. What is the ESR (erythrocyte sedimentation rate), and what does its value signify?

ESR is the rate at which erythrocytes precipitate out of unclotted blood in 1 hour. Inflammation, infections, malignancy, and various collagen vascular diseases increase the ESR because they facilitate erythrocyte aggregation. This affects the rate at which erythrocytes precipitate in a tube (increased aggregation/heaviness = increased rate of descent/sedimentation = increased ESR value).

42. What are some common conditions that lead to an increased ESR?

- Infections
- Inflammatory diseases
- Collagen vascular diseases
- Malignancy
- Anemia

43. What are the clinical applications of the ESR?

ESR is a nonspecific index of inflammation. It should not be used as a screening tool in asymptomatic patients. It is indicated in the diagnosis and monitoring of temporal arteritis and polymyalgia rheumatica. It may also be helpful in monitoring therapy in rheumatoid arthritis, Hodgkin's disease, and other inflammatory disorders. ESR values can increase with age in the normal population, and tend to be slightly higher in females. Normal values are 0 to 15 mm/hr (males) and 0 to 20 mm/hr (females).

44. What are symptoms of hypoglycemia and what is the most common cause of this condition?

Adrenergic and neuroglycopenic derangements occur as a result of hypoglycemia. Symptoms and signs include weakness, sweating, tremors, tachycardia, headache, confusion, seizure, and coma. By definition, blood glucose levels <50 mg/dl are considered hypoglycemic. The most common cause of hypoglycemia is excessive insulin dosage/administration.

45. What three criteria must be met to diagnose hypoglycemia?

- Presence of symptoms (adrenergic and/or neuroglycopenic)
- Low plasma glucose level in a symptomatic patient
- Relief of symptoms after ingestion of carbohydrates

46. What are symptoms of hyperglycemia?

The "3 P's" are used to remember symptoms of hyperglycemia: polydipsia, polyphagia, and polyuria.

47. What are some of the complications of hyperglycemia and long-standing diabetes?

Retinopathy, neuropathy (peripheral and autonomic), nephropathy, and infections are some of the complications.

48. What is the average life span of platelets, and where are they produced?

The life span of platelets is 7 to 10 days. Platelets are produced in the bone marrow from megakaryocytes. Platelets are necessary for blood clotting, and contribute to vascular integrity, adhesion, aggregation, and subsequent platelet plug formation.

49. What are symptoms of thrombocytopenia?

Symptoms include mild to severe hemorrhage, petechiae, purpura, epistaxis, hematuria, bruising, menorrhagia, and gingival bleeding. Platelet counts $>50 \times 10^9$/L are usually adequate to prevent major bleeding. Spontaneous bleeding is not uncommon with counts $<10 \times 10^9$/L.

50. What are the three major causes of thrombocytopenia?

- Splenic sequestration of platelets
- Increased platelet destruction
- Decreased platelet production

Splenic sequestration or hypersplenism can result in pooling of platelets in the spleen and a subsequent decrease in the number of circulating platelets available for clotting.

51. What specific clinical conditions cause thrombocytopenia?

Thrombocytopenia can be caused by idiopathic thrombocytopenic purpura (ITP), anemias (aplastic and hemolytic), massive blood transfusions, pneumonia, infections, drugs, HIV, splenomegaly, disseminated intravascular coagulation (DIC), and thrombotic thrombocytopenic purpura (TTP). Most of these conditions cause platelet injury, platelet consumption, or platelet loss.

52. What is thrombocytosis?

It is increased platelet count, defined as $>400 \times 10^9$/L. This can be a primary (essential thrombocythemia), secondary (e.g., leukemia, myeloma, polycythemia, splenectomy, hemorrhage, infections, or drugs), or transient process (following exercise, stress, or epinephrine injection). Clinically, thrombocytosis can cause thrombosis or bleeding or can remain asymptomatic.

53. What are some basic facts about potassium?

K^+ plays a major role in nerve conduction and muscle function. Total body potassium stores are roughly 3500 mEq. About 90% to 95% of potassium is intracellular and functions as a buffer.

Potassium is the body's major cation. Approximately 5% to 10% of K^+ is extracellular. Routine blood testing measures only the small extracellular portion, and not total body potassium. The majority of K^+ (90%) is excreted by the kidneys, with the remainder lost in stool and sweat.

54. What factors influence K^+ levels?

K^+ levels are influenced by acid-base status, hormone status, renal function, gastrointestinal loss, and nutritional status.

55. What are common causes of hypokalemia?

- Cellular shift (resulting in extracellular to intracellular movement): alkalosis, insulin administration, β-agonists
- Gastrointestinal loss: diarrhea, vomiting, nasogastric (NG) suction, laxative use, fistulas
- Renal loss: diuretic use, magnesium deficiency, renal tubular acidosis, Bartter syndrome
- Sweating, severe burns
- Poor dietary intake, starvation, licorice

56. What is a normal K^+ level?

Normal potassium levels are 3.5 to 5 mEq/L.

57. What are common causes of hyperkalemia?

- Cellular shift (resulting in intracellular to extracellular movement): cell damage (muscle injury, hemolysis, internal bleeding, burns, surgery, acidosis) causes hyperkalemia by releasing/shifting intracellular K^+ into the extracellular space (blood)
- Decreased urinary excretion: renal excretion is the main elimination pathway for potassium; therefore renal failure or decreased urinary K^+ excretion results in hyperkalemia
- Increased potassium intake
- Spurious: spurious causes result from hemolyzed specimen, fist clenching during blood draw, severe thrombocytosis/leukocytosis

58. What are symptoms of hypokalemia and hyperkalemia?

- Hypokalemia—muscle weakness, paralysis, cardiac arrhythmias, ECG changes
- Hyperkalemia—weakness, paresthesias, cardiac arrhythmias, ECG changes

59. What is rheumatoid factor (RF)?

It is an anti-γ-globulin antibody thought to be directed against the Fc portion of the IgG molecule. A large portion of patients with rheumatoid arthritis (RA) are RF positive, but the role RF plays in RA is uncertain. About 25% of patients with rheumatoid arthritis are RF negative, but may become positive later in their disease course. RF is not a screening test for RA. In addition to rheumatoid arthritis, RF can be seen in SLE, chronic inflammatory processes, old age, infections, liver disease, multiple myeloma, sarcoid, and Sjögren's syndrome.

60. How is rheumatoid factor (RF) reported?

It is reported as a titer. Values greater than 1:80 are significant; values of 1:640 and higher can be seen in rheumatoid arthritis. Higher titers can correlate with disease severity/activity.

61. What is the human leukocyte antigen (HLA) test?

HLAs are major histocompatibility antigens that are found on all nucleated cells and detected most easily on lymphocytes. The HLA complex is located on chromosome 6 and affects immune system functions.

62. What is the purpose of HLA testing?

HLA testing determines the degree of histocompatibility between a donor and recipient when organ transplantation is contemplated. The degree of HLA "matching" between donor and recipient will impact graft survival and rejection.

63. What are other functions of HLA testing?

HLA testing is also used in various rheumatologic disorders. The presence of a certain HLA antigen may be associated with an increased susceptibility to a specific disease, but it does not mandate the development of that disease in the patient.

64. List the disease and corresponding HLA antigen.

Disease	HLA Antigen
Ankylosing spondylitis	B27
Reiter syndrome	B27
Multiple sclerosis	B27, Dw2, A3, B18
Myasthenia gravis	B8
Psoriasis	A13, B17
Graves' disease	B27
Rheumatoid arthritis	Dw4, DR4

65. What percentage of patients with ankylosing spondylitis are HLA-B27 positive?

About 90% of patients with ankylosing spondylitis are HLA-B27 positive.

66. What is C-reactive protein (CRP)?

CRP is a protein that is present in the blood during periods of inflammation (infection, tissue damage). Besides blood, it can be found in peritoneal, pleural, synovial, and pericardial fluid. Diseases such as rheumatoid arthritis, SLE, inflammatory bowel disease, bacterial infection, and malignancy result in increased CRP levels.

67. What is a normal value for CRP?

A normal value for CRP is <0.8 mg/dl. The presence of CRP can be detected 16 to 24 hours after the inciting inflammatory event.

68. What is the importance of creatine phosphokinase/creatine kinase (CPK/CK)?

CK is an enzyme found in high levels in skeletal muscle (MM), cardiac muscle (MM and MB), and brain tissue (BB). Tissue injury results in CPK enzyme elevations, and the specific isoenzyme (MM, MB, BB) reflects the affected organ or source.

69. List some of the more common causes of CK-MM (skeletal) elevation.

The MM isoenzyme is found in skeletal muscle. Common causes for elevation include rhabdomyolysis, myositis, crush injury/trauma, polymyositis, dermatomyositis, vigorous exercise, muscular dystrophy, seizures, and IM injection.

70. What are causes of CK-MB elevation?

Myocardial infarction, muscular dystrophy, myocarditis, and cardiac surgery all contribute to CK-MB elevation.

71. What are causes of CK-BB elevation?

CK-BB elevation can be caused by severe brain injury, hyperthermia, Reye's syndrome, and uremia.

72. What are the general functions of sodium?

In general, sodium affects acid-base balance, osmotic pressure balance, and nerve transmission. Sodium concentrations are regulated by the renal system, CNS, and endocrine systems acting in concert. Despite wide variations in sodium intake, serum levels are maintained within a narrow therapeutic range. The normal serum sodium level is 135 to 148 mEq/L. Changes in body water and salt balance are determined/monitored by serum sodium levels.

73. What factors play a role in sodium homeostasis?

Renal blood flow, carbonic anhydrase activity, aldosterone, pituitary hormones, renin, and antidiuretic hormone are important in sodium homeostasis.

74. What are symptoms of hyponatremia?

Manifestations vary with the degree of hyponatremia and the rapidity of onset. Confusion, muscle cramps, lethargy, anorexia, and nausea are seen with moderate hyponatremia or gradual onset of hyponatremia. Severe hyponatremia or rapid onset can lead to seizures or coma.

75. What are causes of hyponatremia?

There are many causes: (1) hypotonic (isovolemic, hypovolemic, or hypervolemic); (2) isotonic; or (3) hypertonic. Within these categories are renal losses (diuretic use, urinary obstruction), extrarenal losses (vomiting, diarrhea, burns, third spacing), adrenal insufficiency, syndrome of inappropriate antidiuretic hormone (SIADH), water intoxication, renal failure, NSAID use, ACE inhibitor use, CHF, nephrosis, cirrhosis, pseudohyponatremia, and hyperglycemia.

76. How are hyponatremia and hypernatremia similar?

The clinical manifestations (confusion, lethargy, seizures, and coma) relate to the degree of hyponatremia or hypernatremia and the rapidity of onset of the electrolyte disturbance.

77. A patient with low serum sodium levels, tachycardia, hypotension, vomiting, diarrhea, and diuretic use has what form of hyponatremia?

This patient is volume depleted and is suffering from hypovolemic hyponatremia. Treatment is isotonic fluid replacement.

78. A patient with low serum sodium levels, edema, CHF, cirrhosis, and renal failure has what form of hyponatremia?

This patient is volume overloaded and is suffering from hypervolemic hyponatremia. Both sodium and water are increased, but water is increased proportionally more than sodium. Treatment is sodium and water restriction, and diuretic therapy.

79. What are causes of hypernatremia?

- Isovolemic (decreased total body water + normal total body sodium levels): diabetes insipidus, skin loss
- Hypervolemic (increased total body water + marked increase in body sodium levels): iatrogenic administration of high sodium solutions, salt intake
- Hypovolemic (loss of body water > loss of body sodium): renal losses, GI losses, respiratory losses, skin losses

80. List some normal laboratory values.

Test	Low Value	High Value
WBC count	<5000/mm^3	>10,000/mm^3
Neutrophils	<55%	>70%
Lymphocytes	>20%	>40%
Monocytes	<2%	>8%
Eosinophils	<1%	>4%
Basophils	<0.5%	>1%
RBC (male)	<4.7 million/mm^3	>6.1 million/mm^3
RBC (female)	<4.2 million/mm^3	>5.4 million/mm^3
MCV	<80 mm^3	>95 mm^3
MCH	<27 pg	>31 pg
MCHC	<32 g/dl	>36 g/dl
Hemoglobin (male)	<14 g/dl	<14 g/dl
Hemoglobin (female)	<12 g/dl	>16 g/dl
Hematocrit (male)	<45%	>52%
Hematocrit (female)	<37%	>47%
Platelets	<150,000 mm^3	>400,000 mm^3
ESR (male)	Up to 15 mm/hr is normal	
ESR (female)	Up to 20 mm/hr is normal	
CPK (male)	<12 units/ml	>70 units/ml
CPK (female)	<10 units/ml	>55 units/ml
ANA	Normal findings are no ANA detected in a titer with a dilution of >1:32	
CRP	—	>1 mg/dl
Rheumatoid factor	Abnormal if present	

81. What do these figures represent?

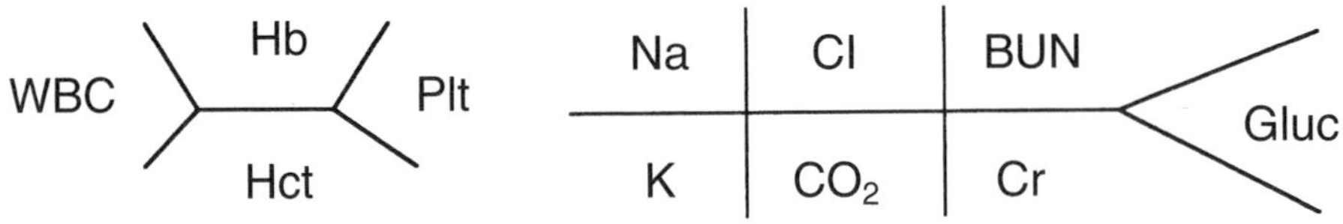

Laboratory values are usually recorded as follows:

- WBC white blood cell count
- Hb hemoglobin level
- Hct hematocrit level
- Plt platelet count
- Na sodium concentration
- K potassium concentration
- Cl chloride concentration
- CO_2 bicarbonate concentration

- BUN blood urea nitrogen level
- Cr creatinine level
- Gluc glucose level

Bibliography

Henry JB: *Clinical diagnosis and management by laboratory methods,* ed 19, Philadelphia, 1996, WB Saunders.
McMorrow ME, Malarkey L: *Laboratory and diagnostic tests: a pocket guide,* Philadelphia, 1998, WB Saunders.
Pagana KD, Pagana TJ: *Mosby's diagnostic and laboratory test reference,* St Louis, 1992, Mosby.
Rave R: *Clinical laboratory medicine: clinical application of laboratory data,* ed 6, St Louis, 1995, Mosby.
Vaughn G: *Understanding and evaluating common laboratory tests,* Stamford, Conn, 1999, Appleton & Lange.

Chapter 19

Clinical Electromyography and Nerve Conduction

Barry L. White, PT, MS, ECS

1. Define the basic nerve conduction study (NCS) terms.

- Latency—this is the time interval between the electric stimulus to excite the nerve and the nerve or muscle response.
- Nerve conduction velocity—the calculated speed or velocity (in meters per second) in which the nerve conducts impulses. It is determined by dividing the distance between two points of stimulation by the latency (time) it took for the nerve impulse to travel between those two points.
- Amplitude—the size of the motor or sensory action potential (measured in microvolts or millivolts). Lower than normal amplitudes often indicate axonal injury or axonal loss disease; a dispersed amplitude may represent demyelination.
- Demyelinating process—the term used to describe a pathologic state of a nerve when its impulses travel at a significantly slower latency or velocity than is normal. When the amplitude is within normal limits, this suggests the existence of a disease process or injury of the myelin.
- Focal demyelinating process—the term given to a nerve injury in which the nerve conduction is determined to be normal distally and proximally to a nerve injury but slow over the segment at which the nerve is injured. This usually has a good prognosis of recovery.

2. Give the normal values of upper limb nerve conduction.

Upper Limb	Distal Latency	Amplitude	Conduction Velocity
Motor nerve	<4.0 ms (8-cm distance)	5-10 mV	50-60 m/sec
Sensory nerve	<3.2-3.4 ms (12-cm distance)	5-50 μV	50 m/sec

3. Give the normal values of lower limb nerve conduction.

Lower Limb	Distal Latency	Amplitude	Conduction Velocity
Motor nerve	<5.2 ms (8-cm distance)	2-10 mV	40-50 m/sec
Sensory nerve	<3.5-4.0 ms (12-cm distance)	5-40 μV	35-40 m/sec

4. Define the common terms used to describe EMG findings that are abnormal.

- Fibrillations and positive sharp waves—indicate spontaneous firing of the muscle fibers within motor units. They most often result from acute or unresolved nerve injury.
- Fasciculations—indicate spontaneous firing of a motor unit. They usually indicate problems in the motor neuron cell body or spinal cord.
- High-frequency discharges—often refer to spontaneous firing of motor units or muscle fibers within a motor unit. They may have many causes.
- Large motor unit potentials (>5 to 7 mV)—after axonal injury, spared motor nerves generate new nerve terminal branches to grow into the adjacent muscle fibers that have been denervated, resulting in a motor unit that now controls more than the average number of muscle fibers. This results in a larger than normal motor unit potential in comparison to its neighbors. This finding usually is a sign of a chronic or long-standing axonal injury.
- Small motor unit potentials (<1 mV)—in myopathy, muscle death results, decreasing the total numbers of muscle fibers within motor units of muscle. A common finding noted in myopathy is that with minimal muscle tension a much greater number of motor units are recruited to compensate for the overall muscle fiber dropout that has occurred. It takes more motor units to produce minimal muscle tension, and the overall amplitude of each motor unit is reduced.

5. What is a motor unit?

A motor unit consists of the anterior horn cell, the nerve fiber with its terminal branches and neuromuscular junctions, and all the muscle fibers that are innervated by those terminal branches of each nerve fiber. It is the anatomic unit of all of the muscle fibers that one motor nerve innervates, which ranges from a few muscle fibers in the eye muscles to thousands of muscle fibers in the calf muscles.

6. Discuss the limitations of clinical EMG, NCS, and somatosensory evoked potential (SSEP) examinations for patients.

EMG and NCS examinations may appear normal when a patient has a clinical presentation of a radiculopathy or other nerve injury in which the nerve injury is so minimal as not to interrupt enough nerve fiber function to be quantifiable or be isolated to a certain level. This is particularly true in nerve injuries that are preganglionic (proximal to the dorsal root ganglion) and involve primarily sensory nerve fibers. In these cases, SSEP is a more effective test because it can evaluate the sensory nerve pathways proximal through the dorsal root ganglion up to the somatosensory cortex of the brain.

7. Because EMG and NCS findings show physiologic function, is there any optimal time frame to perform tests?

Yes. It requires 5 to 10 days for injured nerves to deteriorate completely distal to the suspected lesion. Nerve conduction distal to the lesion may look normal immediately following nerve severance and continue to look relatively normal for up to 3 days. By stimulating proximal to the lesion and recording distal to the lesion, one can show a complete loss of nerve conduction through the severed area. With EMG, it takes 14 to 21 days for degenerative potentials, such as fibrillation potentials and positive sharp waves, to occur; these are the EMG findings that indicate nerve injury. In a completely severed nerve, there are no signs of motor units functioning in the muscles within the injured nerve distribution distal to the nerve lesion. With suspected complete injury, it may be valuable to perform EMG immediately for the purpose of determining whether there are any spared motor units functioning within specific muscles innervated by the nerve.

8. Is there any value in requesting an EMG/NCS evaluation for a patient with a suspected nerve injury during the first 3 weeks of injury?

Yes, to determine if there is total loss of nerve continuity. EMG and NCS evaluations are helpful in showing whether any nerve fibers are spared from injury when clinical evidence is equivocal. NCS performed proximal to the lesion will document the nerve conduction deficit immediately, but will not define the structures (myelin, axon) involved in the injury.

9. Define the classifications of nerve injury that can be documented by EMG and NCS evaluations.

Nerve Injury	Definition	EMG/NCS Findings	Prognosis
Neurapraxia	Conduction block. Often a problem with myelin, which blocks nerve conduction but does not injure actual nerve fibers.	NCS: Shows decreased amplitude of motor or sensory nerve response when stimulated proximal to lesion, which is proportional to number of nerve fibers blocked. EMG: Decreased motor units fire on contraction attempts, which correlates with number of motor nerve fibers continuing to function in incomplete lesion.	Usually recovers within 6 weeks.

continued

continued

Nerve Injury	Definition	EMG/NCS Findings	Prognosis
Axonotmesis	Injury results in nerve degeneration of involved nerve fibers distal to nerve injury and with time regenerates.	NCS: Latencies and calculated velocities may be normal for nerve fibers spared from injury. Amplitude is lower than amplitude of uninvolved side. EMG: *Acute (14-21 days):* Shows fibrillations and positive sharp waves while denervated muscle is at rest. Decreased motor units fire on muscle contractions. *Chronic:* Shows decreased fibrillation potentials and positive sharp waves as spared motor units sprout into denervated muscle fibers.	Nerve fibers regenerate about 1 mm per day or 3 cm per month.
Neurotmesis	Nerve fiber injury results in nerve degeneration of involved fibers distal to nerve injury and does not regenerate because of severity of nerve injury.	Single EMG/NCS examination cannot detect this kind of injury. This injury type can be documented by serial testing. Demonstrates ongoing deficits on EMG/NCS findings that correlate to plateau of function clinically that is less than normal.	No motor or sensory improvement of nerves involved. Best course of action is to salvage functional use of limb.

10. Do the classifications of nerve injuries always fall into a neurapraxia, axonotmesis, or neurotmesis category?

Any nerve injury is most likely a combination of the three injuries, and from EMG and NCS testing the examiner can often determine which one exists predominantly. Through serial clinical evaluations and serial EMG and NCS examinations, the examiner can document more clearly which of the aforementioned classifications best fits the individual patient's injury and if that classification has changed.

11. Can myopathies as well as neuropathies be determined by EMG and NCS findings?

Yes. In many myopathic processes, there are findings of fibrillations and positive sharp waves in the myopathic muscles that are accompanied by an increase in motor units firing on weak contractions, and most often with lower than normal amplitudes. In neuropathic processes with motor axonal loss, there are findings of fibrillations and positive sharp waves in muscles on EMG during the acute stages, which diminish over time. The motor units firing on muscle contractions are fewer than normal, and the amplitudes of the surviving motor units often increase as the spared motor units actually sprout into denervated muscle fibers within their territory. This larger number of muscle fibers within the remodeling survivor motor units creates the larger amplitudes of the motor unit potentials recorded by EMG.

12. Can neuromuscular junction disorders be determined by EMG and NCS findings?

Yes. The neuromuscular disease is shown on sustained contractions recorded by EMG when the motor units drop out quickly. The abnormal neuromuscular junctions can be shown further by repeated stimuli on NCS at rates of 3 per second in which there is a drop in amplitude of >10%. In normal muscle, there is no change in amplitude on repetitive stimulation of rates up to 30 per second.

13. Describe the specific laboratory criteria that need to be met to ensure accurate nerve conduction data.

- Skin temperature—Nerve conduction is relatively slower in cooler temperatures. Skin temperature should be measured from the foot or hand. The ideal temperature is about 32° C. A false-positive result for an abnormal nerve conduction value is possible by conducting studies on a cool limb of undocumented temperature.
- Standardized distal distances—Standardized distance measurements between the distal stimulation point and the recording point for the response should be used because the time for a response to occur varies according to the segmental length between the stimulating and recording electrodes. The longer the distance between the pick-up electrode and the stimulating electrode, the longer the time for a response to occur.

14. What is a somatosensory evoked potential (SSEP) study? When is SSEP appropriate?

SSEP is the study of sensory nerve pathways through the extremity and along the spinal cord to the somatosensory cortex. It is performed by stimulating the nerve most often transcutaneously and picking up the response through multiple recording channels at more proximal segments along the nerve, at one or more sites along the spine, and at the somatosensory cortex. When the clinician determines a weakness or loss of sensation that appears significant and there are signs that the lesion could be of central nervous system origin (spinal cord or brain), use of SSEP is appropriate. Also, one may consider using SSEP when a patient has a significant sensory deficit that appears most likely to be at the nerve root level. SSEP would be more likely to show a nerve root (preganglionic) sensory nerve lesion than EMG and NCS examinations.

15. How is SSEP performed?

The same equipment that is used for EMG and NCS examinations can usually perform SSEP studies. The patient has recording electrodes placed on the extremity and skin over the spine and scalp, and stimulation is given repetitively at a distal site (usually the wrist or ankle) with each of the recording sites' responses averaged. Similar to NCS, the examiner records times of the responses, waveforms of the potentials, and amplitudes. Unique to SSEP, each response is replicated and compared with the contralateral side. Significant side-to-side differences of 3 standard deviations from the laboratory normal responses are considered indicative of a neuronal dysfunction. The site of a specific lesion can be determined by observing where along the distal to proximal nerve conduction an abnormality occurred.

CASE STUDY

A linebacker reports that he received a "stinger" to his right shoulder for the fourth time this season; he demonstrates 3/5 strength in the infraspinatus, deltoids, biceps, and pronator teres without detectable sensory deficits. EMG correlates with the muscle strength grades by demonstrating positive sharp waves in the above listed muscles. Acute denervation is also noted in the cervical paraspinal muscles. There is slight pain (3/10) reported into the right shoulder on cervical rotation to the right. No EMG abnormalities are noted in other muscles sampled throughout the right upper extremity and cervical muscles.

16. At what level does the EMG in this case study demonstrate the lesion?

The lesion is demonstrated to be at the nerve root level and has injured both the posterior rami to the posterior cervical muscles and the C5-C6 myotomes within the anterior rami. This is a nerve root injury that may include some concomitant injury to the upper trunk of the brachial plexus.

17. What category of nerve lesion does the EMG demonstrate on this football player?

The category of nerve lesion that is demonstrated by the EMG is a partial (significant) axonotmesis. Only serial clinical evaluation and EMG will document recovery through regeneration of injured nerve fibers.

18. If no improvement is noted in the follow-up clinical muscle testing or EMG evaluations on this football player, what category of nerve injury would he have?

If no significant improvement occurs over the following 6 weeks to 6 months, the injury would be classified as a neurotmesis.

19. Would the above findings have significant implications in the football player's future in playing football?

The implications are that the football player has sustained probable permanent nerve injury or delayed nerve regeneration and may need to refrain from further contact sports because he has less than normal neurological function to the right shoulder and arm muscles. Further contact sports with that shoulder would subject the shoulder to further injury or further delay in nerve regeneration.

CASE STUDY

A 21-year-old male long jumper arrives at the clinic with a 4-day history of right "foot drop" and paresthesias in the lateral leg and dorsal foot, which reportedly followed a training room treatment of ice application for a lateral distal hamstring strain. Evaluation demonstrates 2/5 strength of the anterior

CASE STUDY *continued*

tibialis, peroneus longus and brevis, extensor hallucis longus, and extensor digitorum longus and brevis. Sensation is decreased to pinprick along the dorsum of the foot. Nerve conduction studies demonstrated a focal conduction block (drop of 60% amplitude) of the deep peroneal nerve isolated to the area just proximal to the fibular head, and there was a concomitant slowing of the nerve conduction velocity to 30m/sec. Nerve conduction through the lower leg was 42m/sec. The superficial peroneal nerve conduction distally was within normal limits. The EMG findings demonstrated a decrease in motor unit firing of the tibialis anterior and extensor digitorum brevis. The short head of the biceps femoris and all tibial nerve innervated muscles tested normal. There were no signs of fibrillation potentials or positive sharp waves found that correlated with the time of the injury.

20. From the information given above, can you classify the category of this injury?

The injury occurred from ice application to the posterior, lateral aspect of the knee. Nerve conduction had confirmed a focal injury to the common peroneal nerve at the site of the reported icing. However, since it takes 14 to 21 days on average for axonal injury to appear on EMG testing in the form of fibrillation potentials and positive sharp waves, the EMG was only effective in demonstrating reduced motor unit activity. The classification of nerve injury cannot be determined at this time.

21. What is the optimal length of time before an EMG exam would be effective for determining the classification of injury to the common peroneal nerve?

The optimal time for a retest of EMG and NCS is another 14 days. Therefore the athlete should be rescheduled for a retest in 14 to 21 days.

A retest 14 days later with EMG/NCS demonstrated slowing of the nerve conduction from the peroneal nerve distally and reduced amplitude of the muscle response to the anterior tibialis and extensor digitorum brevis. The EMG demonstrated positive sharp waves in the common peroneal nerve distribution with reduced motor units upon contraction, which correlated with no change in the muscle grades found during the initial evaluation 2 weeks earlier.

22. Can you categorize the type of nerve injury at this time?

The type of injury is either an axonotmesis or a neurotmesis, which is a conclusion based on the low amplitude on nerve conduction in comparison to the initial exam and the findings of fibrillation potentials and positive sharp waves.

23. Will further evaluation be required to determine which of the two categories of injury the athlete has suffered?

Yes; at least one more EMG/NCS will be required to determine if reinnervation is occurring. The optimal time of the restudy will be every 2 weeks for manual muscle testing, and an EMG/NCS exam will be optimal in 6 weeks, at which time the anterior tibialis and peroneus longus muscles will most likely yield the most appropriate data by EMG. This statement is based on the fact that the nerve will degenerate proximally to distally. Therefore the anterior tibialis will most likely be the first muscle to undergo reinnervation.

CASE STUDY

A 16-year-old female with the history of falling off a horse 4 weeks ago sustained a closed comminuted fracture of the right mid-humerus. She was noted to have weakness of her hand while in her cast. Upon cast removal, she was sent for an EMG/NCS evaluation.

24. What would you expect to find on musculoskeletal evaluation?

Most often with a mid-humerus fracture the radial nerve is injured. This is because it emerges from the neurovascular sheath in the proximal humeral area and is closely adjacent to the humerus, laterally, in the spiral groove at the mid-humerus level.

25. What are the clinical findings that would be expected during musculoskeletal screening of this patient with radial nerve injury?

Weakness should be found in all forearm muscles within the common radial nerve distribution and sensory deficits should exist in the posterior antebrachial cutaneous and superficial radial sensory nerve distributions. This patient had 0/5 strength and absence of sensation to pinprick, light touch, and temperature in the common radial nerve distribution distal to the triceps.

26. What would you expect to find on EMG/NCS examination of this patient with radial nerve injury?

Since this injury occurred 4 weeks before the initial EMG/NCS evaluation, one would expect the following:

- NCS—near-normal amplitudes and nerve conduction values distal to the nerve injury and an absent response of the radial motor values proximal to the nerve lesion if a neurapraxia; low or absent evoked potential amplitudes for both radial motor and sensory nerves if an axonotmesis; if a neurotmesis, same findings as axonotmesis except loss of anatomic continuity of the nerve fibers and extremely poor prognosis; normal findings for the median, ulnar, and musculocutaneous nerves
- EMG—decreased insertional activity on needle insertion and no fibrillation potentials and positive sharp waves at rest, if this were a neurapraxia, but increased insertional activity and both fibrillation potentials and positive sharp waves at rest, if this were either an axonotmesis or a neurotmesis; normal findings for the muscles sampled in the median, ulnar, and musculocutaneous nerve distributions

This patient demonstrated no response on radial motor nerve NCS to the extensor carpi radialis and the extensor pollicis and an equivocal response for the superficial radial sensory nerve NCS to the base of the posterior portion of the thumb. There were fibrillation potentials and positive sharp waves and zero motor unit potentials upon contraction attempts in the radial distribution from the anconeus, brachioradialis, and all muscles distally. There were a few positive sharp waves found in the lateral head of the triceps and mild reduction in motor units firing on contraction attempts, while the medial and long heads of the triceps demonstrated normal insertional activity and resting activity, and motor units firing on contractions of various tensions.

27. Combining the clinical findings and the EMG/NCS data, how would you categorize this patient's injury?

The NCS and EMG findings demonstrate a complete axonal loss injury (axonotmesis or neurotmesis) without sparing of motor function distal to the branch to the long head of the triceps. The patient will require follow-up EMG/NCS examinations if the return of motor function is not clear clinically.

28. At 8 weeks postinjury, a second EMG/NCS does not appear to demonstrate improvement in motor or sensory nerve function. Can you predict what category of nerve lesion now exists?

The category of injury is most likely a neurotmesis and provides the orthopaedic surgeon with evidence that exploratory surgery of the fracture site and the radial nerve in that area may be beneficial for this patient to determine if there is anatomic continuity of the radial nerve. The surgeon may decide to perform a neurolysis or nerve grafting as a result of his direct observation after exposure of the radial nerve NCS testing.

Bibliography

Aminoff M: *Electromyography in clinical practice,* ed 2, New York, 1987, Churchill Livingstone.
Dawson D, Hallett M, Millender L: *Entrapment neuropathies,* ed 2, Boston, 1990, Little Brown.
Dumitru D: *Electrodiagnostic medicine,* Philadelphia, 1995, Hanley & Belfus.
Johnson EW: *Practical electromyography,* ed 2, Baltimore, 1982, Williams & Wilkins.
Kimura J: *Electrodiagnosis in disease of the nerve and muscle,* ed 2, Philadelphia, 1989, FA Davis.
Nelson R, Hayes K, Currier D: *Clinical electrotherapy,* ed 3, Stamford, Conn, 1999, Appleton & Lange.
Oh S: *Clinical electromyography nerve conduction studies,* ed 2, Baltimore, 1993, Williams & Wilkins.
Spinner M: *Injuries to the major branches of peripheral nerves of the forearm,* ed 2, Philadelphia, 1978, WB Saunders.

Chapter 20

Orthopaedic Neurology

Mark Wiegand, PT, PhD

1. What are the common myotomes tested in an upper and a lower quarter screening examination?

Spinal Segment Level	Myotome
C3-4	Shoulder elevation and cervical rotation
C5	Shoulder abductors and external rotators
C6	Elbow flexors and wrist extensors
C7	Elbow extensors and wrist flexors

continued

continued

Spinal Segment Level	Myotome
C8	Thumb and finger extensors
T1	Hand intrinsic muscles
T3-12	Segmental innervation of muscles in thoracic and abdominal walls
L2-3	Hip flexors
L3-4	Knee extensors
L4-5	Ankle dorsiflexors
L5	Great toe extensors, hip abductors
S1	Plantar flexors
S2-3	Foot intrinsic muscles

2. How accurate is weakness of the extensor hallicus longus (EHL) in diagnosing L5 radiculopathy?

Overall clinical accuracy is approximately 60%, with positive and negative predictive values being 0.76 and 0.60, respectively. Other studies reported lower values, but the studies were conducted in populations with a lower prevalence of the disease.

3. What is the best strength test to determine weakness of the quadriceps in patients with known L3-4 radiculopathy?

In L3 and L4 radiculopathy, unilateral quadriceps weakness was best detected by a single leg sit-to-stand test. This may not always be practical; thus testing of the knee extensors in flexion is the next best method, followed by knee extensor strength testing in the knee-extended position.

4. How accurate is muscle strength testing in the diagnosis of cervical radiculopathy?

This type of testing is fairly accurate; muscle weakness associated with cervical radiculopathy has been found to agree with surgical findings approximately 77% of the time.

5. What are the common dermatomes tested in an upper and a lower quarter screening examination?

Spinal Root	Dermatome
C1	Top of head
C2	Side of head
C3-4	Lateral neck and top of shoulder
C5	Lateral shoulder and arm
C6	Lateral forearm, thumb, and index finger
C7	Middle and ring fingers
C8	Ring and little fingers
T1-2	Medial forearm and arm

continued

Spinal Root	Dermatome
L1-2	Groin
L2-3	Anterior and medial thigh
L4	Medial lower leg
L5	Lateral lower leg and dorsum of foot
S1	Posterior lateral thigh and lower leg and lateral foot
S2	Plantar surface of foot
S3	Groin
S4	Perineum region, genitals

6. How accurate is sensory testing in the diagnosis of cervical radiculopathy?

This type of testing is fairly accurate; decreases in sensation associated with cervical radiculopathy have been found to agree with surgical findings approximately 65% of the time.

7. What are commonly tested deep tendon reflexes?

Stretch Reflex	Spinal Root Level
Jaw jerk	Trigeminal nerve **(cranial nerve V)**
Biceps	**C5** (C6)
Brachioradialis	(C5) **C6**
Triceps	**C7** (C8)
Quadriceps femoris	(L3) **L4**
Medial hamstrings, extensor digitorum brevis	**L5**
Achilles tendon	**S1** (S2)

8. How valuable are the Achilles tendon reflex and the Hoffmann reflex in detecting L5/S1 root compression?

The Achilles tendon reflex and the Hoffmann reflex (H-reflex) are not valuable in detecting L5 root compression. However, they are valuable in detecting S1 root compressions. The H-reflex is more accurate than the Achilles tendon reflex.

9. How accurate is reflex testing in the diagnosis of cervical radiculopathy?

Testing accuracy is fair; side to side reflex changes associated with cervical radiculopathy have been found to agree with surgical findings approximately 77% of the time.

10. Classify the cranial nerves, their functions, and how they are tested.

Cranial Nerve (CN)	Function	Test	Clinical Note
I—Olfactory	Smell	Place common strong smells (e.g., coffee, lemon juice, cloves) under each naris (closing untested side).	Smell may be lost posttrauma because of tearing of olfactory stria from cribriform plate of ethmoid bone (seen in whiplash, closed head injury).
II—Optic	Vision	Test visual fields; test visual acuity using a Snellen chart.	Accurate assessment of visual fields greatly aids in localization of neurologic dysfunction. For example, bitemporal hemianopia is a common clinical presentation of tumors within pituitary gland.
III—Oculomotor	Most extraocular muscles, pupil constriction, and lens accommodation	Check pupillary size for symmetry and pupillary light response; both eyes should look forward and move smoothly and symmetrically (no nystagmus). Check ability of subject to track examiner's finger, moving it up, down, and toward midline.	Dysfunction of CN III, IV, or VI produces diplopia with head held in neutral position. Patients often present with cervical deviation to correct diplopia. Cervical deviation may be mistaken for a torticollis deformity.
IV—Trochlear	Superior oblique extraocular muscle (moves eye down and in)	Test subject's ability to move eyes diagonally downward and toward midline.	See CN III.
V—Trigeminal	Sensation from face (including cornea) and motor innervation of muscles of mastication	Perform sensory testing of face; check ability to clench teeth and open mouth. Subject should blink eye with gentle brushing of cornea (tests afferent limb of corneal blink reflex).	An upper motor lesion produces little dysfunction because of bilateral innervation to muscles of mastication. Lower motor neuron lesion results in unilateral paralysis and atrophy of muscles of mastication.
VI—Abducens	Lateral rectus extraocular muscle (moves eye laterally)	Test subject's ability to move eyes away from midline.	See CN III.

continued

Cranial Nerve (CN)	Function	Test	Clinical Note
VII—Facial	Muscles of facial expression, taste, and salivation	Check symmetry and smoothness of facial expressions; both eyes should blink with corneal brushing (efferent limb of corneal blink reflex). Test taste sensation in anterior two thirds of tongue.	Swelling within facial canal results in weakness in ipsilateral facial muscles and loss of taste from ipsilateral anterior two thirds of tongue (Bell's palsy).
VIII—Vestibulo-cochlear	Hearing and vestibular function (balance)	Rub fingers by each ear. Subject should hear equally from both ears. Rinne test and Weber's test can be performed: move head slowly side to side and rotate head (vestibuloocular reflex). Eyes should move in opposite direction of head movement. Check for nystagmus.	Common cause of cochlear damage to this nerve is an acoustic neuroma— a tumor of the Schwann cells that myelinate this nerve.
IX—Glosso-pharyngeal	Gag reflex, swallowing, taste, and salivation	Check gag reflex; check taste sensation in posterior tongue.	Lesions of this nerve seldom occur alone. Sudden pain of unknown cause that begins in throat and radiates down side of neck in front of ear to posterior mandible usually precipitated by swallowing or protrusion of jaw is known as glossopharyngeal neuralgia.
X—Vagus	Phonation, swallowing, thoracic and abdominal viscera regulation	Have subject say "ah"; observe elevation of soft palate.	Lesions result in hoarse voice and difficulty swallowing. Patient often complains of food and fluid regurgitation into nasal cavity.
XI—Accessory	Trapezius and sternocleidomastoid	Test trapezius and sternocleidomastoid muscles.	Usually related to radical neck surgery (as in resection of laryngeal carcinomas) that involves dissection of lymph nodes.

continued

continued

Cranial Nerve (CN)	Function	Test	Clinical Note
XII—Hypo-glossal	Tongue	Stick tongue straight out and observe for symmetric movement of tongue.	Upper motor neuron lesion results in weakness without atrophy and deviation to side opposite lesion. Lower motor neuron lesion results in paralysis and atrophy of tongue muscles on affected side, and tongue deviates to same side as lesion. Common causes are metastatic tumors or cerebral infarction.

11. Define referred pain and radicular pain.

- Referred pain—pain that is felt at a site removed from the source of involvement. It may be caused by irritation of a nerve root or by tissue supplied by the same nerve root. Cardiogenic pain may be referred to the left axilla and left arm region because of the shared sensory distribution of the T2 spinal nerve (intercostobrachial nerve), and spinal segments that receive afferent pain from the gallbladder also receive afferent input from the shoulder region.
- Radicular pain—a specific type of referred pain that is felt in a dermatome, myotome, or sclerotome of an involved peripheral nerve root. Compression of the C5 nerve root may affect sensation on the anterior shoulder.

12. What is a "burner" or "stinger"?

A burner or a stinger is a traction or compression injury to a cervical nerve root or brachial plexus trunk. Often the injury involves the C5 or C6 nerve root or upper trunk of the brachial plexus, with burning, numbness, tingling, or weakness in the distribution of the involved root or trunk. The mechanism of injury can involve distraction of the pectoral girdle from the neck, either through excessive shoulder girdle depression or through forced hyperlateral flexion of the neck. Forced oblique hyperextension of the neck may also cause ipsilateral compression injuries of the cervical nerve roots or upper brachial plexus trunks.

13. Define the terms anesthesia, paresthesia, and dysesthesia.

The root word *-esthesia* means "feeling" or "sensation."

- Anesthesia—the complete lack of sensation in a particular dermatome, peripheral nerve distribution, or region. The prefix *an-* means "none."
- Paresthesia—abnormal sensation, often described as pins and needles. The prefix *para-* means "aside" or "beyond."
- Dysesthesia—unpleasant sensations that occur in response to a usually benign stimulus. The prefix *dys-* generally means "bad." Dysesthesia has been described as "Dante-esque type of pain."

14. What are hypoesthesia and hyperesthesia?

- Hypoesthesia—diminished sensation
- Hyperesthesia—heightened sensation

15. What is a syrinx?

A syrinx is a neuroglial cell–lined, fluid-filled cavity. The Latin word *syrinx* means "tube." When this occurs within the spinal cord, the condition is known as syringomyelia; in the brain stem it is called syringobulbia. The cause of a syrinx is not fully understood; possible mechanisms of pathology are associated with the accumulation of cerebrospinal fluid within the spinal cord or brain stem, genetic malformations, and the proliferation and subsequent regression of embryonic cell rests. The syrinx generally is restricted to the cervical and upper thoracic regions, with extensions into the medulla occurring occasionally.

16. Describe the signs and symptoms of syrinx.

- If the cavity is within the central canal, it will interrupt the decussating spinothalamic tract fibers, and the patient will experience bilateral loss of pain and temperature sensations around the level of the lesion.
- If the cavity extends laterally into the lateral funiculus of the spinal cord, the lateral corticospinal pathway will be involved, with ipsilateral upper motor neuron signs and symptoms.
- Patient symptoms may include gastrointestinal disturbances, including nausea, vomiting, eating disturbances, and weight loss. This is often caused by involvement of neural regions that mediate esophageal reflexes and gastrointestinal reflexes.
- Joint arthropathy may be seen in individuals with syringomyelia. It has been reported that syringomyelia is the second most common cause of Charcot's joint.

17. What is Horner syndrome?

It is a disease in which there is an interruption of sympathetic nervous system innervation to the head and face region. It is usually caused by a brain stem lesion.

18. List signs and symptoms of Horner syndrome.

- Miosis—constricted pupil (from uncompensated parasympathetic nervous system input to pupil)
- Ptosis—drooping of the eyelid (from lost sympathetic innervation of the levator palpebrae superioris tarsal muscle)
- Enophthalmos—eyeball appears to be sunken into its socket
- Anhidrosis—absence of sweat production on affected side of face
- Flushing—increased superficial blood flow on affected side of face

19. List some of the special neurologic tests and explain their clinical importance.

Test	Description	Response	Clinical Importance
Babinski's sign (extensor plantar)	Plantar surface of foot is stroked with key or fingernail in a sweeping motion from posterior and lateral border toward ball of foot.	Extension of great toe, with or without fanning of other toes	Indicates upper motor neuron lesion.

continued

continued

Test	Description	Response	Clinical Importance
Oppenheim reflex	Anterior border of tibia is stroked.	Presence of Babinski's sign	If Babinski's sign present, indicates upper motor neuron lesion.
Hoffmann's sign	Distal phalanx of index, middle, or ring finger is subjected to rapid, gentle stroking.	Reflexive flexion of thumb distal interphalangeal joint or distal interphalangeal joint of any other finger not struck	If present, indicates upper motor neuron lesion.
Bulbocavernous reflex	Dorsum of penis is tapped.	Retraction of bulbocavernous portion of penis and contraction of anal sphincter	Absence of reflex indicates damage to pudendal nerve, sacral autonomic efferent nerves, or upper motor neuron.
Abdominal reflex	Upper or lower abdominal musculature is gently stroked.	Motion of umbilicus toward stroking	Reduction or absence indicates upper motor neuron damage or involvement of pertinent spinal level reflexes (T7-9, upper abdominal region; T11-12, lower abdominal region).
Romberg's sign	Subject stands with feet close together and then closes eyes.	Subject increases sway or falls with eyes closed	Indicates dorsal (sensory) column disease or pathology.
Rapidly alternating movements	Subject performs rapid forearm pronation and supination or ankle plantar flexion and dorsiflexion.	Inability to perform movement (dysdiadochokinesia)	Indicates ipsilateral cerebellar dysfunction, especially lateral hemispheres.
Finger to nose	Subject extends finger away from face and then toward nose, and repeats this movement.	Subject able to perform movement smoothly, correctly estimating distances and location	If movement is not smooth or there is overshooting or undershooting of movement, then may indicate cerebellar dysfunction (asynergy).

20. Who was Babinski?

Joseph Felix François Babinski was a French physician born in Paris in 1857. He trained under the famed neurologist Jean Martin Charcot. Babinski first described the "cutaneous plantar reflex" in 1896. In that paper, he described the existence of a similar response in infants that was present until approximately 7 months of age. Babinski attributed the presence of this reflex in adults to involvement of the pyramidal tract. The Babinski sign is also called the extensor plantar response.

21. Define the terms light touch, two-point discrimination, and stereognosis.

- Light touch—assesses the ability of the patient to perceive the application of soft brushing to the skin. The sensation of light touch is carried by the anterolateral system (spinothalamic) and dorsal column-medial lemniscal system. A person who has complete absence of light touch sensation generally has peripheral nerve or spinal cord damage.
- Two-point discrimination—assesses the ability of the patient to perceive the application of two points of contact applied simultaneously to the skin as one or two points. The determination of this is a function of the density of Merkel receptors in the skin (palm, high density of receptors; back, low density) and the integrity of the dorsal column-medial lemniscal system. Static two-point discrimination sense is transmitted to the spinal cord by slowly adapting large diameter (type I) afferent nerves, while moving two-point discrimination testing evaluates rapidly adapting fibers.
- Stereognosis—the ability to recognize common objects (e.g., keys, coins) placed in the hand without visual clues. If the patient is unable to name the object, and other touch sensory modalities are intact, it suggests damage in the contralateral parietal cortex.

22. What is the inter-rater and intra-rater reliability of:

A. SEMMES-WEINSTEIN MONOFILAMENT TESTING FOR LIGHT TOUCH?

Reports of inter-rater reliability for the assessment of light touch using Semmes-Weinstein monofilaments have ranged from good to only slight or fair, while intra-rater reliability has been assessed as moderate to good. Inconsistency of standardized testing measures and variations in peripheral nerve tested and the presence or absence of pathology in the subject may explain the variation in reports on light touch reliability.

B. VIBRATION SENSIBILITY TESTING?

Vibration testing stimulates Pacinian corpuscles and assesses the function of large diameter rapidly adapting peripheral nerves and the dorsal column-medial lemniscal central pathways. Using mechanical testing devices, the intra-rater reliability of the assessment of vibration sense has been described as good. Moderate reliability has been reported for inter-rater reliability. Age and height were associated with minimal threshold values of the feet but not of the hands as determined through multiple regression analysis.

C. TWO-POINT DISCRIMINATION SENSIBILITY TESTING?

While numerous studies have described the reliability of two-point discrimination testing, interpreting these results to apply them to clinical practice has been hampered by the lack of standardized testing procedures and the inability to quantify subject cognitive function. Reliability testing has ranged from moderate and good to poor. The cooperation of the subject and the ability of the subject to attend to the stimulus have been suggested to influence two-point discrimination measures, as do central training effects.

There appears to be little carry-over between static two-point discrimination tests and function, although moving two-point discrimination testing (which tests rapidly adapting afferent fibers) has been shown to correlate with object identification tests. Likewise, the sensitivity of two-point discrimination testing to detect change over time is poor.

Reports of the reliability of two-point discrimination testing vary according to the age and sex of subjects, the peripheral nerve tested, and whether the subject is symptomatic or asymptomatic. Testing procedures also vary with the starting position (wide or narrow distances), the amount of pressure applied, and the instrument used to apply the stimulus.

It is questionable whether any reliability measures of sensibility can be used as a reference to judge the presence of pathology. It is recommended that results from any sensory testing procedures not be used as the sole means of developing diagnoses of peripheral or central nervous system origin.

Bibliography

Adams RD, Victor M, Ropper AH: *Principles of neurology,* New York, 1997, McGraw-Hill.
Feinberg JH: Burners and stingers, *Phys Med Clin N Am* 11:771-784, 2000.
Gilroy J: *Basic neurology,* ed 3, New York, 2000, McGraw-Hill.
Haymore J: A neuron in a haystack: advanced neurologic assessment, *AACN Clin Issues* 15:568-581, 2004.
Lance JW: The Babinski sign, *J Neurol Neurosurg Psychiatry* 73:360-362, 2002.
Lundborg G, Rosen B: The two-point discrimination tests—time for a re-appraisal? *J Hand Surg (Br)* 29B(5):418-422, 2004.
Lundy-Eckman L: *Neuroscience: fundamentals for rehabilitation,* Philadelphia, 1998, WB Saunders.
Magee DJ: *Orthopedic assessment,* ed 3, Philadelphia, 1997, WB Saunders.
Milhorat TH: Classification of syringomyelia, *Neurosurg Focus* 8:1-6, 2000.
Novak C et al: Establishment of reliability in the evaluation of hand sensibility, *Plast Reconstruct Surg* 93:311-322, 1993.
Peters EW et al: The reliability of assessment of vibration sense, *Acta Neurol Scand* 107:293-298, 2003.
Rainville J et al: Comparison of four tests of quadriceps strength in L3 or L4 radiculopathies, *Spine* 28:2466-2471, 2003.
Rozental TD et al: Intra- and interobserver reliability of sensibility testing in asymptomatic individuals, *Ann Plast Surg* 44:605-609, 2000.
Shy ME et al: Therapeutics and Technology Assessment Subcommittee of the American Academy of Neurology. Quantitative sensory testing, *Neurology* 60:898-904, 2003.
Umphred DA: *Neurological rehabilitation,* ed 2, St Louis, 1990, Mosby.
Viikari-Juntra E, Porras M, Laasonen EM: Validity of clinical tests in the diagnosis of root compression in cervical disc disease, *Spine* 14:253-257, 1989.
Waxman SG: *Correlative neuroanatomy,* ed 23, Stamford, Conn, 1996, Appleton & Lange.
Yoss RE et al: Significance of symptoms and signs in localization of involved root in cervical disc protrusions, *Neurology* 7:673-683, 1999.
Yuras S: Syringomyelia: an expanding problem, *J Am Acad Nurse Pract* 12:22-24, 2000.

Chapter 21

Clinical Research and Data Analysis

Frank B. Underwood, PT, PhD, ECS

1. What is research?

Research is a controlled, systematic approach to obtain an answer to a question. **Experimental research** involves the manipulation of a variable and measurement of the effects of this manipulation. **Nonexperimental research** does not manipulate the environment but may describe the relationship between different variables, obtain information about opinions or policies, or describe current practice. **Basic research** is generally thought of as laboratory-based research, in which the researcher has control over nearly all aspects of the environment and subjects. **Clinical** or **applied research** usually uses entire, intact organisms in a more natural environment.

2. What are variables?

Variables are measurements or phenomena that can assume more than one value or more than one category. A **categorical** or **discrete variable** is one that can assume only certain values and often is **qualitative** (no quantity or numerical value implied). **Continuous variables** are ones that can assume a wide range of possible values and are usually **quantitative** in nature.

3. Define independent variable and dependent variable.

- **Independent variable**—the variable that is manipulated by the researcher
- **Dependent variable**—the variable that is measured by the researcher

Independent variables often are qualitative, and dependent variables usually are quantitative. The different permutations of the independent variable are called **levels.** To be an independent variable, there must be at least two levels; if some aspect of the research has only one possible value or category, it is a **constant.**

4. Describe other types of variables.

Extraneous or **confounding** variables are phenomena that are not of interest to the researcher but may have an effect on the value of the dependent variable. Extraneous variables must be controlled as much as possible, usually by holding some aspect of the research constant. A **covariate** is a phenomenon that affects the dependent variable and is not of interest to the researcher, but that the researcher is unable to control.

5. How accurate are measurements?

The observed measurement of any phenomenon is composed of a **true score** and **error.** Error may be systematic, in which case all scores are increased or decreased by a constant amount, or random. Systematic error generally is the result of using the measurement instrument incorrectly or improper calibration of the instrument. Random error is precisely that—random. Even if the true score is constant, and there is no systematic error, repeated measurements of a phenomenon do not produce identical scores. It is generally assumed that the effects of all of the sources of random error cancel each other, such that the measured score is the best estimate of the true score. If the true score is constant, repeating the measurement and calculating an average score may be a better estimate of the true score. If the true score is labile or is altered as a consequence of the measurement, repeated measurements may reduce the accuracy of the measurement.

6. Define measurement reliability.

Reliability is related to consistency or repeatability. In the absence of a change in the true score, how similar are repeated measurements of the same phenomenon? **Intra-rater reliability** is a measure of how consistent an individual is at measuring a constant phenomenon, **inter-rater reliability** refers to how consistent different individuals are at measuring the same phenomenon, and **instrument reliability** pertains to the tool used to obtain the measurement. If a measurement cannot be performed reliably, it is difficult to ascribe changes in the dependent variable to the effects of the independent variable, rather than measurement error.

7. Describe statistical procedures used to estimate reliability.

The **intraclass correlation coefficient (ICC)**, which is based on an **analysis of variance (ANOVA)** statistical procedure, is a popular means of estimating reliability. A means of measuring absolute concordance is the kappa statistic. In the past, a **Pearson** or **Spearman correlation** procedure often was used to estimate reliability; these procedures are insufficient as measures of reliability because they measure covariance, not agreement.

8. Define measurement validity.

It is an indication of whether the measurement is an accurate representation of the phenomenon of interest. Some clinical measurements have obvious validity. For example, using a **goniometer** to measure the angle between two bones with the joint as the axis is generally accepted as a valid indication of the status of the tissue that limits motion at that joint. For other measurements, the relationship between what is measured and what is inferred from the measurement is more tenuous. To establish the validity of a clinical test, a more direct measurement that is considered a **gold standard** is established. If acceptable numbers of patients with a positive Lachman's test have anterior cruciate ligament tears and those without tears have a negative Lachman's test, the Lachman's test is considered a valid test for anterior cruciate ligament integrity. There is no universal definition of **acceptable numbers;** this is left to the researcher to defend and the clinician to accept or reject.

9. What is a research design?

A research design is a plan or structure of the means used to answer the research question or to gather the information for a nonexperimental study. There are three basic designs for experimental research:

1. A **completely randomized design** uses a single independent variable and assigns different groups of subjects to each level of the independent variable. Because each subject receives only one type of treatment, this design is also called a **between-subjects design.** If the independent variable is the type of brace and there are three levels (i.e., three different braces are being used), then an individual subject would be measured while using only one of the three braces.
2. A **repeated measures design** uses a single independent variable and measures each subject under all levels of the independent variable. If the independent variable is the dosage of a drug and levels are 200, 400, and 600 mg/day, then each subject would be measured while taking each of the three dosages.
3. A **factorial design** uses two or more independent variables. A **completely randomized factorial design** is one in which all of the independent variables are independent factors, meaning an individual subject is measured under only one condition. If the two independent variables are type of brace and dosage of a drug, and there are three levels of each variable, then nine groups of subjects would be studied. A **within-subjects factorial design** measures each subject in all levels of all variables. Using the brace and dosage variables, each subject would be measured with each brace and dosage (e.g., brace A and 200 mg, brace A and 400 mg, brace A and 600 mg). A **mixed factorial design** uses at least one independent factor and at least one repeated factor. If subjects are assigned to only one brace, but are measured with all three drug dosages, the design is mixed.

10. Which descriptive statistics are most useful for describing a set of data?

It depends on the data. If the data are distributed normally, the three measures of central tendency are equal; in this case, the **mean** is most often used to describe the typical performance. If there are a few scores at one extreme or the other in the set of data, the **median** is considered the best measure of central tendency. For example, in the data set 2, 4, 5, 7, 83, the mean is 20.2, and the median is 5; 5 is more descriptive of the typical score than 20.2. The **standard deviation** (or **variance**) is the most descriptive value for the variability of a data set that is distributed normally, and **minimum-maximum** may be the best measure of variability in data sets that are best described with the median.

11. Are the terms normal distribution, bell curve, and gaussian distribution equivalent?

Yes, in that all three terms refer to the shape of a frequency histogram constructed using the scores from any measurement that is the sum of a true score and multiple, small, independent sources of error. Nearly any physiologic or anatomic parameter that is measured in a large group of individuals falls into a **normal distribution.** For example, suppose the maximal aerobic capacity is measured in 500 individuals selected at random. The scores are counted and grouped into increments of 5 (e.g., the number of subjects with a maximal aerobic capacity of 0 to 5, 6 to 10, 11 to 15), and the results are used to construct a bar plot with the increments on the x-axis and the number of individuals in each bin on the y-axis. If the average value was 36, and the standard deviation was 6, the resulting plot might look like the figure. Most scores were between 31 and 35, with fewer scores at each extreme. For example, the number of scores in the 6-10 range is approximately equal to the number of scores in the 51-55 range. In a perfectly normal distribution, 68% of the scores will be found within 1 standard deviation of the mean; in this example, 340 of the 500 scores should be between 26 and 38 (32 ± 6), 95% of the scores will be within 2 standard deviations of the mean, and 99% of the scores will be within 3 standard deviations of the mean.

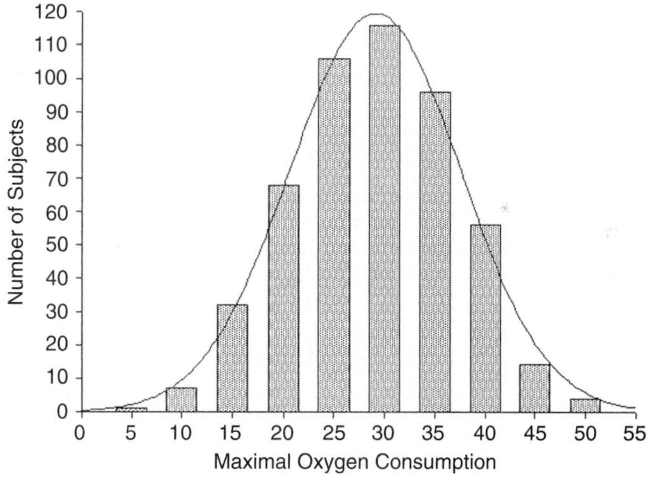

12. Are there distributions other than a normal distribution?

Yes, especially with small samples, **skewed distributions** are possible. A skewed distribution results when there are a few extreme scores at one end or the other of the distribution. For example, if most of the scores are low, but there are a few high scores, the distribution might be similar to the figure. This distribution is skewed to the right by the few extremely high scores. If there are a few extremely low scores, the distribution is skewed to the left. The direction of the skew is determined by drawing (or imagining) a line connecting the top of each bar in the histogram and stating to which side of the plot the tail extends.

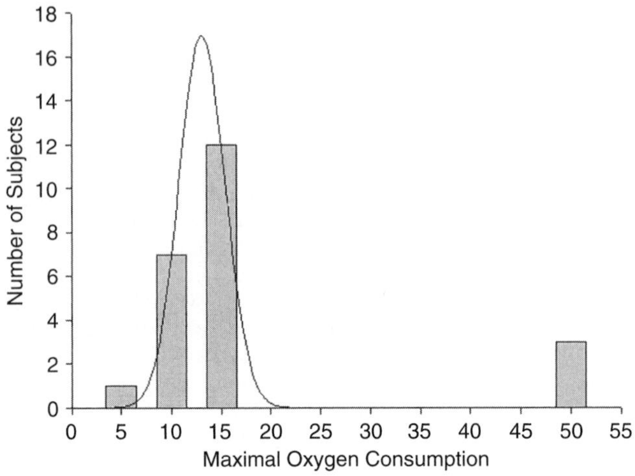

13. Can the same concepts be used with a skewed distribution; that is, are 68% of the scores within 1 standard deviation of the mean?

No. These values hold true only for a normal distribution. In the case of a skewed distribution, the median is a better descriptor of the typical score, and the minimum-maximum better describes the variability in the set of data.

14. What are inferential statistics?

When data are collected, the researcher needs to determine the probability of obtaining a particular set of scores by chance alone. The procedures used to calculate this probability are called **inferential statistics** and are the heart of testing an experimental hypothesis. There are different procedures used based on the research design, the nature of the research question (what the researcher is trying to answer), and the nature of the data.

15. Describe the fundamental concept of inferential statistics.

In the simplest case, consider a randomized design, with a single independent variable having two levels and a single dependent variable. Suppose a researcher posed the following question: What is the effect of adding neural glide techniques for the median nerve to the standard treatment for patients with carpal tunnel syndrome? The independent variable is treatment, and the levels are standard and neural glide. The dependent variable could be number of days until the patient is free of symptoms for 10 consecutive days. A sample of patients with carpal tunnel syndrome is selected at random from the population of patients with carpal tunnel syndrome, and the patients in the sample are assigned at random to one of the two treatment levels. Because the patients have been selected at random from the population, and then assigned at random to one of the two treatment groups, it is a reasonable assumption that the mean and standard deviation for the dependent variable would be the same for both treatment groups if there is no effect of adding neural glide to the standard treatment. All of the subjects are treated until the criterion for discharge is met (i.e., free of symptoms for 10 consecutive days), and the data are summarized. If the standard group recovered in an average of 40 days, with a standard deviation of 7 days, and the neural glide group recovered in 32 days, with a standard deviation of 6 days, did the treatment work? There is a difference in the average days to recovery, but is that difference large enough to conclude that it was due to the neural glide, or could it be attributed to chance alone? Perhaps the subjects in the neural glide group did not have as severe compression of the median nerve at the beginning of the study and recovered more quickly despite the neural glide. The essence of inferential hypothesis testing is to answer the following question: What is the probability of having obtained a difference in days to recovery of this magnitude as a result of random factors? If this probability is low enough, the researcher can conclude that the treatment had a beneficial effect and should become a part of standard practice.

16. How is the correct statistical test chosen?

The short answer is that it depends on the question being asked:

- If the desire is to learn about the association between two variables (e.g., the relationship between thigh girth and knee extensor force), a **correlation coefficient** should be calculated.
- If the question concerns prediction (e.g., if a patient has knee range of motion of 5 to 60 degrees on the second postoperative day, how many days will the patient likely remain in the hospital?), a **regression analysis** is appropriate.
- If the question is whether a treatment has an effect (e.g., does spinal traction reduce the signs and symptoms of a lumbosacral root compression?), a **chi-square,** analysis of variance **(ANOVA),** or ***t*-test,** which is a special case of the ANOVA, is appropriate.

However, because there are different types of data and different types of restrictions placed upon the testing, the answer is more complicated. There are four levels of data: nominal, ordinal, interval, and ratio. Information measured on a nominal scale results in a name only; that is, it does not imply a quantity. Left versus right and red versus blue are examples of nominal data. If a numeral is assigned to information on a nominal scale, a quantity is not implied; if red is coded 1 and blue is coded 2, it does not mean that blue is twice as much as red.

An ordinal scale implies a rank order, with some quantitative value. The person who finishes a race first receives the number 1, meaning this person finished the race in a shorter time than the second-place finisher. However, the amount of time between first and second place is not likely the same as the amount of time between fifth and sixth place.

For statistical purposes, there are no meaningful differences between an interval and a ratio scale; both imply not only a rank order but also an equivalence between points on the scale. The difference between 80 and 95 is the same as the difference between 25 and 40; in both cases, it is 15.

For a correlation study, a **Spearman rho** (for Spearman, who developed the procedure, and rank order) is used for ordinal data. A **Pearson correlation coefficient** is calculated for interval data. In both cases, the coefficient can vary between −1.00 and +1.00. A value of zero means that there is no correlation, and a value of 1.00 signifies the correlation is perfect. If the sign is +, the value of one variable increases as the other increases. If the sign is −, the value of one variable decreases as the other increases.

For experimental studies, those designed to determine if there is a difference, a chi-square is computed for data that are nominal. There is some disagreement regarding the appropriate analysis when the data meet the definition of ordinal or interval. It is almost universally agreed that to perform a traditional ANOVA, the sets of data should have a normal distribution, and the variance of the sets of data should be similar (the definition of similar is usually lacking; a rule of thumb is that the variance of one set should be no more than twice the other set). There are formal tests that can be used to determine whether the data are normally distributed, and whether the variances are equal; these are beyond the scope of this book, and are generally of little or no interest to the clinician. Some authors further state that the data must meet the definition of interval or ratio data; in fact, some researchers ignore the more important requirements of normal distribution and equality of variance and claim that the tests are robust enough that any data on an interval or ratio scale can be analyzed with a traditional ANOVA. However, the scale of the data was not an issue when the traditional ANOVA approach was developed. Therefore if the data are normally distributed, and the variances are equal, then a traditional ANOVA is appropriate, regardless of the scale of the data. Often, especially with the small sample sizes usually used in rehabilitation research, the two requirements of normal distribution and equality of variance are not met, even with ratio data, and a traditional ANOVA is inappropriate.

If the question is whether two groups differ on the dependent variable, and the data are normally distributed with equal variances, a *t*-test is appropriate. The *t*-test is a special case of the ANOVA, developed to make the calculations easier. With software, it is just as easy to use an ANOVA because the information is the same. If there are more than two levels of a single independent variable, or if there is more than one independent variable, the ANOVA can be extended to handle the variables. The type of ANOVA performed is often referred to by the number of rows and columns that are required to represent all of the permutations of the independent variables. A $2 \times 3 \times 2$ ANOVA means that there were three independent variables (because there are three numerals), two of the independent variables had two levels, and the third variable had three levels (the value of the numerals). The exception is a 1×4 ANOVA, which has only one independent variable, with four levels; if the value of one of the numerals is 1, it cannot represent a variable (because, by definition, variables have more than one possible value). If the data are not normally distributed, or the variances are not equal, a nonparametric equivalent is appropriate.

17. Differentiate between parametric and nonparametric statistical procedures.

Parametric statistical procedures are performed on data that have a normal distribution, such as the distribution observed in a **population. Nonparametric procedures** are performed on data that do not have a normal distribution, that is, a skewed distribution, as often is observed in a **sample.** Parametric procedures include the ANOVA and *t*-test, and nonparametric procedures include the chi-square, Kruskal-Wallis, and Spearman rho. As mentioned earlier, some authors add the requirement that the data have the characteristics of an interval or ratio scale in order to conduct parametric procedures, but this is debatable. Nonparametric procedures are often regarded as second-class procedures, used only when the data are extremely skewed. However, nonparametric procedures are nearly as powerful as their parametric equivalents when the data are normally distributed, and more powerful than parametric procedures when the data are skewed. Because of the small sample sizes typically used in orthopaedic and rehabilitation research, nonparametric procedures should likely be used more often.

18. How is the appropriate type of statistical analysis determined?

		Samples Used	
Purpose of Analysis	**Nature of Distribution**	**Independent**	**Related**
Show a difference	Normal	ANOVA	Repeated measures ANOVA
	Skewed	Chi-square for frequency; Mann-Whitney or Kruskal-Wallis	McNemar's for frequency; Wilcoxon signed-rank
Determine degree of association	Normal	Pearson or linear regression	
	Skewed	Contingency coefficient for frequency; Spearman rho	

19. Other than intuition and clinical experience, how can the best clinical tests be identified?

The performance of clinical tests (e.g., straight-leg raise, Lachman test, shoulder impingement tests) can be measured in many ways, some more enlightening than others. The point of a clinical test is to sort patients into two basic categories: those who truly have the disorder and those who truly do not have the disorder. Depending on the situation, disease, dysfunction, or pathology can be substituted for the term disorder.

It is often difficult or hazardous to know with absolute certainty whether a disorder is present. For example, the definitive test for a ruptured anterior cruciate ligament (ACL) is direct visualization of the ligament, with an arthrotomy, arthroscopy, or, potentially, MRI. Obviously, it would be unreasonably hazardous to subject all patients with a clinical history suggestive of an ACL rupture to a surgical procedure, and MRI is expensive. These definitive tests are considered gold standards against which the results of a less invasive or less expensive test are compared.

The typical approach to establishing the performance of a clinical test is to conduct both the clinical test and the definitive test (gold standard) on a group of patients, some of whom have the disorder and some of whom are free of the disorder. Specific values are then calculated, and the clinician can determine how confident one can be in the results of the test. The clinical test is not always what is typically considered a test: It can be a specific question asked during the patient interview (such as "Did you hear a pop before your knee gave way?"), or it can be a combination of tests and interview information, such as whether the straight-leg raise is positive and the patient has pain radiating from the back to the buttock and down the posterior thigh.

20. What is meant by sensitivity, specificity, positive predictive value, and negative predictive value?

These terms are used to describe the usefulness of the clinical tests described above. It is easiest to comprehend these values if a 2 × 2 table is constructed, with the results of the definitive test entered in the columns, and the results of the clinical test entered in the rows. A study conducted by Roach et al. can illustrate the calculation and use of these values. Among other variables, the researchers determined the usefulness of asking patients with degenerative disk disease (DDD) and low back pain whether they also had pain radiating down the lower member; this was the clinical test used to predict the presence of spinal stenosis (the target disorder). Out of 17 patients with the target disorder (spinal stenosis), 16 had a positive clinical test (that is, they had pain radiating down the lower member). Out of 89 patients with DDD and low back pain but without the target disorder, 70 had pain radiating down the lower member. The table illustrates how to calculate the values.

		Reality		
		Stenosis	**No Stenosis**	**Row Total**
Radiating leg pain	Positive	a = 16	b = 70	a + b = 86
	Negative	c = 1	d = 19	c + d = 20
Column total		a + c = 17	b + d = 89	a + b + c + d = 106

Sensitivity is the proportion of patients with a disorder who also have a positive clinical test; it is the probability of having a true-positive test. It is calculated by dividing the number of patients with the target disorder and a positive test by the number of patients with the target disorder: Sensitivity = a ÷ (a + c). Using the example above, 16 ÷ (16 + 1) = 0.94. This means that of 100 patients with stenosis, 94 will have pain radiating down the lower member.

Specificity is the proportion of patients without the disorder who also have a negative clinical test; it is the probability of having a true-negative test. It is calculated by dividing the number of patients without the target disorder and a negative test by the number of patients without the target disorder: Specificity = d ÷ (d + b). Thus 19 ÷ (19 + 70) = 0.21. This means that of 100 patients with DDD but without stenosis, only 21 will not have pain radiating down the lower member.

Sensitivity and specificity deal with reality; they are based on knowing for certain whether the target disorder is present. The reason clinicians use a clinical test in the first place is because they are trying to determine whether the target disorder is present; **reality** usually is unknown.

21. Do other performance characteristics depend on a knowledge of reality?

No. Positive predictive values (PPVs) and negative predictive values (NPVs) deal with the situation of having a patient and the results of a clinical test. This is the usual situation that confronts a clinician.

PPV is the proportion of patients with a positive clinical test who also have the target disorder. It is calculated by dividing the number of patients with a positive clinical test and the target disorder by the total number of patients with a positive clinical test: PPV = a ÷ (a + b) = 16 ÷ (16 + 70) = 0.19. This means that of 100 people with pain radiating down the lower member, only 19 will have stenosis.

NPV is the proportion of patients with a negative clinical test who also do not have the target disorder. It is calculated by dividing the number of patients with a negative clinical test and free of the target disorder by the total number of patients with a negative clinical test: NPV = d ÷ (d + c) = 19 ÷ (19 + 1) = 0.95. This means that of 100 people without pain radiating down the lower member, 95 will not have stenosis.

22. What is the principal drawback to the PPV and NPV?

These values change with changes in the prevalence of the target disorder; if the target disorder is uncommon, there are many more false-positive results, and the PPV goes down. Because the sensitivity and specificity deal with reality, they are not affected by changes in the prevalence of the target disorder.

23. Is there a way to combine the best characteristics of sensitivity, specificity, PPV, and NPV?

Yes; **likelihood ratios** are often considered a useful approach for clinical decision making. Likelihood ratios are expressed as **odds** and are calculated from values used to calculate sensitivity and specificity. The likelihood ratio of a positive test **(LR+)** is the quotient of the sensitivity and the complement of the specificity, i.e., the sensitivity divided by 1 minus the specificity. In the example above, the LR+ is 0.94 ÷ (1 – 0.21), or 1.19. This means that a patient with the target disorder (i.e., stenosis) is 1.19 times more likely to have a positive test (i.e., radiating leg pain) than a patient without the target disorder. Another way of viewing a LR+ value is that it gives the odds that a patient with the target disorder would be expected to have a positive test. A likelihood ratio of 1.00 is of no value; a patient with a positive test is equally likely to have the target disorder as not.

The likelihood ratio of a negative test **(LR–)** is the quotient of the complement of the sensitivity and the specificity, i.e., 1 minus the sensitivity divided by the specificity. In this example, the LR– is 1 – (0.94 ÷ 0.21) = 0.29. This means that a patient with the target disorder (stenosis) is 0.29 times as likely (or only about 3/10 as likely) to have a positive test as a patient without the target disorder. An alternative way of viewing the LR– is to determine the inverse of the LR– (or divide the specificity by the complement of the sensitivity) and use this value to decide how much more likely an individual without the target disorder is to have a negative test than an individual with the target disorder. The reciprocal of 0.29 is 3.5 (or, 0.21 ÷ [1 – 0.94] = 3.5); therefore an individual without stenosis is 3.5 times more likely to have a negative test than an individual with stenosis. Either approach is appropriate, but some clinicians find the second method more intuitive. An LR– value of 1.00 is equivalent to flipping a coin to determine the meaning of a negative test.

24. Define the terms prevalence and incidence.

Prevalence is the proportion of a population who has a particular disorder or condition at a specific point in time. If in a population of 233,658 there are 253 individuals with carpal tunnel syndrome (CTS), the prevalence of CTS is 253 ÷ 233,658 = 0.0010828. Because prevalence typically is a small number, it usually is multiplied by an appropriate constant and expressed as the number of cases per 1000 or 10,000. In this example, the prevalence of CTS would be about 1 per 1000.

Incidence is the rate of development of new cases of a disorder in a particular at-risk population over a given period of time. As with prevalence, the value usually is small and is multiplied by an appropriate constant and expressed as the number of cases per the constant for a given period of time. If a new manufacturing plant opens and employs 2355 people, and 89 people develop CTS during the calendar year from January 1, 1999, to December 31, 1999, the incidence of CTS is (89 ÷ 2355) × 1000 = 38 cases for that 1-year period. One difficulty in calculating incidence is in determining the denominator; it is unlikely that there will be 2355 people employed by the plant on January 1 and December 31. If the population is not constant, the size of the population at some point is selected to represent the size for the entire time period; usually, it is the midpoint of the time period, that is, July 1, 1999, in our example. Another difficulty is in defining the at-risk population. If one is determining the incidence of pregnancy, obviously males, premenarche girls, and postmenopausal women would not be included in the denominator. In the manufacturing plant that employs 2355 people, it may be that only the 985 people who work with impact tools are at risk for CTS.

25. Discuss risk ratios and odds ratios.

These are used to determine how likely it is that an individual with a particular risk factor will or will not develop a disease. The calculation of these ratios is similar to the calculation of likelihood ratios, PPVs, and NPVs. A **risk ratio** is calculated by dividing the incidence for the disorder for one group by the incidence for the disorder for another group; the two groups are considered to be **at risk** or **not at risk.** For example, if the manufacturing plant employs 2355 people and 985 of the employees use impact tools, the following question could be asked: "What is the risk of an employee who uses impact tools developing carpal tunnel syndrome (CTS) as compared to an employee who does not use impact tools?" A 2 × 2 table could be constructed as follows:

		Developed CTS During 1999?		
		Yes	**No**	**Row Total**
Impact tool use?	Yes	a = 297	b = 688	a + b = 985
	No	c = 43	d = 1327	c + d = 1370
Column total		a + c = 340	b + d = 2015	a + b + c + d = 2355

The incidence (expressed as a proportion) of CTS in the at-risk group is a ÷ (a + b) = 297 ÷ 985 = 0.30, and the incidence of CTS in the not-at-risk group is c ÷ (c + d) = 43 ÷ 1370 = 0.03. The risk ratio is then [a ÷ (a + b)] ÷ [c ÷ (c + d)] = 0.30 ÷ 0.03 = 10. An individual who uses impact tools is 10 times more likely to develop CTS as compared to an individual who does not use impact tools. As with PPVs and NPVs, which also are calculated using the data in the rows of the table, the risk ratio is changed easily by changes in the prevalence of the condition; the more rare the disorder, the higher the risk ratio.

An **odds ratio** is calculated using the information in the columns of the table, and similar to sensitivity and specificity, the odds ratio is not changed by changes in prevalence. The odds that someone with CTS uses impact tools is a ÷ c = 297 ÷ 43 = 6.9. The odds that someone without CTS uses impact tools is b ÷ d = 688 ÷ 1327 = 0.52. The odds ratio is (a ÷ c) ÷ (b ÷ d) = 6.9 ÷ 0.52 = 13.3, which means that someone with CTS is 13.3 times more likely to use impact tools. In contrast to the risk ratio, the odds ratio is not changed by changes in prevalence of the disorder.

26. Discuss how a clinician can judge the effectiveness of a treatment or prevention program.

One approach to assessing treatment effectiveness is by using **relative risk reduction (RRR), absolute risk reduction (ARR),** and the **number needed to treat (NNT)** estimates. To illustrate the use of these concepts, consider the effectiveness of an educational program (a back school) for the reduction of the incidence of low back pain (LBP) in an industrial setting. The fundamental question is: Does a back school reduce the rate of LBP, and if so, is it cost-effective? Because a history of LBP before attending the back school is likely to have an impact on the development of LBP during the study period, people enrolled in the study would need to be divided into those with and those without a history of LBP. After completing the back school, the subjects would be followed for a period of time, and the number of cases of LBP that occur among the subjects with and without a history of LBP would be recorded for subjects who had attended and who had not attended the back school. These data along with the calculation of the incidence are used to produce the RRR, ARR, and NNT values:

		Incidence of LBP (As a Proportion)		*RRR*	*ARR*	*NNT*
		Control (C), no back school attendance	**Experimental (E), back school attendance**	**C − E ÷ C**	**C − E**	**1 ÷ C − E**
Prior history of LBP	Yes	0.43	0.17	0.61	0.26	4
	No	0.13	0.06	0.54	0.07	14

The RRR values of 0.61 and 0.54 signify that the risk of developing LBP is reduced by 61% and 54% among individuals with a prior history of LBP and individuals without a prior history of LBP, respectively. What is missing from the RRR is the fact that the ARR for individuals without a history of LBP is relatively trivial. The reciprocal of the ARR yields a value that is potentially useful; the NTT is the number of people who would have to attend the back school to prevent an episode of LBP in one person. Therefore 4 people with a prior history of LBP should be sent to the back school to prevent the development of LBP in 1 person. Of the people who do not have a history of LBP, 14 need to attend the back school to prevent LBP in 1 member of this group. If the decision were made based solely on the RRR, everyone should attend back school. By assessing the NTT values, the decision might be to send anyone with a prior history of LBP to the back school but not the people without a history of LBP.

Bibliography

Glantz SA: *Primer of biostatistics,* ed 4, New York, 1997, McGraw-Hill.

Keppel G: *Design and analysis: a researcher's handbook,* ed 3, Englewood Cliffs, NJ, 1991, Prentice Hall.

Roach KE et al: The sensitivity and specificity of pain response to activity and position in categorizing patients with low back pain, *Phys Ther* 77:730-738, 1997.

Sackett DL et al: *Clinical epidemiology: a basic science for clinical medicine,* ed 2, Boston, 1991, Little Brown.

Chapter 22

Evidence-Based Practice

Britt Smith, PT, MSPT, OCS and
Michael Dohm, MD, FAAOS

1. Define the terms evidence-based medicine (EBM) and evidence-based practice (EBP).

- EBM—the conscientious, explicit, and judicious use of current best evidence in making decisions about the care of individual patients
- EBP—the application of this EBM framework to clinical practice

2. List the components of practicing EBP.

- Asking clear, concise, and relevant questions about one's patients that are readily answerable with a literature search
- Efficiently and effectively searching the available literature for articles that might answer the questions
- Evaluating the merits of the most relevant articles from the search result, and assessing the validity and value of the most important and strongest articles for practice

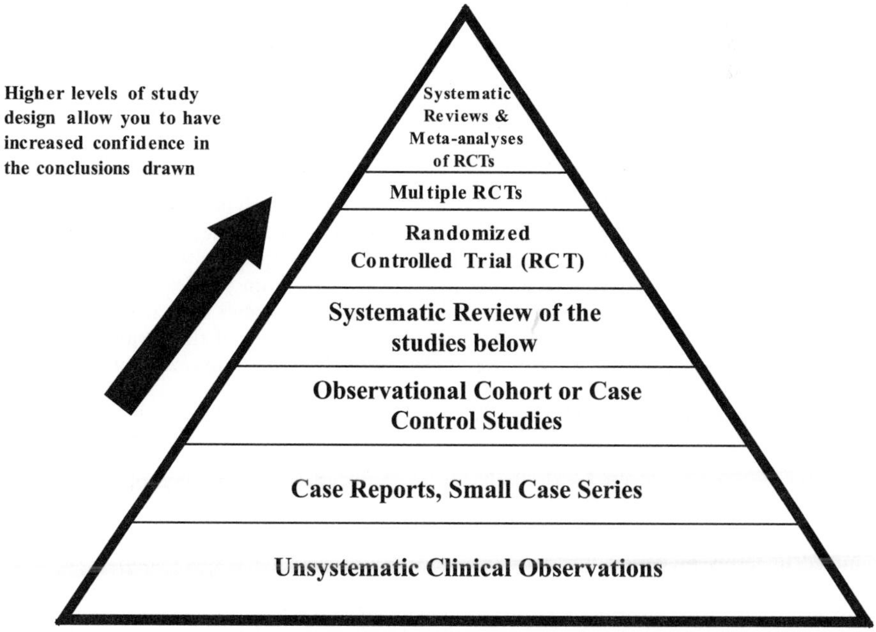

- Implementing the findings in the care of patients by forming a new practice pattern (e.g., consistent and overwhelming evidence against a therapeutic intervention from the literature or no positive effect ever shown) or supporting the practice pattern begun with the patient

3. What are the sources of the hierarchy of evidence?

The hierarchy or "cascade" of evidence suggested by Straus et al. is based on available sources of evidence (see figure).

4. Define the different study types in a hierarchical manner.

- **Randomized controlled trials**—Individuals are selected at a specific time in the history of a diagnosis and randomly allocated to two or more groups; one is an intervention group and the other group is a control, or no intervention, group. Randomization reduces the risk of bias caused by group differences. These studies are sine qua non for evaluating cause-effect and therapeutic efficacy.
- **Cohort study**—Individuals assembled at a specific time in the history of a diagnosis are divided into two groups, and one group receives an intervention and the other does not. Efforts are made to match the groups by characteristics.
- **Case-control study**—This is a retrospective study of patients compared with characteristic-matched subjects who are not ill or have not received an intervention.
- **Case series**—In this expansion of a case study, the investigator describes observations of a series of similar cases.
- **Descriptive study**—This case study is designed to analyze factors important to cause, care, and outcome of the patient's problem. These studies are most important for generating hypotheses.

5. Why are randomized controlled trials considered the strongest methodology in studies of treatment effectiveness?

Randomization of subject assignment helps avoid selection bias in the control and intervention groups by matching of characteristics in the groups. Other research designs in randomized controlled trials that reduce the risks of biases include the blinding of the assignment of interventions to the patients and the provider, if possible (i.e., **double-blinding**); concealment of outcomes; and monitoring for contamination from other interventions. Randomized controlled trials can discern causal relationships with interventions (i.e., treatment) from other causes (e.g., spontaneous recovery) across populations.

6. What is a systematic review?

A systematic review is a thorough review and summary of the research on a particular topic about a clinical problem. The review has a specific methodology that distinguishes it from a general review. Systematic reviews should capture the homogeneity or heterogeneity of the various study methods and designs. The review's conclusions should come from studies that ask the same research questions. Simply comparing the number of positive studies with negative studies is inadequate. Systematic reviews include an assessment of the quality of the various studies and weighting of studies, with higher weight given to larger studies and randomized controlled trials.

7. What is a meta-analysis?

A meta-analysis is a variety of systematic reviews that use statistical techniques to combine and summarize quantitative results for similarly constructed studies. This method of combining the results of many studies allows an estimate of the magnitude of intervention or risk factor effect and subgroup analysis. Meta-analysis requires a high degree of homogeneity among the studies examined in terms of design, methodology, and reporting of data. Meta-analyses should be understood as narrow presentations of relevant research on a particular topic, designed to provide more precisely the positive or negative direction of an effect.

8. Describe resources in the search for evidence to clinically generated questions.

- **Evidence-based journals** (e.g., *ACP Journal Club, Evidence-Based Medicine,* and, in physical therapy, *Physical Therapy in Perspective*) summarize relevant articles.
- Accessing **Internet Web sites** is rapidly becoming the most common approach. Grateful Med and PubMed are available on the Internet along with access to Medline, EMBASE, and other databases.
- A Web site called *Hooked-on-Evidence* has been developed by the American Physical Therapy Association (APTA) to facilitate dissemination of evidence supporting physical therapy practice (http://www.apta.org/hookedonevidence/index.cfm).
- **PEDro** (http://www.pedro.fhs.usyd.edu.au/index.html) was established at the Centre for Evidence-Based Physiotherapy at the University of Sydney, Australia. PEDro is a database of clinical trials to assist in EBP, supplying bibliographic details, abstracts, and quality assessment scores of all published randomized controlled trials in physical therapy.
- The **Cochrane Collaboration** conducts systematic reviews and updates on the effects of health care (http://www.update-software.com/publications/cochrane). Access to the Cochrane Library is available through a subscription service (CD-ROM).

9. List two useful mnemonics for EBP practitioners to filter studies for clinical practice.

- **POEM** (**P**atient-**O**riented **E**vidence that **M**atters)—an article about quality of life, mortality, and morbidity. A POEM may lead a clinician directly to change practice patterns. This evidence is usually foreground knowledge.
- **DOE** (**D**isease-**O**riented **E**vidence)—an article about organ or systemic physiology, biochemistry, pathophysiology, anatomy, or biomechanics (pathomechanics). This is usually background knowledge.

10. What is a gold standard versus a reference standard in a study of a diagnostic test?

A **gold standard test** is a test that is as near as possible to 100% specificity and 100% sensitivity. **Reference standards** are criteria tests that approximate the definitive diagnosis, but are not as accurate as a gold standard test. Reference standards are most often imaging studies (e.g., MRI, ultrasound) or surgical examination (e.g., arthroscopy).

11. What are Bayes' theorems?

In 1763, Sir Thomas Bayes, a British minister and mathematician, proposed a set of theorems to express statistical probabilities. Bayes' theorems, applied to medicine, relate disease prevalence and probability with sensitivity, specificity, and predictive values. The theorems apply to the incidence of the disease in a population, the incidence of a specific clue in a disease, and the incidence of the clue in persons with the disease compared with persons without the disease.

12. Express Bayes' theorems in the form of a simple equation.

Pretest probability + Likelihood ratio = Posttest probability

"What we thought before" + "Test information" = "What we think after"

Pretest odds × Likelihood ratio = Posttest odds

13. List the principal sources for pretest probability.

- The clinician's professional and personal experiences and knowledge
- The patient's history of injury, symptoms, experience, and/or any elements that increase the suspicion of a diagnosis

- Clinical databases on the prevalence of the disease by referral to the clinic
- Published data on regional prevalence of the disease

14. How is the pretest probability determined?

Experienced skilled clinicians rely on personal experience and a cognitive process called **heuristics** or **diagnostic rules of thumb.**

Individual clinicians should develop a sense of their clinic's patient population and prevalence of disease by referral. Remember that *your clinic* has different sources of referrals, different clinical expertise and experiences, and different overall patient population than other clinics.

Pretest probability is also established by mechanism of injury, natural history of humans, and the patient's history. Stratford and Binkley provide an excellent example of a clinician establishing the pretest probability of a meniscus tear based on the clinician's knowledge of mechanism of injury, natural history, and factors from the patient's history. They present three different patients: a 14-year-old female volleyball player with anterior knee pain, a 21-year-old soccer player who twisted her knee while kicking a ball, and a 37-year-old furnace repairman who twisted his knee squatting. The estimated pretest probabilities are 1% in the volleyball player, 50% in the soccer player, and 95% in the furnace repairman:

Pretest odds = prevalence/[1 – prevalence] = pretest probability/[1 – pretest probability]

Soccer player's pretest probability = 50% = 0.50/1 – 0.50 = 1:1 = pretest odds

15. In regard to diagnostic test studies, what is a likelihood ratio?

The likelihood ratio is the likelihood that a test's results would be expected in a patient with the target disorder compared with the likelihood of the results with a patient without the disorder. The relationship of likelihood ratio can be remembered with the mnemonic **WOWO** (**w**ith **o**ver **w**ith**o**ut):

$$\text{Likelihood ratio (LR)} = \frac{\text{Likelihood of a particular test result in someone with disease}}{\text{Likelihood of the same test result in someone without disease}}$$

16. What is the difference between a positive LR and a negative LR?

The positive LR is the probability of a positive test if the disease is present (i.e., Sn) divided by the probability of a negative test if the disease is absent, whereas the negative LR is the probability of a negative test if the disease is present divided by the probability of a negative test if the disease is absent (i.e., Sp).

$$\text{Sn}/100\% - \text{Sp} = \text{LR+}$$

$$100\% - \text{Sn}/\text{Sp} = \text{LR–}$$

17. What are SnNouts and SpPins?

They are mnemonics that have been proposed to help remember the most useful aspects of tests with **moderate to high** sensitivity and specificity.

- SnNout—A test with a high **sensitivity** value (**Sn**) that when negative (**N**) helps to rule out a disease (**out**)
- SpPin—A test with a high **specificity** value (**Sp**) that when positive (**P**) helps to rule in a disease (**in**)

18. What are the advantages of sensitivity, specificity, and likelihood ratios over the concept of predictive values (positive predictive value and negative predictive value [PPV and NPV])?

PPV and NPV are the proportion of persons with a positive (or negative) test result who have (or do not have) a disease. The predictive value is the posttest probability of the disease. The problem with predictive values is that they are variable by the *population prevalence* of a disease or pretest probability of having a disease.

Sensitivity, specificity, and likelihood ratios are properties of the tests themselves and are stable or unchanging by various population risks, prevalence, or pretest probabilities. The advantage lies in the ability to compare tests, or to apply these statistics to various populations without recalculation of the values. PPV and NPV will change; sensitivity, specificity, and likelihood ratios are constants.

19. What is a nomogram?

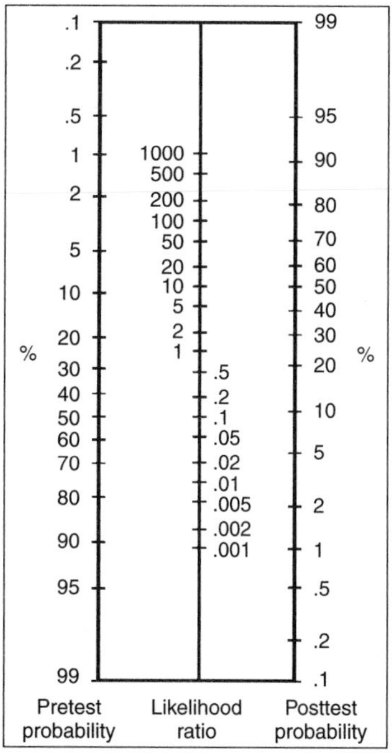

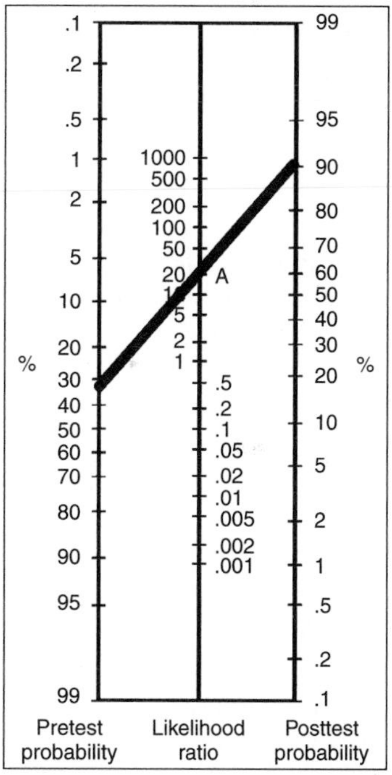

A likelihood ratio nomogram. (*From Straus S et al:* Evidence-based medicine, *ed 3, Edinburgh, 2005, Elsevier.*)

A nomogram is a graphic scale developed to facilitate the calculation of probabilities. The right-hand column is the estimated pretest probability (or prevalence) (30% in example above) of a disorder or condition (e.g., low back pain). The calculated or estimated likelihood ratio (LR+ = 20+) is represented in the middle of the graph (A). The line that projects from the pretest probability to the likelihood ratio ends on the posttest probability (90+%). Thus a nomogram simplifies the estimates of change in certainty of a diagnosis after a test is applied.

20. What is a clinical prediction rule or decision rule?

A clinical prediction rule is a clinical tool that quantifies the contributions of history, physical examination, and basic laboratory testing towards establishing a diagnosis, prognosis, or likely response to treatment in an individual patient.

21. What are some examples of clinical prediction rules (CPRs) for diagnosis?

- Ottawa ankle rule (Stiell et al, 1992)
- Ottawa knee rule (Stiell et al, 1995)
- Canadian C-spine rule (Stiell et al, 2001)
- NEXUS cervical spine study (Hoffman, 1998)

22. What is an example of a CPR for determining the likely response to treatment in an individual patient?

Flynn et al. developed a CPR for predicting which low back pain patients are most likely to benefit from spinal manipulation. The study found that if four of the five following clinical findings were positive the patient would most likely benefit from spinal manipulation (LR+ = 23).

- Episode of pain <16 days
- Pain does not extend below the knee
- FABQ work subscore <19
- Internal rotation of at least one hip >35 degrees
- Stiffness identified at one or more lumbar segment

Bibliography

Childs JD: A clinical prediction rule to identify patients with low back pain most likely to benefit from spinal manipulation: a validation study, *Ann Intern Med* 41:920-928, 2004.

Cutler P: Digits, decimals and doctors. In Cutler P, editor: *Problem solving in clinical medicine, from data to diagnosis,* ed 2, Baltimore, 1984, Williams & Wilkins.

DiFabio RP: What is 'evidence'? *J Orthop Sports Phys Ther* 30:52-55, 2000.

Eddy DM: Evidence-based medicine: a unified approach, *Health Aff (Millwood)* 24:9-17, 2005.

Elstein AS: On the origins and development of evidence-based medicine and medical decision making, *Inflamm Res* 53(suppl 2):S184-189, 2004.

Flynn T: A clinical prediction rule for classifying patients with low back pain who demonstrate short-term improvement with spinal manipulation, *Spine* 27:2835-2843, 2002.

Friedland DJ et al: *Evidence-based medicine: a framework for clinical practice,* Stamford, Conn, 1998, Appleton & Lange.

Guyatt G, Rennie D: *User's guides to the medical literature,* Chicago, Ill, 2004, AMA Press.

Haynes RB: What kind of evidence is it that evidence-based medicine advocates want health care providers and consumers to pay attention to? *BMC Health Serv Res* 2:3, 2002 (Epub 2002 Mar 6).

Herbert R, Moseley A, Sherrington C: PEDro: a database of randomized controlled trials in physiotherapy, *Health Inf Manag* 28:186-188, 1999.

Hoffman JR: Selective cervical spine radiography in blunt trauma: methodology of the National Emergency X-Radiography Utilization Study (NEXUS), *Ann Emerg Med* 32:461-469, 1998.

Maher CG et al: Challenges for evidence-based physical therapy: accessing and interpreting high-quality evidence on therapy, *Phys Ther* 84:644-654, 2004.

Richardson WS: How to practice evidence-based health care: the 6th Rocky Mountain workshop, Vail, Colo, August 1-5, 2004.

Riegelman RK: *Studying a study and testing a test,* ed 4, Philadelphia, 2000, Lippincott Williams & Wilkins.

Sackett D et al: *Evidence-based medicine: how to practice and teach EBM,* ed 3, New York, 2005, Churchill Livingstone.

Stiell IG et al: A study to develop clinical decision rules for the use of radiography in acute ankle injuries, *Ann Emerg Med* 21:384-390, 1992.

Stiell IG et al: Derivation of a decision rule for the use of radiography in acute knee injuries, *Ann Emerg Med* 26:405-413, 1995.

Stiell IG et al: *JAMA* 286:1841-1848, 2001.
Stratford PW, Binkley J: A review of the McMurray test: definition, interpretation and clinical usefulness, *J Orthop Sports Phys Ther* 22:120-128, 1995.

Chapter 23

Sports Medicine

Janice K. Loudon, PT, PhD, ATC

1. How are different degrees of sprains classified?

- **Grade I**—≤25% of ligament tearing, mild pain, and swelling without instability
- **Grade II**—26% to 75% of ligament tearing, moderate pain and swelling, loss of range of motion, and slight instability
- **Grade III**—total disruption of the ligament, resulting in severe pain and swelling, severe loss of range of motion, and joint instability

2. How are brachial plexus lesions classified?

- **Grade I**—neurapraxia characterized by transient loss of motor and sensory nerve conduction with complete recovery in ≤2 weeks
- **Grade II**—significant motor deficits and some sensory deficits lasting at least 2 weeks; full recovery is variable, ranging from 4 to 6 weeks to 1 year (average, 3 months)
- **Grade III**—complete loss of nerve function with motor and sensory deficits lasting for at least 1 year with no appreciable improvement during this time

3. Is it dangerous for the young adolescent to lift weights?

As long as the athlete uses proper technique with supervision and does not maximally lift, injuries should be minimal. The major injuries that occur are **growth plate fractures,** usually resulting from improper execution.

4. Describe a good youth strength training program.

- Phase I: Education—Introduce children to proper exercise technique, strength training guidelines, and safety procedures. Focus is on technique. Begin with 1 set of 10 to 15 repetitions in 2 to 3 nonconsecutive training sessions per week.
- Phase II: Progression—Increase gradually the overload placed on the various muscle groups. This may be achieved by increasing the resistance or the number of repetitions, sets, exercises, or training sessions; 2 to 3 sets of 8 to 12 repetitions may be appropriate. New multijoint exercises may be introduced. Monitor child's response to the exercise session constantly.

- Phase III: Function—Depending on the goal of the workout, the volume of training may increase to 2 to 3 sets of 6 to 8 repetitions on the major muscle groups. If the child is ready, more challenging exercises can be incorporated. Skill technique is still a priority.

5. What is the appropriate initial treatment for someone with an acute sports injury?

The acronym **PRICEMMS** is used to describe the initial care:

- **P** = **Protection** from further injury (e.g., use of crutches)
- **R** = **Rest** from further activity of the injured part, but not complete immobilization of the whole body
- **I** = **Ice** to decrease metabolism and pain
- **C** = **Compression** to minimize swelling
- **E** = **Elevation** to minimize swelling
- **M** = **Modalities,** such as electric stimulation for pain control
- **M** = **Medication,** such as antiinflammatories
- **S** = **Support,** such as taping or bracing

6. List general criteria for return to sport activity.

- Complete resolution of acute signs and symptoms related to the injury
- Full dynamic range of motion of all joints
- Adequate strength and proprioception to be able to perform expected skills
- No alteration in normal mechanics and good sport technique
- Performance of sport-specific activity at or above preinjury level
- Good mental and emotional state for return to sport
- Appropriate cardiovascular (aerobic or anaerobic) condition

7. Describe the miserable malalignment of the lower extremity.

This is the posture used to describe the female athlete with wide hips, femoral anteversion, genu valgum, and overpronation of the foot. This type of posture may predispose the athlete to various knee injuries, such as patellofemoral pain or anterior cruciate ligament sprain.

8. Why do females sustain so many noncontact ACL injuries?

Noncontact injuries to the ACL in the female athlete have increased over the last 20 years. Possible reasons for this increase include both intrinsic and extrinsic factors.

INTRINSIC FACTORS

- Alignment: increase valgus at the knee
- Physiologic rotatory laxity
- ACL size: smaller ligament with less strength
- Notch size and shape: narrower notch or A-shaped
- Hormonal influence: increased laxity during certain portions of the menstrual cycle
- Hyperelasticity in females

EXTRINSIC FACTORS

- Shoe wear
- Training
- Strength: decreased as compared to males
- Motivation

COMBINED

- Proprioception: deficient
- Neuromuscular activation patterns: females have a tendency to fire quads before hamstrings

- Athletic technique: females land from jump with straighter knees
- Ligament dominance: knee ligaments absorb ground reaction force rather than musculature, resulting in valgus stress to knee
- Acquired skill

9. How are contusions treated?

Ice, compression, and active range of motion are used to treat contusions. Treatments such as heat, massage, ultrasound, and passive stretching should be avoided because of the possible development of myositis ossificans.

10. Name the most common mechanisms of injury in football resulting in permanent cervical quadriplegia.

Axial loading in the form of spearing is the most common mechanism. Hyperflexion and hyperextension of the neck also may cause cervical fracture.

11. How is the transmission of pathogens such as HIV and hepatitis prevented?

To prevent transmission of blood-borne pathogens such as HIV, hepatitis B, or hepatitis C, the following specific measures should be followed:

- Pre-event—dressing of all open wounds with occlusive dressings
- Use of gloves, disinfectant, bleach, antiseptic for washing/cleaning surfaces and clothing
- Receptacles for contaminated clothing, bandages, dressing, and needles; must be available on the side of the field of play and in the dressing rooms
- Removal of players from play if active bleeding is present
- Control of bleeding, covering of wound with occlusive dressing, and change of blood-stained clothing before return to play
- Wearing adequate, appropriate protective equipment by players
- Athlete education and empowerment with responsibility to report wounds
- Caregiver precautions including using and changing of gloves between contacts
- Covering of minor cuts and abrasions while on the field
- Airway devices available for use in case of life-threatening emergencies
- Contaminated areas (e.g., mats) wiped down immediately and disinfected with bleach; area should be dry before being reused
- Postevent—wounds should be reviewed and redressed
- Soiled clothing and towels should be washed separately
- All personnel involved in coaching and support of a team should be trained in basic first-aid*

12. List injuries that may occur from a fall on an outstretched hand.

- Distal radial fracture
- Scaphoid fracture
- Perilunate dislocation
- Radial head fracture
- Acromioclavicular separation
- Glenoid labrum tear

13. How can a stress fracture of the femoral neck be identified?

These fractures (**fatigue fractures**) can develop from compression or distraction forces. Fractures resulting from distraction usually appear along the superior cortex of the femoral neck, whereas compressive loads result in fractures to the inferior cortex. Local tenderness at the greater

---

*From American Medical Society for Sports Medicine, American Academy of Sports Medicine: Human immunodeficiency virus and other blood-borne pathogens in sports, joint position statement, *Clin J Sports Med* 5:199-204, 1995.

trochanter may radiate into the inner thigh and groin. Pain is not relieved with a cortisone injection. Internal rotation usually is limited, whereas with trochanteric bursitis external rotation is limited. The athlete may complain of night pain. Radiographs may be normal initially. The most reliable test is a technetium bone scan that reveals a focal **hot spot.**

14. What is the most common athletic injury to the ankle and what structures are involved?

Lateral ligament sprains are the most common ankle injury. The ligaments involved include the anterior talofibular ligament, calcaneofibular ligament, and posterior talofibular ligament. The anterior talofibular ligament is involved in 60% to 70% of all ankle sprains; a combination of the anterior talofibular ligament and calcaneofibular ligament constitutes 20%; and the remaining 10% consists of injury to the syndesmosis, deltoid, or posterior talofibular ligament.

15. Describe three functional tests that can be used to decide return to sport after anterior cruciate ligament injury.

1. **Single-leg hop for distance**—The athlete stands on the test limb behind the starting line. When ready, the athlete is instructed to jump as far as possible, landing on the same limb. The best of three trials is used. The opposite limb is then tested.
2. **Single-leg vertical jump**—The test is begun with determination of the initial reach height of the athlete. The subject stands erect with the dominant side next to the wall. When ready, the athlete jumps off one leg, as high as possible. The difference between the reach height and the jumped height is absolute jump height. The test is then repeated on the opposite side.
3. **Cross-over hop test**—A piece of tape that is 6 m in length is placed on the floor. The subject is instructed to perform four consecutive hops on a single limb, crossing over the center line with each hop. The opposite limb is then tested.

16. What is the limb symmetry index (LSI)?

The LSI is calculated for all three of the tests described in the previous question. The LSI is the involved score divided by the uninvolved score, multiplied by 100. An LSI of 85% is ideal for return to sport.

17. Define proprioceptive training and give examples for lower extremity rehabilitation.

Proprioception is the ability to sense joint position and joint motion; there is a loss of proprioception after joint injury. Exercises include single-leg balancing on a mini trampoline or using a balance or wobble board.

18. List some physiologic changes that occur to the aging athlete.

Age-Related Decreases in Functional Status

System	Function	Decreases
Cardiovascular	Maximal heart rate	10 beats/min per decade
	Resting stroke volume	30% by age 85
	Maximal cardiac output	20-30% by age 65
	Vessel compliance	BP 10-40 mm Hg
Respiratory	Residual volume	30-50% by age 70
	Vital capacity	40-50% by age 70

Age-Related Decreases in Functional Status *continued*

System	Function	Decreases
Nervous	Nerve conduction	1-15% by age 60
	Proprioception and balance	35-40% by age 60
Musculoskeletal	Bone loss	
	>35 years old	1% per year
	>55 years old	3-5% per year
	Muscle strength	20% by age 65
	Flexibility	Degenerative diseases
Metabolic	Maximal oxygen uptake	9% per decade

From Hough DO, Barry HC, Eathrone MD: The mature athlete. In Mellion MB, editor: *Sports medicine secrets,* ed 2, Philadelphia, 1999, pp 47-52, Hanley & Belfus.

19. Are the aforementioned physiologic changes a natural part of aging?

Many of the changes may be caused by inactivity rather than the true aging process. Maintaining a consistent exercise program can combat many of these changes.

20. What value does athletic tape provide to a joint?

The effect of tape application is still being investigated by researchers. Possible explanations include improved joint stability, increased joint proprioception, and prevention of injury. Tape loosens during participation about 20 minutes after its initial application.

21. What are the advantages of using athletic braces, as compared to tape?

Various forms of braces have been used in place of tape because of the ease of application and the long-term reduction in costs. Bracing has been shown to maintain support for extended periods as well as or better than tape.

22. Describe the female athlete triad.

- Amenorrhea
- Eating disorders
- Osteoporosis

Anorexia nervosa and **bulimia nervosa** are the most common eating disorders in females who participate in sports such as gymnastics and distance running. The eating disorders accompanied by heavy training may lead to **amenorrhea** (cessation of menstrual cycle), and eventually the athlete may develop **bone loss** or **osteoporosis.** These athletes then are more susceptible to stress fractures. An eating disorder is a symptom of underlying emotional distress. Eating disorders impair athletic performance.

23. List potential side effects of anabolic-androgenic steroid use.

GENERAL SIDE EFFECTS

- Liver dysfunction
- Hair loss
- Immune system dysfunction
- Kidney malignancy

- Liver cysts
- Decreased high-density lipoproteins
- Increased low-density lipoproteins
- Aggressive behavior
- Depression
- Premature epiphyseal closure in children
- Migraine headaches

IN MALES
- Testicular atrophy
- Prostate gland problems
- Breast development
- Acne
- Abnormally low sperm count

IN FEMALES
- Masculinizing effect
- Menstrual irregularities
- Hirsutism (excessive hair on face and body)
- Deepening of voice

24. List the symptoms, presentation, and treatment of heat exhaustion and heat stroke.

	Symptoms	Mental Status	Rectal Temperature (°F)	Skin	Sweat	Blood Pressure	Treatment
Heat exhaustion	Fatigue, exhaustion	Usually conscious	104	Pale	Perfuse	Narrow pulse pressure	IV fluids, electrolytes, cool with ice
Heat stroke	Disoriented, headache, incoherent	Confused or unconscious	≥105	Flushed	May not be sweating	Low diastolic with wide pulse pressure	IV fluids, cool with ice, transport to hospital

25. What actions can be taken to prevent heat exhaustion and heat stroke?

- Prevention requires careful monitoring of ambient temperature and humidity.
- Regular hydration before, during, and after sports participation is a must.
- Consumption of 8 to 16 ounces of water is required for every 15 minutes of strenuous exercise.
- Rehydration with 24 to 40 ounces of water after exercise is needed.
- Cold water absorbs faster than warm water in the gastrointestinal tract.

26. Is extra protein needed when participating in athletics?

Yes. The recommended dietary allowance (RDA) for sedentary individuals is 0.8 g/kg/day. Endurance athletes require 1.2 to 1.4 g/kg/day, and strength athletes require 1.4 to 1.8 g/kg/day. This protein requirement can be found in a normal diet; extra protein supplements are not necessary. Female athletes and amenorrheic athletes may not consume enough protein.

27. List examples of foods that contain 10 g of protein.

- 50 g of grilled fish
- 35 g of lean beef
- 40 g of turkey
- 2 small eggs
- 300 ml of skim milk
- 3 cups of wheat flake cereal
- 2 cups of cooked pasta
- 2 cups of brown rice
- $\frac{3}{4}$ cup of cooked kidney beans
- 120 g of soybeans
- 60 g of nuts

28. What is glucosamine, and what is it used for?

Glucosamine is a nutritional supplement that has been used for individuals with osteoarthritis. Glucosamine is an essential building block for the synthesis of glucosaminoglycans. Studies have shown that supplementing the body with additional amounts of glucosamine (1500 mg) daily promotes the production of chondrocytes, reduces pain, and increases joint function. In addition to glucosamine, chondroitin sulfate may inhibit several enzymes that degrade articular cartilage. Clinically, chondroitin supplements appear to reduce osteoarthritis symptoms. The American Academy of Orthopaedic Surgeons position statement indicates that there is good evidence that glucosamine and chondroitin sulfate may help symptomatically with no side effects.

29. What is turf toe?

Turf toe is an acute sprain to the first metatarsophalangeal joint. The mechanism usually involves the athlete hyperextending this joint as the foot gets jammed on the artificial turf while trying to push-off.

30. List treatments for turf toe.

- Applying ice
- Strapping the toe
- Using nonsteroidal antiinflammatory drugs

31. What is chronic compartment syndrome?

The lower leg is divided into four compartments that contain muscles plus neurovascular bundles. An increase in volume in the compartment may result from exercising muscles causing excessive pressure within the compartment (preexercise pressure, >15 mm Hg; 1-minute postexercise, >30 mm Hg; 5-minute postexercise, >20 mm Hg; normal values, 5 to 10 mm Hg). Symptoms of chronic compartment syndrome include compartment tightness, which occurs during or after exercise. Swelling may exist as well as paresthesia over the dorsum of the foot.

32. List treatment options for chronic compartment syndrome.

- Fasciotomy
- Training modification
- Icing
- Stretching
- Strengthening
- Biomechanical correction

33. Why might an athlete collapse on the field?

Traumatic

- Head injury
- Spinal cord injury

Nontraumatic

- Cardiac (coronary artery disease, arrhythmia, congenital abnormality)

- Thoracic injury (multiple rib fractures, hemothorax, tension pneumothorax, cardiac tamponade, cardiac contusion)
- Abdominal injury (ruptured viscus)
- Multiple fractures
- Blood loss
- Hyperthermia
- Hypothermia
- Hyponatremia
- Respiratory (asthma, spontaneous pneumothorax, pulmonary embolism)
- Allergic anaphylaxis
- Drug toxicity
- Vasovagal response (faint)
- Postural hypotension
- Hyperventilation
- Hysteria

34. How are concussions classified, and what are the return-to-play guidelines?

Return-to-Play Guidelines

Grade	First Concussion	Second Concussion	Third Concussion
Grade 1 (mild) No loss of consciousness Posttraumatic amnesia <30 min	May return to play if no headaches, dizziness, impaired orientation for 1 week	Return to play in 2 weeks if asymptomatic at that time for 1 week	Terminate season; may return to play next season if asymptomatic
Grade 2 (moderate) Loss of consciousness <5 min Posttraumatic amnesia >30 min to <24 hr	Return to play if asymptomatic for 1 week	Minimum of 1 month before return to play; has to be asymptomatic for 1 week before return	Terminate season; may return to play next season if asymptomatic
Grade 3 (severe) Loss of consciousness >5 min Posttraumatic amnesia >24 hr	Minimum of 1 month before return to play; has to be asymptomatic for 1 week before return	Terminate season; may return to play next season if asymptomatic	

Adapted from Cantu RC, Micheli LJ: *ACSM's guidelines for the team physician,* Philadelphia, 1991, Lea & Febiger.

35. What is exercise-induced asthma (EIA)?

Exercise-induced asthma (EIA) is characterized by a transient narrowing of the airway following intense exercise lasting longer than 10 minutes. This transient narrowing is associated with bronchospasms. EIA is more common in exercises such as long-distance running and cross-country skiing. A positive test for EIA is a >10% decrease of the forced expiratory volume in 1 second (FEV_1). Management of EIA usually involves the use of a β_2-agonist with a mast cell stabilizer before exercising.

SPORTS AT RISK

- Tolerable—archery, baseball, downhill skiing, football, golf, gymnastics, karate, riflery, short-distance running, swimming, tennis, volleyball, wrestling
- Less tolerable—basketball, cross-country skiing, cycling, ice hockey, ice skating, lacrosse, long-distance running, rowing, soccer

Signs and Symptoms

Obvious Signs and Symptoms

- Wheezing
- Difficulty breathing
- Chest tightness
- Coughing
- Problems with prolonged exercise

Subtle Signs and Symptoms

- Stomach pain/nausea
- Fatigue
- Inability to exercise in the cold
- Chest congestion
- Frequent colds
- Dry throat
- Headache

MANAGEMENT

- Pharmacotherapy:
  First line—β-agonist
  Second line—mast cell stabilizers
  Third line—corticosteroids

PREVENTION

- Preactivity (0 to 60 min)—10- to 15-min warm-up
- Short bursts of submaximal activity (5 to 10 min)
- Premedicate 15 to 30 min before practice/event
- Postcompetition—0- to 15-min cool-down

Bibliography

American Academy of Pediatrics: Weight training and weight lifting: information for the pediatrician, *Phys Sportsmed* 11:157-161, 1983.

Andrews JR, Whiteside JA: Common elbow problems in the athlete, *J Orthop Sports Phys Ther* 17:289-295, 1993.

Arnheim DD: *Principles of athletic training,* ed 8, St Louis, 1993, Mosby.

Barber SD et al: Quantitative assessment of functional limitation in normal and anterior cruciate ligament-deficient knees, *Clin Orthop* 255:204-214, 1990.

Cantu RC, Micheli LJ: *ACSM's guidelines for the team physician,* Philadelphia, 1991, Lea & Febiger.

Clancy WG, Brand RI, Bergfield JA: Upper trunk brachial plexus injuries in contact sports, *Am J Sports Med* 5:209-216, 1977.

Daniel DM et al: Quantification of knee stability and function, *Contemp Orthop* 5:83-91, 1982.

Donatelli R, Wooden M: *Orthopaedic physical therapy,* New York, 1989, Churchill Livingstone.

Faigenbaum AD, Bradley DF: Strength training for the young athlete, *Orthop Phys Ther Clin N Am* 7:67-90, 1998.

Halbach JW, Tank RT: The shoulder. In Gould JA, Davies GJ, editors: *Orthopaedic and sports physical therapy,* St Louis, 1985, pp 497-517, Mosby.

Magee DJ: *Orthopedic physical assessment,* Philadelphia, 1992, WB Saunders.

Nirschl R, Pettrone F: Tennis elbow, *J Bone Joint Surg* 61A:835-837, 1979.
Noyes FR, Barber SD, Mangine RE: Abnormal lower limb symmetry determined by function hop tests after anterior cruciate ligament rupture, *Am J Sports Med* 19:513-518, 1991.
Palmer AK, Werner FW: The triangular fibrocartilage complex of the wrist: anatomy and function, *J Hand Surg* 6:153-162, 1981.
Reid DC: *Sports injury: assessment and rehabilitation,* New York, 1992, Churchill Livingstone.
Roy S, Irvin R: *Sports medicine: prevention, evaluation, management, and rehabilitation,* Englewood Cliffs, NJ, 1983, Prentice Hall.
Sargent DA: The physical test of a man, *Am Phys Educ Rev* 26:188-194, 1921.

Chapter 24

Differential Diagnosis and Clinical Reasoning

Fredrick D. Pociask, PT, PhD, OCS, and John R. Krauss, PT, PhD, OCS

1. What is a diagnosis, and what is a differential diagnosis?

A diagnosis is a named category of specific clinical data that labels a condition and provides characteristics of the condition when communicated to health care professionals. A differential diagnosis is a list of possible diagnoses generated from the patient interview and physical examination, listed in order of likelihood from the most likely to the least likely. In general terms, in the context of physical therapy (APTA Guide to PT Practice, 2001) the diagnosis is used to identify "the impact of a condition on function at the level of the system and at the level of the whole person."

2. What are characteristics of visceral symptoms?

- **Location**—Unilateral or bilateral; poorly localized in terms of specific organ or system (e.g., angina)
- **Quality**—Knifelike, boring, deep bone pain, deep aching, cutting, moderate to severe, and/or perceived from the inside out
- **Character**—Symptoms often unrelieved by rest, changes in position, and interventions that would typically affect musculoskeletal disorders. Associated symptoms that do not occur with musculoskeletal disorders can be identified via a careful review of systems.
- **Quantity or severity**—Typically related to exacerbating factors and varies based on organ/organ system and status of disease processes (e.g., dull to sharp or mild to severe)
- **Onset**—Recent or sudden but does not typically present as being chronically observed (i.e., insidious onset often without an attributable mechanism)
- **Duration and frequency**—Constant or intermittent based on organ/system and attributing factors, gradually progressive, cyclical, or symptom may come in waves

- **Aggravating factors**—Differ based on involved organ/system and status of disease processes (e.g., fatty foods will typically aggravate a gallbladder disorder)
- **Relieving factors**—Differ based on involved organ/system and status of disease processes. A specific strategy such as rest may initially relieve symptoms (i.e., pain), but there is typically a recurring progression of increasing frequency, intensity, and/or duration of symptoms.
- **Client's perception of the symptom**—Should be expected to vary between patients and will be influenced by cognitive, affective, cultural, socioeconomic, and environmental factors. For example, patients may self-diagnose, select unwise self-treatments, or perceive certain symptom such as coughing, sweating, or diarrhea as normal and not symptoms of illness.

3. What are somatic disorders?

Somatic disorders are musculoskeletal syndromes in which symptoms are caused by nociceptive stimulation of pain-sensitive structures. The origin of somatic pain is mechanical and/or chemical stimulation of nerve endings. Somatic pain may be either localized to a body region and/or referred to other body regions. Somatic pain and somatic referred pain are typically static, aching in quality, and difficult to point-localize.

4. What are characteristics of somatic symptoms?

- **Location**—Typically unilateral and described as presenting in one joint or in one body region; somatic referred may or may not be present
- **Quality**—Achy, deep, sharp, pulling, sore, stiff, and/or cramping pain
- **Character**—Local tenderness or pain that is attributable to an activity or underlying pathology (e.g., pain exacerbated by overhead activities with secondary impingement tendonosis; morning stiffness with osteoarthritis)
- **Quantity or severity**—Mild to severe
- **Onset**—Sudden or gradual: sudden associated with acute overload stresses and macrotrauma and gradual associated with chronic overloading stresses and repetitive microtrauma
- **Duration and frequency**—Intermittent to constant: usually intermittent with varying intensity based on activity and/or position with mechanical disorders; constant with acute inflammatory disorders. Symptoms may present as chronologically observed, characterized by asymptomatic periods with exacerbations or progressively exacerbated symptoms attributed to causal factors or progression of the underlying disorder.
- **Aggravating factors**—Symptoms are typically exacerbated with specific movement, activities, loading, etc., and the degree of exacerbation is a function of attributing factors or progression of the underlying disorder.
- **Relieving factors**—Relieving factors are typically a function of identifying and managing aggravating factors (e.g., activity modification, rest, pacing, therapeutic interventions, improved self-management, eliminating attributing factors, positioning, relative rest).

5. What are radicular disorders?

A radicular disorder is a neurogenic disorder in which signs and/or symptoms are caused by damage or irritation of the spinal nerves or spinal nerve roots. The origin of signs and symptoms is mechanical and/or chemical and is attributable to a block in conduction rather than stimulation of nerve endings. Radicular disorders produce lower motor neuron lesion signs and symptoms, which include muscle weakness, atrophy, hyporeflexia, and sensory changes such as paraesthesia and/or numbness. A block in conduction itself does not necessarily cause pain in either the spine or the corresponding extremity, but radicular disorders typically occur concurrently with somatic pain disorders.

6. What is a key characteristic of radicular symptoms?

Radicular pain is described as shooting or lacerating and is typically felt in a relatively narrow band about 4 cm wide; it is often combined with other radicular symptoms such as tingling, numbness, and burning sensations.

7. What is the difference between radicular referred symptoms and somatic referred pain accompanying a radicular disorder?

Radicular symptoms result from a block in conduction rather than nociceptive stimulation of pain-sensitive structures (i.e., the spinal nerve or nerve root). Radicular symptoms are typically referred to the distribution supplied by the involved spinal nerve or nerve root, but this assumption must take into consideration the following:

1. The distribution of radicular symptoms is not always distinctive.
2. Radicular pain from a given nerve root does not always follow a consistent distribution.
3. All radicular disorders do not result in referred pain.
4. Radicular symptoms do not always extend to the distal portion of the involved dermatome.

Somatic referred pain is generated by either mechanical or chemical irritation of somatic structures such as the dural lining on the nerve root or the epineurium of the spinal nerve. Like radicular referred pain, somatic referred pain is felt in body regions separate from the irritated structures (e.g., lumbar facet arthrosis can refer pain into the leg).

8. How can the physical therapist distinguish between radicular and somatic pain disorders?

Somatic disorders do not involve neurologic signs and symptoms such as reflexive, sensory, or myotomal changes; positive bowstring tests; and positive dural tensions tests.

SCREENING FOR SYSTEMIC INVOLVEMENT

9. Why do physical therapists need to screen for systemic involvement?

Physical therapists need to screen for systemic or non–physical therapy involvement because many visceral (organ or organ system) diseases mimic orthopaedic symptoms. For example, Jarvik and Deyo (2002) reported that among patients with low back pain being seen in ambulatory primary-care clinics, 4% will have osteoporosis-related fractures, 2% will have spondylolisthesis (forward displacement of a vertebral body) or spondylolysis (fracture of a portion of the vertebra, which may lead to spondylolisthesis), 2% will have visceral disease, 0.7% will have cancer, and 0.5% will have infections. Given the possibility of such disorders, the clinician must promptly screen patients at risk for such medical conditions and make the appropriate referrals.

10. List common body systems and aggregates of signs/symptom that may indicate systemic involvement.

General	Endocrine/Metabolic	Genito-Reproductive	Peripheral Vascular
Appetite	Hot/cold intolerance	Contraceptive measures	Claudication
Weakness	Goiter	Pain	Raynaud's
Fatigue	Irradiation exposure	Mass	Ulcers
Weight loss	Lipid disorder	Lesions	Thrombophlebitis
Fever	Diabetes	Discharge	Varicosities
Chills	Change in physical	Pruritic	**Psychiatric**
Diaphoresis	features	VD	Anxiety
Light-headedness	**ENT**	Sexual dysfunction	Depression
Adenopathy	Infections	Infertility	Treatment
Edema	Hearing loss	Infections	NBD

continued

General
Injuries

Allergic
Food
Seasonal
Bee sting
Hay fever
Asthma
Allergic rhinitis

Breasts
Mass
Tenderness
Discharge
Asymmetry
Gynecomastia
Implants

Cardio-pulmonary
Cough
Expectoration
Hemoptysis
Wheezing asthma
COPD
Infections
Syncope
Dyspnea
Orthopnea PND
Cyanosis
Murmur
Palpitations
Rheumatic fever
Hypertension
Infarction
Tuberculosis
TB skin test

ENT
Vertigo
Tinnitus
Epistaxis
Voice change

Eye
Acuity
Glasses/contacts
Visual fields
Diplopia
Scotoma
Cataracts
Glaucoma
Infections
Pain

Gastrointestinal
Nausea
Vomiting
Dysphagia
Bowel habits
Hernia
Pain
Ulcer history
Gas
Blood
Hemorrhoids
Jaundice
Pancreatitis
Stones

Hematologic
Anemia
Sickle cell
Leukemia
Transfusions
Bruising
Bleeding

Musculoskeletal Pain
Stiffness
Swelling
Weakness
Deformity
Arthritis
Siccus
Neurologic
Paresthesia
Paresis/paralysis
Gait
Headache pain
Head trauma
Unconsciousness
Tremors
Seizures
Speech

Psychiatric
Shy/sensitive
Irritable/irate
Nervous/worry
Life is unpleasant
Cry often

Renal
Dysuria
Urgency
Frequency
Stream
Nocturia
Hematuria
Proteinuria
Pyuria
Nephritis
Infections
Incontinence
Colic/calculi

Skin
Hair and nails
Pruritus
Tumor
Rash
Mole change
Keloid

11. What are examples of common "Red Flags" that typically require physician referral and further investigation?

- Anorexia
- Back and abdominal pain at the same level
- Bilateral symptoms
- Changes in mental status
- Chills
- Constipation

- Diaphoresis (excessive perspiration)
- Diarrhea
- Dyspnea (breathlessness at rest or after mild exertion)
- Early satiety (feeling full after eating)
- Elevated body temperature
- Fecal or urinary incontinence (inability to control bowels or urine)
- Frequency (increased urination)
- Headaches, dizziness, fainting, or falling
- Hematuria (blood in the urine)
- Insidious onset with progression of symptoms
- Melena (blood in feces)
- Nausea
- Night sweats
- Nocturia
- Obvious change in a wart or mole
- Pain at night
- Pain that forces a patient to curl-up into fetal position
- Pain unrelieved by recumbency
- Painless weakness of muscles: more often proximal, but may occur distally
- Poor or delayed healing
- Sacral pain without history of injury
- Skin lesions
- Thickening of a lump
- Unexplained weight loss
- Unusual bleeding, bruising, or discharge
- Unusual vital signs
- Urgency (sudden need to urinate)
- Visual disturbances
- Vomiting
- Weakness and/or fatigue
- Weight loss/gain without explanation

PHYSICAL THERAPY DIFFERENTIATION

12. What are the limitations of a physical therapy diagnosis?

The physical therapy differential diagnosis is often provisional based on further examination, evaluation, trial interventions, patient outcomes, diagnostic imaging, etc. Additionally, it must be specific to diagnostic labels that we can substantiate directly through specific physical therapy tests and measures or indirectly through interpretation of medical tests or procedures and/or through consultation with other medical professionals.

Cardiovascular

13. True or false: Pain referral patterns associated with myocardial infarction are the same for men and women.

False. Symptoms of MI do not always follow the classic pattern, especially in women. Women may experience pain referred into the right shoulder in addition to shortness of breath (sometimes occurring in the middle of the night) and chronic, unexpected fatigue.

14. What are silent heart attacks, and who do they commonly affect?

Silent attacks (painless infarction without acute symptoms) are more common among nonwhites, older adults (>75 years), all smokers, and adults (men and women) with diabetes, presumably because of reduced sensitivity to pain.

15. For myocardial infarctions associated with a blood clot, what time frame for the administration of medications that dissolve clots, promote vasodilation, and reduce infarct size is considered the most crucial?

Administration of medication within the first 70 minutes after the onset of symptoms is associated with improved outcomes.

16. What are typical pain referral patterns for the heart?

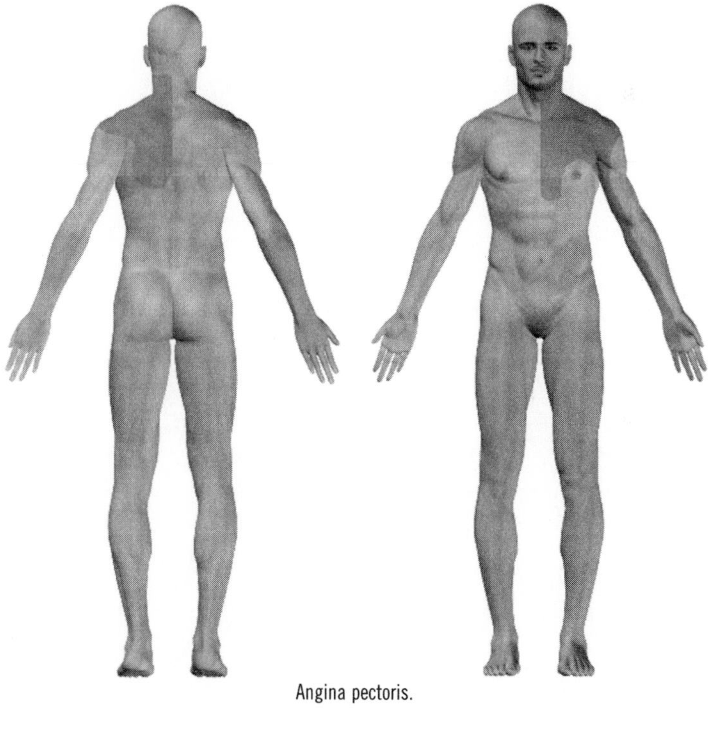

Angina pectoris.

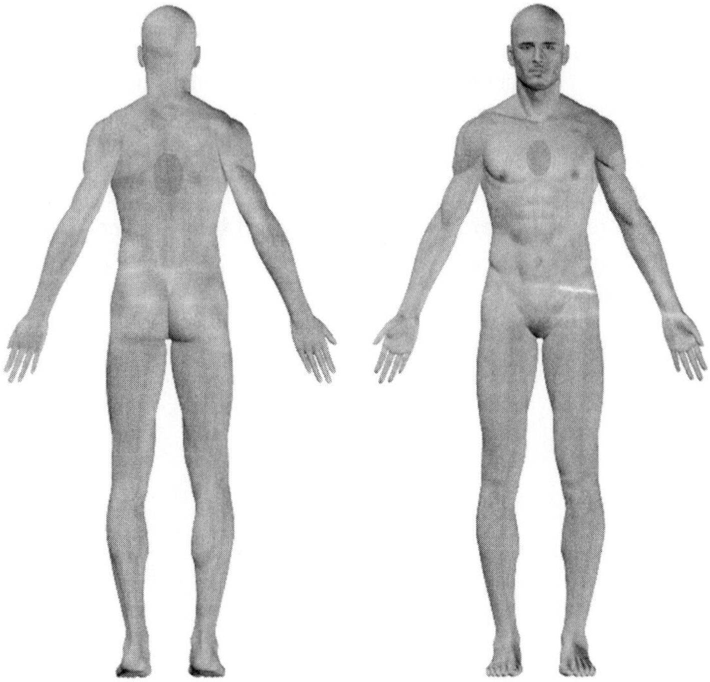

Myocardial infarction.

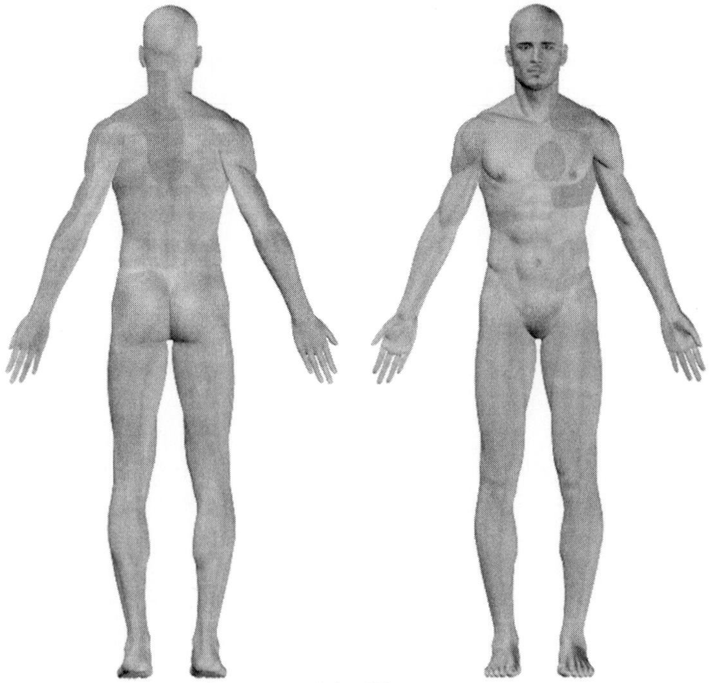

Pericarditis.

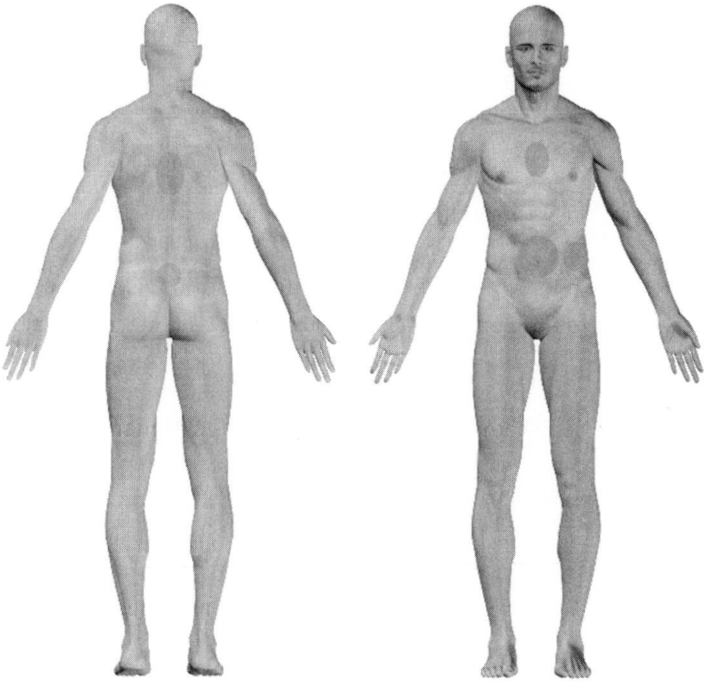

Dissecting aortic aneurysm.

17. What signs and symptoms are commonly associated with cardiac pathology?

- There is a sudden sensation of pressure in the chest that occasionally radiates into the arms, throat, neck, and back.
- Pain is constant, lasting 30 minutes to hours.
- Pain may be accompanied by shortness of breath, pallor, and profuse perspiration.
- Angina pectoralis has similar symptoms to an MI. However, angina pectoralis is less severe, does not last for hours (rarely more than 5 minutes), and is relieved by cessation of all activity and administration of nitrates.
- Symptoms of MI do not always follow the classic pattern, especially in women.
- Two major symptoms in women are shortness of breath (sometimes occurring in the middle of the night) and chronic, unexpected fatigue.
- A typical presentation may include continuous pain in the mid-thoracic spine or interscapular area, neck and shoulder pain, stomach or abdominal pain, nausea, unexplained anxiety, or heartburn that is not altered by antacids.
- Silent attacks (painless infarction without acute symptoms) are more common among nonwhites, older adults (>75 years), all smokers, and adults (men and women) with diabetes, presumably because of reduced sensitivity to pain.
- Nausea and vomiting may occur because of reflex stimulation of vomiting centers by pain fibers.
- Fever may develop in the first 24 hours and persist for 1 week because of inflammatory activity within the myocardium.
- Myocarditis and endocarditis do not produce chest pain, but a chest tightness with breathlessness.

18. What are cardiac red flags?

Pain in the chest lasting longer than 30 minutes, shortness of breath with exertion or when sleeping, increased fatigue, nausea, vomiting, nonproductive cough, nocturia, changes in skin color (bluing or ashen), and onset of pain in the early morning hours are all cardiac red flags.

19. What subjective questions should be asked when cardiac dysfunction is suspected?

- Presence of any red flags as previously described
- Questions about pain, regarding the onset, location, and character of the pain
- Additional information regarding dietary habits, cigarette or alcohol use, and exercise habits
- Questions regarding the use of prescription, over-the-counter, or street drugs; especially antihypertensive medications, β-blockers, calcium channel blockers, digoxin, diuretics, and aspirin/anticoagulants

20. List common musculoskeletal disorders that mimic cardiovascular pain patterns.

Cervical radiculopathy (C8), ulnar nerve injuries, rotator cuff disorders, upper thoracic dysfunction, pectoralis major strain, subacromial bursitis, acromioclavicular arthritis, and temporomandibular (TM) joint pain mimic cardiovascular pain patterns.

Pulmonary

21. Does the following presentation warrant immediate medical care? A patient with a medically diagnosed and properly managed history of emphysema presents with a definitive orthopaedic referral. During the examination the patient demonstrates shortness of breath, wheezing, a barrel chest deformity, and the use of accessory muscles of respiration; the patient also reports that he/she does not tolerate supine positioning.

No; the symptoms are consistent with chronic emphysema.

22. Describe clinical signs and symptoms of acute pleuritis.

Sharp, stabbing substernal pain, especially with exertion, pleural rub on auscultation, and referred upper trapezius and interscapular pain are symptoms of acute pleuritis.

23. A patient reports for an initial evaluation immediately following a motor vehicle accident. Primary complaints include lumbar pain with neurogenic signs and symptoms in an L5 distribution. Additional symptoms include malaise, sharp chest pain, changes in respiratory rate, diminished and rapid pulse rate, decreased blood pressure, and a dry cough. The latter symptoms potentially describe which serious pulmonary disorder?

The examiner should be alert for the presence of a pneumothorax.

24. True or false: Hoarseness of voice and a morning cough are of no diagnostic significance if a patient undergoes regular medical examinations and is able to specifically relate the symptoms to their smoking habit.

False; the above symptoms warrant further investigation.

25. How does pulmonary function change with obstructive and restrictive pulmonary disorders?

- Restrictive—normal expiratory airflow, decreased vital capacity, decreased total lung capacity, decreased residual volume, and decreased Pa_{CO_2}
- Obstructive—reduced airflow with/without changes in vital capacity, increased total lung capacity, increased residual volume, and increased Pa_{CO_2}

26. Given the following information, should a pulmonary condition be suspected as a primary diagnosis? A patient presents with sharp, right lateral thorax pain on inhalation (T4 to T7) secondary to a motor vehicle accident that occurred 5 weeks ago. During sustained inhalation, the symptomatic pain can be eliminated with right side-bending and exacerbated with left side-bending. Additional symptoms include intercostal tenderness and trigger points noted in the involved area of dysfunction.

No; the symptoms appear musculoskeletal in nature as they can be specifically provoked and alleviated with position.

27. What are typical pain referral patterns for the lungs?

Primary pain is typically noted over the midchest or involved lung, and is often greater anterior as opposed to posterior. Referred pain may be noted in the neck, upper trapezius muscles, proximal shoulders, T1/C8 dermatome, along the ribs, and in the upper abdomen.

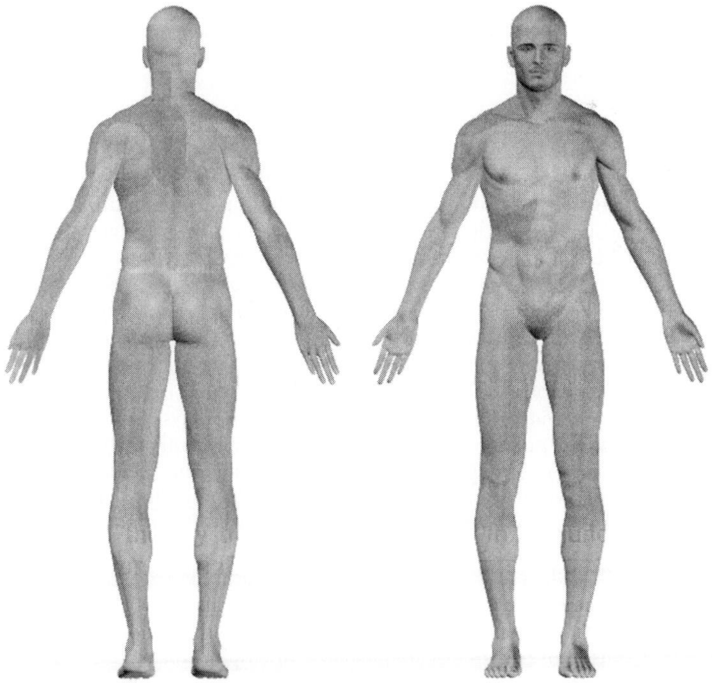

Pain patterns associated with pleuritis.

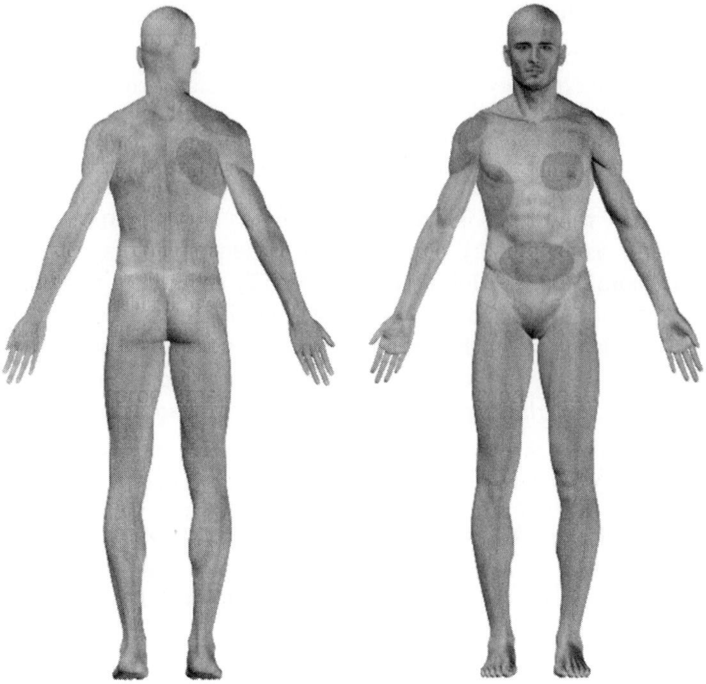

Pain patterns associated with pneumothorax.

28. What signs and symptoms are commonly associated with pulmonary pathology?

- Cough—continuous coughing (possibly indicating an acute or chronic pathology, e.g., respiratory tract infection, allergies, bronchitis, emphysema, COPD, lung cancer), time of day cough (e.g., environmental exposure to an irritant), night cough (e.g., sinusitis or allergies), and early morning cough (e.g., bronchial inflammation secondary to smoking)
- Sputum, including color and odor—clear to white sputum (e.g., cold [viral infection] and bronchitis), purulent yellow or green sputum (e.g., bacterial infections), reddish-brown sputum (e.g., tuberculosis and pneumonia), and pink-foamy sputum (e.g., pulmonary edema)
- Hemoptysis or blood derived from the lungs or bronchial tubes may result from a large number of conditions (e.g., pneumonia, infections, cancer, trauma)
- Shortness of breath without physical exertion or with minimal physical exertion (e.g., bronchitis, emphysema, pneumonia, pulmonary embolism, pleurisy, pneumothorax)
- Cyanosis (e.g., respiratory acidosis, chronic bronchitis, pneumonia, cystic fibrosis)
- Chest pain that occurs with breathing (e.g., pneumonia, pleurisy, lung cancer)
- Changes in respiratory rate or breathing patterns (e.g., acute and chronic bronchitis, respiratory acidosis, emphysema)
- Change in normal breath sounds (e.g., asthma, bronchitis, pneumonia, emphysema, pleurisy, lung cancer, bronchiectasis)
- Chest cavity deformities or compensatory breathing patterns (e.g., a barrel chest deformity and use of accessory muscle of respiration are indicative of emphysema)
- General undiagnosed symptoms of dizziness, fainting, fever, shortness of breath without exertion, cyanosis, night sweats, tachycardia, especially with a positive pulmonary history

29. What are pulmonary red flags?

- Central nervous system symptoms
- Change in normal breath sounds, especially wheezing
- Hemoptysis, especially with a long-term history of smoking
- Pain increased by recumbency or while sleeping, especially if disturbing sleep
- Persistent undiagnosed cough
- Recurrent pulmonary infections
- Sharp pain with breathing, especially on inhalation
- Signs or symptoms of DVT
- Signs or symptoms of insufficient oxygenation or increased carbon dioxide levels
- Splinting used to reduce pain
- Sudden, sharp chest pain with or without trauma combined with changes in respiratory rate, diminished but rapid pulse rate, diminished blood pressure, and changes in respiratory rate
- Undiagnosed neck, shoulder, chest, and arm pain
- Unexplained hoarseness of voice and/or difficulty swallowing
- Unexplained upper extremity weakness
- Unexplained weight loss or gain, especially sudden
- Undiagnosed symptoms of dizziness, fainting, fever, shortness of breath without exertion, cyanosis, night sweats, tachycardia, especially when occurring in a cluster and in combination with specific pulmonary signs and symptoms

30. What subjective questions should be asked when pulmonary dysfunction is suspected?

- Presence of red flags as previously described
- Age (i.e., >35-year-old female/>40-year-old male)
- History of respiratory tract infections, cough, sputum, hemoptysis, dyspnea, infection, fever, chills
- History of smoking
- History of exposure to environmental contaminants
- Personal and family history of cancer
- History of pain exacerbated by inhalation or exhalation (e.g., breathing, coughing)
- History of pain that is provoked or alleviated by lying on one side (e.g., sleeping)
- Female: history of gynecologic care (e.g., self-breast examinations, mammograms)
- History of general self-care and medical management (e.g., last TB test, last chest x-ray, immunizations)

31. List common musculoskeletal disorders that mimic pulmonary pain patterns.

Musculoskeletal disorders mimicking pulmonary pain patterns include cervical radiculopathy (C8, T1), cervical and upper thoracic dysfunction (e.g., arthrosis and spondylosis), rotator cuff disorders, and acromioclavicular arthritis regional muscle dysfunction (e.g., pectoralis major strain, intercostal muscle strain, trigger points).

Integumentary

32. What signs and symptoms are commonly associated with integumentary system pathology?

- Changes in a pigmented mole or benign tumor may indicate a possible malignancy.
- Cyanosis (dark bluish or purplish discoloration of the integument and mucous membranes) may indicate hypoxia or hematologic pathology.
- Edema, if generalized, may indicate cardiovascular, pulmonary, or renal dysfunction; localized edema may indicate infection, inflammation, or sudden change in pressure (i.e., compartment

syndrome). If edema is unilateral, consider a local or peripheral cause; if bilateral, consider a central disorder (e.g., congestive heart failure and renal dysfunction).

- Hyperthermia may indicate localized or systemic infection, inflammation, thermal injury; hyperthyroidism or fever is generalized.
- Hypothermia may indicate arterial insufficiency or shock.
- Jaundice (yellowish discoloration of skin and sclera) may indicate liver disease or hemolytic pathology.
- Paleness of the skin may indicate arterial insufficiency, anemia, or shock.
- Redness of the skin may indicate fever, local infection, local inflammation, carbon monoxide poisoning, or polycythemia.
- Unexplained skin lesions may indicate infection, allergic reaction, parasitic infection, thermal injury, herpes, fungal infection, cancer, or neoplasm.

33. List common nail abnormalities and probable causes.

Suspected Etiology	Nail Characteristics
Addison's disease	Brown band around nail plate
Carbon monoxide poisoning	Red nail bed
Cardiac failure	Red lunula
Chronic renal insufficiency	Brown discoloration of distal one third of nail plate
Cyanosis or hemorrhage	Blue nail bed
Jaundice	Yellow nail bed
Onychomycosis	Brown nail plate
Psoriasis	Yellow nail plate and bed
Superficial onychomycosis	White nail plate
Tetracycline	Yellow nail plate

34. What are integumentary system red flags?

- Sudden enlargement of an existing mole or benign tumor.
- New areas of involvement or spreading of an existing mole or benign tumor.
- Sudden change in color of an existing mole or benign tumor.
- Formation of an irregular border or butterfly appearance to a new or previously existing mole or benign tumor.
- A previously flat mole becomes elevated or raised, especially with irregular borders or notching.
- Irregular or clumping of colors across a new or existing mole or benign tumor (i.e., nonuniform browns and blacks mixed with reds, blues, and/or whites).
- Unexpected, especially sudden changes such as scaling, flaking, drainage, itching, redness, swelling, warmth, point tenderness, or bleeding.

35. What subjective questions should be asked when integumentary system pathology is suspected?

- Presence of any red flags as previously described
- History of drug or topical agent use and self-care
- History of allergies
- History of circulatory or vasospastic disorders
- History of endocrine disorders (e.g., thyroid disease or diabetes)

- History of applicable environmental factors (e.g., exposure to radiation or x-rays, living conditions, dietary habits, occupations, leisure activities, travel, emotional stress; especially changes that occurred before or during identification of possible integumentary involvement)
- History of applicable genetic factors (e.g., family history, gender, age, race)
- History of gynecologic factors (e.g., pregnancy, menstruation, birth control pills)

36. True or false: A deep vein thrombosis will appear cyanotic and present with warmth and tenderness to palpation.

False. The skin may or may not appear cyanotic. Skin may be warm, cool, or normal to palpation. Pain, tenderness or swelling, a positive Homans' sign, and a positive venogram are more definitive in terms of differential diagnosis.

37. True or false: Malignant melanomas arise from melanocytes in moles.

False. About 40% to 50% of malignant melanomas arise from melanocytes in moles; the remainder arise from melanocytes in normal skin.

38. What is the integumentary presentation of herpes zoster (shingles)?

Symptoms of shingles include vesicular eruptions and neuralgic pain in the cutaneous distributions supplied by peripheral nerves.

39. Describe signs and symptoms of dysvascular and neuropathic foot ulcer.

Dysvascular Foot Ulcer	Neuropathic Foot Ulcer
Lesions are painful	Lesions are painless
Irregularly shaped	Circular in shape
Multifocal	Develop over bony plantar regions
Located on toes	Can be associated with callus formation
Located over nonplantar areas	Tend to be clean and nonnecrotic
Lesions are typically necrotic	Ulcer regions are warm and pink
Ulcer regions are typically cool and pale	

40. What are the key characteristics of cellulitis?

Key characteristics include the following: poorly defined and widespread distribution that is red, edematous in appearance, and warm to hot with palpation; often accompanies infections.

Gastrointestinal

41. What is the most common intraabdominal disease referring pain to the musculoskeletal system?

It is ulceration or infection of the mucosal lining of the GI tract.

42. How quickly do drug-induced symptoms occur in the GI tract?

While some medications (e.g., NSAIDs, digitalis, antibiotics) may result in immediate symptoms in patients, it is not uncommon for symptoms to occur as long as 6 to 8 weeks after exposure.

43. What are typical pain patterns for GI pathologies?

- Pain of GI origin can mimic primary musculoskeletal lesions.
- Referral locations can include the following: shoulder, neck, sternum, scapular regions, mid back, low back, hip, pelvis, sacrum.

44. What signs and symptoms are commonly associated with esophageal pathologies?

Diseases affecting the esophagus can cause the following symptoms: (1) dysphagia (sensation of food catching in the throat); (2) odynophagia (pain with swallowing); and (3) a burning sensation beginning at the xiphoid and radiating to the neck and throat (heartburn).

Causes of dysphagia include stricture, inflammation, neurologic conditions (such as stroke, Alzheimer's and Parkinson's disease), drug side effects, and space-occupying lesions. Causes of odynophagia include inflammation, spasm, and viral or fungal infection. Esophageal pain is reported as sharp, knifelike, stabbing, strong, and burning.

45. What signs and symptoms are commonly associated with stomach and duodenal pathologies?

Stomach and duodenal pathologies (peptic ulcers, stomach carcinoma, and Kaposi's sarcoma) may be associated with early satiety, melena (dark, tarry stools), and symptoms associated with eating. Pain is typically described as aching, burning, gnawing, and cramplike. It ranges from mild to severe in intensity and typically comes in waves.

46. What signs and symptoms are commonly associated with small intestine pathologies?

Small intestine pain is described as cramping pain (moderate to severe in intensity), is intermittent in duration, and may be associated with nausea, fever, and diarrhea. Pain relief may not occur after defecation or passing gas.

47. What signs and symptoms are commonly associated with large intestine and colon pathologies?

Large intestine and colon pain is described as a cramping pain, dull in intensity, and steady in duration; it may be associated with bloody diarrhea, increased urgency, or constipation. Pain relief may occur after defecation or passing gas.

48. What signs and symptoms are commonly associated with pancreatic pathologies?

Pancreatic pain is described as a severe, constant pain of sudden onset that is burning or gnawing in quality. Associated signs and symptoms include sudden weight loss, jaundice, nausea and vomiting, light-colored stools, weakness, fever, constipation, flatulence, and tachycardia; it may or may not be related to digestive activities.

49. What are GI red flags?

- Difficulty swallowing
- Pain when swallowing
- Pain associated with eating (immediately or 2 to 3 hours postingestion)
- Changes in frequency and ease of defecation
- Changes in coloration of stools
- Decreased appetite

- Sudden weight loss
- Vomiting
- Gnawing, burning pain
- Migratory arthralgias
- Decreased immune response

50. What subjective questions should be asked when GI pathology is suspected?

- Presence of any red flags as previously described
- History of drug or topical agent use, including self-care
- History of previous gastric or peptic ulcer

51. List common musculoskeletal disorders that mimic GI disorders.

Sports hernia, adductor strain/tear, lumbar disk disease, lumbar facet arthrosis, and symptomatic thoracic movement impairment are all common musculoskeletal disorders mimicking GI disorders.

52. What is McBurney point and what is its significance?

It is a point midway between the umbilicus and the right anterior-superior iliac spine used as a guide to locate the position of the appendix. McBurney point is the most common site of maximum tenderness in acute appendicitis, which is typically determined by the pressure of one finger.

53. List the structures contained in each of the four abdominal quadrants.

Right Upper Quadrant	Left Upper Quadrant
Ascending colon (superior portion)	Descending colon (superior portion)
Duodenum	Jejunum and proximal ileum
Gallbladder	Left colic (hepatic) flexure
Liver (right lobe)	Left kidney
Pancreas (head)	Left suprarenal gland
Right colic (hepatic) flexure	Liver (left lobe)
Right kidney	Pancreas (body and tail portions)
Right suprarenal gland	Spleen
Stomach (pylorus)	Stomach
Transverse colon (right half)	Transverse colon (left half)
Right Lower Quadrant	**Left Lower Quadrant**
Ascending colon (inferior portion)	Descending colon (inferior portion)
Cecum	Left ovary
Ileum	Left spermatic cord (abdominal portion)
Right ovary	Left ureter (abdominal portion)
Right spermatic cord (abdominal portion)	Left uterine tube
Right ureter (abdominal portion)	Sigmoid colon
Right uterine tube	Urinary bladder (only when full)
Urinary bladder (only when full)	Uterus (if enlarged)
Uterus (only one enlarged)	
Vermiform appendix	

Renal

54. List common signs and symptoms associated with chronic renal failure.

Uremia, dizziness, headaches, heart failure, hypertension, ischemic lower extremity pain, muscle cramps, edema, peripheral neuropathy, weakness, decreased endurance, decreased heart rate, decreased blood pressure and hypotension, among others

55. What is the costovertebral angle and what is its significance?

The costovertebral angle is the angle formed on either side of the vertebral column between the last rib and the lumbar vertebrae. Tenderness in this region is indicative of renal disease, and it is a potential site for unintended encroachment on the pleural cavity during surgery.

56. What are the two most common urinary tract infections?

- Cystitis—inflammation and infection of the bladder
- Pyelonephritis—inflammation and infection of one or both kidneys

57. A male patient presents with complaints of low back pain (myalgia and arthralgia) that he attributes to heavy physical labor over the past several weeks. A careful medical screening uncovers concurrent symptoms, which include general malaise, urinary infrequency, urinary urgency, pain with urination, interrupted urine stream, chills, fever, and nocturia. Which renal disorder do the above symptoms best describe?

The symptoms best describe prostatitis of undiagnosed origin.

58. What is a key feature that typically distinguishes a radicular disorder from renal pain?

Renal pain is rarely influenced by changes in spinal posture or movements of the spine.

59. List common "clinically observable" signs and symptoms of chronic renal disease.

Hyperpigmentation, bruising, itching, paleness/anemia, redness of the eyes, shortness of breath, uremic breath, tremors, footdrop, weakness/altered movement patterns, decreased ability to concentrate, lethargy, irritability, and impaired judgment

60. What are typical pain patterns for renal pathologies?

Primary pain is typically noted in a T10 to L1 distribution, in the groin and genital regions. Pain is predominantly in the anterior, lateral, and posterior subcostal regions, and posteriorly in the area of the lower costovertebral articulations. Referred pain may include the abdomen, lumbar "back belt," and ipsilateral shoulder.

61. What signs and symptoms are commonly associated with renal pathologies?

- Bladder and urethra—Sharp and localized upper pelvic, lower abdominal, and back pain; painful spasms of the anal sphincter; involuntary straining and a urgent need to empty the bowel with minimal passage of urine or fecal matter; urinary urgency and burning pain with urination
- Ureter—Severe unilateral or bilateral costovertebral angle pain, painful spasms of the anal sphincter, involuntary straining and a urgent need to empty the bowel with minimal passage of

urine or fecal matter, malaise, vomiting, nausea, abdominal distention, kidney/ureter tenderness, abnormal tenderness, and pain in a T10 to L1 distribution; a lesion outside of the ureter may be provoked with an active contraction of the iliopsoas muscle
- Kidney—Pain in the posterior subcostal region and in the area of the costal-vertebral articulations, posterior to lateral referred pain into abdominal region and groin (usually unilateral), malaise, fever, chills, frequent urination, possible blood in urine, nausea and vomiting, abdominal spasms, abnormal tenderness and pain in a T9 to T10 distribution

62. What are renal red flags?

- Abdominal muscle spasms
- Abdominal splinting
- Abnormal tenderness and pain in a T9 to L1 distribution
- Blood in urine (e.g., brown or red) or clouding of urine
- Changes in sexual function or pain during intercourse
- Changes in urinary patterns and/or urine flow
- Costovertebral angle pain
- Decreased or absent urination
- Dependent edema (moderate to significant)
- Fever and chills
- Genital discharge
- Genital lesions
- Headaches
- Low back and abdominal pain at the same level
- Malaise
- Masses, lesions, or swelling
- Nausea and vomiting
- Pain with urination
- Proximal lateral thigh and/or lower lateral trunk pain
- Shortness of breath
- Shoulder pain (usually with ipsilateral kidney problems)
- Tenesmus

63. What subjective questions should be asked when renal pathology is suspected?

- Presence of red flags as previously described
- Past medical and surgical history (e.g., kidney stones, bladder stones, infections, abdominal injuries, hernias, history of cancer, abdominal surgery, all applicable interventions and outcomes)
- History of abdominal pain (e.g., primary and referred pain, influence of movement and position on pain and referred pain)
- History of proximal lateral thigh and/or lower lateral trunk pain (suspect kidney or ureter)
- History of upper pelvic and lower abdominal pain (suspect bladder and/or urethra)
- History of changes in bowel/bladder function (e.g., increased frequency of urination, suspect infection; decreased flow or trouble initiating flow, suspect urethral obstruction; decreased diameter of flow, suspect urethral obstruction; feeling of bladder fullness after urination, suspect bladder disorder or enlarged prostate; burning pain during or after urination, suspect sexually transmitted disease or lower urinary tract infection; loss of control, suspect incontinence)
- History of nutritional/dietary changes
- History of relevant associated symptoms (e.g., fatigue, nausea, vomiting, vaginal or penile discharge, changes in menstrual cycle and sexual habits as applicable)

64. List common musculoskeletal disorders that mimic renal disorders.

Common musculoskeletal disorders that mimic renal disorders include lower thoracic or lumbar plexus radiculopathy, lumbar and lower thoracic dysfunction (e.g., arthrosis, spondylosis, and costal/costal-vertebral), regional muscle dysfunction (e.g., adductor strain), central nervous system disease, meralgia paresthetica, and trauma.

Hepatic and Biliary

65. What musculoskeletal signs or symptoms may be associated with hepatic and biliary dysfunction?

Bilateral carpal tunnel syndrome accompanied by bilateral tarsal tunnel syndrome is a musculoskeletal sign associated with hepatic and biliary dysfunction.

66. What are typical pain patterns for the hepatic and biliary system?

Pain associated with the liver, gallbladder, and the common bile duct is typically located in the mid-epigastric or right upper quadrant of the abdomen. Musculoskeletal pain referred from the hepatic and biliary systems may be located in the right shoulder, upper trapezius, or right scapular area, or between the scapulae.

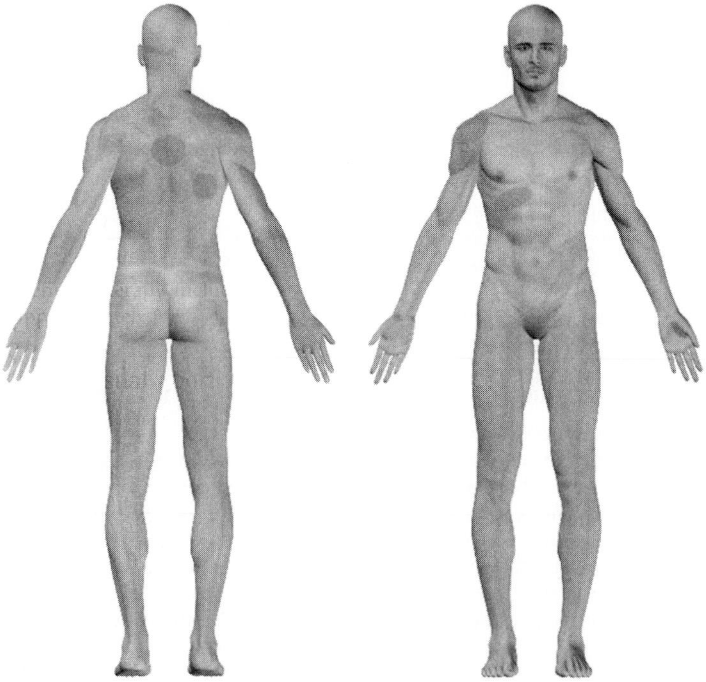

Liver, gallbladder, and common bile duct pain (upper right quadrant) and referred pain patterns (shoulder and scapular regions).

67. What signs and symptoms are commonly associated with hepatic and biliary system pathologies?

In addition to the musculoskeletal pain referral patterns listed previously, patients experiencing hepatic or biliary dysfunction may also demonstrate changes in skin color, as well as neurologic symptoms. Skin changes include yellowing of the skin or sclera of the eyes (jaundice), pallor, and orange or green skin. Neurologic signs and symptoms include confusion, sleep disturbances, muscle tremors, hyperactive reflexes, and asterixis (flapping tremor where the patient is unable to maintain wrist extension with forward flexion of the arms).

68. What are hepatic and biliary system red flags?

- Anorexia, nausea, and vomiting
- Arthralgias
- Dark urine and light-colored or clay-colored feces
- Edema and oliguria (reduced urine secretion in relation to fluid intake)
- Excessive belching
- Extreme fatigue
- Gynecomastia
- Neurologic symptoms (confusion, sleep disturbances, muscle tremors, hyperactive reflexes, asterixis, bilateral carpal/tarsal tunnel syndrome)
- Painful abdominal bloating
- Pallor, yellowing of the eyes or skin
- Right upper quadrant abdominal pain
- Sense of fullness in the abdomen
- Skin changes (jaundice, bruising, spider angioma, palmar erythema)

69. What subjective questions should be asked when hepatic and biliary system pathology is suspected?

- Presence of any red flags as previously described
- Recent changes in bowel and bladder habits
- Exposure to needles (including injection, drug use, acupuncture, tattooing, ear or body piercing, recent operative procedure, hemodialysis), exposure to certain chemicals or medications, severe alcoholism, fever

70. List common musculoskeletal disorders that mimic hepatic and biliary disorders.

Musculoskeletal conditions that may mimic hepatic and biliary pain patterns include symptomatic mid-thoracic hypomobility, rotator cuff dysfunction, subacromial/deltoid bursitis.

Hematology

71. List common disorders of erythrocytes, leukocytes, and platelets.

Erythrocytes	Leukocytes	Platelets
Anemia	Leukemia	Thrombocytosis
Aplastic anemia	Leukocytosis	Thrombopenia
Hemorrhagic anemia	Leukopenia	
Hypochromic (iron deficiency) anemia		
Megaloblastic anemia		
Pernicious anemia		
Polycythemia		
Sickle cell anemia		

72. List signs and symptoms of polycythemia (increased red blood cell mass).

History of headaches, blurred vision, dizziness, fainting, altered mentation, feeling of fullness in the head, altered sensation in the distal extremities, malaise, fatigue, weight loss, easy or unexplained bruising, cyanosis, digital clubbing, and hypertension

73. List common disorders or conditions that elevate red blood cell levels.

Alcoholism, burns, chronic pulmonary disease (e.g., fibrosis), dehydration (e.g., vomiting and diarrhea, burns, or use of diuretics), diminished blood-oxygen tension, heart disease (e.g., cor pulmonale and congenital), liver disease, renal disease, smoking, and exposure to carbon monoxide

74. List signs and symptoms of leukocytosis (increased white blood cell count).

Signs and/or symptoms consistent with local or systemic infection (e.g., fever) and inflammation or trauma

75. List common disorders or conditions that elevate white blood cell levels.

Burns, cancer, immune system responses (e.g., lupus, rheumatoid arthritis), infections, inflammatory responses (e.g., tissue damage), kidney failure, leukemia, lymphoma, malnutrition, multiple myeloma, removal of the spleen, stress (e.g., emotional, physical), and tuberculosis

76. List signs and symptoms of anemia (decreased red blood cell levels).

Pail skin and nails, shortness of breath with little to no exertion (based on degree), heart palpitation, and increased pulse rate; with severe anemia, fatigue, decreased diastolic blood pressure, and changes in mentation

77. List common disorders or conditions that lower red blood cell levels.

Addison's disease, anemia (e.g., blood loss, hemorrhage, pernicious, sickle cell), bone marrow disease, bowel disease, colon cancer, excessive menstrual bleeding, hemolysis, kidney disease, lead poisoning, leukemia, malnutrition, multiple myeloma, stomach ulcers, and vitamin and/or mineral deficiencies (e.g., B_{12}, B_6, folic acid, iron)

78. List signs and symptoms of leukopenia (decreased white blood cell levels).

Cough, sore throat, fever, chills, swelling, ulceration of mucous membranes, increased frequency of urination, painful urination, and persistent infections

79. List common disorders or conditions that lower white blood cell levels.

Alcoholism, aplastic anemia, autoimmune/collagen-vascular diseases (e.g., lupus, AIDS), bone marrow failure, Cushing's syndrome, disorders of the spleen, infections, liver disease, radiation exposure or exposure to toxic chemicals (e.g., chemotherapy), tumors, and viral infections

80. What are hematologic red flags?

- Evidence of platelet disorders (e.g., bleeding with minor to no trauma, multiple petechiae, purpura, severe bruising, nosebleeds, hematemesis, blood in urine or stool, dark tarry stool, excessive menstrual bleeding; especially when undiagnosed, sudden, and/or unexplained)
- Evidence of anemia, especially in the presence of CNS, and cardiopulmonary manifestations
- Undiagnosed muscle and joint pain in patients with a history of hemophilia
- Undiagnosed variations in hematologic values

81. What subjective information should be obtained when hematologic pathologies are suspected?

- Presence of any red flags as previously described
- History of anemia (e.g., excessive bruising or blood loss)
- Medical history including dental procedures (e.g., blood transfusion, hemophilia, hepatitis, genetic, major trauma, cancer)
- Laboratory tests (e.g., hematocrit, platelet count, hemoglobin concentration)
- Surgical history (e.g., transplant surgery, oral surgery, major surgeries)
- History of radiation exposure or exposure to toxic chemicals (e.g., chemotherapy, industrial gases)
- Integumentary changes as described in this chapter including bruising, petechia, and purpura visible through the epidermis, widespread color changes, itching, body temperature, mobility, and turgor

82. List three early signs and symptoms of anemia.

Difficult or labored breathing, weakness, and fatigue

Endocrine and Metabolic Disorders

83. What are two primary life-threatening metabolic conditions that can develop if uncontrolled or untreated diabetes mellitus progresses to a state of severe hyperglycemia?

- Diabetic ketoacidosis
- Hyperglycemic, hyperosmolar, nonketotic coma (HHNC)

84. What two patient types may exhibit orthostatic hypotension because of slight dehydration, especially when intense exercise increases the core body temperature?

Athletes and normal adults

85. What signs and symptoms are commonly associated with endocrine system pathologies?

Neuromusculoskeletal signs and symptoms include muscle weakness, myalgia and fatigue, bilateral carpal tunnel syndrome, periarthritis, chondrocalcinosis, spondyloarthropathy, osteoarthritis, hand stiffness, and pain.

86. What are endocrine system red flags?

DIABETES INSIPIDUS

- Confusion
- Increased frequency of urination (polyuria, nocturia)

SIADH

- Excessive weight gain or loss
- Edema
- Headache, seizures, and muscle cramps
- Vomiting/diarrhea

ADDISON'S DISEASE

- Dark pigmentation of the skin, mucous membranes, and scars
- Hypotension

- Fatigue that improves with rest
- Arthralgias
- Tendon calcification
- Hypoglycemia

CUSHING'S SYNDROME
- Moon face
- Cervicodorsal fat pad
- Protuberant abdomen with accumulation of fatty tissue and stretch marks
- Muscle wasting and weakness
- Kyphosis and back pain secondary to bone loss
- Easy bruising
- Emotional disturbances
- Diabetes mellitus, slow wound healing
- In women: masculinizing effects

GOITER (ENLARGED THYROID)
- Increased neck size
- Hoarseness
- Difficulty breathing and swallowing

HYPERTHYROIDISM
- Proximal weakness, primarily of pelvic girdle and thigh muscles
- >50% of adults over 70: tachycardia, fatigue, and weight loss
- <50 years of age: tachycardia, hyperactive reflexes, increased sweating, heat intolerance, fatigue, tremor, nervousness, polydipsia, weakness, increased appetite, dyspnea, weight loss
- Musculoskeletal symptoms including chronic periarthritis, pain and decreased ROM, periarticular and tendinous calcification

HYPOTHYROIDISM
- Headaches, excessive fatigue, and drowsiness
- Hoarseness and thick, slurred speech
- Intolerance to cold
- Weight gain
- Dryness of skin
- Nails become increasingly thin and brittle
- Menses become irregular
- Myxedema: nonpitting boggy edema around the eyes, hands, feet, and supraclavicular fossae
- Synovial thickening and joint effusion

THYROID CANCERS
- New onset of hoarseness, hemoptysis, elevated blood pressure

87. What red flags are associated with metabolic disorders?

METABOLIC ACIDOSIS
- Headache, drowsiness, lethargy
- Nausea, vomiting, diarrhea
- Muscle twitching
- Convulsions, coma (if severe)
- Rapid, deep breathing (hyperventilation)

METABOLIC ALKALOSIS
- Nausea, prolonged vomiting, diarrhea
- Confusion, irritability, agitation, restlessness

- Muscle twitching, cramping, and weakness
- Paresthesias
- Convulsions, eventual coma
- Slow, shallow breathing

GOUT

- Joint pain and swelling (especially the first metatarsal joint)
- Fever and chills, redness
- Malaise

HEMACHROMATOSIS

- Arthropathy, arthralgias, myalgias
- Progressive weakness
- Bilateral pitting edema (lower extremities)
- Vague abdominal pain
- Hypogonadism (lack of menstrual periods, impotence)
- Congestive heart failure
- Hyperpigmentation of the skin (gray/blue or yellow)
- Loss of body hair
- Diabetes mellitus

OSTEOPOROSIS

- Episodic back pain, kyphosis (dowager's hump)
- Decreased activity tolerance
- Early satiety

OSTEOMALACIA

- Bone pain, skeletal deformities, fractures
- Myalgia, severe muscle weakness

PAGET'S DISEASE

- Headache and dizziness
- Periosteal tenderness, bone fractures, vertebral compression and collapse, deformity (bowing of long bones, increased size and abnormal contour of clavicles, osteoarthritis of adjacent joint, acetabular protrusion, head enlargement)
- Compression neuropathy (spinal stenosis, paresis, paraplegia, and muscle weakness)
- Decreased auditory acuity

88. What subjective information should be obtained when endocrine system pathology is suspected?

- Presence of any red flags as previously described
- Medication use, including use of insulin or cortisol, or excessive use of antacids
- Slow wound healing
- Family history of osteoporosis
- Increase in collar size (goiter growth), difficulty in breathing or swallowing

89. List common musculoskeletal disorders that mimic endocrine system disorders.

Periarthritis and calcific tendonitis of the shoulder is common in endocrine clients and must be ruled out from other musculoskeletal disorders such as rotator cuff dysfunction, rotator cuff tears, slap lesions, labral tears, and subacromial/subdeltoid bursitis.

Immunologic

90. What are the four principal classifications of immunologic disorders?

The four principal classifications are immunodeficiency, hypersensitivity, autoimmunity, and immunoproliferative disorders.

91. Name the only disease known to directly attack the human immune system.

AIDS (acquired immunodeficiency syndrome)

92. How are hypersensitivity disorders classified?

Hypersensitivity disorders are grouped into four types: type I anaphylactic hypersensitivity (allergies), type II hypersensitivity (cytolytic or cytotoxic), type III hypersensitivity (immune complex), and type IV hypersensitivity (cell-mediated or delayed).

93. What neurologic disorders may be associated with immune system dysfunction?

Myasthenia gravis, Guillain-Barré syndrome, and multiple sclerosis are neurologic disorders associated with immune system dysfunction.

94. List examples of autoimmune disorders.

Examples of autoimmune disorders are fibromyalgia syndrome, rheumatoid arthritis, systemic lupus erythematosus, scleroderma, spondyloarthropathy, Reiter syndrome, psoriatic arthritis, Lyme disease, and bacterial arthritis.

95. What signs and symptoms are commonly associated with pathologies of the immunologic system?

AIDS

- Early signs and symptoms include fever, night sweats, fatigue, headache, minor oral infections, cough, shortness of breath, and skin changes (e.g., rash, nail bed changes, dry skin).
- Advanced signs and symptoms include Kaposi's sarcoma and the presence of opportunistic diseases (TB, pneumonia, lymphoma, thrush, herpes 1 and 2).

HYPERSENSITIVITY DISORDERS

- Signs and symptoms may be as minor as sinus drainage to as severe as coma or death of the patient.
- Additional signs and symptoms include nausea, prolonged vomiting, diarrhea; confusion, irritability, agitation, restlessness; muscle twitching, cramping, and weakness; paresthesias; convulsions, eventual coma; and slow, shallow breathing.

NEUROLOGIC DISORDERS

- Signs and symptoms of myasthenia gravis include muscle fatigability and proximal muscle weakness aggravated with exertion, respiratory failure, ptosis, diplopia, dysarthria, and bulbar involvement (alteration in voice quality, dysphagia, nasal regurgitation, choking).
- Signs and symptoms of Guillain-Barré syndrome include muscle weakness (bilateral, progressing from the legs to the arms to the chest and neck), diminished deep tendon reflexes, paresthesias, fever, malaise, and nausea.
- Signs and symptoms of multiple sclerosis include optic neuritis leading to unilateral visual impairment, paresthesia, nystagmus, spasticity or hyperreflexia leading to ataxia

or unsteadiness, vertigo, fatigue, muscle weakness, and bowel and bladder dysfunction. Positive Babinski's sign, positive Lhermitte's sign, and absent abdominal reflex are also present.

AUTOIMMUNE DISORDERS

- Signs and symptoms of fibromyalgia syndrome include fatigue, depression, anxiety, short-term memory loss, decreased attention span, headaches, nocturnal bruxism, myalgia, tender points of palpation, tendonitis, bursitis, morning stiffness, low back pain, subjective swelling, and irritable bowel and bladder symptoms.
- Signs and symptoms of rheumatoid arthritis include swelling in one or more joints, early morning stiffness, recurring joint pain or tenderness, impaired joint motion, joint redness and warmth, unexplained weight loss, and fever or weakness.
- Signs and symptoms of systemic lupus erythematosus include constitutional symptoms, arthralgia, arthritis, skin rashes, anemia, pulmonary and renal disorders, CNS signs and symptoms, hair loss, and mouth, nose, or vaginal ulcers.
- Signs and symptoms of systemic scleroderma include calcinosis (abnormal deposition of calcium salts in tissues, particularly over bony prominences), Raynaud's phenomenon, dysphagia, heartburn, hardening and shrinking of the toes and fingers, and formation of spiderlike hemangiomas in the face and hands.
- Signs and symptoms of spondyloarthropathy include back pain with insidious onset; first episode occurs before age 30, episodes of pain last months, and pain intensifies with rest and decreases with movement.
- Signs and symptoms of ankylosing spondylitis include:
  - Early signs and symptoms—intermittent low-grade fever, fatigue, anemia, anorexia, painful limited spinal motion, loss of spinal motion, inflammation of the iris (iritis or iridocyclitis)
  - Advanced signs and symptoms—constant low back pain, ankylosis of the SI joints and spine, muscle wasting in the shoulder and pelvic girdles, marked cervical kyphosis, decreased chest expansion, arthritis in the extremity joints
- Signs and symptoms of Reiter syndrome include polyarthritis, SI/low back pain, heel pain, plantar fasciitis, low-grade fever, urethritis (precedes other symptoms by 1 to 2 weeks), and bilateral conjunctivitis and iritis.
- Signs and symptoms of psoriatic arthritis include fever, fatigue, dystrophic nail bed changes, polyarthritis, psoriasis, and sore, swollen fingers.
- Signs and symptoms of Lyme disease include rash, flulike symptoms, migratory musculoskeletal pain, severe headaches, numbness, weakness and pain in the extremities, and poor motor coordination.
- Signs and symptoms of bacterial arthritis include fever and chills, rapid onset of mono-articular involvement (knees and shoulders most frequent), joint inflammatory symptoms/signs, restricted motion, local tenosynovitis, and skin lesions near the involved joint.

96. What are immunologic red flags?

In addition to the signs and symptoms described previously, the following red flags should also be screened:

- Development of neurologic symptoms 1 to 3 weeks after an injection (Guillain-Barré syndrome)
- New onset of inflammatory joint pain postoperatively, especially if accompanied by extra-articular signs and symptoms such as rash, diarrhea, urethritis, mouth ulcers, and raised skin patches
- Joint pain preceded or accompanied by skin rash or lesions
- Generalized weakness
- Nail bed changes (e.g., dystrophic nail changes associated with psoriasis, atrophy of the fingertips, calcific nodules, digital cyanosis and tightening of the skin associated with scleroderma)

97. What are other musculoskeletal causes of pain that must be differentially diagnosed from an immunologic disorder?

Because of the multisystem impact of immunologic disorders, it is important that a complete health history is performed to identify if musculoskeletal signs and symptoms are attributable to a mechanical origin, or whether other sources should be investigated. Close cooperation and appropriate comanagement with the referring physician are crucial for the proper management of musculoskeletal cases with suspicious origins.

CLINICAL REASONING

98. Do knowledge, efficiency of data collection, and data interpretation improve with experience?

No. The literature suggests that inadequate knowledge and imprecise data collection improve with increasing clinical experience but data integration and interpretation does not.

99. Why do errors in clinical reasoning occur?

It is well documented that human beings are for the most part noncritical thinkers and that we are prone to deductive and inductive errors in reasoning (i.e., judgment errors). Additionally, the cognitive limitation of human working memory leads us to access simpler rather than more complex cognitive or problem-solving strategies (i.e., shortcuts in reasoning). In actuality, it is likely the combination of judgment errors and reliance on shortcuts in reasoning (e.g., heuristics) that leads to most errors in clinical reasoning. Finally, errors will vary based on the difficulty of the patient case, knowledge of content and context, strategy selection, and integration and interpretation of pertinent patient information.

100. What is deductive reasoning?

Deductive reasoning involves reaching a conclusion based on evidence (i.e., deductive reasoning combines two or more pieces of evidence to reach a conclusion).

101. What are examples of deductive reasoning errors?

Illogical or poor reasoning, persistence of beliefs despite empirical data to the contrary, rationalizing, justifying, and using biases and heuristics to assess information are examples of deductive reasoning errors.

102. What is inductive reasoning?

Inductive reasoning uses specific pieces of evidence (i.e., more than one example) to draw conclusions that are probably, but not necessarily, true (e.g., generalizations, cause and effect, and analogies).

103. What are examples of inductive reasoning errors?

Examples include overconfidence in validity of beliefs, confusion of opinion or anecdotal evidence with truth, overestimation of knowledge, and basing a decision on personal interests.

104. What is iterative hypothesis testing?

Iterative hypothesis testing, as described by Kasper and Harrison, is a process used by medical practitioners to increase the efficiency of the interview process. During this process interview questions are used to confirm or refute the evolving diagnostic hypothesis. Iterative hypothesis testing uses specific questions to probe patient answers. Iterative hypothesis testing does not replace a systematic, thorough, and complete history of present illness, past medical history, review of systems, family history, and the physical examination. Iterative hypothesis testing represents a pattern of application of inductive and deductive reasoning.

105. Give an example of iterative hypothesis testing based on a patient's perception of illness.

The patient presents with a referral that states: "Lumbar pain, Evaluate and Treat." Therapist: "What are you here for today?" Patient: "I have a pinched nerve in my back." Therapist: "Who was the doctor that diagnosed you with this condition?" Patient: "It was not my doctor." Therapist: "I am not certain if I understand; how did you determine that you have a pinched nerve in your back?" Patient: "About a year ago my neighbor had the same pain that I am having and he was diagnosed with a pinched nerve in his back." In this example if the therapist did not test the hypothesis, a serious error could have occurred.

106. List common errors or biases in clinical reasoning and a potential consequence of the error or bias.

Error or Bias	Possible Consequences
Adding pragmatic inferences	Making diagnostic assumptions that result in misdiagnoses or faulty clinical decisions
Confirmation bias (e.g., emphasizing or validating information that supports clinician's favored hypotheses while negating information that does not)	Failure to identify or address competing diagnoses and limiting examination to tests and measures that confirm suspected diagnosis while ignoring evidence and testing that might eliminate diagnosis
Confusing covariance with causality	Presuming that two or more factors are causally related when two factors have been found to covary
Confusions between deductive and inductive logic	Deductive reasoning errors or drawing conclusions that go beyond the information contained in premises (e.g., correct: if A then B, A therefore B; incorrect: if A then B, therefore if B then A); inductive reasoning errors or generalizations based on specific observations that are not based on deductive reasoning (e.g., all A are B $\neq$ all B are A)
Considering too few diagnoses (e.g., hypotheses)	Artificially or prematurely limiting number of plausible diagnoses
Considering too few interventions	Choosing same intervention option when there are additional and alternative options available
Errors in detecting variance	Making a judgment about relationship of two factors without understanding how two factors covary with one another
Failure to sample enough information	Basing clinical decisions on generalizations and limited data and discontinuing search for

continued

continued

Error or Bias	Possible Consequences
	additional diagnoses after anticipated diagnosis is made
Faulty hypotheses testing	Making clinical decisions based on illogical or faulty reasoning processes
Faulty or inadequate knowledge or skill base	Making clinical decisions based on omissions that stem from lack of knowledge or omitting more beneficial interventions secondary to lack of knowledge or skill
Generating a diagnosis based on availability or recall	Overestimating probability of a diagnosis and generating false sense of frequency
Generating a diagnosis based on similarity or pattern recognition	Neglecting prevalence of competing diagnoses
Generating a diagnosis based on patient perception of illness	Type of confirmation bias in which clinician seeks to validate a self-reported patient diagnosis

Bibliogaphy

Addison RG: Chronic pain syndrome, *Am J Med* 77:54-58, 1984.

American Physical Therapy Association: Guide to physical therapist practice: second edition, *Phys Ther* 81:9-746, 2001.

Bogduk N, Twomey LT: *Clinical anatomy of the lumbar spine,* New York, 1987, Churchill Livingstone.

Bordage G: Elaborated knowledge: a key to successful diagnostic thinking, *Acad Med* 69:883-885, 1994.

Boyling JD, Palastanga N, Grieve GP: *Grieve's modern manual therapy: the vertebral column,* ed 2, New York, 1994, Churchill Livingstone.

Edwards I et al: Clinical reasoning strategies in physical therapy, *Phys Ther* 84:312-330, 2004 (discussion 331-335).

Elstein AS: Heuristics and biases: selected errors in clinical reasoning, *Acad Med* 74:791-794, 1999.

Friedman MH et al: Medical student errors in making a diagnosis, *Acad Med* 73(10 suppl):S19-21, 1998.

Gamsa A, Vikis-Freibergs V: Psychological events are both risk factors in, and consequences of, chronic pain, *Pain* 44:271-277, 1991.

Garfin SR et al: Spinal nerve root compression, *Spine* 20:1810-1820, 1995.

Goodman CC, Snyder TEK: *Differential diagnosis in physical therapy,* ed 3, Philadelphia, 2000, WB Saunders.

Groves M, O'Rourke P, Alexander H: The clinical reasoning characteristics of diagnostic experts, *Med Teach* 25:308-313, 2003.

Higgs J, Jones MA: *Clinical reasoning in the health professions,* ed 2, Oxford, 2000, Butterworth-Heinemann.

Holloway PJ: Inductive vs deductive reasoning, *Br Dent J* 188:643-644, 2000.

Jarvik JG, Deyo RA: Diagnostic evaluation of low back pain with emphasis on imaging, *Ann Intern Med* 137:586-597, 2002.

Jarvis C: *Physical examination & health assessment,* ed 4, St Louis, 2004, WB Saunders.

Kasper DL, Harrison TR: *Harrison's' principles of internal medicine,* ed 16, New York, 2005, McGraw-Hill.

Kempainen RR, Migeon MB, Wolf FM: Understanding our mistakes: a primer on errors in clinical reasoning, *Med Teach* 25:177-181, 2003.

Mense S, Simons DG, Russell IJ: *Muscle pain: understanding its nature, diagnosis, and treatment,* Philadelphia, 2001, Lippincott Williams & Wilkins.

Moore KL, Dalley AF: *Clinically oriented anatomy,* ed 4, Philadelphia, 1999, Lippincott Williams & Wilkins.

Nissl J: *Health guide A-Z: complete blood count (CBC) HTML*; December 14, 2004; WebMDHealth (website): http://my.webmd.com/hw/lab_tests/hw4260.asp. Accessed July 29, 2005.

Round A: Introduction to clinical reasoning, *J Eval Clin Pract* 7:109-117, 2001.
Rubin E: *Essential pathology,* ed 3, Philadelphia, 2001, Lippincott.
Seidel HM et al: *Mosby's guide to physical examination,* ed 4, St Louis, 1999, Mosby.
Wall PD, Melzack R, Bonica JJ: *Textbook of pain,* New York, 1984, Churchill Livingstone.
Willis WD, Jr: The pain system: the neural basis of nociceptive transmission in the mammalian nervous system, *Pain Headache* 8:1-346, 1985.

Chapter 25

Pediatric Orthopaedic Physical Therapy

Beth Ennis, PT, EdD, PCS, and Jeffrey D. Placzek, MD, PT

1. List the common developmental milestones.

1. Rolls prone to supine: 4 months
2. Rolls supine to prone: 6 months
3. Sits alone: 6 to 7 months
4. Creeps: 9 months (not *all* children creep)
5. Pulls to stand: 9 to 10 months
6. Cruises: 10 months
7. Walks well: 12 to 14 months
8. Jumps: 2 years
9. Hops: 4 years
10. Skips: 5 years

2. Can young children be taught to use crutches?

Children can learn to use crutches easily, provided the crutches are properly fitted and the child's coordination level is normal. Age is also a factor, because of the development of bilateral coordination. Typically, children can stand on one leg for 4 to 6 seconds at around 4 years of age. Colored yarn or colored dots on the shoe and crutch that are supposed to move together facilitate teaching a 4-point gait pattern to 3- to 5-year-old children.

3. How early can children benefit from using a wheelchair or powered mobility?

For parents who want a convenient way to move the child while shopping, a stroller may be all that is needed, provided it has proper support and does not promote poor positioning. At other times a *properly fitted* wheelchair may be the answer. Some children may need a powered chair, but not if the home has insufficient space to make it useful. Children as young as 18 months of age can be competent, independent users of powered mobility. One consistent movement, such as an eye blink or wrist twitch, and some amount of cognitive ability are all that is needed for power mobility to be attempted.

4. Name the standardized tests commonly used in pediatric physical therapy. When are they useful?

Testing Tool	Areas Evaluated	Ages Evaluated	Type of Tool	Strengths
Denver (DDDST II)	Motor, cognitive, language, social and adaptive	1 week-6.5 years	Screen	Quick and easy to learn
Peabody (PDMS II)	Gross and fine motor	1-72 months	Evaluation	Allows for emerging skills
Bayley II	Motor and cognitive	1-42 months	Evaluation	Considered gold standard
TIME	Motor, functional skills	4 months-3.5 years	Evaluation	Some qualitative assessment; subscales for atypical tone
Bruiniks-Oseretsky	Gross and fine motor, bilateral coordination	4.5-14.5 years	Evaluation	Tests bilateral coordination and balance
WeeFIM	Functional mobility	6 months-8 years	Screen	Used in pediatric rehab settings to document functional progress
PEDI	Functional activities	6 months-7.5 years	Evaluation	Assesses functional skills in children with motor and cognitive disabilities
GMFM	Motor skills	5 months-16 years	Evaluation	Used to document progress in children with CP

CP, Cerebral palsy.

5. When do children develop an adult gait pattern?

Gait laboratory studies show that the normal pattern of adult gait is established at age 3 years, although heel strike is seen as early as 18 months. A stable pattern in the adult mode is present by age 7 years, but stride length continues to increase with increases in height and leg length.

6. What is Gowers' sign or maneuver?

Children with weakness, especially of the quadriceps, use Gowers' maneuver to stand up from the floor. The child rolls prone, gets onto the hands and knees, extends the knees, and uses the hands to "walk up" the legs until the erect position is achieved. Gowers' maneuver is *not* normal and indicates major muscle weakness. Suspect a muscular dystrophy (most commonly Duchenne's disease in males) and refer the child to the appropriate physician immediately.

7. What is the role of physical therapy for children with torticollis?

Children with congenital muscular torticollis demonstrate decreased cervical range of motion in rotation to the same side and lateral flexion to the opposite side of the tight sternocleidomastoid muscle (SCM). Cervical restriction patterns other than the aforementioned pattern may suggest other cervical or neurologic issues. Before treatment, best practice suggests radiologic assessment of the cervical region to rule out any spinal abnormalities, as aggressive range of motion would be contraindicated in these conditions. Treatment for torticollis ranges from aggressive stretching, bracing, and positioning to encouraging active motion and using vision to align the head and body. However, active movement and positioning appear to be the most successful, especially in children with positional torticollis or muscular torticollis. Torticollis with palpable sternomastoid tumor is the most resistant to treatment. Early age at initiation of treatment is also associated with positive results from conservative treatment.

8. What is deformational plagiocephaly?

Deformational plagiocephaly is a flattening of the skull, causing asymmetry in alignment of the ears, orbits, or jaw if the flattening is on one side, or elongation of the skull if the flattening is centrally located. Once evaluation has determined that the change in shape is not caused by premature fusion of the sutures (craniosynostosis), the shape may benefit from remolding using molding helmets or bands. Helmets or bands are generally worn 23 hours a day, for 3 to 6 months, and are fabricated by orthotists. Referral for the helmet should occur at or before 5 months of age, as the use of a helmet is most effective before 1 year of age. Cranial measurements can be used to assess progress, and determine the need for a helmet.

9. Is developmental dysplasia of the hip (DDH) the same as congenital dislocation of the hip (CDH)?

Yes. DDH used to be called CDH, but the newer terminology better describes its dynamic nature. DDH refers to a wide spectrum of hip abnormalities, ranging from complete dislocation of the femoral head to mild acetabular abnormality or laxity of the hip. It is more common in females (in the left lower extremity), in children with a family history of the disorder, and in first-born children. Breech births, decreased uterine space, metatarsus adductus, and torticollis are also associated with DDH.

10. How is DDH treated?

Infants with DDH who are under 6 months of age usually are treated with the Pavlik harness. Treatment for older children varies with age. In children younger than 1½ years, reduction probably will be attempted (with or without prior traction), and older children usually need open surgical reduction, possibly with proximal femoral shortening and a pelvic osteotomy (such as Salter's or Pemberton's procedure).

11. What is the role of physical therapy in the treatment of DDH?

Occasionally, physical therapy will be requested for a child just out of a harness, because of difficulty with prone positioning and active hip extension following prolonged positioning in hip flexion and external rotation. This can limit the development of rolling and transitions in sitting, as well as movement in prone. If an older child is referred, pool therapy or kicking-out exercises in a warm bathtub at home are excellent choices for treatment. Tricycles with adjustable seat heights are also helpful for increasing hip range of motion (ROM) and weight bearing. If a child is treated after age 6, the gluteus medius and maximus have worked at a mechanical disadvantage for a long period, and the child may walk with an abductor lurch or trunk shift. Such walking habits are hard to break without the use of visual feedback (e.g., walking toward a mirror).

12. Describe the classic tests used to evaluate DDH.

- Ortolani sign—The child is supine and the examiner grasps the flexed thigh with thumbs on the inner thigh and fingers on the greater trochanters. As the hip is abducted and the greater trochanter is elevated, a clunk is felt, indicating that the hip is reduced. This test is less sensitive after 2 months of age; mnemonic: Ortolani's = out to in.
- Barlow's Test—Begin this test the same as the Ortolani procedure; adduct the flexed hip and gently push the thigh posteriorly, testing for dislocation. This test is also less sensitive after 2 months of age because of muscular development.
- Galeazzi sign or Allis' sign—This is a test of apparent thigh length. The patient lies supine with hips and knees flexed to 90 degrees. In a positive test, one knee is higher than the other. The results will not be accurate if bilateral DDH is present.

13. What are the components of a clubfoot (talipes equinovarus)?

- Hindfoot varus and equinus
- Supination/adduction of the forefoot
- Medial and plantar rotation of the talus

This can be seen either unilaterally or bilaterally.

14. How are physical therapists involved in treating children with congenital clubfoot?

The best treatment begins as close to birth as possible and consists of repositioning of the foot, either manually or surgically, followed by casting. Forced dorsiflexion by serial casting must be avoided as a rocker-bottom foot may develop. However, splinting in ankle-foot orthosis (AFO), or taping, especially if the infant is in the neonatal intensive care unit with other issues, can be used to gain range of motion and improve positioning. Ponseti's technique of manipulation and casting, followed by Achilles tenotomy if needed, has shown up to 90% success, reducing the need for surgical correction. After surgery or casting/ bracing, the physical therapist may be involved in teaching postoperative exercises to maintain or regain ROM and to regain strength in the muscles of the calf and foot.

15. Describe the normal progression of lower extremity alignment in children.

- Newborns: varus knees
- 18 months: straight knees
- $2\frac{1}{2}$ years: valgus knees
- 4 to 6 years: normal alignment

16. What is brachial plexus palsy (BPP) in infants?

BPP is the term commonly used to describe injury to the brachial plexus during birth. Larger infants (such as those born to mothers with gestational diabetes) are at greater risk, as are breech and assisted (forceps or vacuum) deliveries. Erb-Duchenne palsy (C5, C6) or waiter's tip deformity has the best prognosis, followed by Klumpke's palsy (C8-T1); complete plexus palsy has the worst prognosis. Occasionally, a clavicle fracture accompanies the injury, and should be ruled out.

17. How is BPP treated?

Approximately 80% to 90% of children recover spontaneously, but there are indicators for a better prognosis. Traction injuries tend to recover over time, whereas avulsion injuries are less responsive. If movement is not regained in the first 4 months, the child should be referred for further evaluation and possible surgical intervention. Initial therapy involvement includes positioning to decrease further stretch on the shoulder, and prone-supported weight-bearing activities to stimulate muscle activity. Therapy can also minimize the likelihood of a contracture when the muscles recover to whatever level they can reach.

18. What actions can be taken to make a baby move its arms to test for BPP?

Tactile stimulation along the muscles, stimulation of the grasp reflex, and sharp/dull testing should produce active movement in innervated muscles. The Moro test (dropping the child backward suddenly in a controlled fashion) is often used, but can cause additional tension on the shoulder. If movement does not return after 1 to 2 weeks, EMGs are often used to determine the extent of injury.

19. Can physical therapy to reduce spasticity improve function in children with cerebral palsy?

No scientific evidence indicates that physical therapy can reduce spasticity over the long term. Therapy techniques have been shown to be effective in the short term; however, significant spasticity often needs to be addressed to improve functional independence. However, evidence has shown that therapy to strengthen spastic muscles has a positive effect, and does not negatively influence spasticity. Typical growth and development can also cause changes that shorten spastic muscles and can cause loss of function. This can be addressed by physical therapy.

20. What are some methods of addressing spasticity medically?

Of the various medical treatments for spasticity reduction, the easiest to use is an oral agent such as diazepam (Valium) or oral baclofen. The dosage needed to cross the blood-brain barrier for effectiveness, however, may make the child sleepy. Baclofen delivered intrathecally from a battery-powered pump has helped some children who are severely limited by spasticity, and tends to affect legs more than arms. For children with more localized issues, intramuscular injection of botulinum toxin type A (Botox) prevents the presynaptic release of acetylcholine at the nerve-muscle junction. Often, mild reductions in spasticity can result in improved functional ability.

21. Define osteochondritis dissecans.

Osteochondritis dissecans (OCD) is a necrotic bone lesion with no known cause that may affect subchondral bone and adjacent articular cartilage. It is seen most commonly in the knee (in the intercondylar region of the medial femoral condyle). The ankle and elbow are the other areas that may be affected. Lesions are staged 1 through 4, with stage 1 being a small area of compression and stage 4 having a displaced loose body. It is generally seen in teenagers, but can occur at any age. Patients may have complaints of instability and joint locking.

22. What tests are useful for the diagnosis of osteochondritis dissecans?

The Wilson test may be useful to diagnose OCD of the knee. With the knee flexed to 90 degrees, the tibia is rotated medially. The knee is extended passively while medial tibial rotation is maintained. Pain is detected at about 30 degrees of knee flexion and relieved by lateral tibial rotation. However, it is often diagnosed with radiography.

23. How is osteochondritis dissecans treated?

Immobilization in a cast is a common treatment if the subchondral bone is intact. Children with open epiphyseal plates tend to respond well to 2 to 3 months of casting. Otherwise, a reduction in activity level with gradual increase is indicated. Isometric exercises are indicated during casting, progressing to active exercise to regain full ROM when the cast is removed and finally to resisted strength training and return to full activity. If a loose fragment is present or if the subchondral bone is involved, surgery (usually arthroscopic) is indicated.

24. What is Osgood-Schlatter disease?

Osgood-Schlatter disease involves enlargement and microfractures in the apophysis of the tibial tubercle (where the quadriceps inserts) and is commonly seen in young, highly active adolescent males who are going through a rapid growth spurt. Males are typically affected from ages 13 to 14 years, whereas girls more often have symptoms from the age of 11 or 12. The tibial tubercle is usually prominent and tender. The pain is worsened by squatting, jumping, or kneeling.

25. How is Osgood-Schlatter disease treated?

Treatment is directed at relief of symptoms with heat or ice massage, changes in activity, use of knee pads, and administration of antiinflammatory medication. Splinting is rarely indicated. The condition usually resolves once the tibial tubercle apophysis fuses. While the problem is being treated, flexibility and isometric strengthening exercises for the quadriceps and hamstring muscles may help. Sometimes a separate ossicle (small bone) develops under the patellar tendon and may need to be removed surgically.

26. What is Sinding-Larsen–Johansson syndrome?

Sinding-Larsen–Johansson syndrome is a traction apophysitis at the distal patella pole.

27. What is Legg-Calvé-Perthes (LCP) disease?

LCP disease is idiopathic avascular necrosis (probably episodic) of the femoral head. It is seen most often in children aged 4 to 12 years and affects boys more often than girls (4:1). The disease is bilateral in approximately 12% of cases. The hip progresses from synovitis to an avascular stage to fragmentation to reossification and finally heals within approximately 18 to 24 months following reossification.

28. How is LCP disease treated?

Treatment usually consists of maintaining or regaining hip ROM, especially abduction, to keep the deformable involved segment of the femoral head contained within the acetabulum. How the range of hip abduction should be maintained is controversial. Currently surgery (i.e., Salter's osteotomy of the femur or proximal femoral osteotomy) or bedrest and traction are favored. Abduction bracing, used more commonly in the past, is losing favor. Mild cases in younger children may be treated with physical therapy alone. Postoperative or nonoperative physical therapy involves regaining strength and ROM of the leg and progression from protected weight-bearing with crutches to resumption of full activity.

29. Define Sprengel's deformity. What associated features may be seen?

Sprengel's deformity is a congenital elevation of the scapula, often accompanied by tethering of the scapula to the spinal column by a bony, cartilaginous, or soft tissue band. The deformity leads to limitation of arm abduction. Because the problem originates in the cervical region, children with Sprengel's deformity may have associated congenital anomalies of the cervical spine (Klippel-Fiel syndrome).

30. What type of individual is most likely to suffer from a slipped capital femoral epiphysis?

Obese adolescent males, ages 10 to 16, are most likely to have a "slip" or displacement of the capital (i.e., head or proximal) femoral epiphysis. They present with limping and pain in the distal thigh, or knee. Because of this symptom, the diagnosis is often incorrect as a result of isolated evaluation of the knee. The condition is more common in African Americans and patients with endocrine abnormalities. Slips can be acute or chronic, and patients have limited hip ROM, especially internal rotation. Patients with chronic slips may show shortening of the involved leg. Gait can be waddling in nature with a laterally rotated leg.

31. Describe the treatment of a slipped capital femoral epiphysis.

Treatment usually requires surgical pinning with in-situ screw fixation to stabilize "the slip" and to close the physis. Postoperative physical therapy involves regaining hip ROM, strengthening the lower extremity, especially the hip abductors, and protected partial weight-bearing with crutches. Partial weight-bearing is suggested (even if minimal) because non–weight-bearing requires use of the hip muscles to maintain the leg in the air and puts more stress on the hip than resting the foot on the floor. Chondrolysis and avascular necrosis (AVN) are potential late complications. Attempted reduction of slips increases the rate of AVN.

32. What conditions can affect the young baseball player?

Repetitive stress may cause epiphysiolysis at the proximal humerus (little league shoulder) or stress the medial epicondyle apophysis (little league elbow).

33. What lower extremity changes normally occur with growth?

Femoral anteversion decreases from 40 to 15 degrees at maturity, whereas tibial rotation increases from 5 degrees of external rotation to 15 degrees at maturity.

34. What is a pectus excavatum (cave chest) indicative of in a child?

This is a depression of the sternum, generally related to poor muscle tone and respiratory insufficiency. Abdominal support to improve the effectiveness of the diaphragm could help to decrease the pectus.

35. What is nursemaids' elbow?

Also referred to as pulled elbow, temper tantrum elbow, or supermarket elbow, nursemaids' elbow is subluxation of the radial head from the annular ligament. The mechanism of injury is usually a traction force on the arm, often seen when children are swung by the hands or an arm is jerked rapidly. Radiographs showing displacement of 3 mm or more from the capitellum suggest subluxation. Reduction is achieved with supination. Recurrence rates vary from 5% to 39%.

36. What are growing pains?

While not well-defined, growing pains are nonspecific intermittent pains, usually occurring at night, but often coming and going. They can be in the quads, calves, or other muscle groups, and generally occur during growth spurts. It is hypothesized that they are related to rapid bone growth, and muscle fatigue while trying to accommodate to the new length. It is important to note that physical exam is normal in these children. Generally, slow stretching, warmth, and massage help.

37. How are growth plate fractures classified?

Salter-Harris classification is the most well-defined system for identifying physeal fracture. Additionally, Rang and Ogden have added to this classification.

SALTER-HARRIS CLASSIFICATION
I: Fracture through physis
II: Fracture through physis exits metaphysis
III: Fracture through joint surface, through epiphysis and across physis
IV: One segment including epiphysis, physis, metaphysis
V: Crush injury

RANG CLASSIFICATION
VI: Perichondral ring

OGDEN CLASSIFICATION
VII: Osteochondral fracture
VIII: Metaphysis fracture

Bibliography

California Department of Education: *Guidelines for occupational therapy and physical therapy in California public schools,* Sacramento, Calif, 1996, Bureau of Publications.
Campbell SK, editor: *Physical therapy for children,* ed 2, Philadelphia, 2000, WB Saunders.
Cheng JCY et al: Clinical determinants of the outcome of manual stretching in the treatment of congenital muscular torticollis in infants, *J Bone Joint Surg* 83:679-687, 2004.
Dobbs MB et al: Factors predictive of outcome after use of the Ponseti method for the treatment of idiopathic clubfeet, *J Bone Joint Surg* 86:22-27, 2004.
Dormans JP: *Pediatric orthopedics and sports medicine: the requisites in pediatrics,* St Louis, 2004, Mosby.
Evans AM et al: Prevalance of "Growing Pains" in young children, *J Pediatr* 145:255-258, 2004.
Long TM, Toscano K: *Handbook of pediatric physical therapy,* ed 2, Baltimore, 2002, Lippincott Williams & Wilkins.

Chapter 26

Women's Health Issues

Rebecca G. Stephenson, PT, DPT, MS
Susan Dunn, PT

1. What physiologic changes occur during pregnancy?

Most systems of the body undergo change during the 9 months of pregnancy, including the reproductive, cardiovascular, gastrointestinal, respiratory, and endocrine systems. The breasts and kidneys are also altered as well as the metabolic and dermatologic functions of the body.

2. What are the cardiovascular changes during pregnancy?

Some of the cardiovascular changes during pregnancy are the following: blood volume increases approximately 50%; dilutional anemia occurs because of an initial early increase in plasma volume and a slower initial increase in red cell mass; pulse rate increases 10 to 15 beats/min; chambers of the heart dilate and the position of the heart changes, rotating outward and to the left; stroke volume and cardiac output increase 30% to 50%; blood pressure decreases slightly; venous return to the heart is affected by the increasing size of the uterus (especially in the supine position). In well-conditioned athletes, blood flow to the uterus and heat dissipation may be improved with exercise because of increased blood volume, as compared to sedentary women.

3. What respiratory changes occur during pregnancy?

The overall vital capacity is unchanged; the diaphragm elevates and the rib cage expands and flares; the residual volume decreases and the tidal volume/oxygen consumption increases. The respiratory changes that are occurring with the mother are amplified with the fetus. Therefore if the mother is experiencing a persistent state of hypoxia or acidosis while exercising, the fetus will experience these respiratory changes to a greater degree. It is for this reason that prolonged anaerobic exercise is not recommended, or aerobic exercise that causes dyspnea.

4. What musculoskeletal changes occur during pregnancy?

Posture, gait, and balance are all affected. The center of gravity moves up and forward, causing flexion in the cervical spine and increased lordosis in the lumbar spine. The hormones progesterone and relaxin increase ligamentous and joint laxity. The additional body weight increases the joint forces on the spine. There is an increased risk for sprains, strains, and falls. Active women may want to opt for swimming or low-impact aerobics rather than running and physical sports.

5. What physical therapy techniques are contraindicated in pregnant clients?

A. Deep heat modalities and electrical stimulation
B. Positions that:
- Involve abdominal compression in mid-to-late pregnancy
- Maintain the supine position longer than 3 minutes after the fourth month of pregnancy
- Raise the buttocks higher than the chest
- Strain the pelvic floor and abdominal muscles
- Encourage vigorous stretching of hip adductors
- Involve rapid, uncontrolled bouncing or swinging movements

6. How is the pubic symphysis affected during pregnancy?

Changes begin as early as the tenth to twelfth week of pregnancy. Radiographic evidence has shown changes beginning during the first trimester with maximum relaxation at term. The hormone relaxin has been identified as the major contributor to this response. There is only pain if there is dysfunction within this joint or the pelvic ring. Rupture of the pubic symphysis associated with pregnancy is rare but can occur in late pregnancy or with delivery.

7. What causes back pain during pregnancy?

The hormone relaxin is released by the third month of pregnancy, and under its influence, increased movement is experienced throughout the vertebral spine and pelvis. Many pregnant women complain of low back pain, which often is caused by the many physical changes of pregnancy: added weight, increased lordosis, changes in the center of gravity, loose pelvic ligaments, and poor muscle tone. Back pain may be muscular, mechanical, joint, or diskogenic in origin.

8. Describe diastasis recti abdominis.

Diastasis recti abdominis is the separation of the two recti muscles in the abdomen. It often is undetected in pregnancy and contributes to back pain, which may be the primary problem because the diastasis itself is not painful. During shifts from supine to sitting position, a bulge may be seen along the center of the abdomen.

9. How is diastasis recti diagnosed?

The woman is placed in the supine position with her knees bent and no pillow under her head. The therapist palpates the rectus muscle at the level of the umbilicus while the client is asked to lift her head. The therapist's fingers are horizontal to the rectus muscles, and if they sink into a gap of two or more fingers' width, the test is considered positive for diastasis recti abdominis. Two fingers above and two fingers below the umbilicus are also tested on subsequent head lifts. The width of the gap is defined by the number of fingers inside the gap.

10. What treatments are available for diastasis recti?

Physical therapy cannot correct this problem in pregnancy. Traditional curl-ups and sit-ups should be avoided if the diastasis is larger than two fingers in width. Leg slides and isometric abdominal control help to maintain strength during the pregnancy. Often a low-slung brace worn as an abdominal lift helps to decrease the load on the muscles and alleviates back pain. In the postpartum period, electrical stimulation during curl-ups with approximation of the recti muscles encourages the recti muscles to return to normal length. To approximate the abdominals, the patient can manually press the gap together as she performs a small curl-up. Another option is to take a sheet folded to a width of 12 inches and place it around the waist of the client. Cross the sheet in front of the client and have her hold onto the midpoint of each side of the sheet while she does a curl-up. Actively pulling in the abdominal muscles helps to restore the abdominal wall.

Often the separated muscles approximate in the postpartum period. When the gap is large, as in pregnancies with multiple gestations, the diastasis may not approximate even after 1 year. In such cases, plastic surgery can realign the recti muscles.

11. How soon can a patient begin performing corrective exercises for diastasis recti following a normal vaginal delivery?

In the absence of any complications, the patient can begin these exercises as soon as she feels comfortable, which is usually within 3 days of delivery.

12. Following a normal vaginal delivery, how soon can women begin:

- Pelvic floor exercise/Kegel exercise—This type of exercise should be initiated as soon as possible following a delivery. It can aid in healing, improve circulation to the perineal tissue, aid in the reduction of urinary stress incontinence, and accelerate improvement in muscle tone for tissue that may be experiencing sudden onset of decreased tone and proprioception as a result of the trauma of delivery.
- Aerobic exercise—This can be resumed as soon as the patient feels able. Hormone-induced joint laxity can be present up to 4 to 6 weeks postpartum. If the mother is breast-feeding, this could be longer. Therefore the patient should take precautions to protect joints by not stretching them beyond their physiologic ranges. Hamstrings and adductors should be stretched with caution because of their relationship with the pelvic girdle. The patient should be careful not to promote hypermobility and instability. Lower extremity unilateral weight-bearing exercises can lead to sacroiliac and/or pubic symphysis pain.

13. How soon following a cesarean section can women begin physical therapy/ exercise?

Pelvic floor exercises can begin as soon as the woman is comfortable. Abdominal exercises should not be performed for 6 to 8 weeks following surgery or until cleared by the physician, other than pelvic tilts and abdominal isolation exercises. Aerobic activity can begin with light conditioning when cleared by the surgeon. The activity should not apply unnecessary pull or tension on the abdominal wall incision.

Physical therapists are recommended to follow the American College of Obstetrics and Gynecology Guidelines for exercise when treating a pregnant client. A summary of these guidelines follows:

IN THE ABSENCE OF OTHER MEDICAL OR OBSTETRIC CONDITION/ COMPLICATION:

- Perform 30 minutes (or more) of moderate exercise per day.
- Avoid supine exercise after first trimester.
- Avoid prolonged periods of motionless standing.
- Do not exercise to fatigue/exhaustion.
- Non–weight-bearing exercises (e.g., swimming, cycling) are recommended. Some weight-bearing exercise can be continued during pregnancy if the exercise remains at the prepregnancy intensity.
- Avoid exercise that can challenge balance or involve potential for even mild abdominal trauma.
- Pregnancy requires an additional 300 kcal/day; therefore a woman who is exercising should ensure adequate caloric intake.
- Postpartum exercise should resume gradually as tolerated by the woman's physical capabilities.

CONTRAINDICATIONS TO EXERCISE:

- Pregnancy-induced hypertension
- Preterm rupture of membranes
- Preterm labor during the prior or current pregnancy, or both
- Incompetent cervix or cerclage
- Persistent second- or third-trimester bleeding
- Intrauterine growth retardation

PRECAUTIONS (NEED TO BE CLEARED BY PHYSICIAN):

- Chronic hypertension
- Active thyroid, cardiac, vascular, or pulmonary disease

14. Why are carpal tunnel syndrome and de Quervain tenosynovitis common during pregnancy and in the postpartum period?

Increased fluid and fluid retention are believed to be responsible for the increased prevalence of these disorders. Patients with preeclampsia and hypertension appear to be at higher risk. Postpartum mothers who are nursing will sometimes develop carpal tunnel syndrome, and it is believed to be due to the hormone prolactin and to the upper extremity positioning when feeding the baby. de Quervain tenosynovitis results from compression and irritation of the extensor pollicis brevis and abductor pollicis longus tendons as they pass through the first dorsal compartment of the wrist near the styloid process of the radius. This can be prevalent in the postpartum woman who is breast-feeding as well and appears to be exacerbated with child care activities.

15. What are some of the causes of hip pain in the pregnant patient?

Sacroiliac joint dysfunction, innominate biomechanical dysfunction, leg length discrepancy, greater trochanteric bursitis, piriformis syndrome, osteonecrosis of the femoral head, and transient osteoporosis of the hip are all potential causes of hip pain in the pregnant patient. It is vital that women with osteonecrosis and transient osteoporosis of the hip be identified to avoid the possibility of fracture and subsequent surgery.

16. Describe the structure and function of the pelvic floor.

The pelvic floor refers to the pelvic diaphragm, which arises from the posterior superior pubic rami, inner ischial spines, and obturator fascia. The fibers of the pelvic diaphragm insert around the vaginal and rectal openings at the perineal body. The diaphragm is composed of the coccygeus and levator ani muscles. The pelvic floor creates a sling support for the internal organs and openings for the urethra, vagina, and anus.

17. What causes pelvic floor dysfunction?

Pelvic floor dysfunction can be related to any trauma, surgery, or weakness associated with the pelvis. For example, total hip replacement, episiotomy, vaginal delivery, or back surgery could cause pelvic floor dysfunction. When the normal spine or pelvic mechanics are interrupted or when trauma has occurred to the pelvic floor, the patient can be susceptible to pelvic floor pain or dysfunction. These symptoms can also occur with nerve injury, with aging, or with hormonal changes.

18. How is pelvic floor muscle strength assessed?

Frequently, the patient with gynecologic problems needs a musculoskeletal examination as well as a direct manual exam of the perineum. Pelvic floor dysfunctions and musculoskeletal problems can be treated together. Ask the patient to empty the bladder before the start of the exam. The patient lies supine at the end of the musculoskeletal exam, allowing the clinician to proceed directly to manual exam of the perineum with the patient in the lithotomy position. Explain to the patient the order of the exam and the procedures you will be performing. The specially trained physical therapist can assess the strength and tone of the pelvic floor by palpating on the perineum and inserting sterile, gloved, and lubricated fingers 1 or 2 inches into the vagina. Each therapist must decide whether he or she is qualified to do this assessment and also determine whether it is covered by state practice acts and malpractice insurance carriers.

19. How is the pelvic floor graded?

Grading of the pelvic floor presupposes that the examiner has some experience in grading pelvic floor muscles and can discriminate between the levels of strength. Lab instruction with an experienced clinician is the only way to learn. A suggested method for basic grading is as follows:

- 0—No contraction
- 1—Flicker of contraction
- 2—Weak contraction
- 3—Moderate contraction with pelvic floor lift
- 4—Good contraction with pelvic floor lift
- 5—Strong contraction with pelvic floor lift

20. Define pelvic organ prolapse.

The word *prolapse* is derived from the Latin word *prolapsus* ("to slip" or "fall") and refers to the pelvic organs descending into or through the vagina.

21. How is physical therapy involved in treating pelvic organ prolapse?

Physical therapy has not been proven to improve prolapse because this is an anatomic defect; however, it can reduce symptoms and prevent progression. Physical therapy treatment involves:

- Therapeutic exercises for the pelvic floor for strength and conditioning; can be performed against gravity or with gravity eliminated, depending on the severity of the prolapse and the amount of muscle atrophy
- Abdominal retraining and conditioning for strengthening and stabilization, and for decreasing intraabdominal pressure with activity
- Neuromuscular reeducation/modality intervention as needed, depending on the amount of decreased proprioception evident
- Pessary use and surgical correction

22. What patient population is most at risk for pelvic organ prolapse?

Women who have had vaginal deliveries or a history of chronic constipation or obesity are often implicated as being in the highest risk category for developing pelvic organ prolapse. However, retrospective studies have shown that nulliparous women involved in high-impact sports and repetitive heavy lifting occupations also have a high incidence of pelvic organ prolapse. Abdominal training for women should be monitored so that technique does not increase intraabdominal pressure, and women should be instructed to activate a pelvic floor contraction to counteract pressure changes at the level of the perineum as well.

23. Describe the five types of incontinence.

1. **Stress incontinence**—involuntary loss of urine during physical exertion (e.g., coughing, lifting) in the absence of detrusor contractions
2. **Urge incontinence**—loss of urine with urgency, with active detrusor contractions
3. **Mixed incontinence**—both stress and urge incontinence
4. **Overflow incontinence**—the bladder overfills; an outlet obstruction or underactive detrusor may be present
5. **Reflex incontinence**—present with neurologic lesions; urine leaks without warning

24. Describe physical therapy treatment for incontinence.

Treatment for genuine stress incontinence includes pelvic floor (Kegel) exercise instruction, resistive pelvic floor exercise with vaginal-weighted cones, dietary counseling to avoid diuretics and bladder-irritating substances (e.g., caffeine), biofeedback via air pressure or surface electromyography, and electrical stimulation with in-home or office-unit devices.

25. Is urinary incontinence common in the nulliparous female athlete?

Research has shown that women/girls involved in high-impact sports such as basketball, cheerleading, gymnastics, tennis, and field hockey had occurrences of urinary stress incontinence with sporting activity.

26. What are the expected outcomes of physical therapy for incontinence?

Kegel conducted several studies to assess the efficacy of strengthening pelvic floor musculature to control continence. He showed improvement in three fourths of the women in study samples. In the Kegel or pelvic floor exercise, cortical impulses contract fast-twitch, striated periurethral sphincter muscles via the pudendal nerve. It is theorized that these muscle fibers are able to hypertrophy with prolonged training. No optimal number of repetitions has been standardized, but several protocols have been proposed for strengthening, endurance, and functional retraining. Although early studies suggested isolation of the pubococcygeus muscle was the optimal way to increase its strength, recent studies have reported that overflow contractions through lower extremity and abdominal muscle contractions may enhance pelvic floor muscle training.

27. What medications are used to treat incontinence?

- Tolterodine (Detrol)—antimuscarinic agent; patch
- Oxybutynin chloride (Ditropan)—antimuscarinic agent; pill and patch
- Solifenacin succinate (Vesicare)—new; recently approved antimuscarinic agent
- Darifenacin (Enablex)—new; antimuscarinic agent approved December 2004

28. Define delayed menarche and why this is relevant to physical therapy.

Delayed menarche is lack of menstruation by the age of 16. Studies have shown that there is a strong association between delayed menarche and increased risk of scoliosis and stress fractures with girls involved in high-impact sports (runners, ballet dancers).

29. Define oligomenorrhea and amenorrhea.

Oligomenorrhea is scanty menstruation that can occur with a sudden weight loss of 10 lb, with no regard to the woman's original weight. Amenorrhea is an abnormal cessation of the menses for 3 or more months after menarche has already started.

30. What are some of the causes of oligomenorrhea and amenorrhea?

- Strong emotional disturbance
- Exercise induced—increased endorphins inhibiting hypothalamic function
- Pathologic secondary to disease process
- Dietary—severe weight loss or gain. Typically menses cease when a young woman loses weight to the point at which she is about 85% of her ideal body weight for age and height. Women and girls with a history of anorexia nervosa and/or long-standing amenorrhea are hypoestrogenemic and at high risk for osteopenia/osteoporosis.

31. Define lymphedema.

Lymphedema is the chronic unilateral or bilateral swelling of extremities caused by obstruction, disease, or removal or the lymphatic vessels or nodes. Lymphedema may occur after breast surgery, which may involve removal of part of the breast (lumpectomy), one fourth of the breast (quadrectomy), or the whole breast (mastectomy).

32. Describe the treatment of lymphedema.

Physical therapy involves a combination of range of motion exercises, compression, and various systems of manual lymphatic drainage massage. Compression is achieved with intermittent pneumatic pump, compression garments, or wrapping the extremity with bandages. Ultrasound and myofascial release of the chest wall also promote healing of scars and adhesions. Despite their many variations, all manual lymphatic drainage techniques focus on rate of movement, depth of pressure, area of the body treated, desired direction of lymph flow, and scar tissue.

33. Define the "Female Athlete Triad."

This was initially defined at the Triad Consensus Conference in 1992; it defines the relationship between eating disorders, amenorrhea, and osteoporosis among physically active girls and women.

34. Define osteoporosis.

Osteoporosis is a disease of the bones caused by a thinning of the bone matrix, which results in overall bone loss. Osteoporosis reduces the thickness and strength of the bones and makes them more susceptible to fracture. It is most common in postmenopausal women.

35. How can a female athlete develop osteoporosis?

The female athlete is often under intense pressure to have low body fat percentages to improve performance. The athlete may develop eating disorders to obtain low body fat and, as a result of decreased estrogen levels, then develops amenorrhea and the consequences of osteoporosis (as in postmenopausal women).

36. Describe the common causes of osteoporosis.

Decreased weight-bearing, as in decreased activity, reduces stress on the bones, which triggers calcium resorption and results in bone loss. Risk factors for primary osteoporosis include female sex, Caucasian or Asian descent, early menopause (before age 45), no history of pregnancy, low body weight, family history of osteoporosis, use of steroids and high dosages of thyroid hormones, smoking, excessive alcohol consumption, deficient intake of calcium as a child, and inactivity.

37. What methods are used for the diagnosis of osteoporosis?

Osteoporosis is diagnosed through bone density screening methods: dual-energy x-ray absorptiometry (DXA), which is 90% to 99% accurate; peripheral dual-energy x-ray absorptiometry (pDXA), which is 90% to 99% accurate; single-energy x-ray absorptiometry (SXA), which is 98% to 99% accurate; quantitative ultrasound (QUS); quantitative computed tomography (QCT), which is 85% to 97% accurate; and peripheral quantitative computed tomography (pQCT). These methods measure bone mineral density (BMD) at different sites on the body. Choice of test depends on the anatomic sites available for the study, cost, and accessibility of the technology. All of these tests measure the bone absorption of radiation or high-frequency sound waves, but each uses a different method of measuring energy absorbed by the tissue. The results are expressed as grams of calcium hydroxyapatite per square centimeter of bone cross-section. Normal bone mass is defined by the World Health Organization (WHO) as a T-score above −1; low bone mass as a T-score between −1 and −2.5; and osteoporosis as a T-score at or below −2.5.

38. What are the three types of osteoporosis?

1. Idiopathic osteoporosis
2. Type I or postmenopausal osteoporosis (in women around ages 51 to 75; mostly caused by endocrine changes but also occurs in men)
3. Type II or involutional osteoporosis (may be related to a decrease in vitamin D synthesis within the body; occurs in people over 70, although it begins in the third decade; female-to-male ratio = 2:1)

39. What drugs are commonly used in the treatment of osteoporosis?

A. Bisphosphonates—used for prevention and treatment
- Risedronate (Actonel)
- Alendronate (Fosamax)
- Ibandronate (Boniva)—new; approved for oral use since May 2003. FDA approval for intravenous doses and once monthly dose is still pending.

B. Hormones—used for prevention and treatment
- Conjugated estrogens (Premarin)—used for women with hysterectomy
- Conjugated estrogens with progesterone (Prempro)—used for women with an intact uterus
- Estradiol transdermal (Menostar)—newest; approved June 2004. It is used primarily for prevention.

C. Selective estrogen receptor modulators—act at estrogen receptor sites but not as a hormone; used for prevention and treatment
- Raloxifene (Evista)
- Bazedoxifene—in development. This drug is in stage III studies, both in a singular form and with conjugated estrogens, to provide a two-point approach to osteoporosis.

D. Calcium and vitamin D—1000 mg/day of calcium is recommended for premenopausal women and 1500 mg/day for postmenopausal women, along with 400 to 800 IU/day of vitamin D. Foods are the preferred source of calcium, but additional amounts usually are needed.
E. Calcitonin (Miacalcin)—approved by the FDA for prevention and treatment. This is available as an injection or as a nasal spray. It inhibits bone reabsorption.
F. Fluoride—increases the trabecular bone mass in the spine and pelvis of elderly women. However, it decreases bone mass in the appendicular cortical skeleton, resulting in an increased risk of stress fractures in the upper extremities.
G. Teriparatide (Forteo)—approved by the FDA for treatment in November 2002. It is delivered by daily injection. It is a bone formation agent (all others prevent resorption). This drug also increases osteoblast activity.

40. Are radiographs useful in the diagnosis of osteoporosis?

Radiographs are not sufficient for proper diagnosis of osteoporosis. Bone loss of up to 40% can occur before the loss is visible on radiographs.

41. Why is exercise important in the treatment of osteoporosis?

Weight-bearing exercise stimulates increased bone density and bone growth. Exercise must be maintained, or the positive results of exercise are lost with a return to baseline bone mass. Exercise also improves muscle strength, joint flexibility, function, endurance, balance, gait, and posture. Adults who engage in physical exercise have a faster reaction time than sedentary adults. Reaction time is important in response to loss of balance and prevention of falls. Often falls caused by poor balance result in fractures to the distal radius, vertebrae, or proximal femur. Hip fractures have a high mortality rate.

42. Which bones are most commonly affected?

Type I (postmenopausal) osteoporosis involves excessive and disproportionate trabecular bone loss. It is associated with vertebrae and distal radius fractures. Compression fractures may occur in any vertebrae but usually involve those in the lower thoracic and upper lumbar area.

In **type II** osteoporosis, fractures occur in the upper femur and femoral neck. Type II osteoporosis also may result in multiple wedge-type vertebral fractures, which are not as painful as the crush-type vertebral fractures associated with type I.

43. Describe a physical therapy regimen for osteoporosis.

1. Education—prevention of falls and self-protection during a fall, use of safe body mechanics, modification of lifestyle and diet to minimize risk factors, review of home safety, and consultation with nutritionist for support on dietary needs and supplements
2. Goals to increase activity level throughout the day
3. Self-treatment at home for pain control with heat application, therapeutic exercise, and rest
4. In-office physical therapy treatment with appropriate modalities for acute trauma and pain—heat/cold application, massage therapy, transcutaneous electrical nerve stimulation, electrical stimulation, positioning instruction, fitting of splints or back braces, therapeutic exercise, goal-setting, and planning for progression of disease
5. Increasing activity level with weight-bearing activities and postural correction; objective is to increase stress on the skeleton as much as possible
6. Resistive exercises
7. Balance and coordination exercises with dynamic stabilization of the trunk

44. Why does the risk of heart attack and stroke begin to increase after menopause?

Lower estrogen levels found in postmenopausal women have a negative effect on the cardiovascular system for two reasons: (1) estrogen acts to increase the levels of high-density lipoproteins (HDLs) and decrease the levels of low-density lipoproteins (LDLs); (2) estrogen also helps in inhibiting the deposition of atherosclerotic plaque on the intima of arteries. Consequently, a sedentary lifestyle, poor diet, and poor physical fitness can lead to a higher risk of cardiovascular disease, especially coronary artery disease. Myocardial infarction is the leading cause of death among postmenopausal women.

Bibliography

Benson JT: *Clinical gynecology: urogynecology and reconstructive pelvic surgery,* Philadelphia, 1999, McGraw-Hill.
Goldfarb AF: *Clinical gynecology: pediatric and adolescent gynecology,* Philadelphia, 1998, Current Medicine.
Heckman JD, Sassard R: Current concepts review: musculoskeletal considerations in pregnancy, *J Bone Joint Surg* 11:1720-1730, 1994.
Ireland ML, Nattiv A: *The female athlete,* Philadelphia, 2002, WB Saunders.
Merck & Co: *Bone mineral density testing: a pocket guide to evaluation and reimbursement,* West Point, Pa, 1999, Merck & Co.
Pauls JA: *Therapeutic approaches to women's health: a program of exercise and education,* Frederick, Md, 1996, Aspen Publishers.
Pauls JA, Reed KL: *Quick reference to physical therapy,* Frederick, Md, 1996, Aspen Publishers.
Pemberton J, Swash M, Henry M: *The pelvic floor: its function and disorders,* Philadelphia, 2002, WB Saunders.
Sapsford R, Bullock-Saxton J, Markwell S: *Women's health: a textbook for physiotherapists,* Philadelphia, 1998, WB Saunders.
Schussler B, Laycock J: *Pelvic floor re-education,* New York, 1994, Springer-Verlag.
Stephenson RG, O'Conner LJ: *Obstetric and gynecologic care in physical therapy,* ed 2, Thorofare, NJ, 2000, Slack.
Travell JG, Simons DG: *Myofascial pain and dysfunction: the trigger point manual, the lower extremities,* Philadelphia, 1997, Lippincott Williams & Wilkins.
Wilder E, editor: *The gynecological manual,* Alexandria, Va, 1997, Section of Women's Health of the American Physical Therapy Association.

Chapter 27

Wound Healing and Management

Joseph M. McCulloch, PT, PhD, CWS

1. What is moist wound healing?

Within the microenvironment of a wound, certain conditions provide optimal healing. Proper hydration and adequate perfusion facilitate the formation of granulation tissue and epithelial cell migration. As a result, the wound heals more quickly without the formation of a scab or eschar. Many modern synthetic dressings create just such a moist environment. When the standard "wet-to-dry" gauze dressing is permitted to dry, however, tissue desiccation and a lengthened healing response can result. Select a dressing that creates a moist environment without permitting maceration or desiccation.

2. What is granulation tissue? Is too much a bad thing?

Technically, granulation tissue consists of a gel-like matrix of collagen, hyaluronic acid, and fibronectin in a newly formed vascular network. Granulation tissue nourishes the macrophages and fibroblasts that have migrated into the wound and, as healing continues, provides a substrate for the migration of epidermal cells. Granulation tissue first appears as pale pink buds but later becomes bright red. Excessive granulation tissue, often referred to as "proud flesh," sometimes occurs when no other signs of wound healing are evident. Pressure wraps are used frequently to control this problem. Some clinicians burn the tissue back with silver nitrate, but such a technique is of questionable merit. It serves as an acute injury stimulus, and additional granulation tissue may result.

3. What is meant by mechanical debridement and how effective is it?

Mechanical debridement refers to the removal of devitalized tissue by mechanical means and very broadly includes such techniques as whirlpool, pulsatile lavage with suction, other forms of spray irrigation, and the traditional wet-to-dry dressing. Whirlpool and spray irrigation cleanse the wound but have minimal effect in removing adherent necrotic tissue. Furthermore, whirlpool debridement is fraught with other problems such as the potential for cross-contamination. Pulsatile lavage with suction removes debris more effectively and can deliver a controlled irrigation pressure in a sterile environment. Wet-to-dry dressings provide mechanical debridement by attaching to necrotic tissue and lifting off the tissue at dressing change. This debridement is nonselective, however, and viable tissue can be damaged.

4. Why are wet-to-dry dressings inappropriate for use in current wound care?

In addition to the debridement complications mentioned in the previous question, other problems exist with wet-to-dry dressings. These dressings typically consist of a woven gauze dressing that is applied wet and allowed to dry before removal. The thought behind this type of dressing is that the moisture would initially facilitate the softening of necrotic tissue, which would then stick to the dressing and be removed at the time of dressing change. Anyone who has used such a dressing knows the pain and trauma associated with these dressings becoming adherent to viable tissue and damaging it on removal. In addition, the dryness of the dressing promotes an environment that is conducive only to cell death. As stated previously, moist healing is much preferred and is the standard of care. Additionally, the cotton fibers of the dressing are often left behind in the wound and create a foreign body response.

5. What is enzymatic debridement?

Enzymatic debridement involves the application of a commercially prepared proteolytic enzyme to necrotic tissue to aid in removal. A variety of products are available and include such agents as collagenase, papain, urea, and fibrinolysin. Enzymes are generally used in conjunction with moist wound healing for the best results. Certain pharmaceutical antibacterial preparations, which contain silver or other heavy metals, can interfere with enzyme activity. Care should therefore be taken in combining the two types of therapy in a single treatment. Some commonly used enzymatic debriding agents are Accuzyme, Panafil, and Santyl.

6. What are the advantages and disadvantages of autolytic debridement?

Autolytic debridement implies that the body performs its own cleaning. Synthetic dressings, when appropriately used, can trap endogenous enzymes and other beneficial agents in the wound and provide for adequate debridement. This is a highly selective form of debridement and is very nontraumatic. Though effective, autolytic debridement may take longer to debride a wound than the use of commercial enzyme preparations or more invasive forms of debridement.

7. What are some common topical agents that have been shown to delay healing?

Any agent strong enough to kill bacteria on an inanimate object has the potential to disrupt healing. Some of the more common agents that have unfortunately persisted in the wound care arena include hydrogen peroxide, acetic acid, sodium hypochlorite solution (Dakin's solution), and povidone-iodine. All of these substances, when used at standard clinical strength, have been demonstrated to cause the death of fibroblasts in vitro. If these agents are to be used at all, their use should be very focal in nature. Dakin's solution, for instance, could be applied over necrotic tissue to soften the tissue and aid in debridement. Likewise, acetic acid could be used to help address localized colonization of *Pseudomonas.* In general, however, both agents should be discontinued as soon as the desired results are achieved and not simply used as a moistening agent for gauze.

8. What is the primary difference in the clinical presentation of venous and arterial ulcers?

Although both types of ulcers may occur at varying points along the leg, **venous ulcers** typically are located over the medial malleolar area. They tend to be irregular in shape and possess a good granulation base. Venous ulcers often are associated with lower extremity swelling and generally are quite moist. Brownish staining of the skin caused by the pigment hemosiderin, which is released by lysed red blood cells, suggests a venous ulcer. Patients with venous insufficiency ulcers generally complain of pain after prolonged standing and report relief of pain with leg elevation.

Arterial or ischemic ulcers, on the other hand, are noted most often on the distal aspects of the feet but may occur more proximally, depending on the occluded artery. Arterial ulcers have a punched-out appearance with a pale granulation base. Signs frequently associated with ischemic ulcers include a loss of hair on the extremity, poor capillary refill in the toes, and brittle nails. Patients with ischemic ulcers complain of pain whenever the leg is elevated and frequently hang the leg dependently to reduce symptoms.

9. What system is used to classify pressure ulcers?

The most commonly used classification system for pressure ulcers is the Shea scale, which categorizes ulcers according to the degree of tissue involvement from partial- to full-thickness dermal erosion:

- **Stage 1**—Nonblanchable erythema with intact skin
- **Stage 2**—A partial-thickness lesion with a break in the skin and loss of epidermis
- **Stage 3**—A full-thickness lesion with dermal involvement (no penetration of fascia)
- **Stage 4**—A full-thickness lesion involving the dermis, fascia, and, to varying degrees, underlying muscles, bones, and joints

10. What is meant by reverse-staging of pressure ulcers? Why is it inappropriate?

Reverse-staging implies that as an ulcer heals it moves to the next least involved stage of healing. For example, a stage 4 ulcer would be said to reverse to stage 3, then stage 2, and finally stage 1. This system of reverse-staging, although often required by third-party payors, is inappropriate because once full-thickness involvement has occurred, healing can take place only by wound contraction, scarring, and epithelialization—not by replacement of the original tissue. The dermis cannot regenerate. Reverse-staging is, therefore, an inaccurate description of healing. The more appropriate method is to state that the wound is a "healing stage 4, 3, or 2 pressure ulcer."

11. How are plantar ulcers of the insensate foot staged?

The most frequently used staging system for ulcers of the insensate foot is the Wagner grading system:
- Grade 0—Intact skin
- Grade 1—Superficial ulcer
- Grade 2—Deep ulcer
- Grade 3—Deep, infected ulcer
- Grade 4—Partial foot gangrene
- Grade 5—Full foot gangrene

12. How is total-contact casting of benefit to the healing of a plantar foot ulcer in diabetic patients?

A total-contact cast is a minimally padded, closed-toe plaster cast with a walking heel. Total-contact casting is indicated for Wagner grade 1 and 2 plantar ulcers and works by shifting weight from the plantar ulcer to the arch of the foot and the heel, through the walls of the cast, and to the tibia. Padding is placed over the spine of the tibia, medial and lateral malleoli, navicular prominence, wound, and toes. When properly applied, 30% of the weight-bearing load is transmitted to the cast wall. Total-contact casts are contraindicated in the presence of fluctuating edema, suspected osteomyelitis or other infection, heavily exudating wounds, and claustrophobia. Total-contact casts differ from traditional plaster fracture casts in that minimal padding is used and the toes are completely enclosed. Covering the toes prevents foreign bodies from entering the cast because insensitivity precludes their detection.

13. What are the most common locations for plantar ulcers in patients with diabetes?

The most frequent locations of ulcerations in diabetic patients are the first metatarsal head, fifth metatarsal head, and great toe. These areas are predisposed to ulceration because pressure is shifted distally on the foot secondary to Achilles tendon shortening. Achilles shortening is a common finding in diabetic patients because of changes in the structure of collagen.

14. Define Charcot deformity.

Charcot deformity initially was described in patients with tertiary syphilis but is now seen more commonly in patients with advanced stages of diabetic neuropathy. Although the exact pathogenesis is unknown, vasodilation secondary to autonomic dysfunction is thought to be a major factor. High-velocity blood flow in the insensate extremity leads to demineralization of the bone, and repeated unrecognized microtrauma may initiate the destructive process of fractures and subluxation of the midfoot. Initial signs often mimic cellulitis that is supposedly secondary to an underlying osteomyelitis. Often patients are inappropriately placed on antibiotics. If total-contact casting (see question 12) is not initiated at the early signs of Charcot arthropathy, bony deformities can develop and may lead to pressure points on the feet, which, in turn, ulcerate and create chronic wounds. A common finding in diabetic patients with early Charcot changes is a strong pulse rate with associated diffuse erythema in a nonulcerated foot. Osteomyelitis, on the other hand, is generally associated with a chronic soft tissue ulceration that precedes the bony infection. The preferred diagnostic tests are magnetic resonance imaging and bone biopsy.

15. How are wound care dressings classified? Summarize the types, advantages, and disadvantages of the different types of dressings.

One useful technique is to place the dressings along a continuum from totally occlusive and impermeable to oxygen to nonocclusive and permeable to oxygen. Less occlusive dressings generally tend to be absorptive but require frequent changes because wound fluid may penetrate to the outer dressing wrap. More occlusive dressings are generally designed to be left in place for longer periods (depending on absorbency) and, for that reason, are often helpful in promoting autolytic debridement. The table below provides a classification according to permeability for the major dressing types.

Classification of Dressings

Type	Mechanism of Action	Advantages	Disadvantages	Use	Common Names
Hydrocolloid	Absorbant colloid material and elastomers covered with polyurethane Absorbs Protects	Many are adherent Waterproof Vapor-impermeable Changed infrequently	Bunching and wrinkling Some are malodorous Can promote excessive granulation tissue	Maintains moisture Absorbs limited exudate Promotes autolytic debridement	DuoDerm (ConvaTex, Skillman, NJ); Comfeel (Coloplast, Marietta, Ga); Hydrocol (Bertek, Morgantown, WV)
Hydrogel	Cross-linked polymer gel with high water content Hydrates	Provides moist environment Thermal insulator	Can lead to maceration May be difficult to keep in place	Softening eschar and necrotic tissue Providing moisture to desiccated wound, applied in thin layer	Spenco 2nd Skin (Spenco Medical, Waco, Tex)
Fiber	Carboxymethyl-cellulose Absorbs Gels	Can absorb large amounts of exudate Promotes moist environment	Can dehydrate dry wound	Excellent for exudate absorption in variety of wounds	AQUACEL (ConvaTec, Skillman, NJ)
Alginate	Calcium or calcium-sodium alginate Absorbs	Can absorb moderate amounts of exudate Promotes moist environment Some hemostatic properties	Can dehydrate dry wound	Excellent for exudate absorption in variety of wounds but does not absorb as much as fiber dressing	Sorbsan (Bertek, Morgantown, WVa)

continued

Classification of Dressings *continued*

Type	Mechanism of Action	Advantages	Disadvantages	Use	Common Names
Foam	Highly absorbant polyurethane Absorbs Provides padding	Depending on density can absorb large amounts of exudate over an extended period Promotes moist environment Conforms to odd surfaces	Can lead to wound maceration if too much fluid collects between changes Cannot absorb quickly	Excellent secondary dressing for alginates and fiber dressings	Flexzan (Bertek, Morgantown, WVa); Allevyn (Smith & Nephew, Largo, Fla)
Film	Transparent polymer membrane covered with acrylic adhesive Protective covering	Allows visualization of wound Provides protection against shear Bacterial barrier Good for stage 1 pressure ulcers Clear; can visualize wound	Does not absorb	Used for superficial abrasions Useful as secondary dressing for alginates and fiber dressings	Bioclusive (Johnson & Johnson, Arlington, Tex); OpSite (Smith & Nephew, Largo, Fla)

16. Describe the function of hydrotherapy in wound care.

Hydrotherapy, in the broadest sense, is the use of some form of water or other liquid for therapeutic purposes. For many years, whirlpool was used extensively in wound care to aid in cleansing wounds and burns. More recently, irrigation by other means, especially pulsatile lavage, has gained acceptance. This change is due to understanding of the negative effects of whirlpool, such as high pressure from whirlpool turbines, potential cross-contamination, and edema in dependent limbs. Pulsatile lavage, a form of irrigation that can be delivered at controlled pressures with the use of sterile water or saline as the irrigant, makes cleansing more wound-friendly, especially in clean wounds with beefy red granulation tissue. Whirlpool may be of some assistance in general cleansing in patients with wounds, but it should be avoided in patients with venous insufficiency ulcers because the dependent position and warm water increase venous congestion in the extremity. While whirlpool in general has fallen into disfavor in wound care, there is some discussion of the possible benefits of warm water in stimulating healing. Chronic wound fluid is known to be inhibitory to dermal fibroblasts. When chronic wound fluid is heated to as little as 100° C, however, this inhibition is no longer present. While this does not mean that the moratorium on whirlpool in wound care is over, it certainly provides support for the warming of whatever type of irrigation solution is used in wound cleansing.

17. What is the role of electrical stimulation in wound healing?

Numerous controlled studies have demonstrated the benefits of high-voltage galvanic stimulation (HVGS) in augmenting wound healing. The results have been particularly impressive in the management of pressure ulcers. A meta-analysis performed by Gardner et al. reported on the results of 591 chronic wounds treated with electrical stimulation compared to 212 controls. They noted that, based on the overall rates of healing, electrical stimulation increased the healing rate of chronic wounds by 144%. This has not been the case with electromagnetic therapy, however. A systematic Cochrane review was performed on the role of electromagnetic therapy in promoting wound healing in individuals with pressure ulcers and venous insufficiency ulcers. There was insufficient evidence to advocate the use of electromagnetic therapy in wound healing.

Should electrical stimulation be considered as an adjunct to treatment of a chronic wound, the following technique is suggested. A high-voltage pulsed current stimulator should be used. Treatment should be 45 minutes to 1 hour in length, and the stimulus should be delivered at a frequency of 100 pulses per second at a submotor intensity (enough to produce a tingling paresthesia). Polarity of the active electrode plays an important role. The positive electrode (anode) should be placed over the wound when debridement or epithelialization is the objective. The negative pole (cathode) is used to stimulate production of granulation tissue or to promote antimicrobial or antiinflammatory effects. Typically the wound is filled loosely with saline-moistened gauze, and an aluminum foil electrode, connected to an alligator clip lead wire, is used for conductivity. Make sure that the foil electrode is smaller than the moistened gauze so that no portion of the foil comes in contact with intact skin.

18. What is negative pressure wound therapy and how can it benefit an orthopaedic wound?

Negative pressure wound therapy (NPWT) involves the application of a localized negative pressure to the wound and its margins through a special foam dressing. The dressing is placed in a wound cavity, or over a flap or graft, and is covered with an occlusive film drape. The sealed wound is then connected to a computerized vacuum pump that is set to provide between 75 and 125 mm Hg of negative pressure, either continuously or intermittently, for 48 hours. The system helps to remove fluid from the wound and promote granulation tissue development and wound contraction.

There are limited randomized controlled studies on the effectiveness of NPWT in wound healing. A 2000 Cochrane review indicated that only 2 small trials with a total of 34 patients existed, and the studies provided weak evidence that NPWT was any better than saline-moistened gauze in promoting wound healing. Since this review, several additional studies with small sample sizes have attested to the benefits of NPWT in speeding the healing process. There are, however, in excess of 100 case reports attesting to the benefits of NPWT in wound healing.

NPWT is a great asset to treatment of large skin defects often encountered with traumatic injuries to the extremities or to dehisced surgical wounds. It can be used in conjunction with external fixator devices to minimize dressing changes and accelerate healing.

19. Are any of the topically applied growth factors of benefit in wound healing?

Two growth factor preparations commonly encountered in clinical practice are Procuren and Regranex. Procuren is a platelet-derived growth factor developed from a sample of the patient's own blood. It is marketed for use in the management of chronic nonhealing wounds, but insufficient research supports its effectiveness. The clinical practice guideline from the Agency for Health Care Policy and Research, "Treatment of Pressure Ulcers," concludes that the effectiveness of growth factors has not been sufficiently established to warrant recommendation for use. Regranex (becaplermin) gel, on the other hand, is a recombinant form of platelet-derived growth factor. It has been approved by the Food and Drug Administration for patients with neuropathic ulcers. Controlled clinical trials have demonstrated the effectiveness of Regranex gel in improving the healing rates of diabetic foot ulcers.

Bibliography

Berendt AR, Lipsky B: Is this bone infected or not? Differentiating neuro-osteoarthropathy from osteomyelitis in the diabetic foot, *Curr Diab Rep* 4:424-429, 2004.

Gardner SE et al: Effect of electrical stimulation on chronic wound healing: a meta-analysis, *Wound Repair Regen* 7:495-503, 1999.

Guyton G, Saltzman C: The diabetic foot: basic mechanisms of disease, *J Bone Joint Surg (Am)* 83A: 1084-1096, 2001.

Kloth LC: Electrical stimulation for wound healing: a review of evidence from in vitro studies, animal experiment, and clinical trials, *Lower Extremity Wounds* 4:23-44, 2005.

Kloth L, McCulloch J: *Wound healing: alternatives in management,* ed 3, Philadelphia, 2001, FA Davis.

Krasner D, Rodeheaver G, Sibbald G: *Chronic wound care: a clinical source book for healthcare professionals,* ed 3, Wayne, Pa, 2001, HMP Communications.

McCallon S et al: Vacuum-assisted closure versus saline-moistened gauze in the healing of postoperative diabetic foot wounds, *Ostomy/Wound Management* 46:28-29, 31-22, 34, 2000.

McCulloch J: The integumentary system—repair and management: an overview, *PT—Magazine Phys Ther* 12:52-56, 58, 60-64, 2004.

Patout C Jr et al: A decision pathway for the staged management of foot problems in diabetes mellitus, *Arch Phys Med Rehabil* 82:1724-1728, 2001.

Sheffield P, Smith A, Fife C: *Wound care practice,* Flagstaff, Ariz, 2004, Best Publishing.

Sinacore D: Total contact casting for diabetic neuropathic ulcers, *Phys Ther* 76:296-301, 1996.

Sussman K, Bates-Jensen B, editors: *Wound care: a collaborative practice manual for physical therapists and nurses,* Gaithersburg, Md, 2001, Aspen.

Chapter 28

Management of Chronic Pain

Craig T. Hartrick, MD

1. What is the cost of chronic pain?

The economic cost secondary to lost productivity and health care expenses for all chronic pain approaches $100 billion annually in the United States.

2. Can chronic pain be prevented?

The quality of acute pain management is an important factor in the subsequent development or prevention of chronic pain. Persistent postsurgical pain may be seen in patients in whom lower doses of analgesics were initially prescribed, resulting in ineffective analgesia in the early post-operative days. Nerve block and spinal analgesic techniques can hasten the rehabilitation of orthopaedic patients. Patients receiving multimodal analgesia that includes spinal local anesthetics and spinal opiates have improved health-related quality of life measures for months after surgery when compared to patients receiving intravenous analgesic regimens.

3. Define preemptive analgesia.

Preemptive analgesia may refer to the administration of agents before injury to prevent the ensuing cascade of events that leads to the development of chronic pain.

4. How does the response of the central nervous system contribute to the genesis of chronic pain?

High-intensity noxious stimulation alters central processing of afferent neural information. Studies elucidating the mechanisms for central hypersensitivity have documented a host of neurochemical changes, including enhancement of dorsal horn neuronal activity after repetitive C-fiber barrage (wind-up); receptive field expansion with decreased dorsal horn threshold, resulting in both temporal and spatial summation; and increases in immediate gene and dynorphin expression. Resultant increases in the synthesis of nitric oxide (NO), a highly diffusible gas that freely disperses to surrounding regions of the spinal cord, induce a positive feedback cycle with clinical pain on light touch (allodynia). Spinal cord sensitization leads to increased sensitivity in wide areas surrounding the site of injury (secondary hyperalgesia). This sensitivity interferes with movement and rehabilitation. Further, considerable evidence supports a heritable basis for some neurologic conditions, including neuropathic pain. Susceptible people may be predisposed to the development of chronic pain after trauma, especially in the presence of unrelieved acute pain, where spinal mechanisms (including constitutive cyclooxygenase-2 pathways) participate in the development of a "memory" for pain.

5. Do continuous analgesic infusions prevent early recognition of posttraumatic compartment syndromes?

The pain associated with acute compartment syndrome typically breaks through properly regulated analgesia during brachial plexus infusion or lumbar epidural infusion. Furthermore, if weakness develops during the infusion, the local anesthetic can be withheld to facilitate prompt assessment.

6. If no pain relief is obtained by sympathetic block, can the diagnosis still be sympathetically maintained pain?

Sympathetically maintained pain (SMP) retains clinical utility for its therapeutic implications. It applies to a multitude of posttraumatic pain conditions with both burning pain and allodynia, which are, by definition, relieved by sympathetic block. Dystrophic changes, neural injury, and vasomotor or sudomotor changes are often present but are not required for the diagnosis. Complex regional pain syndrome (CRPS type I, also known as RSD, reflex sympathetic dystrophy; or CRPS type II, also known as causalgia) may be either sympathetically maintained (SMP) or sympathetically independent (SIP).

7. Is chronic neuropathic pain peripheral or central in origin?

Neural injury can alter the tonic level of conduction from the dorsal root ganglia and thus sensitize the nociceptors subserving the cutaneous distributions of the affected nerve root. The spread of sensitization to areas surrounding the injury appears to be mediated in part via wide dynamic range (WDR) neurons in the spinal cord. WDR neurons also appear to be the mediators of SMP. Sensitization of WDR neurons in the spinal cord is termed **wind-up.** Any low-threshold myelinated mechanoreceptor afferent activity converging on the same WDR neurons results in an exaggerated response, such as allodynia. Continuous pain results from sympathetic efferent sensitization of the peripheral sensory receptors, which in turn produces tonic firing of the low-threshold myelinated mechanoreceptors, projecting onto previously sensitized WDR neurons. Thus, a painful cycle involving both peripheral and central components maintains neuropathic pain.

8. Why do muscles ache?

While muscle pain and deep hyperalgesia are associated with a number of conditions as secondary phenomena, they may also be the primary source of pain. Primary nociceptors from muscle tissue are nerve fibers that, unlike rapidly transmitting "sharp" pain pathways, transmit afferent information slowly, thus giving rise to dull, aching pain. A-delta polymodal nociceptors responding to mechanical stimulation (group III) and unmyelinated C-fibers responding to ischemia and chemical stimuli (group IV) give rise to poorly localized, cramping muscle pain. The referred pain from muscle likely represents the extensive involvement of reflex mechanisms in the central nervous system. Hyperalgesia caused by central sensitization may result from activation of *N*-methyl-D-aspartate (NMDA) or other mechanisms of modulation of central synaptic processing.

9. How do trigger points differ from chronic muscle tenderness secondary to fibromyalgia?

Histologic changes associated with trigger points include atrophy of type II muscle fibers, a characteristic "moth-eaten" appearance of type I fibers, and segmental muscle fiber necrosis. Some investigators have noted elastic projections constricting affected muscle fibers. Lipid and glycogen deposition and also abnormal mitochondrial accumulations are seen, resulting in muscular bands that are often clinically palpable. Pain from deep somatic structures is typically dull and diffuse. The ability to localize precise trigger areas decreases with increasing tissue depth. Diffusion and radiation can be indicators of severity. Muscle spasm and tenderness in zones of reference (as distinguished from trigger points) often appear at sites distant from the lesion.

10. What causes trigger points?

The precise mechanism of trigger point generation and perpetuation after trauma is not known. Transient overload of a muscle may cause damage to the sarcoplasmic reticulum. Once the t-tubule system is focally disrupted, localized zones within a muscle remain in a perpetually contracted position because of impaired calcium reuptake.

11. Why are trigger points painful?

After damage to the t-tubule system, stored calcium ions are released into the area of injury. Adenosine triphosphate (ATP) may activate the actin-myosin contractile mechanism focally in the absence of action potentials. A palpable band of electrically silent muscle may result. With calcium reuptake limited, unabated focal contractile activity persists. High levels of metabolic activity, documented by ATP depletion, produce the "hot spots" seen on infrared thermography. Further, because ATP is required for the calcium pump to retrieve calcium into the sarcoplasmic reticulum, depletion of ATP further enhances calcium availability and thus perpetuates contractile activity. Accumulation of metabolic byproducts results in local acidosis, which sensitizes adjacent nociceptors. Likewise, increased calcium may act as a second messenger to induce nociceptive neuronal hypersensitivity. Increased vascular permeability, local vasoconstriction, and reduced tissue oxygenation also contribute to the elaboration of algesic substances, which sensitize peripheral nociceptors. In addition, sensitized dorsal horn cells may cause enlargement of the receptive field, resulting in spreading dysesthesia.

12. Can physical manipulation affect the healing process after muscle injury?

Perpetuation of trigger point activity can be expected until the integrity of the sarcoplasmic reticulum is reestablished or the band is physically lengthened to prevent further interaction of the actin-myosin complex. If the taut muscular band comprising the trigger point can be stretched effectively without inducing reflexive contraction secondary to pain, the reparative process is facilitated.

13. How can trigger points induce sympathetic overactivity?

Sensitized muscle nociceptors may evoke sympathetic hyperactivity. Sympathetic activation may sensitize nociceptors, inducing cyclical reflex mechanisms. The progression from acute post-traumatic muscular pain to chronic myofascial pain probably involves peripheral sensitization of high-threshold mechanoreceptors, recruitment of low-threshold mechanoreceptors, and central sensitization of dorsal horn neurons. Increased sensitivity of muscle vasculature to sympathetic transmitter substances may contribute. Clinically, persistence of trigger point activity can result in sympathetically mediated vasomotor changes. In such cases, sympathetic blockade can assist the manipulative therapy.

14. When does the inflammatory cascade cease to be useful after musculoskeletal injury?

The response to connective tissue injury is divided into stages. The first stage in the healing process is the inflammatory response, which typically extends through the first 2 days. During this phase chemotactic mechanisms induce cell mobilization and infiltration. The second stage lasts from the third day through the fifth and is characterized by ground substance proliferation in preparation for collagen deposition. Collagen formation begins in the third proliferative phase and lasts through the second week after injury. The final stage is the formative stage; from 14 days onward, the cross-linked collagen organizes into functional fibrils in the healed tissue. Persistence of inflammation beyond the initial period is not helpful and contributes to persistence of pain.

15. Can corticosteroids interfere with healing?

The timing of therapeutic intervention affects the quality of the reparative process. Corticosteroid administration in the first 2 weeks can inhibit prostaglandin synthesis, thus interfering with the initial proliferative phases of healing. Corticosteroids should be used with caution in acute strains and only when the joint is to be placed at rest. Furthermore, corticosteroid-induced fluid retention may contribute to tissue swelling. This effect may be most damaging after crush or blunt trauma to an extremity, where additional swelling may predispose to development of a compartment syndrome.

16. Can exercise targeted at specific defects be effective in the treatment of chronic low back pain?

Specific programs designed to strengthen the abdominal and lumbar multifidus muscles proximal to the specific defect as a stabilizing maneuver for symptomatic spondylosis or spondylolisthesis are effective.

17. Which patients with low back pain derive the greatest long-term benefits from physical therapy?

Mechanical low back pain responds favorably to physical therapy interventions, whereas radicular pain does not. The finding that multifidus muscle recovery is not necessarily spontaneous after remission of pain may explain a high level of recurrence of low back pain. Specific physical therapy interventions should include manual therapy techniques based on motion-provoked symptoms.

18. Does evidence support physical therapy for acute low back pain?

According to the Agency for Health Care Policy and Research, physical therapy seems helpful for acute low back problems without radiculopathy when used within the first month of symptoms. If the symptoms persist and no functional improvement has been noted after 1 month, therapy should be stopped and the patient reevaluated. An early return to function is favored over traditional bed rest. Bed rest longer than 4 days is not helpful and may hasten debilitation.

19. Are exercise programs helpful?

Stretching programs that progress to a home training and conditioning program after 3 months of therapy have been successful in reducing pain and disability as well as increasing optimism and self-control. Massage may reduce the overall costs of health care in persistent low back pain. Exercise in association with cognitive retraining, although typically failing to improve the number of patients returning to work, may reduce symptoms and improve coping in patients with chronic spinal pain.

20. Should nerve blocks be used to facilitate physical therapy in patients with chronic pain?

Neural blockade immediately before manipulation of the spine enhances the efficacy of treatment used either alone or sequentially. Denervation of receptive fields related to the innervation of the facet joints may allow improved manipulation by prevention of reflex muscle spasm and guarding during treatment. Precision in blockade is essential to avoid total sensory loss, which may permit dangerous overstretching of the tissues. Cervical epidural hematoma and subluxation with quadriparesis have been reported. Widespread nonspecific blockade may permit stretch beyond safe limits. Careful and specific physical interventions within the physiologic range, combined with blockade limited to specific target elements, are designed to minimize such risks. A prospective, double-blind, placebo-controlled study of patients with whiplash found dramatic long-term relief with radiofrequency lesioning of the cervical facets.

21. When are physical measures needed after trigger point injections?

All trigger point injections should be followed by effective stretch of the treated muscles. Moist heat immediately after treatments helps to minimize local soreness and reflex muscle spasm. Best results are obtained when injections are reserved for patients with acute trigger points that, on physical examination, reproduce the patient's pain and are ineffectively stretched by physical means alone. Injections also should be used in conjunction with a home stretching program to facilitate therapeutic exercises. If more than three injections are required, the search for underlying precipitating factors should be intensified.

22. Why does stretching promote healing of trigger points?

Physical therapy directed specifically at stretch of the trigger points to normal resting length is crucial. This prevents actin-myosin interaction, thereby reducing metabolic activity, and improves local blood flow and tissue oxygenation.

23. What measures effectively facilitate trigger point stretching?

Specific techniques are used to permit passive stretching, including vapocoolant spray, ischemic compression, acupuncture, acupressure, dry-needling, or, most effectively, infiltration with local anesthetic (trigger point injection). Injection relieves pain, relaxes muscles (by blocking ongoing reflex activity), and physically flushes away excessive extracellular calcium, hydrogen ions, and algesic substances. Relaxation and electromyogram biofeedback should be considered adjunctive measures.

24. How can trigger point injections abolish pain at sites distal to the injection?

Afferent pain signals secondary to activation of nociceptors enter the spinal cord through the dorsal root, where communication via internuncial neurons leads to hyperactivity in the anterior and anterolateral horn cells. Hyperactivity results in efferent traffic, causing intensified muscle spasm, vasoconstriction, and referred pain. Neural blockade interrupts this reflex arc. Resultant alterations in central nervous system processing of input from the receptive field may be responsible for the spreading tenderness after injury. This response is terminated by local anesthetic application.

25. What circumstances require the application of regional local anesthetic blockade?

Somatic regional block is used when multiple trigger points in a contiguous region make individual injection impractical or when simultaneous antisympathetic effect is required to increase blood flow or reduce sympathetic activity. Regional sympathetic blockade blocks perpetuating sympathetic activity and improves microcirculation, thus decreasing focal ischemia.

26. Discuss the role of sympathetic blocks.

Sympathetic block, by definition, relieves the pain of SMP. Although repeated sympathetic blockade may reduce or permanently eliminate clinical findings, most neuropathic pains are not sympathetically maintained. In fact, not even all cases of CRPS type I are amenable to sympathectomy. However, when a positive response from sympathetic blockade is obtained, the effect of the block often significantly outlasts the action of the local anesthetic, especially when repeated. Of interest, neural blockade distal to the sympathetic chain is also effective in reducing SMP, presumably because neurogenic block of the affected receptive field reduces the low-threshold mechanoreceptor activity that is stimulated by sympathetic outflow. With time, the plasticity of the central nervous system permits enhanced transmission over previously quiescent pathways. Enhanced transmission contributes to the clinical impression that, in the most chronic cases, peripheral measures are ineffective.

27. What physical therapy treatments are helpful in conjunction with invasive therapy for chronic pain?

Manipulation after facet or medial branch blocks provides a more dramatic result than either treatment used in isolation for the treatment of mechanical spine pain. After initial recovery and application of moist heat, provocative maneuvers are repeated to ensure appropriate blockade. The affected segments are then mobilized manually. Subsequent strengthening, especially of the multifidi when treating pain in the lumbar region, is important after permanent medial branch neurolysis.

The use of spinal cord stimulation in conjunction with physical therapy in the treatment of CRPS results in significantly improved pain and economic outcomes.

28. Is physical therapy important after intradiskal electrothermal therapy?

The relatively new technique of intradiskal electrothermal therapy heats the annular disk in an effort to destroy nociceptors and reorganize collagen fibrils, thus sealing fissures within the disk. Because the collagen helices are rearranged, care must be taken to avoid placing stress on the treated disk until its structural integrity is reestablished. While only patients with annular tears meeting strictly defined criteria are likely to benefit from this procedure, in properly selected candidates the number needed to treat (NNT) for 75% pain relief was 5, with 40% of all patients achieving at least 50% relief. Physical therapy, beginning at 6 weeks after the procedure, must be introduced gradually and designed to enhance lower extremity flexibility and truncal stabilization.

29. What exercise programs are effective in chronic pain patients?

Exercises designed for specific impairments, behavioral techniques that promote wellness behaviors and extinguish pain behaviors, and administration of nonsteroidal antiinflammatory drugs and antidepressants are appropriate treatments for chronic pain. Success has been reported with the following paradigm:

- Week 1: Comprehensive evaluation, home stretching program, orientation to program
- Weeks 2 and 3: 2 hours of physical therapy 3 times/week (1 hour of stretching, 1 hour of strengthening)
- Weeks 4-8: 45 minutes of stretching, 1 hour of strengthening, and 1 hour of aerobic training 3 times/week.

Quantification of function biweekly and at program completion is recommended. Compliance, behavioral problems, and treatment goals should be discussed biweekly at case conference. Individualized written recommendations for exercises at home or at a fitness facility should be provided at the end of the program.

30. What are the essential elements in the physical therapist's evaluation of patients with chronic pain?

Serious underlying spinal conditions, such as fracture, tumor, infection, or cauda equina syndrome, must be ruled out. Features that should raise the index of suspicion include presentation under age 20 or over age 55; violent trauma; constant, progressive, nonmechanical pain; thoracic pain; past history of carcinoma; use of systemic steroids; drug abuse; HIV infection; systemic unhealthiness; precipitous or unexplained weight loss; persisting severe restriction of lumbar flexion; and widespread neurologic symptoms. Cauda equina syndrome may present with difficulty with micturition; loss of anal sphincter tone or fecal incontinence; saddle anesthesia about the anus, perineum, or genitals; widespread or progressive motor weakness in the legs; gait disturbance; or a sensory level of hypesthesia.

31. Can disparity between self-report and objective measures be documented?

Inconsistencies in the evaluation should be documented. Waddell signs, which are associated with inconsistent and unreliable self-reports, include superficial nonanatomic tenderness; pain with axial loading on top of the head; increasing back pain or twisting torso as a unit; discrepancy between straight leg raising in sitting and lying positions; nonphysiologic regional disturbances in sensation, pain distribution, or weakness; and excessive verbalization, facial grimacing, and other pain behaviors out of proportion to test stimulus and physical findings. The presence of three or more Waddell signs predicts treatment failure. Although Waddell signs predict poor outcome acutely, they are not necessarily negative predictors in an interdisciplinary context.

32. Which medications are appropriate for chronic pain?

Medications for neuropathic pain are administered by oral, topical/transdermal, IV regional, intraspinal, and nerve-blocking techniques. The oral route is by far the most common. Oral tricyclic antidepressants are standard therapy for chronic pain.

Agent	Indication	Mechanism
Tricyclic antidepressants (e.g., amitriptyline [Elavil])	Neuropathic pain, depression, myofascial pain	Multiple, including central inhibition of 5-HT and NE reuptake
Anticonvulsants Gabapentin (Neurontin)	Neuropathic pain	Multiple, including NA channel inhibition, reduced spontaneous depolarization
Clonazepam (Klonopin)	Neuropathic pain, panic attacks, anxiety states	GABA agonist
Capsaicinoids (e.g., capsaicin [Zostrix])	Neuropathic pain after sever nerve injury	Depletion of substance P
Muscle relaxants (e.g., baclofen [Lioresal]	Spasticity after spinal cord injury; myofascial component	GABA agonist
NMDA receptor antagonists (e.g., ketamine [Ketalar])	Posttraumatic, myofascial neuropathic pain; opioid tolerance	Glutamate receptor antagonism
Local anesthetic derivatives (e.g., mexiletine [Mexitil])	Neuropathic pain with C-fiber hyperactivity, neural injury or neuroma with mechanical hypersensitivity, allodynia	Na channel blockade, reduce spontaneous depolarization
Antihypertensives (e.g., clonidine [Catapres TTS])	Neuropathic pain with hyperpathia/allodynia	α_2-adrenergic agonist
Opioids (e.g., oxycodone [Oxycontin])	Nociceptive pain uncontrolled by other measures in patients at low psychological risk for addiction	Opiate receptor agonists
Nonsteroidal antiinflammatory drugs (e.g., celecoxib [Celebrex])	Neuropathic and myofascial pain	Cyclo-oxygenase inhibition blocks prostaglandin synthesis

5-HT, 5-Hydroxytryptamine; *NE,* norepinephrine; *Na,* sodium; *GABA,* gamma-aminobutyric acid.

33. Discuss the role of perineural steroids in pain management.

Epidural steroid injections are an option for short-term relief of radicular pain after failure of conservative treatment and as a means of avoiding surgery. Evidence-based meta-analysis of epidural steroid studies provides conflicting results. While the Oxford group reported efficacy with an NNT of 7.3 for greater than 75% relief at up to 60 days and an NNT of 13 for greater than 50% relief at up to 12 months, the Cochrane group found no such evidence. In a randomized, controlled trial, the transforaminal approach to epidural steroid injection has been reported to eliminate the need for surgery in 50% of patients with radicular pain emanating from one to two spinal levels.

Bibliography

Bigos S et al: *Acute low back problems in adults,* Clinical Practice Guideline No. 14, AHCPR Publication No. 95-0642, Rockville, Md, 1994, Agency for Health Care Policy and Research, U.S. Department of Health and Human Services.

Boersma K et al: Lowering fear-avoidance and enhancing function through exposure in vivo: a multiple baseline study across six patients with back pain, *Pain* 108:8-16, 2004.

Capdevila X et al: Effects of perioperative analgesic techniques on the surgical outcome and duration of rehabilitation after major knee surgery, *Anesthesiology* 91:8-15, 1999.

Carli F et al: Epidural analgesia enhances functional exercise capacity and health-related quality of life after colonic surgery, *Anesthesiology* 97:540-549, 2002.

Cherkin DC et al: A review of the evidence for the effectiveness, safety, and cost of acupuncture, massage therapy, and spinal manipulation for back pain, *Ann Intern Med* 138:898-906, 2003.

Dreyfus P, Michaelsen M, Horn M: MUJA: manipulation under joint anesthesia/analgesia: a treatment approach for recalcitrant low back pain of synovial joint origin, *J Manipul Physiol Ther* 18:537-546, 1995.

Gam AN et al: Treatment of myofascial trigger-points with ultrasound combined with massage and exercise: a randomized controlled trial, *Pain* 77:73-79, 1998.

Greenough CG, Fraser RD: Assessment of outcome in patients with low-back pain, *Spine* 17:36-41, 1992.

Hartrick CT: Managing the difficult pain patient. In Raj PP, Niv D, editors: *Management of pain: a world perspective,* Bologna, Italy, 1995, pp 330-334, Moduzzi.

Hartrick CT: Pain due to trauma including sports injuries, *Pain digest* 8:237-259, 1998.

Hartrick CT: Screening instruments predict long-term response to epidural steroids, *J Contemp Neurol* 3:1-6, 1998.

Hartrick CT: Multimodal postoperative pain management, *Am J Health Syst Pharm* 61:S4-10, 2004.

Hartrick CT, Kovan JP, Naismith P: Outcome prediction following sympathetic block for complex regional pain syndrome, *Pain practice* 4:222-228, 2004.

Kemler MA, Furnee CA: Economic evaluation of spinal cord stimulation for chronic reflex sympathetic dystrophy, *Neurology* 59:1203-1209, 2002.

Kuukkanen T, Malkia E: Muscular performance after a 3 month progressive physical exercise program and 9 month follow-up in subjects with low back pain: a controlled study, *Scand J Med Sci Sports* 6:112-121, 1996.

Malkia E, Ljunggren AE: Exercise programs for subjects with low back disorders, *Scand J Med Sci Sports* 6:73-81, 1996.

Nelemans PJ et al: Injection therapy for subacute and chronic benign low back pain, *Spine* 26:501-515, 2001 (*Cochrane Database Syst Rev* 2:CD001824, 2000).

Nelson L, Aspergren D, Bova C: The use of epidural steroid injection and manipulation on patients with chronic low back pain, *J Manipul Physiol Ther* 20:263-266, 1997.

O'Sullivan PB, Twomey LT, Allison GT: Evaluation of specific stabilizing exercise in the treatment of chronic low back pain with radiologic diagnosis of spondylolysis or spondylolithesis, *Spine* 22:2959-2967, 1997.

Pauza KJ et al: A randomized, placebo-controlled trial of intradiscal electrothermal therapy for the treatment of discogenic low back pain, *Spine J* 4:27-35, 2004.

Polatin PB et al: A prospective study of Waddell signs in patients with chronic low back pain, *Spine* 22:1618-1621, 1997.

Riew K et al: The effect of nerve-root injections on the need for operative treatment of lumbar radicular pain. A prospective, randomized, controlled, double-blind study, *J Bone Joint Surg Am* 82:1589-1593, 2000.

Chapter 29

Headache

Brian T. Pagett, PT, MPT, and Edward M. Lichten, MD

1. Describe the basic categories of headache and their clinical presentation.

The International Headache Society (IHS) classification defines and categorizes each headache clearly with diagnostic criteria. However, because of considerable symptomatic overlap and common features, the differential diagnosis is difficult (see table).

2. Who is at risk for cervical headache?

Women are three times more likely than men to suffer from cervical headache. Women in managerial or professional occupations are more susceptible to headache than women in either clerical or blue-collar occupations.

3. Describe the symptoms of cervical headache.

Although symptom location may vary widely, prevalent sites of pain are retro-orbital, frontal, temporal, and occipital areas of the head. Usually suboccipital pain and neck pain also are present. These symptoms have strong tendencies to be unilateral with no changing of sides. Other studies report bilateral symptoms, although they are rare. Pain is described as an ache or dull, boring pain that varies in intensity from low-grade to severe. At times throbbing or pulsing pain may be reported, but typically in migraine headaches with the throbbing coinciding with the pulse. Associated symptoms include nausea, vomiting, phonophobia and photophobia, visual disturbances (blurred vision, spots, flashing lights), difficulty in swallowing, dizziness, light-headedness, general irritability, and inability to concentrate. Symptoms are ipsilateral with pain. Headache pain is often present on awakening and may worsen progressively with increased activity levels. Other patients may have an onset of symptoms during or toward the end of the day, with neck pain as a warning sign.

4. How are cervical headaches precipitated?

Cervical headache commonly is precipitated or intensified mechanically by sustained neck flexion while working at a desk, typing, studying, driving a car, or reading. Often patients have difficulty in identifying specific aggravating factors. Although stress, tension, anxiety, and depression also may be provocative factors, they are common to other headache types. Cervical spine pathology may trigger muscle contraction (tension), or, conversely, tension may provoke existing pathology to produce headache. It is easy for patients to blame stresses in their life as a causative factor, but millions of people with significant stress or tension in their lives are symptom-free. Thus musculoskeletal causes of headache should not be ruled out.

5. Discuss the neuroanatomic basis for cervicogenic headache.

Afferent fibers from the trigeminal nerve (cranial nerve V), which carries pain and temperature information for the head region, descend through the medulla oblongata and into the gray matter of the spinal cord as far as C3 and occasionally C4. Afferent fibers from the C1-C3 spinal nerves

Four Types of Headache

	Migraine	Tension	Cluster	Cervical/Cervicogenic
Gender and age	Women > men	Women > men	Men > women	Women > men
Area of symptoms	Unilateral, temporal, frontal, or retro-orbital May change sides	Muscle of head, periorbital, temporal, and occipital; cervical symptoms may be present Bilateral	Frontal, retro-orbital, temporal, occipital Possible neck symptoms, but mild compared with head pain Unilateral; may change sides	Unilateral pain usually starting in sub-occipital neck region and radiating to frontal, retro-orbital, temporal, occipital regions May be bilateral Does not change sides
Quality of symptoms	Throbbing, pounding Moderate-to-severe intensity	Dull, aching quality Tight band or heavy weight on head Moderate-to-severe intensity	Severe, intense, burning, piercing, nonthrobbing; ocular symptoms and pressure retro-orbitally Typically excruciating	Dull ache or boring pain; stabbing, shooting deep pain may be present At times may be throbbing Can reach moderate-to-severe intensity
Associated symptoms	Nausea, vomiting, photo-phobia, phonophobia No specificity to side of pain and neurologic symptoms	Nausea, vomiting, and photophobia	Nausea, vomiting, photophobia, lacrimation, rhinorrhea, ptosis, miosis, nasal congestion, flushed face, bradycardia	Nausea, vomiting, phonophobia, photophobia, blurred vision, difficulty with swallowing Ipsilateral to side of pain
Frequency and duration	4-72 hr, generally < 24 hr 1 per yr-several per wk	May occur daily (few hr-few days) Chronic (semicontinuous or 2-3/wk)	15 min-2 hr 1-8/day for ½ to 3 mo; chronic up to 1 yr Remission for 6 mo-2 yr	Daily or at least 2-3 times/wk 3-24 hr
Precipitating and relieving factors	Stress Food sensitivity Bright lights, exertion, noise Women: menstruation	Stress or tension	Neck movements may trigger headaches	May be triggered by head position or movement Sustained neck postures Sometimes unknown precipitating pattern Stress or tension may increase headache Facet or GON blocks relieve pain
Time and mode of onset	Very rapid; patient awakens with headache, warning or aura of focal neurologic symptoms before headache	Patient awakens with headache less frequently	Neck movements may trigger headaches	May be present when patient awakens and worsen as day progresses: activity-dependent

Adapted from Smith KL, Horn C: Cervicogenic headache. Part I: An anatomic and clinical overview. *J Man Manipul Ther* 5:158-170, 1997.

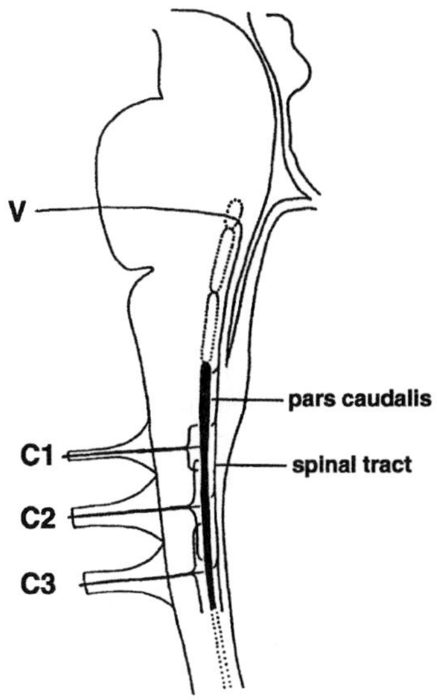

Trigeminocervical nucleus. *(From Bogduk N: Cervical causes of headache and dizziness. In* Grieve's modern manual therapy, *Edinburgh, 1994, pp 317-331, Churchill Livingstone.)*

synapse at the segment at which they enter the spinal cord and send collateral branches to superior and inferior segments. Within this column of the spinal cord, the gray matter that receives both trigeminal and cervical afferents is called the **trigeminocervical nucleus.** This combined nucleus is essentially the nociceptive nucleus of the head, throat, and upper neck. The convergence of afferents constitutes the basis for referred pain in the head and upper neck. If afferents in the trigeminocervical nucleus that otherwise innervate the back portions of the head also receive upper cervical vertebral afferents, nociceptive upper cervical stimulation may be interpreted as arising in the head. All afferents converging on the trigeminocervical nucleus may refer pain to other structures that also synapse in the same nucleus.

6. Which structures facilitate synapsis of afferent information to the trigeminocervical nucleus?

Structures include all of the articular, muscular, and neural structures of the cervical spine from C0 to C3; the upper portion of the vertebral artery; the temporomandibular joint; the posterior cranial fossa/upper spinal cord dura mater; and cranial nerves V, VII, IX, and X.

7. Describe the anatomy of the posterior neck musculature, C2 sensory nerve root, and occipital notch.

Seven layers of muscles attach to the cervical vertebrae and the skull in the posterior neck region. From superficial to deepest, they are the trapezius, splenius capitis, longissimus capitis, semispinalis capitis, obliquus capitis, splenius cervicis, and multifidus. The dorsal root of C2-C3 courses under the obliquus capitis and through the splenius capitis and trapezius muscles before traversing the occipital notch and onto the scalp. The occipital nerve and the deep cervical artery and vein course through the muscles approximately 2 to 3 cm lateral to the midline at the level of the free edge of the posterior skull. The palpated notch on the skull edge is called the occipital notch.

8. What do cervical radiographs show in patients with headache?

Conventional radiographic studies comparing patients with cervical headache and controls found no significant differences. However, one study using computer-based analysis of median tomograms in maximal cervical flexion and extension found significant segmental hypomobility of the craniocervical joints from C0 to C2—most pronounced at C0/C1. In addition, the study found impaired overall mobility of the superior cervical spine from C0 to C5.

9. What roles do MRI studies of the cervical spine have in patients with cervicogenic headache?

None. Studies with MRI scans of patients with cervicogenic headache versus controls have shown no significant pathologic conditions of the cervical spine, although they do remain important in determining underlying pathologic conditions that may require surgery or other aggressive interventions.

10. What is the gold standard for diagnosis of cervical headache?

A C2 nerve blockade or joint block on the symptomatic side can be used for diagnosis as well as therapeutic purposes. Patients generally report reduction of pain or complete resolution of symptoms if the block was successfully targeted. However, studies report no long-lasting therapeutic effect or even remission of pain. The pain cycle has been broken, but the underlying functional problem still exists, whether it be posture, cervical strength, cervical mobility, or myofascial problems.

11. How do poor posture and muscle impairment contribute to cervical headache?

Faulty postural habits can lead to abnormal stresses in the cervical and upper thoracic spine. In particular, forward head posture affects the biomechanics of the head and neck region, putting greater stress on muscles that function as stabilizers of the head. If forward head posture is maintained, it becomes fixed through adaptive shortening in upper cervical joints and posterior superficial and deep myofascial structures. Studies have shown that headache patients exhibit abnormal responses to passive stretching of the upper trapezius, levator scapulae, and short upper cervical extensor muscles. In addition, isometric strength and endurance tests have shown that the upper cervical flexors are significantly weaker in patients with headache compared with asymptomatic controls.

12. What types of physical therapy are useful in reduction of cervical headache?

The goal of physical therapy is to address objective findings of the evaluation. If faulty posture patterns are found, the therapist most likely will find impaired mobility in the upper cervical spine and subsequent forward shoulders with general weakness in the posterior shoulder girdle musculature. Initially, the therapist must correct myofascial and joint restrictions in the cervical and thoracic regions, generally with mobilization and manipulation of affected areas. Modalities that help to relax the patient and provide therapeutic effect *before* mobilization include moist heat, ultrasound, massage, and cervical traction. Other important aspects are postural correction and reeducation by encouraging axial extension and shoulder retraction. Reinforce the importance of posture maintenance to reverse the pain cycle that results from strain on joints and various soft tissues of the cervical spine.

13. What exercises are believed to be of most benefit for the headache patient?

Stretching and exercise should target muscles of the upper quadrant with extensibility losses and weakness. Stretching should focus on posterior neck superficial and deep muscles, including the upper trapezius, levator scapulae, musculi scalenus, sternocleidomastoid, suboccipitals, and pectorals. Strengthening exercises should help to maintain gains in joint mobility after mobilization and stretching by focusing on the trapezius, rhomboids, and deep cervical flexors. A good reinforcement for stretching is a well-balanced home program, which should be done at least two times a day.

14. What does the evidence illustrate regarding manipulative therapy and/or therapeutic exercise for cervicogenic headache?

Studies show evidence that both specific therapeutic exercise and manipulative therapy are effective for cervicogenic headache. Benefits included a reduction in all of the following: headache frequency and intensity, neck pain, disability, and medication intake. Jull et al. provided evidence of a long-term treatment effect over a 12-month period. Their multicenter, randomized controlled study used a manipulative regimen described by Maitland, including low-velocity cervical joint mobilizations and/or high-velocity manipulations. The exercise program involved low load exercise directed to reeducate muscle control of the cervicoscapular region specifically targeting the deep neck flexors, postural correction exercises, and muscle lengthening as needed. It is believed that long-term effectiveness is concurrent with consistent use of a home exercise program and postural pattern awareness.

15. What other instructions are given to patients with cervicogenic headache?

The headache sufferer must be weaned off all caffeine-containing over-the-counter medications and all caffeine-containing products, including coffee, tea, cola, Excedrin, phenacetin, aspirin, Fiorinal, Cafergot, Midrin, Norgesic Forte, Esgic, and the triptan preparations.

16. What is the physician's role in the treatment of cervicogenic headaches?

The general practitioner, anesthesiologist, or orthopaedist can perform occipital nerve blocks. This procedure involves injecting a mixture of 5 ml of 0.25% marcaine (anesthetic) and 1 ml (4 mg) of dexamethasone (steroid) into the left and right occipital notches to block muscle spasms and irritation of the C2 dorsal root (occipital nerve).

17. After a successful occipital block, what are the steps for treatment?

Repeat the occipital nerve blocks as frequently as necessary to keep the patient pain-free (usually every 2 to 4 days for 2 to 3 weeks). The patient must stop or rapidly wean off all caffeine products immediately. A physical therapy program increases mobility in the cervical spine, improves posture, and strengthens the trapezoid and posterior neck musculature.

18. Define temporal arteritis.

Temporal arteritis (also known as cranial arteritis and giant cell arteritis) refers to inflammation of the cranial arteries. It may be limited to the cranial vessels or affect arteries throughout the body. It is associated with polyarteritis nodosa, connective tissue disease, and hypersensitivity angiitis. The intense headache pain is associated with advanced age in both men and women. Most patients have significant pain with mastication and palpation of the superficial temporalis artery. Treatment is directed at reducing the inflammatory reaction.

19. What is trigeminal neuralgia?

Trigeminal neuralgia (tic douloureux) is an episodic, recurrent, unilateral pain syndrome of adults. The female-to-male ratio of occurrence is 2:1, and the pain is more often right sided. It affects branches of the fifth cranial nerve: face, jaw, and, less often, forehead. Slight stimulation of the trigger zones in the midface, near the nose, can provoke an attack. The pain is of high intensity and jabbing; it lasts for seconds and is followed first by relief and then by repeated attacks. Surgical therapies are rarely successful. Tegretol has been found to be the most successful oral treatment.

20. What is the difference between common migraine and classic migraine?

The IHS classification of migraine differentiates migraine without aura (common migraine, hemicrania simplex) from migraine with aura (classic migraine). **Common migraine** is defined as (1) headache attack lasting 4 to 72 hours, (2) pain that is usually unilateral with a pulsating quality of moderate-to-severe intensity that limits normal activity, and (3) pain made worse by activity. Other criteria associated with common migraine but not mandatory for diagnosis are nausea, vomiting, photophobia, and phonophobia. Migraine by definition has no underlying neurologic disease and has occurred more than once.

Classic migraine includes the above criteria plus (1) a fully reversible aura, indicating brain stem dysfunction, and (2) onset of severe pain within 60 minutes of the aura. The aura (warning) develops over more than 4 minutes and never lasts more than 60 minutes. The aura may include visual disturbances such as scotoma (wavy lines), blind spots, and even complete blindness. Paralysis or numbness on one side of the body (**hemiplegic migraine**) is an extreme case. No underlying neurologic disease is present.

21. How does caffeine contribute to analgesic rebound?

Most head pain is due to cervicogenic causes. However, most physicians and laypersons focus on migraine, which is relieved temporarily by Excedrin and caffeine. However, when these products are used repeatedly, the body develops a tolerance for caffeine, just as it does for so many other pain medications. Consequently, the patient's pain returns when the effect of the caffeine wears off. Physicians who fail to recognize that caffeine contributes to analgesic rebound headaches may prescribe a vasoconstrictive agent such as Fiorinal, Norgesic Forte, or Esgic, all of which contain caffeine or have caffeine-like effects. They trigger rebound headaches that are by nature cervicogenic and must be treated as such.

22. What is the usual preventive medication for migraine?

Standard preventive therapy includes propranolol (Inderal) and amitriptyline (Elavil), which is effective for approximately 50% of women.

23. What is the usual abortive therapy for migraine?

Most physicians prescribe a vasoconstrictive agent to interrupt the pulsating pain of migraine. The original medication, Cafergot, is available as a rectal suppository and as sublingual and oral tablets. Midrin sometimes is used for repeated dosing. Recently therapy has shifted to the triptans, which block serotonin receptors from propagating the painful vasospasm. Examples include sumatriptan, Amerge, Zomig, and Maxalt. Sumatriptan preparations include intramuscular injections, nasal sprays, and oral tablets. Maxalt is the only sublingual preparation. If migraine fails to respond to the drugs, injections of dihydroergotamine-45 may be needed. This medication is given intramuscularly or by slow intravenous push every 8 hours. If additional therapy is needed in an emergency setting, IV hydrocortisone and Reglan are prescribed. The addition of oral or intramuscular Ativan may break an otherwise intractable migraine (see table).

24. Is manipulation effective for migraine headache?

Manipulation is likely as effective as amitriptyline for the prophylactic treatment of migraine headache.

25. Is massage or manipulation more effective for cervicogenic headache?

There is moderate evidence to support that manipulation is more effective than massage for cervicogenic headache.

26. Does aerobic exercise decrease migraines?

Long-term aerobic exercise decreases the severity, frequency, and duration of migraines, possibly because of increased nitric oxide production.

27. Can physical therapy decrease dizziness?

Patients with migraine-related vestibulopathy report decreased falls, improved physical performance levels, and decreased dizziness after vestibular physical therapy.

Bibliography

Bogduk N: Anatomy and physiology of headache, *Biomed Pharmacother* 49:435-445, 1995.

Bronfort G et al: Efficacy of spinal manipulation for chronic headache: a systematic review, *J Manipul Physiol Ther* 24:457-466, 2001.

Coskun O et al: Magnetic resonance imaging of patients with cervicogenic headache, *Cephalalgia* 23:842-845, 2003.

Gawel MJ, Rothbart PJ: Occipital nerve block in the management of headache and cervical pain, *Cephalalgia* 12:9-13, 1992.

Grimmer K: Relationship between occupation and episodes of headache that match cervical origin pain patterns, *J Occup Environ Med* 35:929-935, 1993.

Haughie LJ, Fiebert IM, Roach KE: Relationship of forward head posture and cervical backward bending to neck pain, *J Manual Manipul Ther* 3:91-97, 1995.

Jull GA: Headaches associated with the cervical spine—a clinical review. In Grieve GP, editor: *Modern manual therapy of the vertebral column,* New York, 1986, pp 322-329, Churchill Livingstone.

Jull GA: Cervical headache: a review. In Grieve GP, editor: *Modern manual therapy,* New York, 1988, pp 333-347, Churchill Livingstone.

Jull GA et al: Further clinical clarification of the muscle dysfunction in cervical headache, *Cephalalgia* 19:179-185, 1999.

Jull GA et al: A randomized controlled trial of exercise and manipulative therapy for cervicogenic headache, *Spine* 27:1835-1843, 2002.

Lichten EM et al: Efficacy of danazol in the control of hormonal migraine, *J Reprod Med* 36:419-424, 1991.

Lichten EM et al: The confirmation of a biochemical marker for women's hormonal migraine: the depo-estradiol challenge test, *Headache* 36:367-371, 1996.

Lichten EM: *US doctor on the internet* (website): www.usdoctor.com/headache.htm. Accessed January 10, 2005.

Narin SO et al: The effects of exercise and exercise-related changes in blood nitric oxide level on migraine headache, *Clin Rehabil* 17:624-630, 2003.

Non-invasive physical treatments for chronic/recurrent headache, *Cochrane Database Syst Rev* (3):CD001878, 2004.

Peterson SM: Articular and muscular impairments in cervicogenic headache: a case report, *J Orthop Sports Phys Ther* 33:21-30, 2003.

Pfaffenrath V, Dandekar R, Pöllmann W: Cervicogenic headache: the clinical picture, radiological findings and hypotheses on its pathophysiology, *Headache* 27:495-499, 1987.

Pfaffenrath V et al: Cervicogenic headache: results of computer-based measurements of cervical spine mobility in 15 patients, *Cephalalgia* 8:45-48, 1988.

Placzek JD et al: The influence of the cervical spine on chronic headache in women: a pilot study, *J Manual Manipul Ther* 7:33-39, 1999.

Pöllmann W, Keidel M, Pfaffenrath V: Headache and the cervical spine: a critical review, *Cephalalgia* 17:801-816, 1997.

Schoensee SK et al: The effect of mobilization on cervical headaches, *J Orthop Sports Phys Ther* 21:184-196, 1995.

Smith KL, Horn C: Cervicogenic headache. Part 1: An anatomic and clinical overview, *J Manual Manipul Ther* 5:158-170, 1997.

Watson DH, Trott PH: Cervical headache: an investigation of natural head posture and upper cervical flexor muscle performance, *Cephalalgia* 13:272-284, 1993.

Whitney SL et al: Physical therapy for migraine-related vestibulopathy and vestibular dysfunction with history of migraine, *Laryngoscope* 110:1528-1534, 2000.

Pharmaceutical Treatment of Migraine

Drug Name	Brand Name	Headache Type	Mechanism	Dosage	Contraindications
Acetaminophen	Tylenol	All		Oral: 625 mg	Liver disease
Amitriptyline	Elavil	Migraine	Antidepressant with sedative effects Interferes with reuptake of norepinephrine	Oral: 10-100 mg daily IM: 20-30 mg 4 times/day	Adding MAO inhibitors may precipitate hyperpyretic crises, convulsions, and death.
Aspirin		All types		Oral: 5-10 grains	Peptic ulcers or coagulation abnormalities
Barbituates	Phenobarbital	Tension-type	Sedative, hypnotics	Oral: 10-30 mg 1-4 times/day	Habit-forming, porphyria, liver dysfunction
Belladonna	Bellatal/ Donnatal	Tension-type	Muscle relaxation	Oral: 1 every 12 hr	Glaucoma, obstructive uropathy, toxic megacolon
Caffeine		Migraine	Muscle constriction		
Carbamazepine	Tegretol	Trigeminal neuralgia	Unknown	Oral: 200-600 mg/day	Erythromycin, warfarin, Danazol
Clonidine	Catapres	Migraine	Centrally acting alpha-antagonist	Oral: 1 twice daily Patch: TTS 1	Digitalis, calcium, and beta blockade
Codeine				Oral: 3-60 mg 4 times/day	
Corticosteroids	Prednisone	All	Anti-inflammatory	Oral: Medrol dosepak	Infection
Cyproheptadine	Periactin	Migraine	Serotonin and histamine antagonist	Oral: 4 mg 4 times/day	MAO inhibitors, obstructive prostate
Cyclobenzaprine	Flexeril	Tension-type	Relieves skeletal muscle spasm	Oral: 10 mg 3 times/day	MAO inhibitors, hyperthyroidism
Diazepam	Valium	All	Acts on limbic system (calming)	Oral: 2-10 mg 4 times/day IM: 2 mg	Drug addiction, drowsiness
Dihydroergotamine	DHE-45	Migraine	Alpha-adrenergic blocking agent; serotonin antagonist	IM or IV: 1 mg in 1 ml every 8 hr	Numbness of finger and toes; avoid BP medications
Diphenylhydantoin	Dilantin	All	Antiepileptic drug, CNS effects	Oral: 100 mg 3 times/day	Many interactions (see PDR)
Ergotamine tartrate	Cafergot, Wigraine	Migraine	Alpha-adrenergic blocking agent	Oral: 2 tablets at onset; 1 per ½ hr	Vomiting numbness, cyanosis

Pharmaceutical Treatment of Migraine *continued*

Drug Name	Brand Name	Headache Type	Mechanism	Dosage	Contraindications
Estrogen	Estrace, Climara	Hormonal migraine	Stabilizes estradiol level	Oral: Estrace 1 mg daily week before, after start of menses	Thrombophlebitis, estrogen-dependent tumors
Ibuprofen	Motrin	All	Pain relief	Oral: 800 mg 3 times/day Topical: 20% 3 times/day	GI bleed, CNS symptoms
Indomethacin	Indocin	Temporal arteritis	Nonsteroidal anti-inflammatory drug	Oral: 50-100 mg 3 times/day	GI bleed; avoid digoxin, triamterene
Isometheptene mucate	Midrin	Migraine	Sympathomimetic amine (vasoconstriction)	Oral: 1-2 caps every 4 hr; maximum: 8/day	Glaucoma, congestive heart failure, renal disease, and MAO inhibitors
Lithium	Eskalith	Chronic headache	Alters sodium transport For manic and manic-depressed patients	Oral: 450 mg twice daily	Diarrhea, ataxia: avoid NSAIDs, ACE inhibitors, diuretics, SSRIs
MAO inhibitor	Nardil: phenelyzine sulfate	All headaches	MAO inhibitor, hydrazine derivative	Oral: 15 mg 3 times/day	Severe reactions with SSRIs, tyramine
Methylsergide	Sansert	Cluster headaches	Vasoconstrictive agent; antagonist to serotonin	Oral: 4-8 mg/stop for 3-4 wk every 6 mo	Retroperitoneal fibrosis, renal stenosis
Propranolol	Inderal	Migraine	Synthetic beta-adrenergic receptor blocking agent	Oral: 10-40 mg twice daily	Avoid Haldol, calcium channel blockade, reserpine
Sumatriptan	Imitres, Amerge	Migraine	Selective serotonin receptor agonist	IM: 6 mg, maximum: 12 mg/24 hr Oral: 50 mg NS: 20 mg	Heart attacks, asthma attack, strokes
	Zomig, Maxalt	Migraine	Selective serotonin receptor agonist	Oral: Zomig has 2.5- and 5-mg tablets; Maxalt: sublingual 10-mg tablets	Same symptoms but less severity compared with IM

CNS, Central nervous system; *MAO,* monoamine oxidase; *IM,* intramuscularly; *BP,* blood pressure; *PDR,* Physicians' Desk Reference; *GI,* gastrointestinal; *CHF,* congestive heart failure; *ACE,* angiotensin-converting enzyme; *NSAID,* nonsteroidal antiinflammatory drug; *SSRIs,* selective serotonin reuptake inhibitors; *NS,* nasal spray.

Chapter 30

Functional Capacity Testing and Industrial Injury Treatment

Susan J. Isernhagen, PT

1. Define functional capacity evaluation.

The American Physical Therapy Association (APTA) defines functional capacity evaluation (FCE) as an objective measure of a client's safe, functional abilities compared with the physical demands of work.

2. When should functional capacity examinations be performed?

In early stages, when the injury is acute or subacute, the therapist would choose to test the functions that do not involve the healing area and limit testing of items that would be contraindicated because of acuity. Many job functions do not involve the injured part, so the end result is still a list of functions the worker can perform safely. As healing continues and function improves, additional job functions are added until the worker has been evaluated as capable of full duty. For workers who are past the subacute stage and have been off work an extended period of time, testing should be performed as soon as possible also. The sooner the referral and the functional capacity examination, the less the likelihood of disability.

3. How is a functional capacity examination used?

A functional capacity examination provides the decision maker specific information about return-to-work decisions. Outcomes also include specific job placement or job modification, disability evaluations, and determinations of work capability. It also is used as an entrance examination for work rehabilitation and provides excellent information for case management and case closure.

4. What are typical components of a functional capacity examination?

The components most often used follow U.S. Department of Labor definitions and include lifting, carrying, pushing, pulling, gripping, pinching, hand coordination, reaching, bending, climbing, walking, standing, sitting, and balancing.

5. What other areas are covered?

For chronic cases, referrers are also interested in the level of effort or cooperation. Items that measure effort level, consistency of performance, and behaviors are often added. Information regarding whether pain interferes with the effort levels is often included.

6. Does a functional capacity examination have a role in legal disability cases?

The functional capacity examination plays a pivotal role, because it is the only definitive test that measures actual work function. In a typical court hearing, the physician testifies first about the medical status, diagnosis, and prognosis of the worker. The physical therapist then testifies about the outcome of impairments. In other words, what functional capacity does the worker retain and how does it relate to work activities? Often the third expert is the vocational evaluator, who identifies what jobs are within the person's safe physical capabilities.

7. How should pain be reported in a functional capacity examination?

The functional capacity examination is a test of function, but safety is also a prime factor. Pain itself is not a contraindication to testing. The most relevant aspect of the pain report is change in the initial level or area of discomfort during a test. The therapist with a background in pathology helps to determine how the pain is interpreted and relates it to function.

8. Could a client stop performing in a functional capacity exam if he/she did not want to participate?

Consent forms and instructions should indicate that the client is aware of his/her ability to refuse a test or test completion. While effort should be made to make the client feel safe and informed, it remains the right of the client to decline a test or test completion. The documentation would merely state that the test was not completed. Clients are more likely to use full effort when there is a good rapport between the evaluator and the client.

9. Is there a role for functional testing in the hiring of an employee?

Employers are interested in hiring and placing people who can perform the essential functions of the job. If there is a job function description, a job-related test can be developed. This would be used after an offer of employment is given. Applicants are tested on their physical ability to do the job-related test items. The therapist performs the tests, and the employer makes the hiring decision.

10. Distinguish between work conditioning and work hardening.

The APTA states that **work conditioning** is a specific work-related, intensive, goal-oriented treatment that focuses on strength, endurance, movement, flexibility, motor control, and cardiopulmonary functions. **Work hardening** is a broader rehabilitation program, which is interdisciplinary in nature. In addition to what is covered in work conditioning, behavioral and vocational functions also are addressed.

11. What are the eligibility requirements for work conditioning or work hardening?

According to the APTA guidelines, the worker must have the following:

- A job goal
- Stated or demonstrated willingness to participate
- A physical or functional deficit that interferes with work
- A point of resolution after the initial injury at which time participation in the program would not create harm

12. How does a therapist obtain cooperation from a client who is not working toward the program goals?

This common issue is handled by working with the client during admission. The preceding "rules" are discussed. The worker/client often signs a contract that indicates he/she will work toward the program goals. The program is the client's "job," and the client must often clock in and out. The client completes the daily work with self-responsibility, although the therapist and supportive staff are available to help. The focus is on the worker getting better and not on "treatment." Progress must be made, or the program will be terminated. The goals are reached when the worker/client is work-ready.

13. If a worker cannot meet the physical demands of work after a functional capacity examination or work rehabilitation program, what are the options?

Matching the worker to the work through work rehabilitation improves functional capacity. Modifying a job with adaptive equipment, assistive devices, or teamwork is also an option. In addition, possibilities for other jobs can be explored by comparing the abilities of the worker with the demands of other job descriptions.

14. What are the major outcome measures for work rehabilitation?

Outcome measures include return-to-work information as well as demographic and performance information gained from the test or program. Outcome data include return-to-work information such as:

- Same or different employer
- Previous or different job
- Full time or part time
- Time of safe return to work

15. What are the reliability and validity of a functional capacity evaluation?

Test-retest reliability and predictive validity of the material-handling aspect of the Isernhagen work system functional capacity evaluation were found to be acceptable. Ceiling and criterion tests reveal acceptable test-retest reliability of most, but not all, tests. An interclass correlation coefficient (ICC) ≥0.75, a Kappa value ≥0.60, and a percentage of absolute agreement ≥80% were demonstrated. Concurrent validity and reliability of other functional capacity systems such as the Ergos work simulator, Ergo-kit, and Blankenship method are currently not available in the literature.

16. After a well-structured work hardening/work conditioning (WH/WC) program, what is the success rate of returning clients to work in any capacity?

- Overall return to work—83%
- Return to work: same job, same employer—73%
- Return to work: different job, same employer—14%
- Return to work: different job, different employer—13%

17. How long does it take to perform, interpret, and document a functional capacity examination?

Functional capacity examinations take 4 to 6 hours to perform and interpret. The length depends on whether it is a full or a modified FCE (e.g., upper extremity). In addition to total hours, the test may be conducted over 1 or 2 days. The total time generally does not vary from 4 to 6 hours whether it is performed on 1 or 2 days.

18. What is the average cost of a functional capacity examination?

The average cost of a 4- to 6-hour functional capacity examination ranges between $400 and $900 in the United States.

19. How should a therapist evaluate the advantages and disadvantages of proprietary functional capacity examinations?

- Is the functional capacity examination standardized?
- Does it explain full policies and procedures for performing the test?
- Is training in the system part of the purchase of the program? (In the United States, referral sources request such training so that all therapists conducting functional capacity examinations have been trained in the particular system that they use.)
- Have outcome studies been done to verify that the functional capacity examination is useful to return patients to work?
- Have reliability studies been done on the test or important test components?

- Has the predictive validity been established by identifying whether the FCE capacities hold true in actual return to work?
- Does the functional capacity examination meet the requirements of disability insurance companies?
- Will the medical/legal credibility and history of the functional capacity examination stand up in court?
- Is the functional capacity examination reliant on dynamic work tests rather than static isometric tests?
- Is the functional capacity examination infused with safety parameters?
- Is the report format clear and easy to read?

Bibliography

American Physical Therapy Association: *Guidelines for programs for injured workers: work conditioning and work hardening,* Alexandria, Va, 1998, American Physical Therapy Association.
American Physical Therapy Association: *Guidelines for physical therapy management of the acutely injured worker,* Alexandria, Va, 2006, American Physical Therapy Association.
American Physical Therapy Association: *Occupational health guidelines: evaluating functional capacity,* Alexandria, Va, 1997, American Physical Therapy Association.
Brouwer S et al: Comparing self-report, clinical examination and functional testing to measure work limitations in chronic low back pain, *Disabil Rehabil* (accepted for publication).
Gassoway J, Flory V: Prework screen: is it helpful in reducing injuries and costs?, *WORK* 15:101-106, 2000.
Gouttebarge V et al: Reliability and validity of functional capacity evaluation methods: a systematic review with reference to Blankenship system, Ergos work simulator, Ergo-Kit and Isernhagen work system, *Int Arch Occup Environ Health* 77:527-537, 2004.
Gross DP, Battie MC: Reliability of safe maximum lifting determinations of a functional capacity evaluation, *Phys Ther* 82:364-371, 2002.
Isernhagen SJ: *The comprehensive guide to work injury management,* Gaithersburg, Md, 1995, Aspen.
Isernhagen SJ, Hart DL, Matheson LN: Reliability of independent observer judgments of level of lift effort in a kinesiophysical functional capacity evaluation, *WORK* 12:145-150, 1999.
Lemstra M, Olszynski WP: The effectiveness of standard care, early intervention and occupational management in workers compensation claims, *Spine* 25:299, 2003.
Lindstrom I et al: The effect of graded activity on patients with subacute low back pain: a randomized prospective clinical study with an operant conditioning behavioral approach, *Phys Ther* 72:279-293, 1992.
Loisel P et al: Management of occupational back pain: the Sherbrooke model: results of a pilot and feasibility study, *Occup Environ Med* 51:597, 1994.
Loisel P et al: A population-based, randomized clinical trial on back pain management, *Spine* 22:2911, 1997.
Loisel P et al: Cost-benefit and cost-effectiveness of a disability prevention model for back pain management: six year follow-up study, *Occup Environ Med* 59:807, 2002.
Matheson LN, Isernhagen SJ, Hart DL: Relationships among lifting ability, grip force, and return to work, *Phys Ther* 82:249-256, 2002.
Nassau D: The effects of pre-work functional screening on lowering an employee's injury rate, medical costs and lost work days, *Spine* 24:269-274, 1999.
Ostelo R et al: Rehabilitation following first time lumbar disc surgery, *Spine* 28:209-218, 2003.
Reneman MF et al: Concurrent validity of questionnaire and performance-based disability measurements in patients with chronic non-specific low back pain, *J Occup Rehabil* 12:119-130, 2002.
Reneman MF et al: Test-retest reliability of the Isernhagen Work Systems functional capacity evaluation in healthy adults, *J Occup Rehabil* 14:295-305, 2004.
Reneman MF et al: Testing lifting capacity: validity of determining effort level by means of observation, *Spine* 30:E40-46, 2005.
Saunders RL, Beissner KL, McManis BG: Estimates of weight that subjects can lift frequently in functional capacity evaluations, *Phys Ther* 77:1717-1728, 1997.
Stall JB et al: Return to work interventions for low back pain: a descriptive review of contents and concepts of working mechanisms, *Sports Med* 43:251-267, 2002.
Vance SR, Brown AM: Onsite medical care and physical therapy impact. In Isernhagen S, editor: *The comprehensive guide to work injury management,* Gaithersburg, Md, 1995, pp 269-276, Aspen.

Chapter 31

Anatomy Mnemonics

[†]*Edward G. Tracy, PhD*

1. What is a mnemonic?

Named after Mnemosyne, the Greek goddess of memory, mnemonics simply means "memory aid." It is a learning device in which we relate a collection of hard facts to a known word, sequence of letters or numbers, or a rhyme in an effort to recall the facts accurately and sequentially. In human anatomy, there are thousands of facts to learn, and it is the volume of such facts that becomes the challenge and hence the beauty of mnemonics.

2. Can I make up my own mnemonics?

Yes. You have poetic license to construct your own mnemonics based on things you encounter in your own life.

3. What is the military saying for shoulder muscles?

"Lady between two majors." "Lady" is actually "lati" because we are referring to latissimus dorsi. The majors are pectoralis major and teres major. The proximal end of the humerus presents crests for its two tubercles, the greater and lesser. Inserting onto the crest of the greater tubercle is the pectoralis major. Inserting onto the crest of the lesser tubercle is the teres major. Latissimus dorsi inserts into the intertubercular groove between the two tubercles, hence "lady (lati) between two majors."

4. What is SALSAP?

The axillary artery is the continuation of the subclavian artery as it passes the lateral edge of the first rib. It courses obliquely through the axilla behind the pectoralis minor, which divides it into three parts (as blood flows, before-behind-after the muscle for parts one-two-three, respectively). At the lower border of the teres major, it becomes the brachial artery. Of its six branches, the first comes from part one, two branches from part two, and three branches from part three (as easy as 1, 2, 3!). SALSAP reminds us of these six branches:

- **S**upreme thoracic
- **A**cromiothoracic (or thoracoacromial) trunk
- **L**ateral thoracic
- **S**ubscapular
- **A**nterior circumflex humeral
- **P**osterior circumflex humeral

[†]In memory of Edward G. Tracy, beloved husband and father—a cherished professor of anatomy whose charismatic ways taught and inspired thousands of physical therapy, occupational therapy, and medical students over the past three decades.

5. How do elephants serve as a memory tool?

An elephant has a trunk, and the thoracoacromial trunk is a true **trunk**—a short vessel that quickly divides into three or more branches. In addition, an elephant is a **pa**chy**d**erm, which can help you remember this arterial trunk's four branches:
- **P**ectoral
- **A**cromial
- **C**lavicular
- **D**eltoid

6. What does B + B = A mean?

This "formula" describes the fact that, although there is a defined point where the axillary artery becomes the brachial artery (lower border of teres major), no such similar landmark exists at a point where the axillary vein begins. The origin and termination of blood vessels in a limb are always based on blood flow; therefore veins will begin distally and terminate proximally. Wherever a basilic vein (B) joins a brachial vein (B), the axillary vein (A) begins.

7. How can the arrangement of structures in the cubital fossa be remembered?

This triangular fossa in front of the elbow is bounded by the brachioradialis, pronator teres, and a line through the humeral epicondyles. Within this fossa from lateral to medial are TAN:
- T—Tendon of biceps brachii as it inserts onto the radius
- A—Artery, specifically the termination of the brachial artery as it bifurcates into the radial and ulnar arteries
- N—Nerve, the median nerve, which within the fossa gives rise to the anterior interosseous nerve

The direction from lateral to medial, if forgotten, is recalled easily because the tendon and artery are both palpable, and feeling them will indicate the direction. The most medial structure is the median nerve; this is a common site for stimulating the median nerve in nerve conduction studies relative to carpal tunnel syndrome.

8. What is the area code for carpal country?

The number ("area code") 921 reminds us of the carpal canal contents:
- 9 tendons—There are 4 tendons from flexor digitorum profundus and 4 tendons from flexor digitorum superficialis plus the lone tendon from flexor pollicis longus.
- 2 bursae—One large bursa called the ulnar bursa surrounds the 8 digitorum tendons and is thus sometimes called the common synovial sheath. The smaller radial bursa surrounds only the flexor pollicis longus. Bursae are small fascial sacs elongated along tendons to minimize friction when the tendons slide.
- 1 nerve—The median nerve; this is the nerve compressed in carpal tunnel syndrome.

9. Is it true that the most risqué mnemonics relate to the carpal bones?

The mnemonics are:
- Send Lucy To Paris To Tame Carnal Hunger
- Some Lovers Try Positions That They Can't Handle

The carpal bones are arranged in two rows of four bones. In the proximal row, from lateral to medial they are:
- Scaphoid
- Lunate
- Triangular (or Triquetral)
- Pisiform

From lateral to medial in the distal row they are:
- Trapezium

- Trapezoid
- Capitate
- Hamate

10. Moving on to the thorax, if I go cruising in my VAN, where would I be?

The arteries, veins, and nerves of the thoracic wall share the name intercostal. The arteries branch off the aorta, the veins return blood to the inferior vena cava via the azygos system of veins, and the nerves are the ventral rami of the thoracic spinal nerves (although T7-T11 are properly called thoracoabdominal nerves and T12 the subcostal nerve). As these structures course forward on the thoracic wall, they occupy a groove at the lower edge of the rib called a costal groove. Within this groove the structures from superior to inferior are in the VAN arrangement—**V**ein, **A**rtery, **N**erve.

11. Is LARP a radio station in California?

LARP refers to the twisting of the right and left vagus nerves as they course onto the esophagus after passing the heart. The anterior and posterior vagal trunks come from the left and right vagi, respectively, hence LARP—**L**eft **A**nterior **R**ight **P**osterior.

12. How many birds reside in the (thoracic) cage?

The thoracic wall, with its 24 ribs and sternum, has been likened to a birdcage. One can see inside the cage through the ribs like one can view the inside of a birdcage. With a stretch of the imagination and slight mispronunciation of the named structures, there are four birds of the thoracic cage. Remember the duck lies between two gooses (azygos and esophagus).

- Esophagus, or esopha-*goose*
- Vagus (nerve), or va-*goose*
- Azygos (system of veins), or azy-*goose*
- Thoracic duct, or thoracic *duck*

13. What does the formula S + S = P mean?

The large portal vein that carries nutrient-rich blood from the intestines to the liver is formed by two veins that both begin with "s." Hence this formula states that when the **s**plenic vein joins the **s**uperior mesenteric vein, the **p**ortal vein is formed.

14. What does SCALP tell you about the head and neck?

SCALP can be used to remember the scalp's five layers, which from superficial to deep are:

- **S**kin—This layer is covered with hairs, the follicles of which extend to deeper layers.
- **C**lose subcutaneous tissue—It is called "close" because of its tightness and the fact that it binds skin to the aponeurosis.
- **A**poneurosis, specifically the galea aponeurotica—This is a flat tendon between the frontalis muscle in the forehead and the occipitalis muscle posteriorly (the term *epicranius* can be used for this entire layer).
- **L**oose subaponeurotic layer—This is a layer of loose connective tissue that allows the first three layers to move as a group. It is also called the "dangerous layer" because infections can spread through it.
- **P**ericranium—This is the periosteum on the outside of the cranial bone.

15. Is there an easy way to remember the terminal branches of the facial nerve?

Two Zebras Bit My Cat. The five terminal branches of the facial nerve originate from the facial plexus embedded within the parotid gland:

- **T**emporal—to muscles of the eye and forehead
- **Z**ygomatic—to muscles of the eye and upper lip

- **B**uccal—to muscles of the cheek and upper lip
- **M**arginal mandibular—to muscles of the lower lip
- **C**ervical—to the neck muscle, platysma

16. What can help me remember the cranial nerves?

On Old Olympus' Towering Top, A Finn And German Viewed Some Hops. This is a classic mnemonic for the 12 cranial nerves (usually indicated by Roman numerals), and they match up as follows:

I. **O**lfactory, sensory to the nasal mucosa
II. **O**ptic, sensory to the eye
III. **O**culomotor, motor to the eye
IV. **T**rochlear, motor to the superior oblique muscle
V. **T**rigeminal, sensory and motor to the face through its three divisions (ophthalmic, maxillary, mandibular)
VI. **A**bducent, motor to the lateral rectus muscle
VII. **F**acial, ends up in the parotid gland (see question 15)
VIII. **A**uditory or **A**coustic (or vestibulocochlear), sensory to the ear
IX. **G**lossopharyngeal, sensory to the tongue and motor to the stylo-pharyngeus
X. **V**agus, sensory and parasympathetic to head, neck, thoracic, and abdomen
XI. **S**pinal accessory, both sensory and motor to trapezius and sternomastoid muscles
XII. **H**ypoglossal, motor to the tongue

Regarding fiber content, the 12 cranial nerves follow the following saying, with S = sensory, M = motor, and B = both sensory and motor (again, the capital letters are the 12 nerves in sequence): Some Say Marry Money. But My Brother Say Marry Money, Bad Business (Some-Olfactor-Sensory, Say-Optic-Sensory, Marry-Oculomotor-Motor, etc.).

17. What is the formula for remembering the nerve supply to the seven muscles of the orbit?

For the cranial nerves to the muscles that move the eyeball, the formula is:

$$LR_6(SO_4)_3$$

The lateral rectus (LR) is supplied by the sixth nerve—abducens; the superior oblique (SO) by the fourth nerve—trochlear; and the remaining five muscles (superior rectus, medial rectus, inferior rectus, inferior oblique, levator labii superioris) by the third nerve—oculomotor.

18. Are there any slick mnemonics for the back and lower limbs?

Not slick, but SLIC. The largest deep back muscle that is concerned with posture is termed the erector spinae or sacrospinalis. This muscle consists of three longitudinal columns of muscle that, from medial to lateral, are the **s**pinalis, **l**ongissimus, and **i**liocostalis.

19. Is poetry ever used to assist in recall of anatomic facts?

Mnemonics can on occasion be in the form of poems. The intervertebral disks that separate vertebral bodies help bind the vertebral canal anteriorly. Each disk consists of the outer, tough fibrous annulus fibrosus and the inner, semigelatinous nucleus pulposus. Hence the poem:

Said the nucleus pulposus to the annulus fibrosus,
"Why do you hold me so tight?"
"If I didn't, you would fall into the vertebral canal,
And then you would be out of sight."

20. What does the phrase "say grace before tea" stand for?

The pes anserina ("foot of the goose") on the medial side of the knee is formed by three tendons that insert from anterior to posterior in this order: sartorius, gracilis, semitendinosus. This arrangement can be recalled by the letters in the mnemonic Say Grace before Tea for **s**artorius, **g**racilis, and semi**t**endinosus.

21. Who are Tom, Dick, and Harry?

On the medial side of the ankle lies the flexor retinaculum, which with the tarsal bones forms the tarsal tunnel. Through this tunnel will pass three tendons (tibialis posterior, flexor hallucis longus, flexor digitorum longus) and vessels and nerves (posterior tibial artery and tibial nerve) that can be recalled by Tom, Dick, and Harry. The association from anterior to posterior is **T**ibialis posterior, flexor **D**igitorum longus, posterior tibial **A**rtery, tibial **N**erve and flexor **H**allucis longus, respectively.

22. What are the branches of the brachial plexus from lateral to medial? Remember, "My Aunt Ravaged My Uncle."

- Musculocutaneous
- Axillary
- Radial
- Median
- Ulnar

23. What nerve roots comprise the long thoracic nerve that innervates the serratus anterior?

C5, 6, 7—Raise your arms to heaven.

24. What is the innervation of the pectoral muscles? Remember, "Lateral is less and medial is more."

The lateral pectoral nerve innervates the pectoralis major only, and the medial pectoral nerve innervates both pectoralis major and pectoralis minor. Remember, these are named for the cord from which they are derived.

25. How do you remember the results of peroneal and tibial nerve injury? Remember "PED and TIP"

- **P**eroneal—**E**verts and **D**orsiflexes; loss = drop foot.
- **T**ibial—**I**nverts and **P**lantar flexes; loss = can't walk on TIP toes.

26. What is the relationship of the suprascapular artery and nerve at the suprascapular notch?

The Army (artery) travels over the bridge, and the Navy (nerve) travels under.

Chapter 32

Nutrition

Victoria L. Veigl, PT, PhD

1. Briefly describe the Zone diet. How does this diet claim to control weight?

The Zone diet consists of eating foods that have a low glycemic index (such as vegetables) and limiting consumption of foods with a high glycemic index (such as starches and grains). Intake of vitamins and minerals that can be found in vegetables and fruits is also encouraged. Fats that are consumed should be monounsaturated. The diet is considered to consist of a moderate amount of carbohydrate (40% of calories), a moderate amount of fat (30% of calories), and a moderate amount of protein (30% of calories). Proteins should be eaten with each meal and snack. Carbohydrate portions should be twice the size of protein portions. The dieter should never exceed more than 5 hours without eating a meal or snack.

The Zone diet claims that weight can be controlled by limiting the amount of insulin in the blood. This is accomplished by choosing the appropriate carbohydrates to eat and by consuming the correct ratio of proteins, carbohydrates, and fats. The diet increases the loss of body fat, resulting in decreased weight. The protein/carbohydrate ratio described by the Zone diet promotes the production of eicosanoids, which accelerate the use of stored body fat. The diet also claims to decrease the risk of cardiovascular disease and improve a multitude of chronic disease conditions including chronic fatigue, arthritis, diabetes, depression, and cancer.

2. Describe the Ornish low-fat diet. How does this diet claim to control weight?

The Ornish diet is a vegetarian diet based mainly on vegetables, fruits, whole grains, and beans. No animal products are eaten except moderate amounts of egg whites and nonfat dairy products. It consists of 10% fat, mainly polyunsaturated and monosaturated; 70% to 75% carbohydrates, mainly complex; 15% to 20% protein; and 5 mg of cholesterol per day. According to Ornish, people lose weight on his diet for several reasons: (1) it takes more calories to metabolize complex carbohydrates than simple carbohydrates; (2) metabolic rate may increase on the diet; (3) people consume fewer calories when eating complex carbohydrates because they are more filling. Meat and animal products contain protein, but they also contain saturated fats and cholesterol. Obtaining protein from plants rather than meat or animal products helps to avoid saturated fats and cholesterol. Ornish claims that his diet is the most effective diet for lowering cholesterol, preventing heart disease, reducing symptoms of type 2 diabetes, and decreasing the risk of developing many cancers.

3. What are possible problems that may result from being on a very low fat diet?

Very low fat diets (approximately 16 g of fat, 10% of calories from fat) may lead to insufficient amounts of essential fatty acids. Individuals with low HDL, high triglyceride, and high insulin levels may have these abnormalities amplified with these diets. Some studies have found very low fat diets to be low in vitamins E and B_{12} and in zinc, but these reports are inconsistent.

4. Briefly describe the Atkins diet. How does this diet claim to control weight?

The Atkins diet is a low-carbohydrate, high-protein, ketotic diet; it is divided into four stages. The most restrictive stage limits carbohydrate consumption to 20 g/day. Other stages allow between 25 and 90 g/day. Most nutritionists recommend about 300 g/day. The diet does not restrict protein, fat, or calories, but many dieters have suppressed appetite and decrease their caloric intake. Several dietary supplements are included, such as vitamins and minerals, especially antioxidants, trace minerals, and essential fatty acids.

Atkins claims that his diet mobilizes fat more than any other diet, is the easiest diet for maintenance of weight loss, and is a high-energy diet that makes people feel good. He believes that most obesity is caused by metabolic imbalances resulting from carbohydrate consumption.

5. According to most traditional nutritional professionals, why do high-protein and high-fat diets cause weight loss?

Fewer calories are consumed on high-protein and high-fat diets because proteins and fats are more filling than simple carbohydrates. The fewer calories you consume, the more weight you lose. Much of the initial weight loss is due to water loss from naturesis. Additional water loss occurs when glycogen is converted to glucose. This conversion must occur to maintain blood sugar levels. In subsequent weeks, weight loss is from body fat, at a rate of 1 to 2 lb per week. This rate is similar to that obtained with other types of low caloric diets.

6. What are the possible side effects of a high-protein, high-fat diet?

Some authors report few side effects of a high-protein, high-fat diet, while others report several significant side effects, including the following: high-protein, high-fat diets cause the liver and kidneys to work harder to metabolize and excrete excessive nitrogen, which may result in organ failure. Excessive water loss may cause dehydration and orthostatic hypotension. The dosages of certain medications may need to be adjusted to compensate for diuresis. There may be an increased risk of osteoporosis caused by calcium loss that occurs with excess water loss. Evidence suggests that high-protein diets are associated with certain cancers and heart disease. Vitamins and minerals found in carbohydrates may be deficient unless supplements are taken. Lowered glycogen stores may cause problems for long-distance runners.

7. Is there a difference between the Atkins, Ornish, Weight Watchers, and Zone diets in the effectiveness of reducing the risk of heart disease?

This is a very controversial question, but a comparison study done by Dansinger et al. showed that all of these diets significantly reduced the low-density lipoprotein/high-density lipoprotein cholesterol ratio by approximately 10% after 1 year. There was no significant difference between diets, but there was a significant correlation with the amount of weight loss. The Atkins and Zone diets tended to lower triglyceride levels more, while the Weight Watchers and Ornish diets lowered low-density lipoprotein levels more.

8. Is there a difference in the adherence rates between the Atkins, Ornish, Weight Watchers, and Zone diets?

Few studies have compared adherence rates of various diets. Dansinger et al. have shown that there was no significant difference in the adherence rates of the more extreme Atkins and Ornish diets compared to the moderate Zone and Weight Watchers diets after 1 year, but there was a trend toward better adherence in the moderate diets. The average adherence rate for all the diets combined was only 58%. This rather low adherence rate is the major cause for the lack of long-term success with all these diets.

9. What are the typical components of an American diet?

Most Americans consume a diet consisting of 35% fat, 50% carbohydrates, and 15% protein.

10. What type of diet is most effective for long-term weight loss?

There are widely varying opinions on which diet is most effective for long-term weight loss. Most scientifically controlled studies indicate diets that reduce caloric intake are most effective for long-term weight loss and body fat reduction regardless of the macronutrient composition. Dansinger found no significant difference in weight loss after 1 year between individuals on the Atkins, Ornish, Weight Watchers, or Zone diet. Weight loss will occur if the number of calories consumed is less than the number of calories expended. For most people the caloric deficit should be about 1000 kcal/day. If physical activity is not increased, a diet of approximately 1400 to 1500 kcal/day seems to be optimal.

11. Can blood pressure be lowered by reducing salt intake in people with normal blood pressure and in hypertensive individuals?

Studies have shown that a modest reduction in daily salt intake (4.4 to 4.6 g/day) for 4 or more weeks results in a decrease in systolic pressure of almost 5 mm Hg and a drop of almost 3 mm Hg in diastolic pressure for hypertensive individuals. Systolic pressure decreases approximately 2 mm Hg and diastolic pressure decreases almost 1 mm Hg in normotensive individuals. There seems to be a correlation between the magnitude of salt reduction and the drop in blood pressure.

12. Does soy protein decrease the risk of developing cardiovascular disease?

A meta-analysis concluded that consumption of soy protein in place of animal protein significantly lowers blood levels of total cholesterol, LDL, and triglycerides without affecting HDL levels. This is especially true in subjects with baseline cholesterol levels greater than 240 mg/dl. The FDA has approved that foods containing more than 6.25 g of soy protein per serving may be labeled as reducing the risk of heart disease, assuming 25 g of soy protein intake daily.

13. Do antioxidant supplements decrease the risk of developing cardiovascular disease?

There is insufficient evidence for recommending the use of antioxidant supplements for decreasing the risk of developing cardiovascular disease. Observational studies involving consumption of foods rich in vitamin E have shown an association with lower disease risk. Similar studies using foods rich in vitamin C have not been as consistent. However, direct evidence that the decrease in disease was due to the antioxidants has not been shown for either vitamin. A few observational studies using vitamin E supplements have reported inconsistent results. No randomized trial studies have been done. Trials using β-carotene supplements have not shown any benefits and in some cases caused increased risk of cancer.

14. Do folic acid, vitamin B_6, and vitamin B_{12} decrease the risk of developing cardiovascular disease?

Case-control and prospective studies have shown that lower levels of folic acid and vitamin B_6 have been associated with coronary artery disease but low levels of vitamin B_{12} have not been associated with vascular disease. However, randomized trial studies have not been conducted to determine a cause and effect relationship between high folic acid and vitamin B_6 consumption and decreased risk of cardiovascular disease.

15. Does omega-3 fatty acid consumption alter mortality or the prevalence of cardiovascular events or cancer?

Several studies have reported beneficial effects of increased omega-3 fatty acid intake in patients with coronary artery disease, including reduction in plasma triglyceride levels, and a decrease in death rates. However, meta-analysis of several randomized control trials found no clear evidence that dietary or supplemental omega-3 fatty acids from fish or plants alter mortality, cardiovascular events, or cancers in individuals with cardiovascular disease or those at high risk of developing cardiovascular disease, or in the general population. These analyses also found no increased risks of mortality, cancers, or stroke as a result of consuming omega-3 supplements or increasing omega-3 fatty acid intake in the diet. Individuals who have previously had a myocardial infarction are therefore encouraged to consume more omega-3 fatty acids. However, people who have angina but no previous myocardial infarction and also the general public are not advised to increase their consumption of omega-3 fatty acids.

16. Do folate supplements decrease the prevalence of neural tube defects?

Yes; there is a significant reduction in the prevalence of neural tube defects when folate supplements are taken before and during the first 2 months of pregnancy.

17. Do folic acid supplements with or without vitamin B_{12} supplements improve cognitive function or mood?

Although studies are limited, there is no evidence that folic acid with or without vitamin B_{12} improves cognitive function or mood in normal or cognitively impaired older adults. Folic acid with vitamin B_{12} has been shown to reduce serum levels of the amino acid homocysteine. Elevated homocysteine levels have been linked to increased risk of developing dementia and DVT.

18. Does dietary fiber decrease the incidence of colorectal adenomas and carcinomas?

Currently there is no evidence that increased dietary fiber intake will reduce the incidence or recurrence of adenomatous polyps within a 2- to 4-year period.

19. Do calcium supplements increase bone density in postmenopausal women?

Calcium supplements appear to increase bone density between 1.6% and 2%. There is a trend toward reduction in vertebral fractures associated with this increase, but evidence is not clear regarding a reduction in nonvertebral fractures.

20. What dietary guidelines does the American Heart Association recommend?

The American Heart Association recommends:

1. Consume at least 5 daily servings of fruits and vegetables.
2. Eat at least 6 daily servings of grain products, including whole grains.
3. Eat fish at least twice a week, particularly fatty fish.
4. Use fat-free and low-fat milk products, legumes, skinless poultry, and lean meats.
5. Choose fats and oils with 2 g or less saturated fat per tablespoon, such as liquid and tub margarines and canola, olive, corn, safflower, and soybean oils.
6. Limit intake of foods high in calories or low in nutrition, such as soft drinks and candy.
7. Limit foods high in saturated fat (less than 10% of total calories), trans fat (less than 3% of total calories), and/or cholesterol (less than 300 mg/day for general public, 200 mg/day for those with heart disease or diabetes), such as full-fat milk products, tropical oils, partially hydrogenated vegetable oils, and egg yolks.
8. Use less than 6 g (about 1 teaspoon) of salt per day.

9. If you drink alcohol, limit intake to 1 drink (½ oz of pure alcohol) per day for women and 2 drinks per day for men.
10. To maintain weight, balance the number of calories consumed with the number you use each day.
11. Walk or perform other activities for at least 30 minutes every day.

21. How should the daily-recommended percentages of carbohydrate, fat, and protein intake be altered during heavy training?

In a training athlete, the percentage of carbohydrates should be higher, the percentage of fats should be lower, and the percentage of protein should be the same as for a sedentary person. Carbohydrates are the primary nutrient used during prolonged, moderate-to-high intensity exercise.

22. Should athletes consume additional protein when they are in training?

The current recommended daily allowance for protein in sedentary people is 0.8 g of protein/kg of body weight/day. Several investigators have shown that athletes require more protein. Recommended amounts range from 1.2 to 1.8 g/kg/day for aerobic and resistance trained athletes. People just beginning an exercise program should use the upper end of this range. Because the average North American diet consists of 1.9 g/kg/day, additional protein usually is not necessary.

23. Does carbohydrate consumption affect the amount of muscle growth?

Yes; carbohydrate consumption causes an increase in the release of insulin, which stimulates muscle synthesis. Testosterone levels, which also stimulate muscle synthesis, appear to be highest when the ratio of carbohydrate to protein intake is 4 to 1. Maximal muscle growth seems to occur when protein intake is 1.7 to 1.8 g of protein/kg of body weight/day, energy intake is sufficient to prevent weight loss, and carbohydrate intake is 60% to 65% of nutrient intake. Consuming a carbohydrate with protein beverage after resistance exercise may enhance recovery or reduce muscle breakdown.

24. What is the primary factor that determines whether carbohydrates, fats, or proteins are metabolized during a bout of exercise?

The availability of oxygen is the main factor that determines whether fats or carbohydrates are metabolized. The more limited the supply of oxygen, the more carbohydrates will be metabolized. Less oxygen is needed for carbohydrate metabolism than for fat metabolism. More calories per liter of oxygen are produced from carbohydrates, and oxidation of carbohydrates occurs more quickly. During high-intensity exercise, therefore, carbohydrates are the prominent fuel source. As exercise intensity decreases, oxygen becomes more readily available, carbohydrate metabolism decreases, and fat metabolism increases. However, the duration of exercise also contributes to the type of fuel used. The longer the duration of exercise, the greater the contribution of fat. Under normal circumstances, proteins provide only 5% to 10% of the fuel source during exercise. The contribution is directly proportional to the intensity and duration of exercise. The increase in protein utilization with prolonged exercise seems to be related to glycogen stores. As glycogen stores are depleted, the body becomes more dependent on protein for energy production.

25. Do creatine supplements improve an athlete's performance?

Most studies agree that creatine supplements are beneficial for short-duration, repetitive bursts of intense exercise. Kreider has shown that short-term creatine supplementation (15 to 25 g/day for 5 to 7 days) improves maximal power and strength by 5% to 15%, work performed during sets of maximal effort muscle contractions by 5% to 15%, single-effort sprint performance by 1% to 5%, and work performed during repetitive sprint performance by 5% to 15%. Long-term supplementation (15 to 25 g/day for 5 to 7 days and 2 to 25 g/day for 7 to 84 days) also results in significantly greater gains in strength, sprint performance, and fat-free mass. The most popular dosage is a loading phase of 0.3 g/kg/day for 5 to 7 days and a maintenance dosage of 0.03 g/kg/day. Creatine supplements do not appear to improve longer duration, aerobic exercise performance.

26. What are the side effects of creatine supplementation?

The only negative side effect reported in scientific studies is weight gain. When creatine supplements are taken, endogenous synthesis decreases; it returns when creatine is removed from the diet. Supplements may increase stress on the liver and kidneys, but this theory has not been confirmed. Anecdotal evidence suggests an increased prevalence of muscle cramps and strains, minor gastrointestinal distress, and nausea, but no scientific studies validate such reports. Further research clearly is needed.

Bibliography

American Heart Association Dietary Guidelines: *Circulation* 102:2284-2299, 2000.

Asano TK: Dietary fiber for the prevention of colorectal adenomas and carcinomas, *Cochrane Database Syst Rev* (1):CD003430.DOI:10.1002/14651858.CD003430, 2002.

Atkins RC: *New diet revolution,* New York, 1992, Avon Books.

Beckles-Willson NNR, Elliott T, Everard MML: Omega-3 fatty acids (from fish oils) for cystic fibrosis, *Cochrane Database Syst Rev* (3):CD002201.DOI:10.1002/14651858.CD002201, 2002.

Berning JR, Steen SN, editors: *Nutrition for sport and exercise,* ed 2, Gaithersburg, Md, 1998, Aspen.

Blackburn GL, Phillips JC, Morreale S: Physician's guide to popular low carbohydrate weight-loss diets, *Cleve Clin J Med* 68:761-778, 2001.

Dansinger MI et al: Comparison of the Atkins, Ornish, Weight Watchers, and Zone Diets for weight loss and heart disease risk reduction, *JAMA* 293:43-53, 2005.

Fouque D et al: Low protein diets for chronic renal failure in non-diabetic adults, *Cochrane Database Syst Rev* (4):CD001892.DOI:10.1002/14651858.CD001892, 2002.

Freedman MR, King J, Kennedy E: Popular diets: a scientific review, executive summary, *Obesity Res* 9:1S-5S, 2001.

Hasson SM, editor: *Clinical exercise physiology,* St Louis, 1994, Mosby.

He FJ, MacGregor GA: Effect of longer-term modest salt reduction on blood pressure, *Cochrane Database Syst Rev* (1):DC004937.DOI:10.1002/14651858.CD004937, 2004.

Hooper L et al: Omega-3 fatty acids for prevention and treatment of cardiovascular disease, *Cochrane Database Syst Rev* (4):CD003177/pub2.DOI:10.1002/14651858.CD003177.pub2, 2004.

Kreider R: Creatine supplementation: analysis of ergogenic value, medical safety, and concerns, *J Exercise Physiol* 1:1-12, 1999.

Lumley J et al: Periconceptional supplementation with folate and multivitamins for preventing neural tube defects, *Cochrane Database Syst Rev* (3):DC001056.DOI:10.1002/14651858.CD001056, 2001.

Malouf R, Grimley Evans J, Areosa Sastre A: Folic acid with or without vitamin B_{12} for cognition and dementia, *Cochrane Database Syst Rev* (4):CD004514.DOI:10.1002/1465158.CD004514, 2003.

Ornish D: *Dr. Dean Ornish's program for reversing heart disease,* New York, 1990, Ballantine Books.

Robergs RA, Roberts SO: *Exercise physiology: exercise, performance, and clinical applications,* St Louis, 1997, Mosby.

Roberts DC: Quick weight loss: sorting fad from fact, *Med J Aust* 175:637-640, 2001.

Sears B, Lawren B: *Enter The Zone,* New York, 1995, HarperCollins.

Sommerfield T, Hiatt WR: Omega-3 fatty acids for intermittent claudication, *Cochrane Database Syst Rev* (1):CD003833.pub2.DOI:10.1002/14651858.CD003833.pub2, 2004.

Stein K: High-protein, low-carbohydrate diets: do they work?, *J Am Dietetic Assoc* 100:760-761, 2000.

Tarnopolsky MA et al: Evaluation of protein requirements for trained athletes, *J Appl Physiol* 73:1986-1995, 1992.

Volek JS: Enhancing exercise performance: nutritional implications. In Garrett W, Kirkendall DT, editors: *Exercise in sport science,* Philadelphia, 2000, pp 471-485, Williams & Wilkins.

Wells SB et al: The Osteoporosis Methodology Group and the Osteoporosis Research Advisory Group: calcium supplementation on bone loss in postmenopausal women, *Cochrane Database Syst Rev* (1):CD004526.pub2.DOI:10.1002/14651858.CD004526.pub2, 2004.

Wheeler KB, Lombardo JA, editor: Nutritional aspects of exercise, *Clin Sports Med* 18:469-701, 1999.

Chapter 33

Spinal Exercise Programs

Robert C. Rinke, PT, DC, FAAOMPT

1. What is the current information on the scope of low back problems?

At least 80% of the general population will suffer back pain at some time in their lives. Traditional teaching was that 90% of low back pain (LBP) patients would recover within 6 weeks, but recent natural history studies suggest that this is overly optimistic. McGorry reported that two thirds of the people who have had back pain in the past can be expected to have some symptoms every year; 70% of patients who have acute back pain will suffer three or more recurrences, and 20% of patients with LBP will continue to have some back symptoms over long periods of their lives. Recent estimates show that 25% of working men experience back pain each year; over time, eventually 4% change jobs. Those off work longer than 6 months have a 50% chance of returning to work; after 1 year, the chance decreases to 20%. Virtually no one returns to the work force after 2 years off work. The cost is enormous and in the United States is estimated at over $14 billion annually. Back injuries account for at least one fifth of all work-related injuries and approximately one third of all compensable claims. However, it is estimated that <10% of patients account for approximately 90% of the total costs.

2. Do patients with back pain have weaker spinal musculature?

In general, patients with acute back pain show little deficit in muscle power. However, patients with chronic low back pain typically demonstrate weak abdominal and extensor muscles with predominance of back extensor weakness. Normally trunk extensors are 30% stronger than trunk flexors. This ratio may be reversed in patients with chronic low back pain.

3. What is the rationale behind Williams' flexion exercises?

Williams believed that the basic cause of all back pain is the stress induced on the intervertebral disk by poor posture. He theorized that the lordotic lumbar spine placed inordinate strain on the posterior elements of the intravertebral disk and caused its premature dysfunction. He was concerned about the lack of flexion in daily activities in the accumulation of extension forces that hurt the disk.

4. What are the goals of Williams' flexion exercises?

The goals of these exercises are to open the intravertebral foramina and stretch the back extensors, hip flexors, and facets; to strengthen the abdominal and gluteal muscles; and to mobilize the lumbosacral junction.

5. List the core exercises of Williams' flexion program.

Pelvic tilts, knee-to-chest exercises, hip flexor stretching, and crunches are the core exercises.

6. Explain McKenzie's extension philosophy.

McKenzie also believes that the disk is the primary cause of back pain but that flexion, not extension, is the culprit. According to McKenzie, prolonged sitting in flexed positions and lack of extension are the two factors predisposing to back pain. The accumulation of flexion forces causes early dysfunction in the posterior elements of the disk.

7. Describe McKenzie's classification of lumbar disorders.

- Postural syndrome—Sedentary occupation, age <30 years, midline pain, no referred pain, no pain induction by movement, possible hypermobility, pain with prolonged positioning
- Dysfunction syndrome—Usually >30 years old (unless trauma is involved), often sedentary occupation, local pain at end of range movements, restricted range of motion with shortened soft tissues
- Derangement syndrome—Typically 20 to 55 years old, sudden onset (from hours to 1 to 2 days), possible radiation of pain, paresthesias, migrating pain, often constant pain exacerbated with certain movements, possible postural deformity

8. Describe the typical treatment for postural syndrome.

Postural correction advice, use of a lumbar roll, and active and passive extension exercises are the suggested treatment for postural syndrome.

9. What is the typical treatment for dysfunction syndrome?

Dysfunction syndrome is typically treated by postural education; flexion, extension, and/or lateral deviation stretching and correction; and mobilization or manipulation into restricted ROM.

10. What is the typical treatment for derangement syndrome?

Reduction of derangement, maintenance of reduction, recovery of full function, prevention of recurrence, postural education, repeated extension in prone or standing position, and use of lumbar supports are all used to treat derangement syndrome. Lateral deviation may need to be corrected to maintain reduction. Add extension and rotation mobilization to regain movement and decrease pain as well as extension manipulation, if necessary. When pain is intermittent, add flexion exercises in recumbent position, and progress to weight-bearing. Always follow flexion exercises with extension.

11. Which are more effective—extension or flexion exercises?

Studies of the extension versus flexion approach appear inconclusive. Compared with patients educated in a mini back school, McKenzie's patients initially showed greater improvement, but little difference was found at 5-year follow-up. The McKenzie method was found effective in assisting resolution of the lateral shift but ineffective in improving clinical condition. When flexion exercise was compared with extension exercise, no differences were found in increasing coronal and transverse mobility, but flexion was more helpful in increasing sagittal mobility. Another study, however, showed a clear patient preference for extension movements and positions (40%) over flexion (7%). Finally, an extension and flexion exercise program in conjunction with manipulation was found to be quite effective in helping low back pain sufferers. The exercise program should be based on each patient's needs for flexion and/or extension in combination with manipulation.

12. What is the reliability of McKenzie evaluation techniques?

Inter-tester reliability was quite poor for the McKenzie classifications and did not improve with postgraduate training in the McKenzie methods. Inter-tester reliability in detecting the presence and direction of the lateral shift also was very poor, but better results were obtained with a positive slide-glide test to assess the relevance of lateral shifts to pain complaints.

13. What is the role of aquatic exercise?

Clinically, aquatic exercise has proved helpful for load-sensitive patients because exercise in water reduces compression, increases resistance to movement, and may increase aerobic capacity. Load clinically appears to make important contributions to disk and joint dysfunction as well as degenerative changes. However, there are two randomized controlled trials (RCTs) that have evaluated hydrotherapy for chronic LBP, both finding no difference between hydrotherapy and control treatment, and no studies assess its efficacy in the treatment of acute LBP.

14. Define functional range.

The spine has optimal positions in which it functions most efficiently, but these positions vary with physical condition and stresses. In general, there is no one "best" position for all functional tasks. Often the preferred position is near the midrange of all available movements, but this must not be confused with the spine's mythical "neutral" position. According to Morgan, the functional range is quite simply "the most stable and asymptomatic position of the spine for the task at hand."

15. Describe an alternate method for classification of low back syndromes.

- Flexion bias preferred
- Extension bias preferred
- Weight-bearing intolerance
- Intolerance of static postures
- Irritability

16. What special considerations should be kept in mind when training begins?

- Because of limited tolerance for weight-bearing or vertical loading, patients should limit weight-bearing exercise time and continue exercising in the recombinant, semirecumbent, and even antigravity positions. Increase weight-bearing as tolerance increases.
- Control the amount of movement. Starting with isometric exercises may be necessary. Gradual progression can relieve pain and spasm. Additional specific techniques are also available.
- Control the direction of movement initially to sagittal and frontal planes. Torsional or oblique movements are most difficult to perform. Symptoms can be avoided with good trunk control. After control is achieved in cardinal planes and the condition is stable, movements around combined axes in multiple planes may be attempted.
- Progress movement complexity from large, gross, and simple to smaller, isolated, and complex.
- Beginning exercise in stable positions allows increased intensity and decreases the risk of aggravation. Progress to exercise and unstable positions and/or unstable surfaces (e.g., balls, foam rollers, balance boards).
- Exercise while compensating for other areas of the body. Many patients also have problems with shoulders, knees, or ankles.

17. How can movements be limited and controlled (stabilization)?

- Passive prepositioning uses body and limb placement to maintain a particular spinal position or to avoid movement into a painful range or position. Minimal muscular effort is required.
- Active prepositioning uses primarily muscle activity to maintain an overcorrected spinal position.
- Dynamic control continually alters muscle activity to accommodate varying demands and loads.
- Transitional control involves a change in the primary muscle stabilizers from agonist to antagonist. In reaching from below the waist to overhead, a change from extension stabilizers to flexion stabilizers often is required to protect the low back.

18. How is the intensity of exercise increased?

Traditionally, exercise intensity has been increased by adding repetitions and resistance. However, intensity also can be improved by challenging the balance and coordination demanded by the exercise. Continuing an exercise for a longer time challenges endurance; an increasing amount of movement and speed adds intensity. Efficient and effective exercise trains the patient at maximal intensity in all physical skills.

19. What are the implications of weak multifidi in relation to LBP?

Back extensor weakness has been shown to be a risk factor in the incidence of LBP. Multiple studies show the multifidus to be the largest, most medial, and most used extensor muscle group. It contributes nearly 70% of the stiffness resulting from muscle contraction in the neutral zone of the lumbar spine, where the spine is least stiff. Danneels et al. demonstrated multifidus cross-sectional area wasting in LBP patients. Selective training of these muscles significantly increases cross-sectional area and is meaningful in the prevention and rehabilitation of chronic LBP.

20. How does instruction in body mechanics and home exercise, such as provided in many back schools, compare to more intensive, specific, physical therapist supervised exercise programs?

Changing long-standing habits with better biomechanical technique requires time, multiple repetitions, and a high degree of attention to detail. Rarely will the patient achieve this level of improvement without supervision and reinstruction. In their RCT, O'Sullivan et al. found significant improvements in pain and disability that were maintained at 30-month follow-up visits in patients provided with a supervised exercise program. The exercise group had an average pain score of 59/100 at baseline that reduced to 23/100 at the 30-month follow-up, whereas the group who was managed by their general practitioner had no meaningful reduction in pain (baseline score, 53/100; 30-month follow-up score, 52/100).

21. Are intensive exercise programs more effective than gentle programs?

Current evidence now shows that intensive exercise programs are more effective in reducing pain and increasing mobility and function than gentle programs. Intensive programs consist of specific exercises directed at specific muscle groups, movements, and control. Gentle programs are those where the patient is encouraged to gradually resume normal daily activities as tolerated and begin a gradual general exercise program such as walking or swimming.

22. Can exercise treatments be functionally helpful and cost effective and enhance future quality of life?

A recent study appears to be the first to show convincingly that exercise can be a part of a physical therapy treatment regimen that both is cost effective and shows statistically significant improvement in function, pain, disability, physical and mental aspects of quality of life, and beliefs about back pain. Patients with chronic low back pain were trained how to activate their multifidus and transverse abdominis muscles. The Roland disability index improved an average of 50% and the Oswestry disability index improved an average of 25%. In 2002 Bogduk reviewed RCTs and systematic reviews of the efficacy of various therapies for chronic LBP. No data from RCTs support any efficacy for surgery, spinal cord stimulation, or use of epidural steroids and intraspinal opioids. The best studies have failed to show any efficacy greater than that of placebo for acupuncture, injection of tender points, traction, and epidurolysis. The only treatment shown in a controlled trial to have produced substantial and lasting reductions in chronic LBP was specific exercises designed to coactivate abdominal and multifidus muscles. Bogduk found only specific exercises designed to coactivate these muscles hold the promise of substantial and sustained reductions in back pain.

23. Are there similar effects of multifidus weakness and benefit from specific exercise in people with chronic neck pain?

Ylinen studied patients with chronic neck pain who were put on exercise programs and followed up 12 months later. There was a 70% to 100% improvement noted in terms of decreased pain and disability following the training program. Both specific strength training and endurance training for 12 months were effective for decreasing pain and disability in patients with chronic neck pain.

Bibliography

Ariyoshi M et al: Efficacy of aquatic exercises for patients with low back pain, *Kurume Med J* 46:91-96, 1999.

Bogduk N, McGuirk B: *Medical management of acute and chronic low back pain: an evidence-based approach,* Amsterdam, 2002, pp 143-161, Elsevier.

Danneels LA et al: CT imaging of trunk muscles in chronic LBP patients and healthy control subjects, *Eur Spine J* 9:266-272, 2000.

Danneels LA et al: Effects of three different training modalities on the cross-sectional area of the lumbar multifidus muscle in patients with chronic LBP, *Br J Sports Med* 35:186-191, 2001.

Delitto A et al: Evidence for use of an extension-mobilization category in acute low back syndrome: a prescriptive validation pilot study, *Phys Ther* 73:216-222, discussion 223-228, 1993.

Ebenbichler GR et al: Sensory-motor control of the lower back: implications for rehabilitation, *Med Sci Sports Exercise* 33:1889-1898, 2001.

Elnaggar IM et al: Effects of spinal flexion and extension exercises on low back pain and spinal mobility in chronic mechanical low back pain patients, *Spine* 16:967-972, 1991.

Frost H et al: Randomized controlled trial for evaluation of fitness programs with chronic low back pain, *BMJ* 310:151-154, 1995.

Lee JH et al: Trunk muscle weakness as a risk factor for low back pain: a 5-year prospective study, *Spine* 24:54-57, 1999.

Liddle SD et al: Exercise and chronic LBP: What works? *Pain* 107:176-190, 2004.

Maher CG: Effective physical treatment for chronic low back pain, *Orthop Clin North Am* 35:57-64, 2004.

McGorry RW et al: Meteorlogical conditions and self-report of low back pain, *Spine* 23:2096-2102, 1998.

McKenzie RA: *The lumbar spine: mechanical diagnosis and therapy,* Waikanae, New Zealand, 1981, Spinal Publications.

Morgan D: Concepts in functional training and postural stabilization for the low-back-injured, *Top Acute Care Trauma Rehabil* 2:8-17, 1988.

Nadler SF: Nonpharmacologic management of pain, *J Am Osteopath Assoc* 104:S6-12, 2004.

O'Sullivan P, Twomey L, Allison G: Evaluation of specific stabilizing exercise in the treatment of chronic low back pain with radiologic diagnosis of spondylolysis or spondylolisthesis, *Spine* 22:2959-2967, 1997.

Riddle DL, Rothstein JM: Anicteric tester reliability of McKenzie's classifications of the syndrome types present in patients with low back pain, *Spine* 18:1333-1344, 1993.

Shaughnessy M, Caulfield B: A pilot study to investigate the effect of lumbar stabilization exercise training on functional ability and quality-of-life in patients with chronic LBP, *Int J Rehabil Res* 27:297-301, 2004.

Stankovic R, Johnell O: Conservative treatment of acute low back pain: a prospective randomized trial: McKenzie method of treatment versus patient education in "mini back school", *Spine* 15:120-123, 1990.

Stankovic R, Johnell O: Conservative treatment of acute low back pain: a 5-year follow-up study of two methods of treatment, *Spine* 20:469-472, 1995.

Sufka A et al: Centralization of low back pain and perceived functional outcome, *J Orthop Sports Phys Ther* 27:205-212, 1998.

Ylinen J et al: Active neck muscle training in the treatment of chronic neck pain in women, *JAMA* 289: 2509-2516; 2003.

Chapter 34

Isokinetic Testing and Exercise

George J. Davies, PT, DPT, MEd,
Christopher J. Durall, PT, DPT, MS,
James W. Matheson, PT, MS, SCS, and Patricia Wilder, PT, PhD

1. What do isokinetic devices do?

Isokinetic devices provide a resistance that accommodates to the torque (force times perpendicular distance) applied by an individual to maintain a constant, preselected angular velocity.

2. What are the advantages of isokinetic devices?

- Because of the accommodating resistance, a muscle can be challenged to its maximal capacity through an entire range of motion (physiologic Blix curve).
- Muscle groups can be isolated for testing and exercising.
- Resistance that accommodates to pain and fatigue provides an inherent safety factor.
- Reliable objective data may be obtained for documentation.
- Exercise is possible at different angular velocities through a velocity spectrum.
- It is possible to train at high angular velocities to increase muscle power, quickness of muscle force development, time rate of torque development, or torque acceleration energy. These muscle performance characteristics are important for functional activities.
- Computerized feedback allows an exerciser to improve torque control accuracy.
- The reciprocal innervation time of agonist and antagonist muscle contractions can be decreased.
- Joint compressive forces decrease with higher angular velocities. Bernoulli's principle states that the faster the movement of a surface (articular surface) over a fluid (synovial fluid), the lower the surface pressures.
- There is a 30 deg/sec physiologic (strengthening) overflow to slower angular velocities with isokinetic resistance.
- There is a 30-degree range of motion strengthening overflow during performance of short-arc exercises.
- Real-time feedback is available to the patient for motivation during exercise.

3. What are the contraindications to isokinetic testing or exercising?

ABSOLUTE CONTRAINDICATIONS

- Acute strain (musculotendinous unit) or sprain (noncontractile tissue)
- Soft-tissue healing constraints (e.g., immediately after surgery)
- Severe pain
- Extremely limited range of motion (ROM)
- Severe effusion
- Joint instability

RELATIVE CONTRAINDICATIONS

- Subacute strain or chronic third-degree sprain
- Pain
- Partially limited ROM
- Effusion
- Joint laxity

4. When is it safe to perform isokinetic testing after surgical repair?

Generally, isokinetic testing may be performed safely when postsurgical soft-tissue healing is complete. The table lists approximate healing times and recommended testing criteria for several common surgical repairs. However, we strongly recommend consulting with the referring surgeon to establish testing criteria.

Approximate Healing Times and Testing Criteria for Common Surgical Repairs

Surgical Repair	Approximate Healing Time	Testing Criteria
ACL (patellar tendon graft)	8-12 weeks	Full AROM; KT scores WNL
ACL (semitendinosis graft)	12-16 weeks	Full AROM; KT scores WNL
PCL	12 weeks	Full AROM; KT scores WNL
Rotator cuff tear		
Small tear	12-16 weeks	Full AROM; healthy tissue
Medium tear	16-24 weeks	Full AROM; healthy tissue
Large tear	24 weeks	Full AROM; healthy tissue
Capsular shift	12 weeks	Full AROM
Lateral ankle reconstruction	8-12 weeks	Full AROM
Achilles tendon rupture	16-24 weeks	Full AROM

ACL, Anterior cruciate ligament; *PCL,* posterior cruciate ligament; *AROM,* active range of motion; *WNL,* within normal limits; *KT,* KT-1000 knee ligament arthrometer (MEDmetric Corp, San Diego, Calif).

5. What parameters are commonly used for assessment of isokinetic data?

- Peak torque—the maximal torque value on the parabolic torque curve (A)
- Angle-specific torque—the torque value at a specific point (angle) in the range of motion (B)
- Time rate of torque development (TRTD) to peak torque—the elapsed time from the onset of torque production to the peak torque (C)
- TRTD to a predetermined torque value—the elapsed time from the onset of torque production to a predetermined level of torque
- TRTD to a predetermined time—the torque developed in a specific time interval
- TRTD to a specific point in the ROM—the elapsed time to reach a specific point in the ROM
- Torque acceleration energy (TAE)—the total work performed in the first 0.125 sec; a measure of the "explosiveness" of a muscle contraction (D)
- ROM—measured in degrees with an electrogoniometer
- Reciprocal innervation time—the time interval from cessation of the agonistic contraction to the initiation of the antagonistic contraction (E)
- Force decay rate—the downslope of the torque curve; in general, the downslope should be straight or convex; if it is concave, the patient probably had difficulty with producing torque at the end ROM (F)
- Total work—the total volume of work under the torque curve, regardless of speed, range of motion, or time (G)
- Average power—the total work divided by the work time

6. How are isokinetic data commonly interpreted and analyzed?

- Bilateral comparison—the analysis of torque values of one extremity relative to the other extremity; probably the most common comparison; differences >10% to 15% indicate significant asymmetry

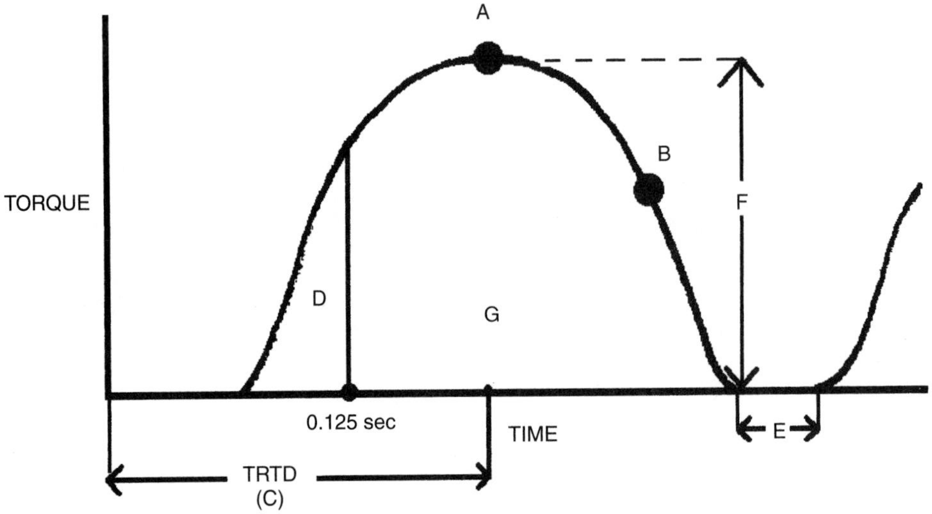

Common parameters for assessment of isokinetic data.

- Unilateral ratios—the comparison of agonist and antagonist muscle torques; this measure is particularly important to assess with velocity spectrum testing because the ratios change through different angular velocities in many muscle groups
- Torque to body weight—the analysis of torque values relative to body weight; used to normalize muscle performance relative to size
- Total leg (TLS)/total arm (TAS) strength—the summation of torque values for individual components of the leg or arm, respectively
- Comparison with normative data—the analysis of torque values relative to published normative data for specific populations

7. Describe the evaluation of isokinetic data relative to normative data.

Descriptive normative data for different populations may be used as another guideline for testing and rehabilitation. The table provides descriptive normative data for peak torques relative to body weight and unilateral agonist/antagonist ratios for several commonly tested muscle pairs. Normative data are particularly useful when a patient has bilateral injuries and bilateral comparison is not a useful measure. Examples of commonly used normative data are included in the table.

Normative Test Data on Cybex

	Speed (degrees/sec)		
Shoulder (modified neutral)	**60**	**180**	**300**
Male			
External rotation (% BWT)	13	10	6
Internal rotation (% BWT)	22	18	14
ER/IR ratio (%)	59	56	43

Normative Test Data on Cybex *continued*

	Speed (degrees/sec)				
Shoulder (modified neutral)	**60**	**180**	**300**		
Female					
External rotation (% BWT)	9	6	3		
Internal rotation (% BWT)	15	12	9		
ER/IR ratio (%)	60	50	33		
Shoulder 90/90	**60**	**180**	**300**		
Male					
External rotation (% BWT)	15-20	13-18	11-16		
Internal rotation (% BWT)	25-30	22-27	19-24		
ER/IR ratio (%)	60-69	60-69	60-69		
Knee extension/flexion	**60**	**180**	**300**		
Male					
Quadriceps (% BWT)	100	75	50		
Hamstrings (% BWT)	60-69	35-47	25-37		
Quadriceps/hamstring ratio (%)	60-69	70-79	85-95		
Female					
Quadriceps (% BWT)	90	65	40		
Hamstrings (% BWT)	60	35	25		
Quadriceps/hamstring ratio (%)	60-69	70-79	85-95		
Ankle inversion/eversion	**60**	**120**			
Inversion (% BWT)	12	10			
Eversion (% BWT)	11	9			
Inversion/eversion ratio (%)	91	90			
Ankle plantar flexion/dorsiflexion	**30**	**60**	**90**	**120**	**180**
Male					
Plantar flexion (% BWT)	70-75	65	51	38	24
Dorsiflexion (% BWT)	16	12		9	8
PF/DF ratio (%)	20-25	25		33-40	33-50
Female					
Plantar flexion (% BWT)	60-65	50		40	22
Dorsiflexion (% BWT)	14	12		8	6
PF/DF ratio (%)	20-25	25		33-40	33-50

ER, External rotation; *IR*, internal rotation; *BWT*, body weight; *PF*, plantar flexion; *DF*, dorsiflexion.

8. Can the isokinetic dynamometer pick up differences between the ACL-deficient knee and the healthy knee?

Yes; injured knees present higher oscillations and more unstable mechanical output as demonstrated by greater frequency content asymmetry for both knee flexion and extension.

9. Discuss the correlation between isokinetic testing and manual muscle testing.

Wilk and Andrews compared the results of knee extension manual muscle testing (MMT) and isokinetic open kinetic chain (OKC) knee extension/flexion in 175 patients after knee arthroscopy. All 175 patients had normal MMT scores, but isokinetic testing revealed bilateral deficits of 21% at 180 deg/sec and 16% at 300 deg/sec. Ellenbecker reported bilateral deficits of the shoulder internal and external rotators ranging from 13% to 28% with isokinetic testing in subjects with normal-grade (5/5) MMT. Isokinetic devices can measure subtle differences in strength that may not be evident with MMT.

10. What is the correlation between isokinetic testing and functional performance?

The research is divided, although most studies indicate that a correlation exists. Only Anderson et al. and Greenberger and Paterno have reported that no correlation is evident.

Relationship between Isokinetic Testing and Functional Performance

Reference	Groups Compared	Isokinetic Test	Functional Test(s)	Significance
Barber et al.	Normals ACL-deficient	60 deg/sec knee extension	Single-leg hop for distance	$p \leq 0.01$
Noyes et al.	Normals ACL-deficient	60 deg/sec knee extension 300 deg/sec knee extension	Single-leg timed hop for distance	Statistical trend was found with 60 deg/sec quadriceps scores and hop tests; trends were not apparent at 300 deg/sec
Sachs et al.	Postoperative ACL	60 deg/sec knee extension and flexion	Single-leg hop for distance	Quadriceps and hamstring peak torque indices correlated with mean hop index
Wilk et al.	Postoperative ACL	180, 300, and 450 deg/sec knee extension and flexion	Single-leg hop for distance Single-leg timed hop Single-leg crossover triple hop for distance	Positive correlation was found between knee extension peak torque (180 and 300 deg/sec) and subjective knee scores of function and hop tests

ACL, Anterior cruciate ligament.

11. How can isokinetic testing be integrated in a rehabilitation functional testing algorithm?

Davies created the Functional Testing Algorithm (FTA), which consists of a series of progressively challenging tests. The FTA can be used to assess patient progress and determine readiness to return to activity. With serial reassessments, the clinician can update and customize the clinical rehabilitation program and home exercise program and plan appropriately for discharge. Specific criteria have been established for testing progression within the FTA (see table).

DAVIES' FUNCTIONAL TESTING ALGORITHM

- Basic measurements (e.g., visual analog pain scales, anthropometric measurements, goniometric measurements)
- KT 1000 testing for injuries of the anterior and posterior cruciate ligaments
- Kinesthetic, proprioceptive, and balance testing
- Closed kinetic chain (CKC) supine isokinetic testing
- OKC isokinetic testing
- CKC squat isokinetic testing
- Functional jump test
- Functional hop test
- Lower extremity functional test
- Specific testing for activities of daily living, vocation, and sports
- Discharge and return to activity

Empirical Guidelines for Patient Progression in the Functional Testing Algorithm

Tests	Empirical Guidelines
Sport-specific testing (SST)	
Lower extremity function test (LEFT)	Female: 2:00 min Male: 1:30 min
Functional hop test (FHT)	<15% bilateral comparison and normals
Functional jump test (FJT)	<20% compared with body height and normals
CKC isokinetic testing (standing)	<20% bilateral comparison
OKC isokinetic testing	<20% bilateral comparison
CKC isokinetic testing (supine)	<30% bilateral comparison
Digital balance evaluation (DBE)	<0.6
KT	<3 mm bilateral comparison
Basic objective measurements	<10% bilateral comparison
Subjective status	Pain <3 (analog pain scale 0-10)

CKC, Closed kinetic chain; *OKC,* open kinetic chain; *KT,* KT-1000 knee ligament arthrometer.

12. Is isokinetic exercise beneficial?

Numerous published studies demonstrate the efficacy of isokinetic exercise in improving muscle performance. Timm conducted a comprehensive study of 5381 patients over a 5-year period to evaluate the effectiveness of rehabilitation programs after knee surgery. He found that people who performed isokinetic exercises were discharged to resume normal activity earlier than people who performed isometrics or isotonics.

13. Discuss the use of a short-arc spectrum isokinetic rehabilitation program.

Short-arc exercise is used when full ROM is contraindicated. It is difficult to accelerate an isokinetic dynamometer to angular velocities in excess of 180 deg/sec in a short arc of motion; angular velocities ≤180 deg/sec avoid free-limb acceleration. Angular velocities slower than 60 deg/sec should be avoided because increased joint compressive forces, abnormally slow motor patterns, and pain inhibition may occur. Angular velocities in multiples of 30 deg/sec should be used because of the physiologic overflow to slower angular velocities.

14. How can the principle of physiologic overflow with isokinetic exercise be applied in rehabilitation?

Increases in strength are fairly velocity-specific, but with isokinetic exercise a 30 deg/sec physiologic overflow occurs at each angular velocity to slower velocities. Therefore it is not necessary to exercise at each angular velocity in a chosen velocity spectrum. Instead, incremental velocities of 30 deg/sec may be used. Isokinetic exercise also produces a physiologic ROM overflow of 30 degrees. For example, a patient with shoulder pain during 90 to 120 degrees of elevation can perform short-arc isokinetic exercises at 60 to 90 degrees and at 120 to 150 degrees and still experience strength gains within the painful arc.

15. Does isolated OKC isokinetic training improve functional performance?

Ellenbecker, Davies, and Rowinski found that performing isolated kinetic OKC rotator cuff muscle exercise increased tennis serve velocity. Mont et al. and Trieber reported similar results. These studies indicate that isolating individual components of the kinetic chain (particularly when they are critical functional components) can positively affect functional performance.

16. What does the evidence show regarding the use of open kinetic chain (isolated joint exercises) or isokinetics in regard to rehabilitation of patients with patellofemoral pain syndromes (PFPS)/anterior knee pain syndromes?

Witvrouw et al. have demonstrated that there is no statistically significant difference in most pain or functional measures between the OKC and CKC groups for rehabilitation of anterior knee pain.

17. What does the evidence demonstrate regarding the use of open kinetic chain (isolated joint exercises) or isokinetics and development of knee pain in patients during the rehabilitation program following ACL reconstructions?

Morrisey et al. divided patients who had ACL reconstructions into an OKC or a CKC rehabilitation program. Morrisey et al. concluded that "OKC and CKC leg extensor training in the early period after ACL reconstruction do not differ in their immediate effects on anterior knee pain."

18. What does the recent evidence demonstrate in regard to the use of open kinetic chain (OKC) (isolated joint exercises) or isokinetics for rehabilitation of patients with ACL reconstructions? What are the effects of the exercises on the graft?

Bennyon et al. used a dynamic variable reluctance transducer (DVRT) that was actually sewn onto the ACL ligament, and then subjects were asked to perform a series of exercises and the strain on the ACL was measured in vivo. OKC knee flexion (100 degrees) to extension (0 degrees) in an unloaded condition created a 3.5% strain on the ACL. CKC squats from extension (0 degrees) to flexion (100 degrees) produced a 3.6% strain on the ACL. CKC squats using a sport cord from extension (0 degrees) to flexion (100 degrees) produced a 4.0% strain on the ACL. In their conclusions, Beynnon et al. speculated that "it might not be valid to designate CKC or OKC activities as 'Safe' or 'Unsafe' with respect to rehabilitation of the injured ACL or healing graft."

19. Do OKC exercises actually stress the graft where it could compromise long-term healing and maturation?

Additional research by Fleming et al. evaluated the strain on the ACL using a similar methodology as described in the previous study. The results demonstrated the following responses regarding the ACL strain:

- Isometric hamstrings at 30/60/90 degrees—0.0%
- Quadriceps and hamstrings (Q & H) co-contraction at 90 degrees—0.0%
- Q & H co-contraction at 60 degrees—0.0%
- Q isometrics at 90 degrees—0.0%
- Q isometrics at 60 degrees—0.0%
- PROM flexion-extension—0.1%
- Q & H co-contraction at 30 degrees—0.4%
- Isometric hamstrings at 15 degrees—0.6%
- Stationary cycling—1.7%
- Anterior drawer at 90 degrees (150 N of anterior shear load)—1.8%
- Stair climbing—2.7%
- Isometric Q at 30 degrees (30 N-m extension torque)—2.7%
- Q & H co-contraction at 15 degrees—2.8%
- Active flexion to extension—2.8%
- Squatting—3.6%
- Lachman's test at 30 degrees (150 N of anterior shear load)—3.7%
- Active flexion to extension with 45-N boot—3.8%
- Squatting with sports cord—4.0%
- Isometric Q at 15 degrees (30 N-m extension torque)—4.4%

20. What do the evidence-based outcome studies demonstrate in regard to using OKC or CKC ACL rehabilitation programs?

Hooper et al. demonstrated no clinically significant differences in the functional improvement resulting from OKC or CKC exercises in the early period after ACL repair.

Mikkelsen et al. demonstrated that there were no significant differences in hamstring torques between the OKC group versus the OKC combined with CKC group. The integrated rehabilitation group (OKC and CKC) did have statistically significant increases in the quadriceps torque. Furthermore, the OKC/CKC group had a significant number of patients returning to sports at the same level as before the surgery. The OKC/CKC group who returned to the same level of sports participation as before the surgery also returned 2 months earlier than those with CKC exercises only.

Bibliography

Andersen MA et al: The relationship among isometric, isotonic and isokinetic concentric and eccentric quadriceps and hamstring force and three components of athletic performance, *J Orthop Sports Phys Ther* 14:114-120, 1991.

Barber SD et al: Quantitative assessment of functional limitations in normal and anterior cruciate ligament-deficient knees, *Clin Orthop Rel Res* 255:204-214, 1990.

Barber SD et al: Rehabilitation after ACL reconstruction: functional testing, *Orthopaedics* 15:969-974, 1992.

Beynnon BD et al: The strain behavior of the ACL during squatting and active flexion and extension, *Am J Sports Med* 25: 823-829, 1997.

Davies GJ: *A compendium of isokinetics in clinical usage,* ed 4, Onalaska, Wis, 1992, S&S Publishers.
Davies GJ, Heiderscheit BC: Reliability of the Lido Linea closed kinetic chain isokinetic dynamometer, *J Orthop Sports Phys Ther* 25:133-136, 1996.
Ellenbecker TS: Muscular strength relationship between normal grade manual muscle testing and isokinetic measurements of the shoulder internal and external rotators, *Isokin Exercise Sci* 6:51-56, 1996.
Fleming BC et al: The strain behavior of the anterior cruciate ligament during stair climbing: an in-vivo study, *Arthroscopy* 15:185-191, 1999.
Hislop H, Perrine JJ: The isokinetic concept of exercise, *Phys Ther* 47:114-117, 1967.
Hooper DM et al: Open and closed kinetic chain exercises in the early period after ACL reconstruction, *Am J Sports Med* 29:167-174, 2001.
Mikkelsen C et al: Closed kinetic chain alone compared to open and closed kinetic chain exercises for quadriceps strengthening after anterior cruciate ligament reconstruction with respect to return to sports: a prospective matched follow-up study, *Knee Surg Sports Traumatol Arthrosc* 8:337-342, 2000.
Mont MA et al: Isokinetic concentric versus eccentric training of the shoulder rotators with functional evaluation of performance enhancement in elite tennis players, *Am J Sports Med* 22:513-517, 1994.
Morrissey MC et al: Effects of distally fixated (CKC) vs nondistally fixated (OKC) leg extensor resistance training on knee pain in the early period after ACL reconstruction, *Phys Ther* 82:35-43, 2002.
Noyes FR, Barber SD, Mangine RE: Abnormal lower limb symmetry determined by functional hop tests after anterior cruciate ligament rupture, *Am J Sports Med* 19:513-518, 1991.
Ross MD et al: Implementation of open and closed kinetic chain quadriceps strengthening exercises after anterior cruciate ligament reconstruction, *J Strength Cond Res* 15:466-473, 2001.
Sachs RA et al: Patellofemoral problems after anterior cruciate ligament reconstruction, *Am J Sports Med* 17:760-764, 1989.
Snyder-Mackler L et al: Strength of the quadriceps femoris muscle and functional recovery after reconstruction of the anterior cruciate ligament: a prospective, randomized clinical trial of electrical stimulation, *J Bone Joint Surg Am* 77:1166-1173, 1995.
Tegner Y et al: Performance test to monitor rehabilitation and evaluate anterior cruciate ligament injuries, *Am J Sports Med* 14:156-159, 1986.
Timm KE: Post surgical knee rehabilitation: a five-year study of four methods and 5,381 patients, *Am J Sports Med* 16:463-468, 1988.
Treiber FA et al: Effects of theraband and lightweight dumbbell training on shoulder rotation torque and serve performance in college tennis players, *Am J Sports Med* 26:510-515, 1998.
Wilk KE et al: The correlation between subjective knee assessments, isokinetic muscle testing and functional hop testing in ACL reconstructed knees, *J Orthop Sports Phys Ther* 20:60-73, 1994.
Witvrouw E: Open versus closed kinetic chain exercises in patellofemoral pain. A 5-year prospective randomized study, *Am J Sports Med* 32:1122-1130, 2004.
Witvrouw E et al: Open versus closed kinetic chain exercises in patellofemoral pain: a prospective randomized study, *Am J Sports Med* 28:687-695, 2000.

Chapter 35

Exercise in Aging and Disease

Patricia Douglas Gillette, PT, PhD

1. Explain the increasing emphasis on older adults in health care.

The process of aging is associated with significant functional declines, physical disability, dependence, and greater use of health care services. The elderly are the fastest growing segment of the population, in part because people are living longer and in part because the "baby boom" generation reaches retirement age in 2011. In 1990 the elderly accounted for approximately 12.5% of the population and approximately one third of all U.S. health care costs. By the year 2030, 20% of the population (about 70 million) will be elderly, more than twice the number in 1998. The "young old" are defined as 65 to 74 years, the "middle old" as 75 to 84 years, and the "old old" or "frail elderly" as 85 years or older. The frail elderly population is growing at the fastest rate.

2. Summarize the health status of older adults. What are the three most frequently occurring medical conditions?

Twenty-seven percent of elders report that they are in fair or poor health compared with 9% of the general population. Most older persons have at least one chronic condition; the number and incidence of chronic conditions and the severity of disability increase with age. From 1994 to 1995, over half of the older population reported one or more disabilities. Approximately one third of the disabilities involved difficulty in performing basic activities of daily living (ADLs), such as walking, or instrumental activities of daily living (IADLs), such as housekeeping or preparing meals. Nonetheless, most elderly people continue to live at home; approximately 4.5% reside in nursing homes. The most common cause of death in the elderly is cardiovascular disease, followed by cancer. However, the most common medical conditions inflicting the elderly are hypertension, arthritis symptoms, and heart disease.

3. What risk factors are associated with the increased incidence of falls in the elderly?

In people over the age of 65 years, falls are the leading cause of death from injury and the sixth leading cause of death overall. Thirty percent of community-living elders and nearly 50% of institutionalized elderly people fall each year. Hip fractures are one of the most disabling consequences of falling; hip and other fractures occur in about 5% of falls. Falls are a contributing factor in about 40% of all nursing home admissions. Risk factors associated with falling include muscle weakness, arthritis, impaired vision, cognitive impairment, depression, polypharmacy, and balance and gait abnormalities, including slower ambulation speeds. Other risk factors are poor nutrition, environmental hazards, decreased financial resources, and lack of a social support system.

4. List the three most common fractures in older adults. What causes them?

1. Vertebral (compression) fractures (>700,000 annually)
2. Proximal femur (>300,000 annually)
3. Distal radius (>250,000 annually)

Most fractures in older adults are secondary to osteoporosis or cancer, rather than a result of high-impact trauma such as an automobile accident.

5. Can exercise reduce the risk of falling?

Yes, but it is difficult to determine the relative contribution or type of exercise for decreasing the risk of falls because many studies incorporated exercise into a multifaceted treatment approach. However, individualized exercise programs carried out by a trained health professional can reduce falls in community-dwelling older adults. Group exercise of tai chi (dynamic balance exercises) in older adults decreased risk and fear of falling. Exercise appears to be beneficial in decreasing fall risks in older adults with muscle weakness, decreased flexibility, and/or impaired balance.

6. What medications are associated with an increased risk of falling?

Antidepressants and sedatives have been most commonly implicated, but antihypertensive medications also are frequently linked with falling. In nursing homes, a significant number of falls have been associated with orthostatic hypotension, an adverse side effect of many cardiovascular medications.

7. Define orthostatic hypotension.

- Decrease >20 mm Hg in systolic blood pressure and >10 mm Hg in diastolic pressure in moving from supine to standing position, accompanied by an increase in heart rate ≥10%
- Systolic blood pressure <90 mm Hg

Associated signs and symptoms may include tachycardia, pallor, dizziness, faintness, weakness, or syncope.

8. What type of exercise can be performed in bed to reverse the effects of orthostatic hypotension?

No type of exercise in the supine position is an effective treatment for orthostatic hypotension.

9. Describe physical therapy interventions for orthostatic hypotension.

Treatment strategies include progressive elevation of the head of the bed, dangling one extremity over the edge of the bed, progressive sitting on the edge of the bed with active lower extremity exercise, deep breathing, and progressive sitting out of bed with the lower extremities progressed to a dependent position. Elastic stockings should be worn over the lower extremities. Elevating the head of the bed by 5 to 20 degrees during sleep also is recommended.

10. What physiologic changes occur with bed rest and/or immobility?

Every major organ system is adversely affected by bed rest; physiologic changes can begin within 24 hours. In the elderly hospitalized population, a significant loss of functional abilities occurs within 2 days of bed rest.

Pathophysiologic Alterations Due to Immobility

Musculoskeletal	Cardiopulmonary
Decreased range of motion	Decreased ventilation
Decreased joint flexibility	Orthostatic hypotension
Loss of muscular endurance (deconditioning)	Increased resting heart rate
Loss of muscular strength (muscular atrophy)	Increased cardiac output

Pathophysiologic Alterations Due to Immobility ***continued***

Musculoskeletal	**Cardiopulmonary**
Development of contractures	Deterioration of respiratory system
Loss of bone strength	Atelectasis
Loss of bone mass	Aspiration pneumonia
Skin	**Genitourinary**
Development of pressure sores	Urinary tract infection
Skin atrophy	Urinary retention
Skin tears	Bladder calculi
Psychologic/Neurologic	**Metabolic**
Depression	Negative balance
Decreased perceptual ability	Loss of calcium
Social isolation	
Learned helplessness	
Altered sleep patterns, anxiety, irritability, hostility	

Adapted from Thompson LV: Iatrogenic effects. In Kaufmann TL, editor: *Geriatric rehabilitation manual,* New York, 1999, pp 318-324, Churchill Livingstone.

11. List strategies for minimizing the negative consequences of bed rest.*

- Minimize duration of bed rest.
- Avoid strict bed rest unless absolutely necessary.
- Allow bathroom privileges or use of a bedside commode.
- Let the patient stand 30 to 60 seconds during transfers (bed to chair).
- Encourage the wearing of street clothes.
- Encourage taking meals at a table.
- Encourage walking to hospital appointments.
- Encourage passes out of the hospital on evenings and weekends.
- Involve physical therapy, occupational therapy, and restorative nursing.
- Encourage daily exercises as a basis of good care.
- Use protective splinting.

12. Describe the musculoskeletal effects of aging.

Decline in muscle mass begins during the third decade of life and accelerates after the age of 50. Total loss of muscle mass ranges from a 10% to a 40% decrease in cross-sectional area, with selective atrophy of fast-twitch type II fibers. Both slow-twitch type I fibers and fast-twitch type II fibers are reduced in number. Muscle strength decreases on the average by 8% per decade, beginning during the third decade of life, with a total loss of 40% to 50% by the age of 80. After the age of 35, bone loss is approximately 0.5% per year for males and 1% per year for females; in immediately postmenopausal women, bone loss is about 4% per year for 5 years. Up to 30% of total bone loss may occur. The amount of collagen increases within the soft tissues, but collagen

*Adapted from Thompson LV: Iatrogenic effects. In Kaufmann TL, editor: *Geriatric rehabilitation manual,* New York, 1999, pp 318-324, Churchill Livingstone.

becomes less extensible because of increased numbers of cross-links or bonds and loss of water content. At age 70, joint range of motion is decreased by an average of 20% to 30%. These adverse musculoskeletal effects of aging can greatly affect mobility and may lead to functional declines, frailty, and, ultimately, loss of independent living.

13. What muscle groups are often weak in the elderly?

In general, trunk and lower extremity muscles are affected to a greater extent than upper extremity muscles. With inactivity, the postural, antigravity muscles such as the quadriceps, gluteals, erector spinae, and gastrocnemius-soleus are affected the most. These muscle groups are important for upright posture, locomotion, and functional independence.

14. What musculoskeletal effects of aging can be reversed or attenuated with exercise?

Exercise has a positive effect on muscle mass, muscle strength, range of motion and flexibility, and bone mass in older adults. Bone mass may be increased 5% to 10% by following an appropriate exercise program and maintaining proper calcium and estrogen levels.

15. Is exercise-induced muscle hypertrophy possible in elderly people?

Yes, but earlier studies of the effects of resistive exercise in older adults did not find significant increases in muscle mass or hypertrophy, probably because the exercise stimulus intensity was too low. Recent studies have shown that older adults can increase muscle mass much like young adults if the exercise stimulus is sufficient.

16. Summarize the recommended protocol for resistance training in older adults.

The American College of Sports Medicine (ACSM) recommends that healthy adults perform muscle strengthening exercises 2 to 3 times per week at an intensity level that fatigues the muscle within 8 to 12 repetitions. The higher the intensity and volume of training, the greater the increase in strength. Fiatarone et al. first showed that frail, institutionalized elders (72 to 98 years old) could safely perform progressive resistive training at intensities of 80% of one repetition maximum (1 RM), 3 sets of 8 repetitions, 3 times/week, and make significant gains in muscle strength. Exercise should begin at a lower intensity (30% to 50% of 1 RM) and progress gradually to the higher intensity over several weeks. In general, significant strength gains are made in older adults within 12 weeks of high-intensity (>70% 1 RM) resistance training, whereas younger people see significant strength gains in 6 to 8 weeks. Strengthening programs should emphasize muscle groups that are often weak in the elderly population and necessary for maintenance of independent living.

17. When is heavy resistance exercise not recommended in older adults?

Porter and Vandervoot determined that participation in heavy resistance exercise should be avoided or limited in older adults with a history of hypertension, acute or "unstable cardiovascular disease, unstable chronic conditions (e.g., uncontrolled diabetes mellitus), recent bone or joint injury, recent surgery, or any condition that prevents strong muscular contractions." Blood pressure and heart rate should be monitored before, during, and after exercise. Elderly people should be taught proper breathing techniques and avoid breath-holding.

18. Summarize the recommendations for strength training in older adults with hypertension.

- Resting systolic blood pressure ≥160 mm Hg and diastolic blood pressure ≥100 mm Hg are relative contraindications.
- Aerobic exercise training should be the first priority.

- Use a resistance of 3% to 60% of 1 RM or low-to-moderate weight loads.
- The rate of perceived exertion should not be higher than 11 to 13 on the 20-point Borg scale (fairly light to somewhat hard).
- Avoid static hand-gripping and breath-holding.
- Use a rest interval ≥30 seconds between stations.
- Increase resistance only after 12 to 15 repetitions can be performed comfortably per station.
- Discontinue this or any exercise with onset of abnormal signs or symptoms, such as dizziness, unusual shortness of breath, angina-type discomfort, abnormal heart rhythm, cold sweat, confusion, excessive fatigue, or incoordination.

19. List the absolute contraindications for exercise in older adults.*

- Severe coronary artery disease with unstable angina pectoris
- Acute myocardial infarction (<2 days after infarction)
- Severe valvular heart disease
- Rapid or prolonged atrial or ventricular arrhythmias/tachycardias
- Third-degree heart block
- New electrocardiographic signs or symptoms of myocardial ischemia
- Decompensated congestive heart failure with respiratory rate >45 breaths/min
- Uncontrolled hypertension
- Resting systolic blood pressure >200 mm Hg, diastolic blood pressure >105 mm Hg
- Profound orthostatic hypotension
- Hypoadaptive systolic blood pressure response to exercise
- Acute myocarditis
- Acute thrombophlebitis
- Acute pulmonary embolism (<2 days after event)
- Partial pressure of oxygen in arterial blood <60%, or oxygen saturation <86%
- Acute hypoglycemia or uncontrolled diabetes
- Known or suspected dissecting aneurysm
- Any profound symptom (nausea, dyspnea, light-headedness)
- Significant emotional distress

20. Can elderly people improve aerobic capacity with endurance training?

Yes; improvements of 10% to 30% can be seen, the same as in younger adults. The amount of improvement in maximal volume of oxygen consumption ($\dot{V}O_2max$) depends on baseline fitness level and training intensity (American College of Sports Medicine, 1998).

21. Summarize the recommendations for aerobic exercise in older adults.

The ACSM recommends aerobic training 3 to 5 days/week for a minimum of 20 to 30 minutes at a target heart rate of 55% to 90% of the age-predicted maximal heart rate for healthy adults. The age-predicted maximal heart rate is estimated by subtracting age from 220. Exercise should include warm-up and cool-down periods. For older adults, the aerobic training session should be performed at a lower intensity: 50% to 70% of maximal heart rate or 11 to 13 on the Borg perceived exertion scale. People who are severely deconditioned should start at a lower intensity and may need to exercise several times during the day to reach a total of 20 minutes of activity daily. Walking is one of the best modes of aerobic exercise in older adults because it is functional, provides weight-bearing stimulus to the lower extremities, and requires no equipment.

---

*Adapted from Cahalin LP: Cardiac muscle dysfunction. In Hillegass EA, Sadowsky HS, editors: *Essentials of cardiopulmonary physical therapy,* Philadelphia, 1994, WB Saunders.

22. Can exercise improve functional outcomes in older adults?

Yes; many studies incorporating exercises of strengthening, stretching, flexibility, and balance have shown improvement in physical performance measures such as balance, stair-climbing power, ability to rise from a chair, gait speed, or risk of falls.

23. Can exercise reduce mortality and increase life expectancy?

Studies have shown that men engaged in regular vigorous exercise increased life expectancy by up to 2 years.

24. What are the primary risk factors for cardiovascular disease? Why is this important information for orthopaedic specialists?

Hypertension (blood pressure ≥140/90 mm Hg), cigarette smoking, hyperlipidemia (cholesterol >200 mg/dl), diabetes mellitus, and positive family history of cardiovascular disease are primary risk factors. Others include age, male gender, obesity, sedentary lifestyle, and stress. A patient may complain of diffuse pain that at first glance appears to be musculoskeletal in origin but turns out to be cardiac-related. Patients referred to physical therapy with the primary diagnosis of an orthopaedic dysfunction should be screened for underlying cardiovascular risk factors if exercise is a planned intervention.

25. What are appropriate cardiovascular responses to aerobic or dynamic exercise?

Symptoms and vital signs should be assessed before, during, and after exercise in the position of the exercise. For example, if walking is the form of exercise, vital signs should be taken at rest in the standing position for accurate comparison. Abnormal hemodynamic effects include failure of the systolic blood pressure to increase with an increase in workload, a decrease in the systolic blood pressure or heart rate with an increase in workload, and an excessive increase in the systolic or diastolic blood pressure with exercise. Diastolic blood pressure should stay the same or slightly decrease. Failure of systolic blood pressure to increase with increasing workloads or a drop >20 mm Hg may indicate a decrease in cardiac output and correlate with myocardial ischemia or left ventricular dysfunction.

26. How should a person taking β-blocker medication be monitored during exercise?

β-Blockers decrease the workload of the heart by decreasing heart rate and contractility, and thus blood pressure at rest; that is, they blunt the body's response to exercise. Therefore blood pressure and heart rate measurements during exercise may not be a true measure of exercise effort. Patient symptoms and rating of perceived exertion are more helpful in evaluating tolerance to exercise. An exercise performance test is needed to prescribe exercise accurately. Calculating a target heart rate from the age-predicted maximal heart rate is inappropriate in patients taking β-blocker medication.

27. How should a person with a pacemaker be monitored during exercise?

People with pacemakers can benefit from exercise training. Warm-up and cool-down periods should be longer for people with fixed-rate pacemakers, and exercise intensity must be monitored by methods other than pulse-counting (e.g., patient symptoms, rating of perceived exertion, blood pressure measurements). Abnormal exercise response or unusual symptoms such as dyspnea, dizziness, or syncope should be reported immediately to a physician.

28. How can one distinguish general musculoskeletal chest pain from cardiac ischemic pain?*

---

*Adapted from Irwin S, Blessey RL: Patient evaluation. In Irwin S, Tecklin JS, editors: *Cardiopulmonary physical therapy,* ed 3, St Louis, 1996, Mosby.

ANGINA

- Stable angina begins at the same heart rate and blood pressure and is relieved by rest or nitroglycerin.
- Angina is relieved by nitroglycerin.
- Angina pain is not palpable.
- Angina is associated with diaphoresis, shortness of breath, and feelings of doom.
- Angina often is associated with electrocardiographic changes of ST-segment depression.

CHEST WALL PAIN

- Nitroglycerin generally has no effect on chest wall pain.
- Chest wall pain can occur at any time and last for hours.
- Chest wall pain often is accompanied by muscle soreness, joint soreness, or deep breaths and evoked by palpation.
- Minimal additional symptoms are associated with chest wall pain.
- No ST-segment depression is seen on the electrocardiogram.

29. Can a patient experience a heart attack without the usual symptoms?

Yes. Sometimes heart attacks are silent. The patient does not experience chest pain but may complain of shortness of breath, weakness, and fatigue or flu-like symptoms. Because diabetic patients may have autonomic neuropathy, they may have no symptoms at all.

30. What are the exercise recommendations for patients with heart failure (HF)?

In the past, physical activity was restricted for patients with HF. In the past 15 years, however, research studies have shown that exercise can improve exercise tolerance and quality of life without adversely affecting ventricular function. Exercise guidelines for persons with HF are difficult to implement because the patient's condition frequently changes, but exercise can be done safely in selected patients. Patients should be assessed thoroughly before exercise, and vital signs and symptoms should be monitored closely during exercise. A relative contraindication for exercise is uncompensated HF. Compensated HF is determined clinically (for noninvasively monitored patients) by the ability to speak comfortably with a respiratory rate <30 breaths/min, less than moderate fatigue, crackles in less than one half of the lungs, and a resting heart rate <120 beats/min. Exercise should be terminated if the patient experiences marked dyspnea (inability to converse comfortably), extreme fatigue, abnormal hemodynamic effects, development of a third heart sound, increase in crackles, arrhythmias, or evidence of myocardial ischemia. Because persons with HF are generally quite deconditioned, a low level of effort may be sufficient to induce positive physiologic changes.

31. What types of exercise are recommended for patients with chronic primary or secondary pulmonary disease? Discuss the outcomes of such exercise.

Patients with pulmonary disease may benefit from breathing exercises, coughing techniques, cardiopulmonary endurance training, strength training, flexibility, respiratory muscle training, and relaxation exercises/techniques. Other components of rehabilitation should include airway clearance techniques, energy conservation/ventilatory strategy training, and patient education.

Improvements	No Improvements
Frequency of hospitalizations	Lung function
Functional level (ADLs)	Heart function
Quality of life	Maximal aerobic capacity

continued

Improvements	No Improvements
Psychological status	Mortality rate
Respiratory symptoms	
Respiratory muscle function	
Symptom-limited exercise capacity	

Adapted from Barr RN: Pulmonary rehabilitation. In Hillegass EA, Sadowsky HS, editors: *Essentials of cardiopulmonary physical therapy,* ed 2, Philadelphia, 2001, p 728, WB Saunders.
ADLs, Activities of daily living.

32. What is metabolic syndrome?

It is a combination of symptoms that helps to identify individuals who are at increased risk for a cardiovascular event and/or diabetes. The National Cholesterol Education Program's Adult Treatment Panel III requires that individuals have three out of the following five clinical findings for a positive diagnosis:

1. Increased abdominal circumference
2. Elevated levels of triglycerides
3. Low HDL levels
4. Elevated fasting blood glucose levels
5. High blood pressure

33. What type of physical activity or exercise is recommended for people with type 2 diabetes mellitus?

Within appropriate serum glucose levels, cardiovascular endurance exercise and resistance training exercise are recommended. Both can help control blood glucose levels by increased glucose utilization and improved insulin resistance, but these effects are lost after a few days of inactivity. Regular physical activity can lower blood pressure, improve lipid profile, and reduce emotional stress, which will reduce the overall risk of cardiovascular disease. Aerobic activity should be at the low to moderate intensity level and performed a minimum of 3 to 5 days/week with a goal of expending a minimum of 1000 kcal/week.

34. What exercise machines are recommended for home use in patients with osteoporosis?

The National Osteoporosis Foundation recommends exercise that promotes weight-bearing and impact through the lower extremities, such as brisk walking. Home exercise machines are recommended only as an adjunct to an existing exercise program. Treadmills offer a greater weight-bearing stimulus and impact than stair-climbers, and stair-climbers offer more impact than cross-country ski machines. Elliptical walkers and recumbent or stationary bicycles offer the least amount of weight-bearing and little or no impact through the lower extremities.

35. What are exercise concerns when prescribing exercise for the obese patient?

Many obese patients may have undiagnosed comorbidities (for example, heart disease or diabetes), orthopaedic limitations to weight-bearing exercises, heat intolerance, and low aerobic fitness level.

36. What are the most common causes of sports injuries in the older athlete?

Acute muscle injuries and overuse injuries in the lower extremities are the most frequent causes of sports injuries in the older adult. The knee is the most commonly injured body part in older athletes.

37. Is exercise recommended for patients with cancer?

In general, yes. Cancer and the adverse effects of treatment can cause generalized weakness and debilitation. Muscle strengthening and endurance exercise help to offset these effects. Because cancer and its treatment can affect response to exercise, all persons should be medically screened before participation in an exercise program. If the patient receives chemotherapy or radiation therapy or if the cancer involves the hematologic system, additional specific criteria should be assessed before treatment. Winningham's contraindications for aerobic exercise in patients receiving chemotherapy are platelet counts <50,000/ml, hemoglobin level <10 g/ml, white blood cell count <3000/ml, and absolute granulocyte count <500/µl. Immunosuppressed patients should be monitored closely during exercise for abnormal signs and symptoms of cardiopulmonary compromise. For patients unable to participate in aerobic exercises because of excessive fatigue, frequent short bouts of intermittent exercise may be indicated. Depending on the stage or severity of the disease, other therapeutic exercise treatments or interventions, such as functional training or energy conservation techniques, may be warranted.

38. Is exercise beneficial in older persons with cognitive impairment or dementia?

Yes; it can improve fitness, functional abilities, mental function, and behavior.

Bibliography

Administration on Aging, U.S. Department of Health and Human Services, *A profile of older Americans: 2004* (serial online): http://www.aarp.org/research/reference/statistics/aresearch-import-519.html. Accessed March 14, 2006.

American College of Sports Medicine: The recommended quantity and quality of exercise for developing and maintaining cardiorespiratory and muscular fitness, and flexibility in healthy adults, *Med Sci Sports Exercise* 30:975-991, 1998.

American College of Sports Medicine: Position stand on exercise and physical activity for older adults, *Med Sci Sports Exercise* 30:992-1008, 1998.

American College of Sports Medicine: Position stand on exercise and type 2 diabetes, *Med Sci Sports Exercise* 32:1345-1360, 2000.

American Geriatric Society, British Geriatric Society, and American Academy of Orthopaedic Surgeons Panel on Falls Prevention: Guideline for the prevention of falls in older persons, *J Am Geriatric Soc* 49:664-672, 2001.

Brown M, Holloszy JO: Effects of a low-intensity exercise program on selected physical performance characteristics of 60- to 70-year olds, *Aging* 3:129-139, 1991.

Cahalin LP: Heart failure, *Phys Ther* 76:516-533, 1996.

Fiatarone MA et al: High-intensity strength training in nonagenarians, *JAMA* 263:3029-3034, 1990.

Frontera WR, Dawson DM, Slovik DM, editors: *Exercise in rehabiltation medicine,* Champaign, Ill, 1999, Human Kinetics.

Goodman CC, Fuller KS, Boissonnault WG, editors: *Pathology: implications for the physical therapist,* Philadelphia, 2003, WB Saunders.

Heyn P, Abreu BC, Ottenbacher, KJ: The effects of exercise training on elderly persons with cognitive impairment and dementia: a meta-analysis, *Arch Phys Med Rehabil* 85:1694-1704, 2004.

Hillegass EA, Sadowsky HS, editors: *Essentials of cardiopulmonary physical therapy,* ed 2, Philadelphia, 2001, WB Saunders.

Irwin S, Blessey RL: Patient evaluation. In Irwin S, Tecklin JS, editors: *Cardiopulmonary physical therapy,* ed 3, St Louis, 1996, Mosby.

Kallinen M, Markku A: Aging, physical activity and sports injuries. An overview of common sports injuries in the elderly, *Sports Med* 20:41-52, 1995.

Kaufmann TL, editor: *Geriatric rehabilitation manual,* New York, 1999, Churchill Livingstone.
Morris M, Schoo A: *Optimizing exercise and physical activity in older people,* London, 2004, Buttermann Heinemann.
National Osteoporosis Foundation. Available at: http://www.nof.org/osteoporosis/diseasefacts.htm. Accessed March 7, 2005.
Porter MM, Vandervoot AA: High-intensity strength training for the older adult—a review, *Top Geriatric Rehabil* 10:61-74, 1995.
Sherrington C, Lord SR, Finch CF: Physical activity interventions to prevent falls among older people: update of the evidence, *J Sci Med Sport* 7(1):supplement 43-51, 2004.
Tinetti ME, Speechley M, Ginter SF: Risk factors among elderly persons living in the community, *N Engl J Med* 319:1701-1707, 1988.
Topp R et al: The effect of a 12-week dynamic resistance strength training program on gait velocity and balance of older adults, *Gerontologist* 33:501-506, 1993.
Wagh A, Stone NJ: Treatment of metabolic syndrome, *Expert Rev Cardiovasc Ther* 2(2):213-238, 2004.
Winningham ML, MacVicar MG, Burke CA: Exercise for cancer patients: guidelines and precautions, *Physician Sportsmed* 14:125-134, 1986.

Chapter 36

Orthopaedic Radiology

Kathleen A. Brindle, MD, and
*Timothy J. Brindle, PT, PhD, ATC**

1. Are x-rays dangerous?

In general, x-rays are not dangerous. Radiation exposure from a single x-ray of an extremity is 0.01 millisievert (mSv). Exposure from a chest x-ray is 0.02 mSv and from a lumbar spine/pelvic x-ray is 1.3 mSv. To put this in context, most people are exposed to a certain amount of radiation from the environment each day; an extremity x-ray is equivalent to one-half day of exposure, whereas chest and lumbar spine/pelvic x-rays are equivalent to 1 and 65 days of exposure, respectively.

2. How is an x-ray different from an arthrogram?

An arthrogram is an x-ray with a contrast material to examine soft tissue structure. The contrast material is commonly radiopaque iodine or gadolinium. The contrast material is injected into the joint typically to determine if there is disruption of the joint capsule, thus evaluating the soft tissue structure of the joint.

---

*The opinions presented in this chapter reflect the views of the authors and not those of the National Institutes of Health or the U.S. Public Health Service.

3. What are the ABC's of reading a radiograph?

- A—Alignment: view the joint surfaces for congruency and alignment. For example, the shoulder, a ball-and-socket joint, should demonstrate the ball of the humeral head aligned within the cup of the glenoid fossa. Deviation from this normal anatomic alignment could indicate a minor subluxation or a major dislocation.
- B—Bone density: observe the general bone density and look for distinct cortical edges. A loss of the distinct cortical edges may indicate loss of bone mass. Next, observe the local bone density. Look for areas of increased density that would indicate sclerosis. Also, observe texture abnormalities of the bone. When the mineralization of a bone is changed, the trabeculae can appear thin, delicate, coarsened, fluffy, or smudged.
- C—Cartilage: although cartilage is not directly seen with x-rays, inspecting the region in which cartilage lies can indicate possible problems with cartilage. Narrowed joint space (the area between articulating bones) can indicate arthritis whereas widened joint space can be indicative of joint effusion or a genetic/metabolic condition such as acromegaly or chondrocalcinosis.
- S—Soft tissue: typically swelling can be observed with x-rays, but is a nonspecific finding. Other soft tissue findings can be the presence of gas following surgery or trauma, calcification, and an abnormal soft tissue mass such as a hematoma, abscess, or tumor.

4. How many views are typically ordered to diagnose injuries?

The minimum number of films needed is usually two—the anteroposterior (AP) view and the lateral view. More often three views are obtained. An oblique view is often included because bones that overlap in either an AP or a lateral view can mask subtle fracture lines.

5. What are CT scans?

Computed axial tomography scans, also called CT scans or CAT scans, were developed jointly in 1972 by Sir Godfrey Newbold Hounsfield in the UK and Dr. Allan Cormack in the United States, based on mathematical reconstruction of multiple axial slices of x-rays surrounding the body part to be imaged. CT scans provide between 200 and 300 shades of gray as compared with x-rays, which produce 20 to 30 shades of gray. All images are collected in the axial plane and then mathematically reconstructed to provide other views, such as coronal, sagittal, or 3-D images.

6. What is diagnostic ultrasound?

Ultrasound images are generated from sound waves that bounce off tissues back to the transducer, generating contrast between the different types of tissue. Originally developed in the 1950s to provide gray scale images of cardiac valve motion, ultrasound is now commonly used in obstetrics to image the developing fetus. Recent advances allow for greater resolution with reconstructed 3-D and 4-D images, creating videos of the moving fetus.

7. Is diagnostic ultrasound dangerous?

No; diagnostic ultrasound has much lower energy than therapeutic ultrasound. However, the effect of long-term, repeated exposure is in debate.

8. How is diagnostic ultrasound different from therapeutic ultrasound?

Therapeutic ultrasound is typically delivered at 1 to 2 W/cm^2, while diagnostic ultrasound is typically of much lower intensity, $<0.1\ W/cm^2$. Therapeutic ultrasound is typically performed at 1 or 3 MHz. Diagnostic ultrasound is usually conducted at 5 to 10 MHz.

9. Can ultrasound visualize the musculoskeletal system?

Advancements over the last decade have increased the resolution great enough to visualize musculoskeletal injuries and observe individual muscle fibers. The cost for ultrasound units is a fraction of that for magnetic resonance imaging units, making ultrasound less expensive. In fact, diagnostic ultrasound is the soft tissue image modality of choice in underdeveloped countries.

10. What are the advantages and disadvantages of ultrasound as an imaging modality?

Ultrasound is quick, readily available, and inexpensive and does not expose the patient to radiation. However, ultrasound is highly operator-dependent, meaning that the skill of the technician administering the exam could enhance or degrade the accuracy of this type of imaging modality.

11. How does MRI obtain images?

An MRI image is based on tissues responses to multiple magnetic fields. The magnetic field knocks the tissue off its aligned position, and the tissue responds based on its water content, or more specifically hydrogen ion concentration. In other words, it is a matter of lining up the molecules (B_0) and then knocking them down (B_1).

The image is generated by how fast tissue responds to being knocked down. The time it takes to return to the upright position generates the T_1 signal, also called the spin-lattice relaxation time, and the time it takes to return to moving at its natural frequency generates the T_2 signal, or the spin-spin relaxation time.

12. What are the characteristics of the T_1 image?

T_1-weighted images show fat and blood as white, muscle tissue as gray, and edema, tumors, and cerebrospinal fluid (CSF) as black.

13. What are the characteristics of a T_2 image?

T_2-weighted images show CSF, edema, and tumors as white, muscle as gray, and fat, cartilage, and tendons as black.

14. Is exposure to the magnetic fields of MRI dangerous?

Magnetic fields of 1.5 and 3 T are generally not thought to be dangerous because of the relatively short exposure times experienced by patients. However, it is unknown at what exposure level (intensity or duration) magnetic fields become more dangerous. Therefore in relatively healthy populations the only contraindication for MRI is pregnancy because of the unknown effects of magnetic fields on the developing fetus.

15. Should people with metal implants or electronic implants be excluded from MRIs?

Metal implants can severely degrade an image, which renders MRI useless and warrants the use of other imaging studies for these types of patients. The farther away the metal is from the area being scanned, the less the effect. Therefore metal implants in the lower extremity should not affect an MRI conducted on the brain. Ferrous metal implants are considered a contraindication for MRI. Magnetic fields can also interfere with electronics and pose a risk to patients with electronic implants.

16. What is an MRI arthrogram?

It is similar to an x-ray and CT arthrogram in that contrast material (gadolinium) is injected to enhance the contrast between soft tissue.

17. What is the most valuable MRI sequence for assessing pathology?

A T_2-weighted image is probably the most useful sequence to assess abnormalities on MRI. The reason for this is that fluid is bright and therefore stands out on T_2-weighted images. Most pathologic processes (trauma, infection, tumors) lead to increased fluid content in tissues and therefore are bright on a T_2-weighted image.

18. Are MRIs best for evaluating soft tissue injuries?

Yes; however, there are circumstances when MRIs might not be needed or warranted. In addition, multiple imaging planes increase scanning time and can cause patients to become claustrophobic. It is necessary for the radiologist to have an idea of what to look for so that the proper sequences can be conducted to image the correct anatomic region. For example, the ACL is best imaged in the sagittal plane where the full length of the ligament can be seen to assess its integrity.

19. What is the appearance of a normal ligament or tendon on MRI?

Both ligaments and tendons should be dark in all imaging sequences. Sometimes striations can be seen within these structures on MRI. The anterior cruciate ligament and the quadriceps and triceps tendons are examples where a striated appearance can be seen.

20. What is a PET scan?

A positron emission tomography, or PET, scan is a diagnostic exam that is the acquisition of positrons from a radioactive substance administered to the patient. It is used most commonly to detect cancer and examine the effects of cancer by characterizing biochemical changes in the body. Patients are given a radioactive or tagged substance, usually glucose, before the examination. The tagged glucose will accumulate in areas representing biologic activity, differentiating it from areas that demonstrated greater uptake of glucose, such as a cancerous tumor. This is typically described as a hot spot. PET scans are also used to evaluate brain and heart function. Radiation doses are very small and short-lived, and will not affect normal body processes. Pregnant women should not undergo this type of study.

21. What is a bone scan?

A bone scan or scintigraphy involves the injection of a slightly radioactive tracer (technetium-99m) into a vein to evaluate biophysiologic aspects of bone and disease. Bone scans are helpful in identifying stress fractures very early, before the onset of architectural changes in the bone. They are also valuable for detecting bone infections, arthritis, metabolic disorders such as Paget's disease, and cancers that can spread to bones. The amount of radioactive material is small and eliminated quickly. Complications are rare; however, pregnant women are not candidates for this procedure.

22. When will a stress fracture become visible on a plain film?

A stress fracture will not be visible on x-ray until approximately 7 to 14 days after the injury. An example of a second metatarsal stress fracture is provided with plain film radiographs.

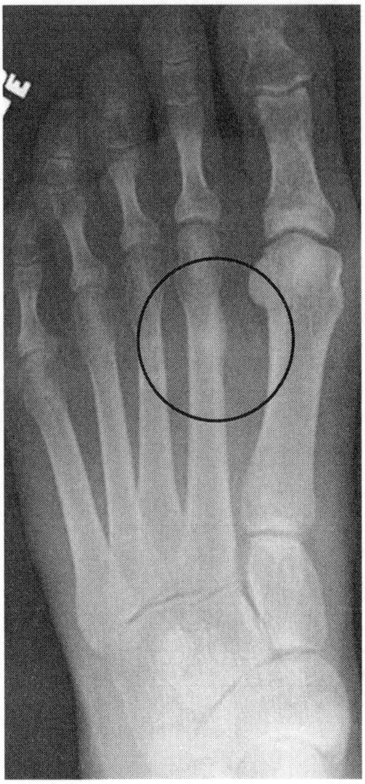

AP view of the foot demonstrates callus formation along the medial aspect of the distal second metatarsal, compatible with a healing stress fracture.

23. What is the x-ray appearance of a stress fracture?

Radiographic abnormalities can include a subtle thin radiolucent line through the cortex, a focal band of sclerosis, or periosteal cortical thickening.

24. What is the appearance of a stress fracture on MRI?

On MRI stress fractures appear as a linear zone of dark signal (the fracture) with a broader, poorly defined area of abnormal signal that represents edema in the bone.

25. What is patella alta and how is it diagnosed on radiographs?

Patella alta is a condition in which the patella is more superiorly displaced than normal. This can be seen with clinical observations or can also be examined radiographically with the Insall-Salvati ratio. The Insall-Salvati ratio is measured with the knee flexed 30 degrees on a lateral knee radiograph and is calculated as the length of the patella over the length of the patella tendon. Normally, this ratio is 1; a 20% deviation indicates patella alta.

26. What is a sulcus angle?

The sulcus angle is used to quantify the angle of the femoral sulcus, in which the patella sits. The sulcus angle is generated from a Merchant's view radiograph, where the knee is flexed 30 degrees and the image demonstrates the patella sitting in its femoral sulcus. The angle is defined by the highest and lowest point of the medial and lateral intercondylar sulci. A sulcus angle >140 degrees indicates a shallower intercondylar sulcus and is suggestive of patellofemoral problems.

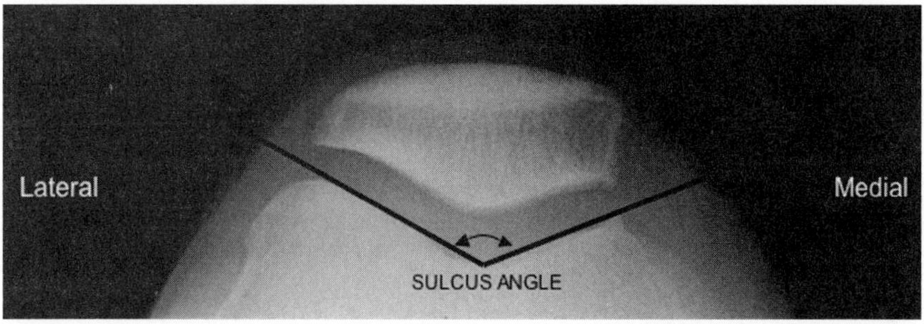

Merchant's view of the knee. The lateral facet of the patella is longer than the medial facet of the patella. Thus on this image lateral is to the left and medial to the right. Measurement of the sulcus angle is demonstrated. In this patient it measures 130 degrees.

27. Is osteoporosis detectable on x-ray, and, if so, what is its appearance?

Yes; it is visible. However, it is visible only after a 30% to 50% loss of bone. Plain film radiographs typically show "picture framing," where the cortex is sharp but the trabeculae are decreased. The vertebral bodies appear as an "empty box," because of increased density of the vertebral endplates. The vertebral bodies also show concavity and will demonstrate compression fractures with more severe cases of osteoporosis. Compression fractures are typically viewed as a wedge-shaped deformity of the vertebral body with loss of vertebral body height.

28. What are a delayed union and a nonunion?

Delayed fracture healing occurs when healing is slower than expected (16 to 18 weeks), while nonunion occurs when healing is delayed for longer than 6 months. Nonunion fractures may be broadly classified as atrophic or hypertrophic. Atrophic nonunions typically require stabilization and bone grafting whereas hypertrophic nonunions may require stabilization only.

29. What is spondylolysis and how is it diagnosed radiographically?

Spondylolysis is a bony defect in the pars interarticularis caused by a chronic stress fracture; it is typically seen at the L5 vertebra in adolescent athletes. With oblique plain film radiographs, a collar or radiolucency is seen around the pars interarticularis, reminiscent of a dog collar. Spondylolisthesis occurs with a bilateral pars interarticularis defect, and there is slippage of one vertebral body on another because of the loss of stability provided by the bony architecture.

30. How is scoliosis measured radiographically?

It is measured on a posteroanterior (PA) film of the entire spine obtained with the patient in a standing position without shoes. The standard method of measuring scoliosis uses the Cobb method.

Lines are drawn along the superior endplate and the inferior endplate of the highest and lowest vertebrae involved in the curvature. The angle subtended by lines drawn perpendicular to these two lines forms the Cobb angle.

31. How is alignment of the cervical spine evaluated?

Three imaginary smooth curved lines can be drawn on a lateral view of the cervical spine to assess alignment. The lines are drawn along the anterior aspects of the vertebral bodies, the posterior aspects of the vertebral bodies, and the spinolaminar line. A fourth line can be drawn along the posterior aspects of the C2 to C7 spinous processes, though even in normal patients this line may not be smooth and contiguous. In the setting of trauma, any malalignment of the first three lines should be considered evidence of fracture or ligamentous injury.

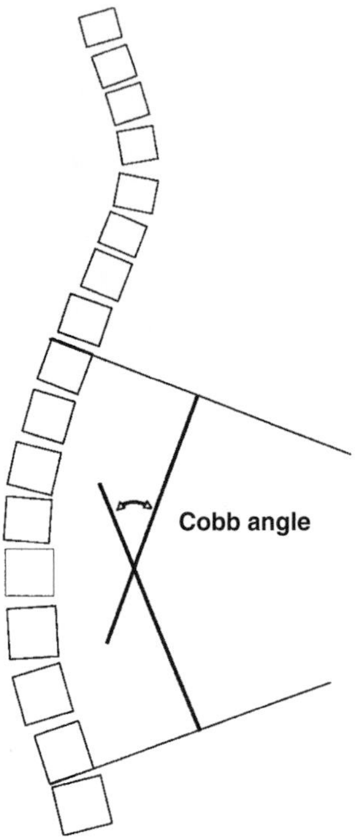

AP view of the thoracolumbar spine. The scoliosis in the lower spine is measured using the Cobb angle.

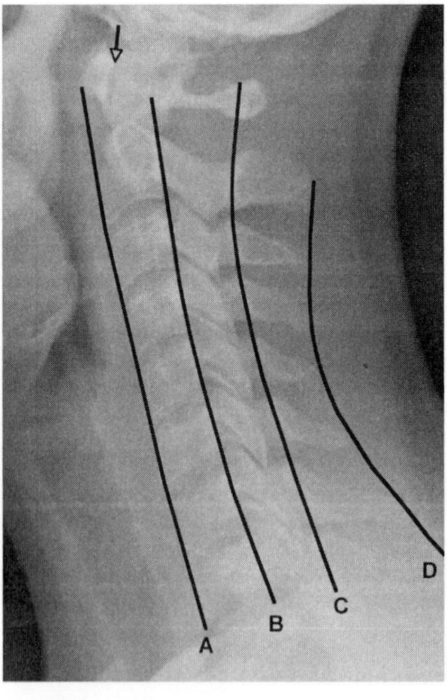

Lateral view of the cervical spine depicting the **(A)** anterior spinal line, **(B)** posterior spinal line, **(C)** spinolaminar line, and **(D)** spinous process line. Note the predental space (*arrow*). It is normal in this adult patient, measuring less than 3 mm.

32. When is the predental space considered abnormal?

The predental space (or atlantodental interval) is the space between the odontoid process and the anterior aspect of the ring of C1 (see figure). It is evaluated on the lateral radiograph of the cervical spine. The predental space is abnormal when it measures greater than 3 mm in adults and 5 mm in children. An increased atlantodental interval indicates atlantoaxial instability caused by rupture of the transverse ligament.

33. What is the normal thickness of the prevertebral soft tissues in the cervical spine?

Hematoma and edema of the soft tissues secondary to trauma can cause thickening of the soft tissues on the lateral radiograph of the cervical spine. Anterior to the C2 vertebral body, the soft tissues should not normally measure more than 7 mm. Anterior to C7, the prevertebral soft tissues can normally measure up to 22 mm.

34. How is basilar invagination diagnosed radiographically?

Basilar invagination or cranial settling is the protrusion of the odontoid process into the foramen magnum. Several lines can be drawn on a lateral radiograph of the cervical spine to assess the occipitocervical junction:

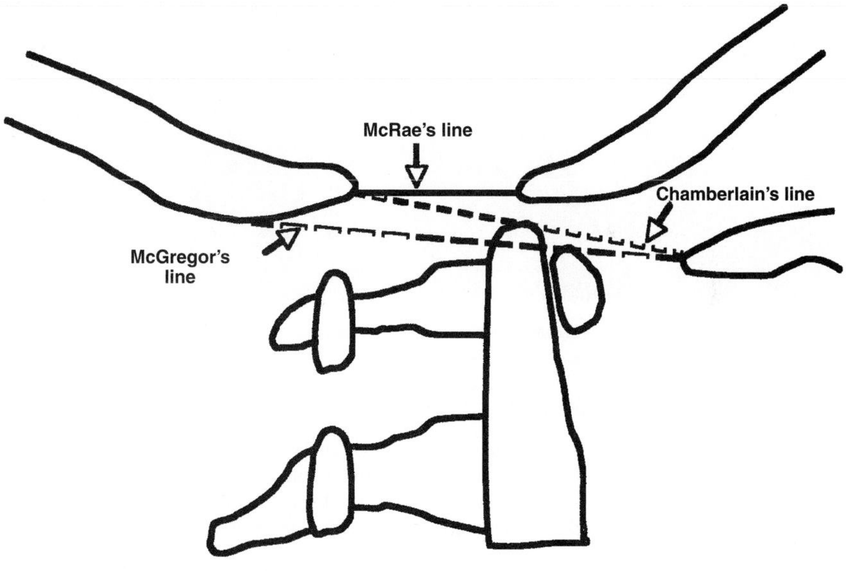

Lateral view of the occipitocervical junction demonstrating Chamberlain's line, McRae's line, and McGregor's line.

- Chamberlain's line—This line is drawn from the superior aspect of the posterior hard palate to the posterior margin of the foramen magnum. The tip of the odontoid process should not be more than 3 mm above this line. If it is, basilar invagination is present.
- McRae's line—This line defines the foramen magnum opening. The tip of the odontoid process should normally be below this line.
- McGregor's line—This is a line drawn from the superior portion of the posterior hard palate to the lowest portion of the occipital skull. Cranial settling exists when the tip of the dens is more than 4.5 mm above this line.

35. What is the anterior humeral line?

This line is drawn along the anterior cortex of the humerus on a lateral radiograph of the elbow. Extension of the anterior humeral line through the elbow joint intersects the middle one third of the capitellum in the normal situation. The anterior humeral line is useful in the diagnosis of subtle nondisplaced supracondylar fractures of the distal humerus in children. This line will pass through the anterior one third of the capitellum or even anterior to the capitellum when a supracondylar fracture is present.

36. What is the radiocapitellar line?

This line is important in the assessment of radial head dislocations. Normally, the proximal extension of a line drawn along the center of the proximal radial shaft should intersect the capitellum regardless of the radiographic view. This will not hold true in the presence of a radial head dislocation.

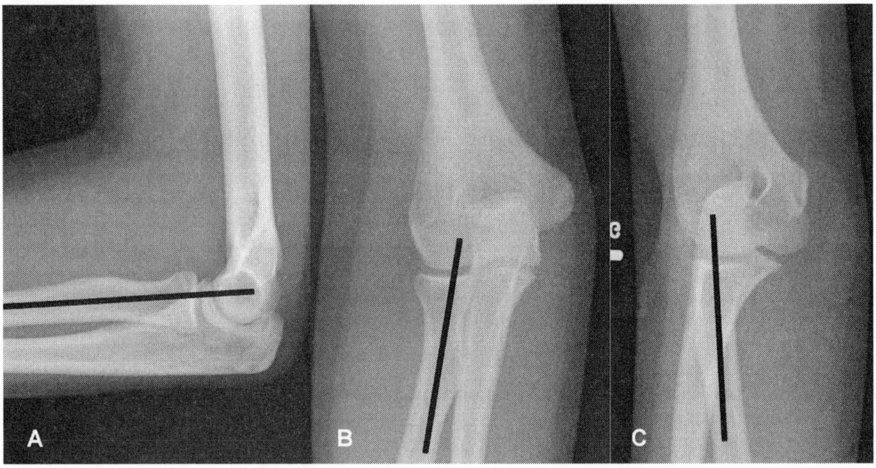

(A) Lateral, **(B)** AP, and **(C)** oblique views of a normal elbow demonstrating the radiocapitellar line. The line bisecting the proximal radial shaft intersects the capitellum on all three views.

37. What is ulnar variance?

Ulnar variance refers to the position of the distal articular surface of the ulna relative to the radius. Ulna neutral exists when the radius and ulna are of equal length.

In this situation, 80% of the axial load across the wrist is transmitted through the radius and 20% through the ulna. Ulnar variance is negative if the articular surface of the ulna is proximal to that of the radius.

Positive ulnar variance exists when the ulna is longer than the radius. With negative ulnar variance, less stress is borne by the ulna; conversely, with positive ulnar variance, the stress borne by the distal ulna increases.

38. What are some of the common radiographic measurements made on wrist x-rays?

- Scapholunate angle—the angle formed by lines drawn through the long axis of the scaphoid and the axis of the lunate on a lateral view of the wrist. In normal individuals the scapholunate angle measures between 30 and 60 degrees. Ligament injuries and fractures can lead to carpal collapse patterns that result in an abnormally increased or decreased scapholunate angle.

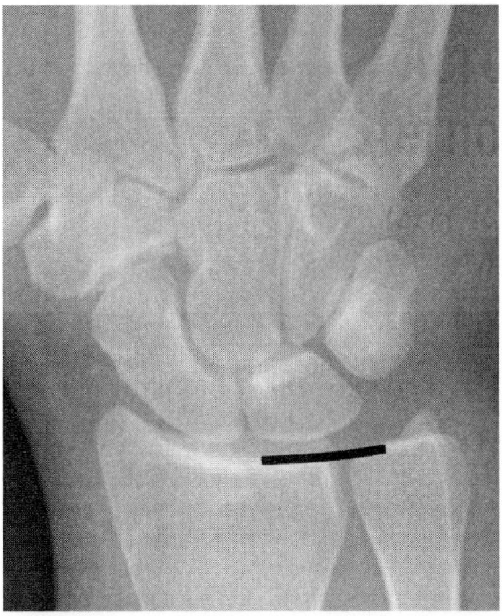

PA view of the wrist in a patient who is ulnar neutral. The radius and ulna are of equal length.

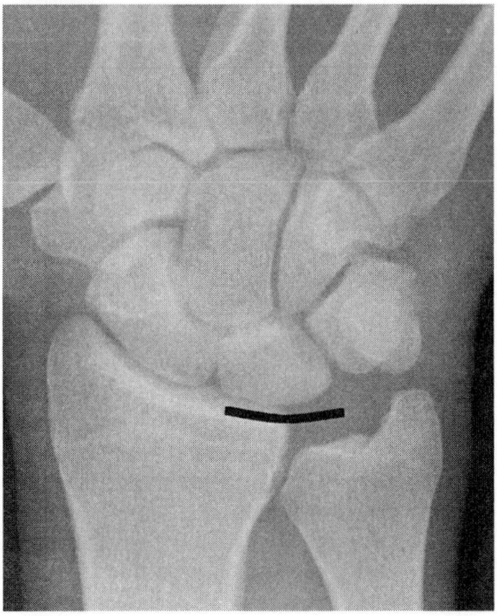

PA view of the wrist demonstrating negative ulnar variance. The ulna is shorter than the radius.

- Capitolunate angle—the intersection of lines drawn through the long axis of the capitate and the axis of the lunate on a lateral x-ray. Normally the capitolunate angles measures less than 20 degrees. An increase in this angle can be seen with carpal instability.
- Radial inclination—drawn on a PA view of the wrist. This is the angle formed by a line drawn perpendicular to the long axis of the radius and a line drawn from medial to lateral along the distal edge of the radius. Normal radial inclination is approximately 23 degrees.
- Palmar tilt—drawn similar to the angle of radial inclination except on a lateral view of the wrist. The first line is perpendicular to the long axis of the radius. The second line extends along the distal aspect of the radius, bridging the volar and dorsal edges. A measurement of 10 to 15 degrees is considered normal.

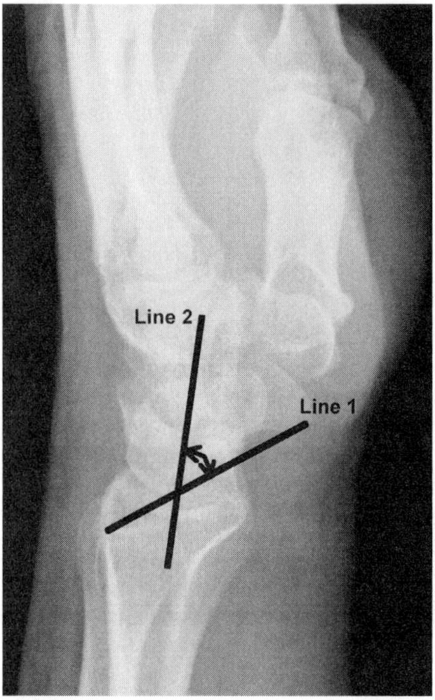

Lateral view of the wrist depicting the scapholunate angle. Line 1 is drawn along the long axis of the scaphoid while line 2 is drawn through the lunate. Normally, the angle measures between 30 and 60 degrees.

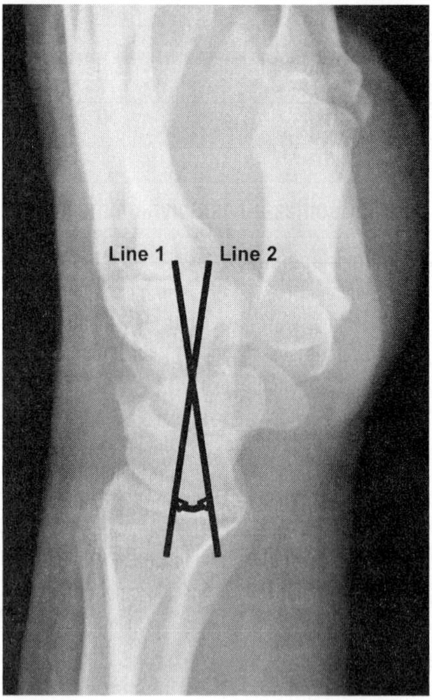

Lateral view of the wrist depicting the capitolunate angle. Line 1 is drawn along the long axis of the capitate while line 2 is drawn through the lunate. Normally, the angle measures less than 20 degrees.

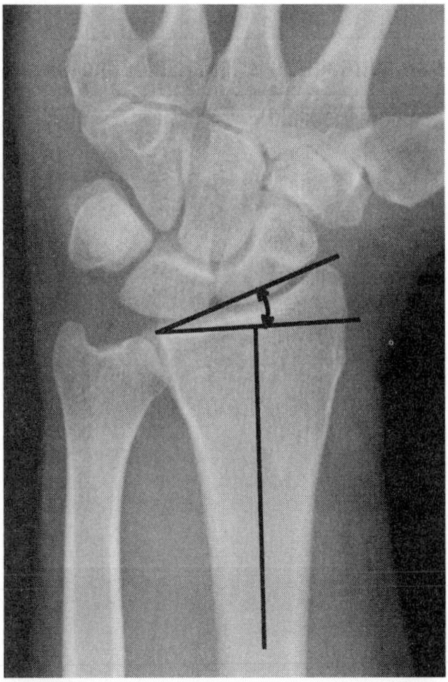

PA view of the wrist demonstrating the normal angle of radial inclination.

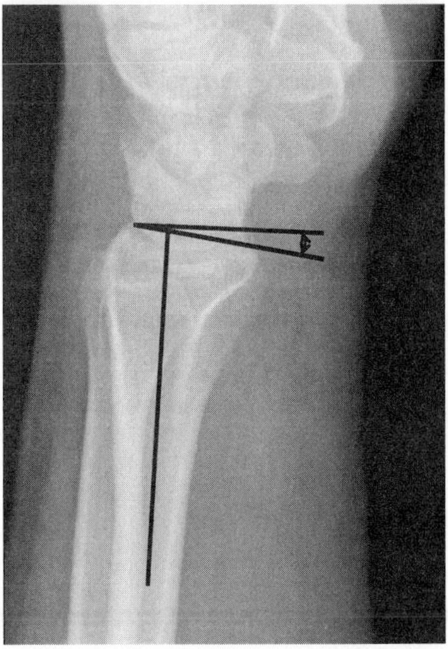

Lateral view of the wrist demonstrating normal volar tilt of the distal radius.

39. What are the carpal arcs?

Drawn on a PA view of the wrist, three distinct parallel arcs help define the normal articular relationships of the carpal bones. Arc 1 follows the proximal surfaces of the bones in the proximal row of the carpus. Arc 2 is formed by a line drawn along the distal margins of these same bones. A line is drawn along the proximal surfaces of the capitate and hamate to form arc 3. Subluxation or dislocation of a carpal bone will disrupt these normally smooth and parallel arcs.

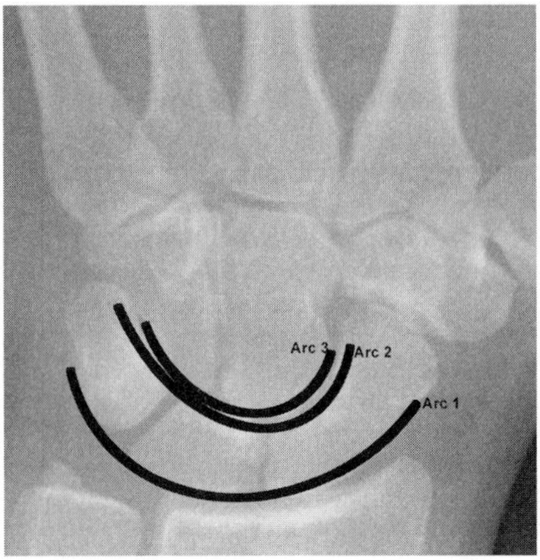

PA view of the wrist with the three carpal arcs shown.

40. What radiographic lines and angles can be used in the diagnosis of developmental dysplasia of the hip (DDH)?

- Hilgenreiner's line—This is a horizontal line drawn through the triradiate cartilage.
- Perkin's line—This line is drawn vertically along the lateral rim of the acetabulum.

The intersection of Hilgenreiner's line and Perkin's line divides the hip into four quadrants. The femoral head ossification center should normally be within the inner lower quadrant. With hip dislocation or DDH, the femoral ossific nucleus will be outside this area.

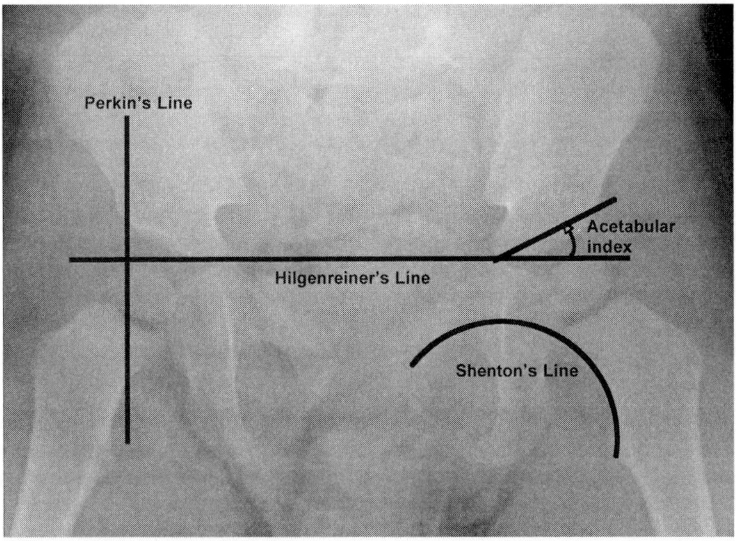

Anteroposterior view of a normal pediatric hip. Perkin's line, Hilgenreiner's line, Shenton's line, and the acetabular index are shown. Note that a major portion of the femoral head ossification center is located in the inner lower quadrant of the intersection of Perkin's and Hilgenreiner's lines.

- Shenton's line—This smooth curved line is drawn between the medial femoral neck and the superior portion of the obturator foramen. This line may be broken or discontinuous in DDH or hip dislocation.
- Acetabular index—This is a measure of the slope of the acetabular roof. The angle is formed by the intersection of Hilgenreiner's line with a line drawn through the lateral margin of the acetabular roof. It varies with age. At birth the angle normally measures between 18 and 36 degrees. Acetabular dysplasia is suggested when the acetabular index is increased.
- Wiberg's center-edge angle (CE angle)—This angle is formed by a vertical line drawn superiorly from the center of the femoral head and a line drawn from the center of the femoral head to the lateral margin of the acetabular roof. It is an indication of acetabular depth. The CE angle is normal when it measures 20 to 40 degrees. The angle is decreased in dysplastic hips.

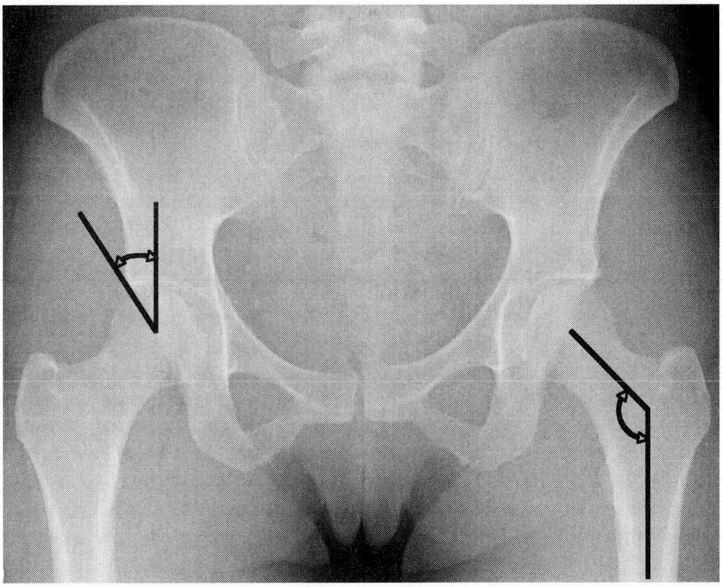

AP view of an adult pelvis with a normal center-edge angle shown on the right and a normal neck-shaft angle on the left.

41. What is the femoral neck-shaft angle?

The intersection of lines drawn through the axis of the femoral neck and femoral shaft forms this angle. It measures approximately 150 degrees at birth and normally decreases with age. The neck-shaft angle measures 120 to 130 degrees in adults. A decrease in the neck-shaft angle is termed coxa vara while an increase in this angle represents coxa valga.

42. How does an osteochondral lesion of the lateral femoral condyle appear on radiographs?

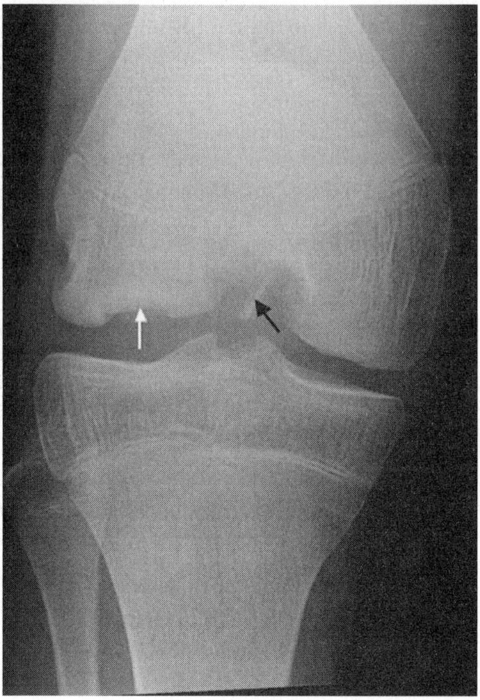

Tunnel view of the knee. There is deformity along the articular surface of the lateral femoral condyle (*thin white arrow*). There is a lucent defect with sclerosis (increased whiteness) in the surrounding bone. This is compatible with osteochondritis dessicans. A free fragment is seen in the notch (*thin black arrow*). Note that the physes are still open in this teenager.

43. How does an anterior dislocation of the shoulder appear on a radiograph?

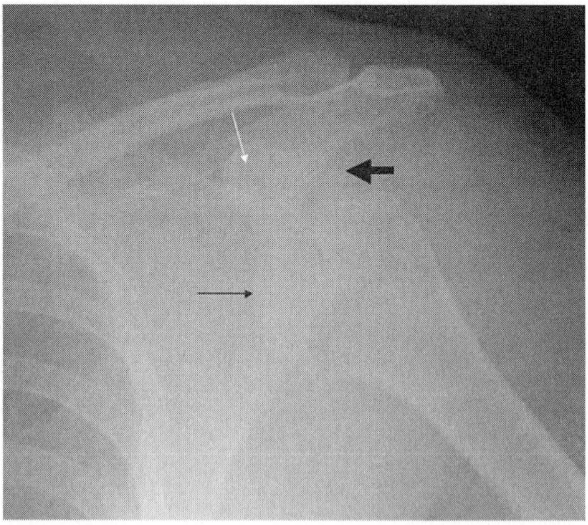

AP view of the shoulder in a patient with an anterior dislocation. While the anterior location of the humeral head (thin black arrow) relative to the glenoid (thick black arrow) cannot be detected on this view, the position of the humeral head below the coracoid process (thin white arrow) and medial and inferior to the glenoid is classic for this type of dislocation.

44. How does a normal ACL appear on MRI?

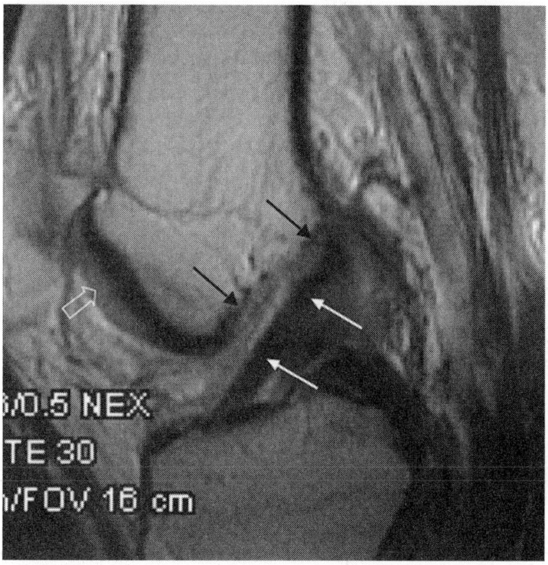

Sagittal proton density images demonstrating a normal ACL. A black signal is seen throughout the ACL as it extends from the femur to the proximal tibia (*white arrows*). The course of the ACL should parallel the posterior aspect of the intercondylar notch of the femur (*black arrows*). This is called Blumensaat's line. Note the normal gray cartilage at the anterior aspect of the distal femur (*open white arrow*).

45. How does a ruptured ACL appear on MRI?

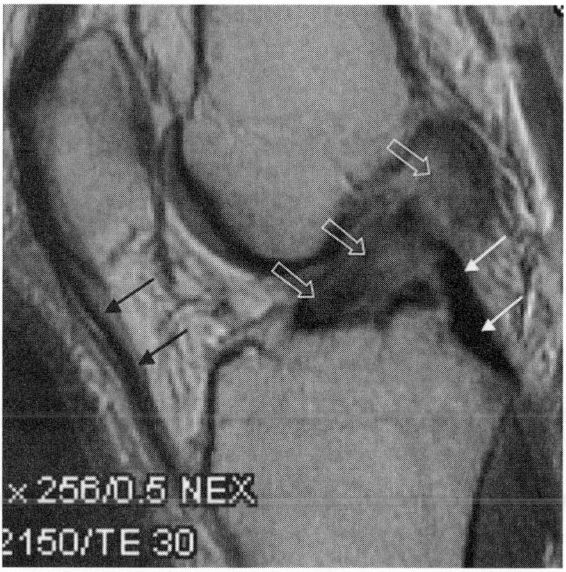

Sagittal proton density MR image of the knee. Normal tendons are black or low-signal on MRI. Note the normal patella tendon anteriorly (*thin black arrows*). The posterior cruciate ligament (PCL) is also normal (*thin white arrows*). Only the inferior portion of the PCL is seen on this image. The anterior cruciate ligament (ACL) is abnormal. There is an amorphous intermediate or grayish signal where the normal ACL should be (*open white arrows*). Only the inferior aspect of the ACL contains the normal black signal.

46. How does a greater tuberosity fracture appear on MRI?

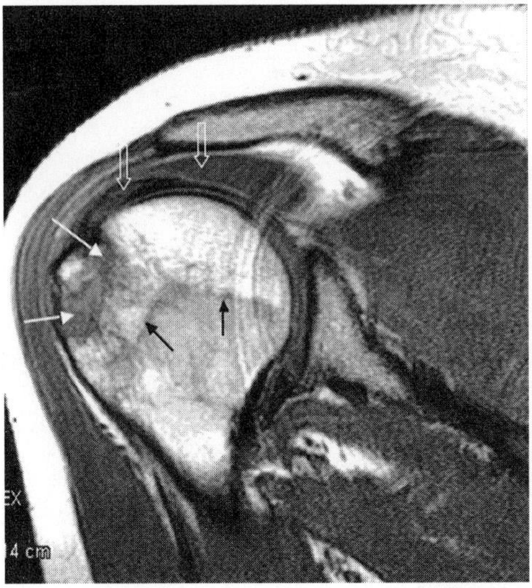

Coronal oblique T_1-weighted MR image of the shoulder. The subcutaneous fat and the fat in bone marrow are normally white or high-signal on a T_1-weighted image. In the region of the greater tuberosity, there is a gray signal in the bone marrow with black lines running through it (*white arrows*). This is compatible with a fracture and surrounding bone marrow edema, confirming the finding seen on the previous x-ray. The black line below the fracture is the normal physeal remnant (*black arrows*). Note the normal supraspinatus muscle and tendon just above the humeral head (*open white arrows*).

Bibliography

Curry TS, Dowdey JE, Murry RC: *Christensen's physics of diagnostic radiology,* ed 4, Philadelphia, 1990, Lea & Febiger.

Hak DJ, Gautsch TL: A review of radiographic lines and angles used in orthopedics, *Am J Orthoped* 24:590-601, 1995.

Halpern B et al: *Imaging in musculoskeletal and sports medicine,* Malden, Mass, 1997, Blackwell.

Kaplan PA et al: *Musculoskeletal MRI,* Philadelphia, 2001, WB Saunders.

Luhmann SJ et al: Magnetic resonance imaging of the knee in children and adolescents: its role in clinical decision-making, *J Bone Joint Surg Am* 87:497-502, 2005.

Resnick D: *Bone and joint imaging,* Philadelphia, 2005, Elsevier Saunders.

Resnick D, Kang HF: *Internal derangement of joints,* Philadelphia, 1997, WB Saunders.

Rogers LF: *Radiology of skeletal trauma,* New York, 2002, Churchill Livingstone.

Section V

The Shoulder

Chapter 37

Functional Anatomy of the Shoulder

Matthew A. Kippe, MD, and J. Michael Wiater, MD

1. Name the origins, insertions, innervation, and actions of all muscles that attach to the scapula.

There are 17 muscles attached to the scapula. The following table summarizes the origins, insertions, innervation, and action of each.

Muscle	Origin	Insertion	Innervation	Action
Subscapularis	Subscapularis fossa	Lesser tuberosity of humerus	Upper and lower subscapular nerve	Glenohumeral head depressor; extension, adduction, and medial rotation of humerus
Supraspinatus	Supraspinatus fossa	Superior facet on greater tuberosity	Suprascapular nerve	Abduction, stabilization of glenohumeral joint
Infraspinatus	Infraspinatus fossa	Middle facet on greater tuberosity	Suprascapular nerve	Extension and external rotation
Teres minor	Superior part of lateral border of scapula	Inferior facet on greater tuberosity	Axillary nerve	Extension and external rotation
Teres major	Dorsal surface of inferior angle of scapula	Medial lip of intertubercular groove of humerus	Lower subscapular nerve	Adducts and internally rotates arm
Serratus anterior	External surfaces of lateral parts of ribs 1-8	Anterior surface of medial border of scapula	Long thoracic Nerve	Protracts and rotates scapula and holds it against thoracic wall
Latissimus dorsi	Spinous processes of inferior 6 thoracic vertebrae, thoracolumbar fascia, iliac crest, and inferior 3 ribs	Floor of intertubercular groove of humerus	Thoracodorsal nerve	Extends, adducts, and internally rotates humerus

continued

continued

Muscle	Origin	Insertion	Innervation	Action
Deltoid	Lateral one third of clavicle, acromion, and spine of scapula	Deltoid tuberosity of humerus	Axillary nerve	Flexes, abducts, and extends arm
Trapezius	Spinous processes of cervical and thoracic vertebrae	Scapula and acromion	Spinal accessory nerve and branches of ansa cervicalis	Elevates, retracts, and rotates scapula
Levator scapula	Posterior tubercles of transverse processes of C1-C4 vertebrae	Superior part of medial border of scapula	Dorsal scapular nerve	Elevates scapula and tilts glenoid cavity inferiorly by rotating scapula
Rhomboids	Ligamentum nuchae and spinous processes of C7-T5	Medial border of scapula from level of spine to inferior angle	Dorsal scapular nerve	Retracts scapula and rotates it to depress glenoid cavity
Triceps	Superior one third of posterior and lateral surface of humerus, infraglenoid tubercle	Supraposterior surface of olecranon process of ulna and deep fascia of forearm	Radial nerve	Extends forearm at elbow; extension of arm at shoulder
Pectoralis minor	Ribs 3-5 near their costal cartilages	Medial border and superior surface of coracoid process of scapula	Medial pectoral nerve	Stabilizes scapula by drawing it inferiorly and anteriorly against thoracic wall
Coraco-brachialis	Tip of coracoid process of scapula	Middle medial border of humerus	Musculo-cutaneous nerve	Horizontal flexion and adduction of humerus at shoulder
Biceps brachii	Tip of coracoid and supraglenoid tubercle of scapula	Tuberosity of radius and lacertus fibrosis	Musculo-cutaneous nerve	Supinates forearm and when supine flexes forearm
Omohyoid	Superior border of scapula and suprascapular ligament	Inferior border of hyoid bone	Ansa cervicalis	Functions in swallowing and phonation

2. What is the normal scapulohumeral rhythm?

Normal scapulohumeral rhythm, as initially described by Codman in 1934, refers to the steady and continuous motion that occurs simultaneously at the scapulohumeral and scapulothoracic articulations during elevation of the arm. If the shoulder joint is abnormal, the scapula moves haltingly on the chest wall and not in concert with the glenohumeral joint. Although the relative motion of the glenohumeral joint to the scapulothoracic joint varies among individuals and at different ranges of the shoulder (1.25 to 1-4.3 to 1), the average is approximately 2 to 1.

3. Describe the gliding movements at the shoulder.

During rotational motion of the shoulder, obligate translation of the humeral head is a result of the asymmetrical tightening and loosening of the capsuloligamentous structures. Anterior translation of the humeral head occurs with forward elevation beyond 55 degrees, and posterior translation occurs with extension >35 degrees. Surgical tightening of the posterior capsule or rotator interval tissue results in increased obligate anterior translation during forward elevation. Conversely, excessively tight anterior instability repairs shift the humeral head and joint contact point posteriorly. These findings illustrate that tightness in one direction can lead to instability in the opposite direction. During elevation the humeral head moves superiorly, approximately 3 mm at the beginning of elevation, and then rotates in place with little excursion.

4. What are the normal strength ratios of the shoulder?

- Internal to external rotation: 3 to 2
- Adduction to abduction: 2 to 1
- Extension to flexion: 5 to 4

Women have approximately 45% to 65% of the shoulder strength of men.

5. Which glenohumeral ligament plays an important role in limiting external rotation with the arm at the side and is frequently contracted in shoulders with adhesive capsulitis?

The coracohumeral ligament limits external rotation with the arm at the side. It arises from the lateral aspect of the coracoid process and inserts into the rotator interval capsular tissue. This ligament is thickened and contracted in frozen shoulders and frequently needs to be released to regain full external rotation.

6. What is the rotator interval?

The rotator interval, as originally described by Neer, is the capsular tissue in the interval between the subscapularis and supraspinatus tendons. The rotator interval is composed of parts of the supraspinatus and subscapularis tendons, the coracohumeral ligament, and the superior glenohumeral ligament. These structures contribute to stability of the shoulder by limiting inferior translation and external rotation with the arm adducted as well as posterior translation when the arm is forward flexed, adducted, and internally rotated. The more medial part of the interval primarily limits inferior translation and to a lesser extent external rotation, while the lateral part of the interval primarily limits external rotation in the adducted arm. Pathologic rotator interval tissue can play a significant role in limiting motion, particularly external rotation, in the setting of adhesive capsulitis. At the opposite end of the spectrum, deficient or attenuated rotator interval tissue may be associated with recurrent anteroinferior or multidirectional instability of the shoulder.

7. What are the four parts of the proximal humerus?

The proximal humerus is composed of four distinct anatomic segments: (1) the shaft of the humerus, (2) the greater tuberosity, (3) the lesser tuberosity, and (4) the articular or head segment. These segments correspond to the four ossification centers of the proximal humerus. The shaft of the humerus connects with the proximal humerus at the surgical neck, just below the tuberosities. The anatomic neck is above the tuberosities, between the articular margin and the attachment of the articular capsule. The greater tuberosity has three facets for the attachment of the supraspinatus, infraspinatus, and teres minor muscles. The lesser tuberosity is the site of insertion of the subscapularis muscle. The four parts of the proximal humerus are common sites of fractures, especially in older patients with osteopenic bone, and form the basis for the Neer classification of proximal humerus fractures.

8. Describe the layers of the rotator cuff.

A five-layer structure has been described for the superior rotator cuff and capsule as the tendons insert onto the greater tuberosity of the humerus. Variation in tissue properties and loads among layers may contribute to shear forces along these planes, which may be a factor in the initiation of rotator cuff tears. At the bursal surface, **layer 1** is composed of a superficial portion of the coracohumeral ligament. **Layer 2** is made up of closely packed parallel bundles of collagen fibers, running from the muscle bellies to the greater tuberosity. This layer is probably the primary load-carrying portion of the rotator cuff. **Layer 3** has smaller fascicles and a more random orientation. **Layer 4** is composed of loose connective tissue and bands of collagen that run perpendicular to the longitudinal orientation of the cuff tendon. This layer also contains the deep extent of the coracohumeral ligament and contains a transverse band or cable that may function to distribute forces along the rotator cuff insertion. **Layer 5** is the true capsular layer.

9. What are the basic biomechanical functions of the rotator cuff?

The rotator cuff acts to provide stability through force couples and aid in motion about the glenohumeral joint. The rotator cuff has a humeral head depressing effect that counteracts the superior pull of the deltoid muscle. The rotator cuff acts multiaxially during motion to maintain proper position of the humeral head within the glenoid.

10. Describe the anatomy of the supraspinatus tendon and its clinical significance.

There are two muscle bellies, anterior and posterior. The anterior muscle belly is larger and pulls through a smaller tendon area. Thus the anterior tendon stress is significantly greater than the posterior tendon stress, and rotator cuff tendon repairs should incorporate the anterior tendon whenever possible, as it acts as the primary contractile unit.

11. Describe the role of the long head of the biceps.

Opinions vary considerably. Some investigators suggest that it is a vestigial structure, whereas others believe that it plays a crucial role in shoulder stability. Dynamic cadaveric and in vivo electromyographic studies have shown that the long head of the biceps may contribute to anterior stability of the shoulder by decreasing translation of the humeral head and may have a humeral head–depressing effect in the presence of a large rotator cuff tear by restraining superior migration of the humeral head. Elbow flexion strength can decrease by as much as 30% after a tear of the long head of the biceps. Supination decreases by an average of 10% to 20%. Abduction strength may decrease 20% after a tear of the long head of the biceps secondary to the loss of its stabilizing function.

12. What is the role of the bicipital groove in anterosuperior shoulder pain?

The differential diagnosis of anterosuperior shoulder pain can include impingement syndrome, rotator cuff pathology, acromioclavicular joint pain, instability, and biceps tendon disease. Furthermore, there is a positive association between radiographic degenerative changes of the bicipital groove and anterosuperior shoulder pain. Studies have shown there is an increased incidence of bicipital tendon disease in patients with degenerative changes in the bicipital groove. These degenerative changes include stenosis and osteophyte formation, which has been correlated to biceps tendon disease via ultrasonography.

13. Describe the most common variations of the labral origin of the bicep anchor.

Forty to sixty percent of the biceps tendon origin is from the supraglenoid tubercle, while the remaining fibers originate from the superior glenoid labrum. There is considerable variability in the attachment to the superior labrum. The most common variation is an equal contribution of anterior and posterior labral attachment. The next most common is attachment mostly posterior, but with a small contribution to the anterior labrum. The third most common variation consists of an entirely posterior attachment. Finally, the least common labral attachment is mostly anterior, but with a small contribution to the posterior labrum.

14. What is the quadrangular space? Which structures pass through it?

The quadrangular space is an anatomic interval formed by the shaft of the humerus laterally, the long head of the triceps medially, the teres minor muscle superiorly, and the teres major muscle inferiorly. Through it pass the axillary nerve and the posterior humeral circumflex artery.

15. What is the triangular space? Which structure passes through it?

The triangular space is an anatomic interval medial to the quadrangular space. Its borders are formed by the long head of the triceps laterally, the teres minor superiorly, and the teres major inferiorly. The circumflex scapular artery, a branch of the scapular artery, passes through the triangular space.

16. How is glenohumeral joint stability maintained?

Stability of the glenohumeral joint depends on both static and dynamic stabilizers of the shoulder joint. The static or passive stabilizers of the shoulder joint include the glenohumeral joint capsule and ligaments. These structures are normally lax during the mid range of motion and tighten at the extremes of motion, serving as passive checkreins to excessive glenohumeral translation. The dynamic stabilizers include primarily the rotator cuff and deltoid muscles, although all glenohumeral muscles contribute to stability to some degree. The dynamic stabilizers make the greatest contribution to stability within the functional mid range of motion by actively contracting and keeping the humeral head centered in the glenoid fossa, producing a concavity-compression effect. They lose their effectiveness as they are stretched beyond their functional length at the extremes of motion.

17. Which structure is the most important static restraint to anterior glenohumeral translation in the 90-degree abducted-externally rotated position?

Most traumatic shoulder dislocations are anterior and occur with the arm in the extreme abducted and externally rotated position. Cadaveric ligament-cutting studies have shown that different regions of the glenohumeral capsule and ligament complex are placed on stretch, depending on the position of the arm. The anterior band of the inferior glenohumeral ligament is the principal static restraint to the anterior translation of the humeral head with the arm in the 90-degree abducted-externally rotated position. The middle glenohumeral ligament is a significant restraint to anterior translation in the mid range of shoulder elevation. The superior glenohumeral ligament appears to prevent excessive external rotation and inferior translation with the arm at the side.

18. What is a Bankart lesion?

A Bankart lesion represents a lesion of the glenoid labrum corresponding to the detachment of the anchoring point of the anterior band of the inferior glenohumeral ligament and middle glenohumeral ligament from the glenoid rim. It is the result of a traumatic anterior dislocation of the glenohumeral joint.

19. What is a HAGL lesion?

A HAGL lesion represents an uncommon avulsion of the humeral attachment of the glenohumeral ligament because of glenohumeral dislocation; it is analogous to the more common avulsion of the glenoid attachment of the glenohumeral ligament, or Bankart lesion.

20. What is a Hill-Sachs lesion and how does it relate to recurrent anterior shoulder instability?

A Hill-Sachs lesion represents an impression fracture of the posterolateral margin of the humeral head caused by impaction on the rim of the glenoid during an anterior shoulder dislocation. Large Hill-Sachs lesions involving more than 30% of the humeral articular surface can contribute to recurrent shoulder instability.

21. What is the biomechanical function of the clavicle?

The clavicle functions as a strut between the shoulder girdle and axial skeleton. By maintaining the upper extremity away from the midline, the clavicle improves the biomechanical efficiency of the axiohumeral muscles. As a result, the muscles do not expend their energy pulling the shoulder medially but rather create motion at the glenohumeral joint.

22. Describe the origin, insertion, innervation, and function of the subclavius muscle.

The subclavius muscle has a tendinous origin from the first rib and inserts on the inferior surface of the middle third of the clavicle. It receives innervation from the nerve to the subclavius, a branch of the superior trunk of the brachial plexus with contributions from C5 and C6. The function of the subclavius muscle is to stabilize the sternoclavicular joint during strenuous activity.

23. Name the primary arterial supply to the humeral head.

The ascending branch of the anterior humeral circumflex artery supplies most of the blood to the humeral head. This branch ascends the bicipital groove with the long head of the biceps tendon, entering the bone near the articular margin. The remainder of the blood supply to the head comes from branches of the posterior humeral circumflex artery and from branches within the rotator cuff tendon insertions.

24. Describe the course of the suprascapular nerve.

The suprascapular nerve arises from the upper trunk of the brachial plexus. It courses posteriorly to the suprascapular notch of the scapula, accompanied by the suprascapular artery. The nerve passes through the notch deep to the transverse scapular ligament, whereas the artery passes over the ligament. The suprascapular nerve then travels deep to the supraspinatus, which it innervates. Next, it passes through the spinoglenoid notch at the base of the spine of the scapula before it continues deep to the infraspinatus, which it also innervates. Articular sensory branches are given off to the acromioclavicular and glenohumeral joints along the course of the nerve. Compression of the suprascapular nerve can occur at the suprascapular or spinoglenoid notches, producing posterior shoulder pain and weakness.

25. Which neurovascular structure is at greatest risk during anterior shoulder surgery? Describe the course and branches of this structure.

The structure at greatest risk during this surgery is the axillary nerve, which traverses posteriorly from the posterior cord of the brachial plexus to innervate the deltoid and teres minor muscles. With the posterior humeral circumflex artery, it passes below the inferior border of the subscapularis and travels along the inferior glenohumeral joint capsule, with which it is intimately associated. While passing through the quadrangular space, the axillary nerve will divide into four branches—motor branches to the anterior and posterior portions of the deltoid muscle, a sensory branch (superior lateral brachial cutaneous nerve), and a motor branch to the teres minor muscle. Careless surgical dissection of the subscapularis or anterior capsule can result in injury to the axillary nerve or one of its branches.

26. Which nerve lies superficial in the posterior cervical triangle and is susceptible to injury?

Cranial nerve XI (spinal accessory nerve) travels through the posterior cervical triangle just below the cervical fascia. The posterior cervical triangle is bordered by the sternocleidomastoid anteriorly, the trapezius posteriorly, and the clavicle inferiorly. The spinal accessory nerve may be injured iatrogenically, most commonly during cervical lymph node biopsy, or by direct trauma. Injury to the spinal accessory nerve, which innervates the trapezius, leads to drooping of the shoulder, an asymmetric neckline, pain, and weakness in elevation of the arm.

27. Injury to which nerve causes classic medial scapular winging?

Injury to the long thoracic nerve leads to paralysis of the serratus anterior muscle. Winging of the scapula results because the medial border of the scapula is no longer closely opposed to the thoracic cage.

28. Describe the course of the musculocutaneous nerve.

The musculocutaneous nerve is a terminal branch of the lateral cord of the brachial plexus with contributions from C5, C6, and C7. It penetrates the muscle belly of the coracobrachialis and sends off motor branches, providing innervation. It then travels into the brachium between the brachialis and biceps brachii muscles, innervating both. Its terminal sensory branch emerges between the brachialis and brachioradialis muscles and travels into the forearm as the lateral antebrachial cutaneous nerve.

29. Describe the basic structure of the brachial plexus.

The brachial plexus, which provides sensory and motor innervation to the upper extremity and shoulder girdle, receives contributions from spinal nerves C5-C8 and T1. Inconstant innervation

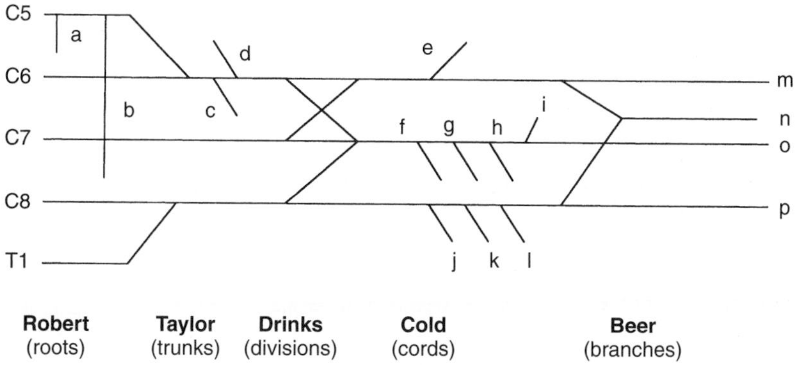

The brachial plexus. *a,* Dorsal scapular; *b,* long thoracic; *c,* suprascapular; *d,* nerve to subclavius; *e,* lateral pectoral; *f,* upper subscapular; *g,* thoracodorsal; *h,* lower subscapular; *i,* axillary; *j,* medial pectoral; *k,* medial brachial cutaneous; *l,* medial antebrachial cutaneous; *m,* musculocutaneous; *n,* median; *o,* radial; *p,* ulnar.

is received from C3 and C4. The five roots from the ventral rami of C5-T1 coalesce to form three trunks (superior, middle, and inferior). The three trunks divide to produce three anterior and three posterior divisions. The divisions combine into the three cords of the brachial plexus (lateral, posterior, and medial). Finally, the cords end in the terminal branches, which are the musculocutaneous, axillary, radial, median, and ulnar nerves. A helpful mnemonic to remember the order of the components of the brachial plexus (roots, trunks, divisions, cords, branches) is **R**obert **T**aylor **D**rinks **C**old **B**eer.

30. Where is the center of rotation of the normal glenohumeral joint? Where is the center of rotation in the severely cuff-deficient glenohumeral joint?

The center of rotation in the normal glenohumeral joint is at the center of the humeral head at the mid glenoid level. In a severely rotator cuff deficient glenohumeral joint, the head of the humerus migrates superiorly and medially secondary to the unopposed pull of the deltoid and the loss of the humeral head–depressing function of the rotator cuff. As a result, the center of rotation migrates superiorly. When the humeral head is no longer centered in the glenoid cavity because of abnormal force couples and loss of the glenohumeral fulcrum, the deltoid is at a mechanical disadvantage and limited abduction results.

31. What are the most frequently occurring anatomic variations of the coracoacromial (CA) ligament?

Variations include quadrangular (48%), Y shape (42%), broader lateral and thinner medial band, broad-banded (8%), and multiple bands (2%).

32. Is the acromial attachment of the coracoacromial ligament and anterior deltoid preserved during arthroscopic acromioplasty?

In most cases, the acromial attachment of the CA ligament is released during an arthroscopic acromioplasty, as it can be an impinging structure and often has calcification, or enthesopathy, within it contributing to anterior acromial spur formation. The overlying deltoid inserting into the anterior part of the acromion remains attached by a bridge of tissue composed of periosteum and deltoid tendon.

33. Describe the three most common normal variations in labral anatomy.

The three most common variations are the following: (1) the presence of a sublabral foramen, defined as the sulcus between a well-developed anterosuperior portion of the labrum and glenoid articular cartilage; (2) the presence of a sublabral foramen and a cordlike middle glenohumeral ligament; (3) the complete absence of labral tissue at the anterosuperior aspect of the labrum in association with a cordlike middle glenohumeral ligament attached to the superior part of the labrum at the base of the biceps (Buford complex).

34. Describe the anatomy of the pectoralis major tendon including the insertion and anatomy of the medial and lateral pectoral nerves as they relate to the insertion of the tendon.

The width of the insertion of the pectoralis major insertion is approximately 6 cm. The insertion is broad on the undersurface of the tendon and small on the anterior surface. The sternal head spirals into its insertion to form the posterior lamina, and the clavicular head remains anterior as it inserts into the humerus to form the anterior lamina.

The medial pectoral nerve enters the pectoralis major approximately 12 cm from its lateral humeral insertion and 2 cm from its inferior edge. The lateral pectoral nerve inserts approximately 12.5 cm from its humeral insertion. The medial pectoral nerve's insertion into the pectoralis major is inferior to the lateral pectoral nerve's insertion. The lateral pectoral nerve passes medial to the pectoralis minor before entering the pectoralis major whereas the medial pectoral nerve passes through or lateral to the pectoralis minor before entering the pectoralis major.

35. Describe the anatomy of the deltoid insertion.

The anterior, middle, and posterior deltoid muscle fibers enter into the deltoid insertion in a V-shaped tendinous confluence. This consists of a broad posterior band and a narrow separate anterior band. The anterior band accounts for approximately one fifth of the insertion. The insertion can be extremely close to the pectoralis major insertion, and in some cases nearly apposed to each other. The average distance from the axillary nerve is approximately 5.6 cm anteriorly and 4.5 cm posteriorly.

36. What are the main stabilizers of the AC joint and in which direction do they resist displacement?

The acromioclavicular ligament and joint capsule acts as a primary constraint for posterior displacement of the clavicle and posterior axial rotation. The conoid ligament plays a primary role in constraining anterior and superior rotation as well as anterior and superior displacement of the clavicle. The trapezoid ligament contributes to constraint for both horizontal and vertical displacement primarily when the clavicle moves in axial compression toward the acromion.

37. What is the average proximal humerus articular version relative to the trans-epicondylar axis of the distal humerus?

Average proximal humerus articular version is 30 degrees of retroversion.

38. What is the normal version or tilt angle of the glenoid?

Normal glenoid version is approximately 8 degrees of retroversion. The clinical significance is that increased retroversion places the patient at increased risk for posterior instability.

39. Is there a relationship between glenoid inclination and rotator cuff tears/instability?

Yes. Preliminary studies have demonstrated that increasing superior inclination of the glenoid significantly reduces the amount of force required for superior humeral head migration. This suggests that more upward-facing glenoids may increase the risk for superior humeral translation, which has been shown to contribute to the development of rotator cuff disease. Increased glenoid retroversion has been shown to increase the risk for posterior instability.

Bibliography

American Academy of Orthopaedic Surgeons: *OKU Shoulder and Elbow 2*, Rosemont, Calif, 2002, AAOS.

Ball CM et al: The posterior branch of the axillary nerve: an anatomic study, *J Bone Joint Surg* 85A:1497-1501, 2003.

Bankart ASB: Recurrent or habitual dislocation of the shoulder joint, *BMJ* 2:1132-1133, 1923.

Clark JM, Harryman DT II: Tendons, ligaments and capsule of the rotator cuff, *J Bone Joint Surg* 74A:713-725, 1992.

Cole BJ, Warner JP: Anatomy, biomechanics, and pathophysiology of glenohumeral instability. In Iannotti JP, Williams GR: *Disorders of the shoulder: diagnosis and management,* Baltimore, Md, 1999, pp 207-232, Lippincott Williams & Wilkins.

Flatow EL: Shoulder anatomy and biomechanics. In Post M et al, editors: *The shoulder: operative technique,* Baltimore, Md, 1998, pp 1-42, Williams & Wilkins.

Harryman DT II et al: Translation of the humeral head on the glenoid with passive glenohumeral motion, *J Bone Joint Surg* 72A:1334-1343, 1990.

Hunt JL, Moore RJ, Krishnan J: The fate of the coracoacromial ligament in arthroscopic acromioplasty: an anatomical study, *J Shoulder Elbow Surg* 9:491-494, 2000.
Jost B, Kocj PP, Gerber C: Anatomy and functional aspects of the rotator interval, *J Shoulder Elbow Surg* 9:336-341, 2000.
Klepps SJ et al: Anatomic evaluation of the subcoracoid pectoralis major transfer in human cadavers, *J Shoulder Elbow Surg* 10:453-459, 2001.
Laing PG: The arterial supply of the adult humerus, *J Bone Joint Surg* 38A:1105-1116, 1956.
Neer CS II: Anterior acromioplasty for the chronic impingement syndrome in the shoulder, *J Bone Joint Surg* 54A:41-50, 1972.
Pfahler M, Branner S, Refior HJ: The role of the bicipital groove in tendopathy of the long biceps tendon, *J Shoulder Elbow Surg* 8:419-424, 1999.
Pieper H et al: Anatomic variation of the coracoacromial ligament: a macroscopic and microscopic cadaveric study, *J Shoulder Elbow Surg* 6:291-296, 1997.
Price MR, Tillett ED, Acland RD: Determining the relationship of the axillary nerve to the shoulder joint capsule from an arthroscopic perspective, *J Bone Joint Surg* 86A:2135-2142, 2004.
Roh MS et al: Anterior and posterior musculotendinous anatomy of the supraspinatus, *J Shoulder Elbow Surg* 9:436-440, 2000.
Sarrafian SK: Gross and functional anatomy of the shoulder, *Clin Orthop* 173:11-19, 1983.
Turkel SJ et al: Stabilizing mechanisms preventing anterior dislocation of the glenohumeral joint, *J Bone Joint Surg* 63A:1208-1217, 1981.
Vangsness CT et al: The origin of the long head of the biceps from the scapula and glenoid labrum, *J Bone Joint Surg [Br]* 76-b:951-954, 1994.
Von Schroeder H, Kuiper SD, Botte MJ: Osseous anatomy of the scapula, *Clin Orthop Relat Res* 383:131-139, 2001.
Wong AS et al: The effect of glenoid inclination on superior humeral head migration, *J Shoulder Elbow Surg* 12:360-364, 2003.

Chapter 38

Shoulder Impingement and Rotator Cuff Tears

David A. Boyce, PT, EdD, OCS, and
Joseph A. Brosky, Jr., PT, MS, SCS

1. What are the prevalence and natural history of rotator cuff disease?

Prevalence data deemed from cadaver investigations range from 7% to 40%. Recent MRI and ultrasound investigations of asymptomatic subjects demonstrate the prevalence of rotator cuff tears to range from 13% to 34%. The prevalence ranges from 51% to 54% in 60- to 80-year-old subjects. Patients with a rotator cuff tear who are asymptomatic have a 51% chance of becoming symptomatic in the future.

2. Define os acromiale.

Os acromiale, or unfused acromial epiphysis, is the failure of the distal end of the acromion to ossify. Ossification usually occurs between 18 and 25 years of age. Os acromiale is often bilateral and may be seen in up to 8% of the normal population. The four presentations of os acromiale (pre, meso, meta, and basi) involve the acromion to greater or lesser degrees. An os acromiale may project into the rotator cuff outlet, decreasing its total area, and is thought to be associated with rotator cuff pathology.

3. What are the three morphologic types of the acromion?

Bigliani classified the acromion according to its shape. **Type I** acromion is flat (17% incidence); **type II** (43% incidence) curves downward into the rotator cuff outlet; and **type III** (40% incidence) is hooked downward into the rotator cuff outlet. Of patients with rotator cuff tears, 70% have type III acromion, 27% have type II, and 3% have type I. Types II and III decrease the area of the rotator cuff outlet and can traumatize the superior surface of the rotator cuff tendons.

4. Are types II and III acromia acquired or developmental?

It has been proposed that acromial hooks lie within the coracoacromial ligament and are actually traction spurs. Whenever the humeral head is pressed upward against the coracoacromial arch, it places a traction load on the distal lateral acromion, and a traction spur forms in response to the loading. It is similar to traction spurs that form on the calcaneus at the attachment of the plantar fascia.

5. Describe Neer's classification of rotator cuff pathology.

- Stage I—edema and hemorrhage. Patients usually are less than 25 years old and have pain with activity that usually resolves with rest. The condition is reversible, and treatment is conservative (relative rest and medication).
- Stage II—fibrosis and tendinitis. Patients typically are between 25 and 40 years old and experience recurrent pain with activity that does not always abate with rest. According to Neer, subacromial decompression should be considered if conservative treatment fails.
- Stage III—bone spur and tendon rupture. Patients typically are older than 40 years and have a history of progressive disability that has led to a tear of the rotator cuff. Rotator cuff repair is advised.
- Stage IV—cuff tear arthropathy. Patients typically are older than 60 years and have a history of progressive disability with a torn rotator cuff. Clinical management consists of rotator cuff repair, hemi-arthroplasty, or total shoulder replacement.

6. Describe the coracoacromial arch and its clinical importance.

The coracoacromial arch consists of the coracoacromial ligament, which spans the distance between the coracoid and acromion of the scapula. The ligament provides a protective covering over the subacromial bursa and rotator cuff tendons and restricts excessive superior humeral head migration. Clinically the coracoacromial ligament has been associated with rotator cuff pathology (especially in overhead athletes). During humeral elevation and internal rotation, the greater tuberosity and the attached rotator cuff tendons can be compressed against the arch. Repetitive compression may traumatize the rotator cuff tendons and lead to pathology.

7. What is a partial-thickness rotator cuff tear (tensile failure of the rotator cuff)?

The rotator cuff degenerates naturally with increasing age, especially after the third decade of life. Degeneration or tensile failure of the rotator cuff begins deep within the tissue near the undersurface attachment of the tuberosity. With time it may extend outward until it becomes a full-thickness tear. Partial-thickness tears of the rotator cuff also may occur on the bursal side of the cuff, most commonly near the insertion.

8. Do partial-thickness tears heal or progress to full-thickness tears?

Partial-thickness tears attempt to heal, but in most instances they progress to full-thickness tears. Matsen describes why partial-thickness rotator cuff tears eventually progress to full-thickness tears:

- Ruptured fibers can no longer sustain a load; thus increased loads are placed on neighboring fibers, making them more susceptible to rupture.
- Disruption of the tendon fibers also disrupts local blood supply within the tendon, thus inducing ischemia.
- Disrupted tendon fibers are exposed to joint fluid, which has a lytic effect on tendons that impairs the healing process.
- When tendon heals, the scar tissue that replaces the ruptured tendon fibers does not have the same tensile strength as the original tissue; thus it is at increased risk of failure.
- Once the tear becomes full thickness, loads that normally are distributed through the entire intact tendon often are transmitted at the torn margins of the rotator cuff tendon. This process produces a "zipper effect" and extends or unzips the tendon from the tuberosity.

9. What is an undersurface rotator cuff tear?

Undersurface rotator cuff tears are caused by rupture of the deep tissues of the rotator cuff that attach to the tuberosity. Undersurface tears, in fact, are partial-thickness tears of the rotator cuff on the articular surface. They can result from the natural degenerative process that affects the shoulder but often are noted in younger overhead athletes. Undersurface tearing in overhead athletes is thought to result from repetitive eccentric tensile loading (i.e., deceleration of the throwing arm).

10. What is rotator cuff arthropathy?

With massive tearing of the rotator cuff, cuff tendons slide off the humeral head. These tendons, which once served as humeral head depressors, now act as humeral head elevators and promote superior translation of the humeral head. The result is excessive wear and degeneration on both the humeral head and the undersurface of the acromion. If allowed to progress, the degeneration of the glenohumeral joint can become so significant and painful that a hemi-arthroplasty or total shoulder replacement is indicated. In severe cases of rotator cuff arthropathy, radiographs can aid in the diagnosis before surgery. Radiographs reveal sclerosis of the undersurface of the acromion ("eyebrow sign") secondary to prolonged bone-on-bone contact (humeral head in contact with undersurface of acromion) and cystic changes of the greater tuberosity.

11. When are acromioplasty and subacromial decompression required? What are the two types?

The typical patient requiring acromioplasty and decompression is between 25 and 40 years of age, experiences recurrent pain with activity that does not always abate with rest, and has failed conservative treatment (physical therapy, medications). The two types of acromioplasty and decompression are open and arthroscopic. Some surgeons believe that a more complete decompression is accomplished with the open technique. In addition, if a large rotator cuff tear is encountered during the open procedure, it can be repaired with relative ease, whereas arthroscopic repair of a large rotator cuff tear is difficult and technically demanding.

12. Should the coracoacromial ligament be released during subacromial decompression?

The coracoacromial ligament is a static stabilizer that limits superior humeral head translation. Release of the ligament contributes to increased superior humeral head migration and degenerative processes in shoulders with a massive rotator cuff tear. Thus some surgeons believe in retaining the coracoacromial ligament and preserving the arch to limit more severe superior humeral head migration, which may lead or contribute to rotator cuff arthropathy.

13. What is the Mumford procedure?

The Mumford procedure is an excision of the distal 2 cm of the clavicle. Mumford originally intended the surgery to provide pain relief for patients suffering from acromioclavicular dislocation. Distal clavicle excision often is performed during acromioplasty and subacromial decompression to allow even greater rotator cuff decompression. The acromioclavicular joint no longer exists, however; distal stability of the scapula is maintained through the intact costoclavicular ligaments (conoid and trapezoid).

14. What are the primary rotator cuff exercises?

The primary or "core" rotator cuff exercises involve the **SITS** muscles:

- Supraspinatus—**Scaption** is best described as abduction in the plane of the scapula. Another form of this exercise is prone scaption, in which the patient lies prone and performs scaption from 90 degrees of elevation to approximately 120 to 150 degrees.
  Infraspinatus—**External rotation** can be performed in many different positions, such as standing or side-lying.
- Teres minor—**Prone extension with external rotation** is preferred. The teres minor is also an external rotator but seems to have greater electromyographic activity when external rotation is combined with glenohumeral extension. The patient lies prone, with the arm hanging off the table, and then extends the shoulder level with the horizon while maintaining the shoulder in external rotation.
- Subscapularis—**Internal rotation** can be performed in many different positions, such as standing or side-lying.

Exercise of the SITS muscles alone does not include all muscles that contribute to optimal dynamic shoulder function. The therapist also should address the axioscapular (e.g., serratus anterior) and the axiohumeral (e.g., pectoralis major) muscle groups.

15. What rotator cuff exercises result in the greatest electromyographic (EMG) activity of the supraspinatus, infraspinatus, and teres minor?

Side-lying external rotation results in the greatest EMG activity of the infraspinatus and teres minor (62% maximum voluntary contraction [MVC]); supraspinatus activity was greatest during prone scaption with external rotation (82% MVC). However, prone scaption is considered an advanced exercise position for the supraspinatus and judgment must be exercised when prescribing this exercise.

16. What is *primary* rotator cuff impingement?

Primary impingement is a mechanical impingement of the rotator cuff beneath the coracoacromial arch and typically results from subacromial overcrowding. Factors related to primary impingement involve abnormal structural characteristics (e.g., congenital anomalies of the osseous structures of the acromioclavicular [AC] joint, coracoid process, or greater tuberosity of the humerus) or tendon thickening attributable to calcific deposits, trauma, or surgery.

17. What is *secondary* rotator cuff impingement?

Secondary rotator cuff impingement is a relative decrease in the subacromial space caused by microinstability of the glenohumeral joint or scapulothoracic instability. Attempts by the active restraints of the glenohumeral joint to compensate for the loss of the passive restraint function of the joint capsule and ligaments result in eventual fatigue and abnormal translation of the humeral head, leading to mechanical impingement of the rotator cuff by the coracoacromial arch.

18. What is posterior (internal) impingement?

Posterior impingement often is seen in overhead athletes, such as throwers, swimmers, and tennis players. It occurs when the arm is in an elevated and externally rotated position (similar to the cocking phase in throwing). The infraspinatus and supraspinatus muscles are pinched between the posterior superior aspect of the glenoid when the upper limb is in the cocked position. The lesion occurs on the undersurface rather than the bursal side of the rotator cuff. In addition, this form of impingement is thought to be associated with anterior instability.

19. What are the typical age, gender, and occupation of patients with rotator cuff tears?

The frequency of rotator cuff tears increases significantly with age. Tears become increasingly more common after the age of 40. Occupations or activities that predispose the rotator cuff to pathology require excessive and repetitive overhead motions. Sports that involve throwing or repetitive overhead motions (e.g., baseball pitching, tennis, swimming) also have a high prevalence of rotator cuff injuries. However, most cuff defects have a degenerative etiology. Neer reported that 40% of patients with cuff defects never performed strenuous physical work, and many heavy laborers never develop cuff defects. Fifty percent of patients with rotator cuff tears had no recollection of shoulder trauma. A high incidence (70%) of rotator cuff defects occurs in sedentary people doing light work; two thirds of cases occur in males.

20. Do shoulder dislocations lead to rotator cuff tears?

Rotator cuff tears may occur with anterior and inferior glenohumeral dislocations. The frequency of rotator cuff tears accompanying glenohumeral dislocations increases with advancing age and has been reported to exceed 30% in patients over 40 and 80% in patients over 60 years of age.

21. What classification system is used to describe the extent or size of a rotator cuff tear?

According to the grading system adopted by the American Academy of Orthopedic Surgeons, a small tear is <1 cm, a medium tear is 1 to 3 cm, a large tear is 3 to 5 cm, and a massive tear is >5 cm.

22. Do full-thickness rotator cuff tears heal?

No. Although primary healing of a full-thickness tear is unlikely, the results of nonoperative management of patients with full-thickness rotator cuff defects have demonstrated various degrees of improvement (33% to 90%) in pain and overall function. Partial-thickness tears may progress to full-thickness tears if left untreated, with deterioration in function over time.

23. Describe the typical physical therapy protocol for patients with rotator cuff repair.

Rehabilitation after rotator cuff repair depends on the following factors: size of the tear, quality of the tissue, method/type of surgical repair, age of the patient, chronicity of the condition, and occupation and/or desired activities. The typical acromioplasty and open cuff repair is followed by a short period of immobilization with or without an abduction pillow—1 to 6 weeks, depending on the size of the tear and quality of repair. Early passive motion exercises (flexion, abduction, external rotation), including pendulum exercises and pulleys, begin within the first few post-operative days to prevent adhesions and loss of motion. Scapulothoracic, cervical, and elbow, wrist, and hand range of motion (ROM) exercises should be incorporated immediately. Submaximal isometrics for shoulder internal/external rotators, flexors, and abductors may begin at 3 to 4 weeks. Active assisted ROM exercises should be progressed, delaying active abduction for up to 6 to 8 weeks. Care should be taken to ensure that exercises are performed in the scapular plane whenever possible. Full ROM should be restored by 8 to 10 weeks. Rhythmic stabilization of the scapulothoracic and glenohumeral joints is incorporated later and progresses as tolerated to promote dynamic stabilization. Strengthening typically progresses from supine to side-lying, sitting, and standing. Isotonic exercises via small handheld weights or elastic tubing typically begins in 4 to 6 weeks. Further progression and rehabilitation should be based on the needs of the individual patient.

24. How is the Neer impingement test performed?

With the patient sitting or standing, the examiner places one hand posteriorly over the scapula and grasps the patient's elbow. With the patient's scapula stabilized, the shoulder is maximally passively flexed overhead, compressing the greater tuberosity against the anteroinferior border of the acromion. Shoulder pain and apprehension indicate a positive sign—involvement most likely of the supraspinatus and possibly of the long head of the biceps tendon.

25. How is the Hawkins-Kennedy impingement test performed?

With the patient sitting or standing and the upper extremities relaxed, the examiner forward flexes the shoulder to 90 degrees and then forcibly internally rotates the shoulder. This action pushes the supraspinatus tendon against the anterior surface of the coracoacromial arch. A positive finding is denoted by pain and apprehension.

26. Describe the reverse impingement sign.

In the presence of a positive painful arc or pain with external rotation, the patient lies supine. The examiner pushes the humeral head inferiorly while simultaneously abducting and externally rotating the shoulder. The test is considered positive for mechanical impingement if the pain is decreased or abolished.

27. Describe the cross-over impingement test.

With the patient seated, the examiner places one hand over the posterior aspect of the scapula to stabilize the trunk and with the other hand grasps the patient's elbow. With the trunk stabilized, the examiner maximally adducts the shoulder horizontally. Superior shoulder pain indicates acromioclavicular joint pathology, whereas anterior shoulder pain may indicate subscapularis, supraspinatus, and/or long head of the biceps tendon pathology. Posterior shoulder pain may indicate pathology of the infraspinatus, teres minor, and/or posterior joint capsule.

28. What is the painful arc sign?

A painful arc refers to a particular ROM that is painful. Usually it is preceded and followed by normal, pain-free ROM and indicates mechanical compression of pain-sensitive tissue such as the supraspinatus or infraspinatus tendon, subacromial bursa, or bicipital tendon. The most common range for a painful arc is 60 to 120 degrees of humeral elevation.

29. How is the supraspinatus or empty can test performed?

The patient stands with both shoulders abducted to 90 degrees, in the scapular plane (horizontally adducted 30 degrees), and internally rotated in such a position that the thumbs point toward the floor. The examiner applies resistance against abduction. Pain and/or weakness indicates a tear of the supraspinatus or injury to the suprascapular nerve.

30. Describe the drop-arm test.

With the patient standing or sitting, the examiner passively places the involved shoulder in 90 degrees of abduction, asking the patient to lower the arm slowly to the side. A positive sign, defined as inability to lower the arm slowly to the side or reproduction of significant pain, indicates a tear in the rotator cuff.

31. What is the lift-off sign?

Standing with the dorsum of the hand placed against the back pocket, the patient lifts the hand away from the back. Inability to perform this task or pain may indicate a lesion of the subscapularis. This maneuver also can produce abnormal scapular motion, indicating scapular instability, and is used to assess rhomboid muscle strength.

32. Describe the drop sign.

The examiner places the patient's arm in 90 degrees of elbow flexion, 90 degrees of abduction, and almost full external rotation. When the arm is released, the patient is asked to maintain the same position. A drop or lag indicates infraspinatus attenuation or insufficiency related to weakness often related to tearing.

33. What are the lag signs of the shoulder?

- **External rotation lag sign**—The examiner places the patient's arm passively in 90 degrees of elbow flexion, 20 degrees of shoulder elevation (in scapular plane), and nearly full external rotation. The examiner then lets go of the wrist support while supporting the elbow. The test is positive for supraspinatus or infraspinatus pathology if the patient cannot maintain the position. The lag is recorded to the nearest 5 degrees.
- **Internal rotation lag sign**—The patient's elbow is passively flexed 90 degrees, the shoulder is held in 20 degrees of extension and 20 degrees of elevation, and the arm is placed behind the patient's back. The hand is passively lifted off the back, and support is maintained on the elbow but released from the wrist. Lag is recorded to the nearest 5 degrees and indicates subscapularis tearing.

34. What are the sensitivity and specificity of the various tests for rotator cuff pathology?

Test	Sensitivity (%)	Specificity (%)
Neer impingement test	89	25
Hawkins-Kennedy impingement test	92	25
Cross-over test	82	28
Painful arc sign	33	81
Drop-arm test	8	97
Jobe	84	58
Lift-off sign	62	100
Internal rotation lag test	97	96
External rotation lag test	70	100
Drop sign	20	100
Yergason's test	37	86
Speed's test (palm-up test)	69	56

35. Can the supraspinatus manual muscle test predict the size of a rotator cuff tear?

Yes, especially as it relates to large and massive rotator cuff tears. Large and massive rotator cuff tears result in approximately a 50% reduction in strength when compared to the noninvolved side (testing performed in 10 degrees of shoulder abduction with focus on the supraspinatus).

36. How accurate is a clinical examination of the shoulder in predicting rotator cuff pathology?

The sensitivity of a clinical exam of the shoulder (which includes the use of various shoulder-special tests) is approximately 91% with a specificity of 75%. Data that assist in the specific diagnosis of a rotator cuff tear are age of the patient (>40 years), previous trauma (minor), and degenerative changes on radiologic examination. Thus a good clinical examination is accurate and more cost-effective than a battery of radiologic studies in diagnosing rotator cuff pathology.

37. What clinical tests are most predictive for a rotator cuff tear?

According to Murrell and Walton, three simple tests are highly predictive of rotator cuff tear: supraspinatus weakness, weakness in external rotation, and impingement sign. When all three of these clinical tests were positive, or if two tests were positive and the patient was aged 60 or older, the individual had a 98% chance of having a rotator cuff tear. Furthermore, the investigators reported that any patient with a positive drop-arm sign also has a 98% chance of rotator cuff tear. If none of the aforementioned clinical features are present, the chance of rotator cuff tear diminishes to only 5%. The predictive influence of clustering these three clinical tests is comparable to the best results for magnetic resonance imaging and ultrasonography, and as suggested by the investigators, easier to perform and more cost-effective.

38. Which imaging study—plain radiographs, arthrography, or ultrasonography—is more accurate in diagnosing a rotator cuff tear?

- **Standard radiographs** reveal bony avulsions, calcific deposits, sclerotic areas, traction spurs, and other conditions associated with rotator cuff pathology, such as AC arthritis, calcific tendinitis, tuberosity displacement, and upward displacement of the head of the humerus in relation to the glenoid and the acromion.
- The **single contrast arthrogram** has been considered the gold standard technique for the diagnosis of rotator cuff tears. Recent literature suggests that the arthrogram has an accuracy of 82%. In addition, it has a sensitivity of 50% and specificity of 96% when used to evaluate full-thickness rotator cuff tears. Other research has reported the arthrogram to have a 0 to 8% probability of a false negative.
- **Ultrasonography,** when performed by experienced clinicians, can reveal noninvasively and non-radiographically not only rotator cuff integrity but also the thickness and location of the tear(s). The diagnostic sensitivity (98%) and specificity (91%) of ultrasonography have been compared with surgical findings. Matsen et al. suggest that expert ultrasonography provides the most efficient and cost-effective method for imaging of rotator cuff tendons.

39. Are there radiographic findings associated with symptomatic rotator cuff tears?

Pearsall et al. documented rotator cuff tears (n = 40) with asymptomatic age-matched controls (n = 84) using three views: acromioclavicular joint view, AP view with 30 degrees of external rotation, and supraspinatus outlet view. They reported that subjects with rotator cuff tear demonstrate radiographic findings (e.g., greater tuberosity sclerosis, osteophytes, subchondral cysts, and osteolysis) that are not observed in asymptomatic individuals. They also noted that in patients with small to moderate rotator cuff tears, acromial morphology and spurring were not predictive of a full-thickness rotator cuff tear.

40. How accurate is magnetic resonance imaging (MRI) at determining a rotator cuff tear?

Although commonly used, MRI is controversial. Recent literature has reported 78% accuracy, 81% sensitivity, and 78% specificity in determining full-thickness rotator cuff tears. Other researchers have reported an accuracy of 80% and sensitivity and specificity values of 92% and 93%, respectively. MRI appears to be slightly less accurate than arthrography. However, arthrography is not as good at imaging partial-thickness rotator cuff tears, whereas an MRI in the hands of a trained individual can provide valuable information about extent, location, and classification of rotator cuff pathology.

41. What are the outcomes of rehabilitation for rotator cuff disease?

Early surgical intervention is recommended in patients with rotator cuff disease who have greater than 12 months' duration of symptoms, severe functional impairment, or a confirmed rotator cuff tear greater than 1 cm. All other patients should undergo a minimum of 18 months of conservative management, including NSAIDs, physical therapy, and subacromial injection. Of these patients, 76% can anticipate a good or excellent result in 6 to 12 months. Of patients with impingement syndrome without rotator cuff tear, 85% will experience a good or excellent result with conservative management of at least 18 months.

42. What are the expected ROM, strength, pain, and function of a patient with rotator cuff repair at 1 and 5 years?

Problems with analyzing outcomes after rotator cuff repair are due to variable accuracy in describing preoperative functional levels, extent and location of the tears, tissue quality, follow-up schedule, and postoperative functional status. Cofield's investigations describing the outcomes of rotator cuff repair reported improvements in pain (averaging 87%) and patient overall satisfaction rates of 77%. Hawkins et al. reported pain relief in 86% of patients; 78% were able to perform activities of daily living (ADLs) above the level of the shoulder after repair compared with only 16% before repair. Neer et al. reported excellent (77%) or satisfactory (14%) results in 91% of patients (n = 233) after rotator cuff repair at an average follow-up of 4.6 years. Gore et al. reported subjective improvement in 95% of patients (n = 63), including significant pain relief and minimal-to-no limitations in ADL function at an average follow-up of 5.5 years. In the same series, flexion ROM averaged 126 degrees actively and 147 degrees passively. Matsen et al. reported that patients with intact repairs at 5-year follow-up averaged flexion of 132 degrees, external rotation (at 90 degrees of abduction) of 71 degrees, and functional internal rotation to T7. At least 12 months is required to restore strength after rotator cuff repair; the most significant increases are noted 6 to 12 months after surgery. Walker et al. reported that isokinetic abductor strength returned to 80% of normal (uninvolved shoulder) and external rotation to 90% of normal after 1 year. Rokito et al., reporting isokinetic torques after rotator cuff repair at 1 year, demonstrated side-to-side comparisons (involved/uninvolved) for flexion, abduction, and external rotation of 84%, 90%, and 91%, respectively. Brems et al. reported that the strength of the external rotators of the repaired shoulder was 71% of the uninvolved shoulder.

43. What percentage of patients undergoing rotator cuff repair have a favorable outcome?

Favorable outcomes after rotator cuff repair include reduction in pain and increases in strength, ROM, and ADL function. Favorable outcomes are achieved in more than 75% of patients undergoing rotator cuff repair. However, some studies have reported satisfactory results in upward of 90% of patients.

44. What is the clinical outcome of a patient suffering structural failure of a rotator cuff repair?

Jost et al. reported that patients who ruptured a repaired rotator cuff reported a subjective shoulder outcome score of approximately 75% of the normal study. Fifty-five percent of the subjects reported that they were very satisfied, 30% were satisfied, and 15% were disappointed with the outcome.

45. Does open or arthroscopic acromioplasty provide a better result?

According to Van Holsbeeck et al. patients receiving open or arthroscopic acromioplasty demonstrated no significant difference at a 2-year follow-up. However, Hawkins has reported 87% satisfaction with open acromioplasty versus 40% satisfaction with arthroscopic technique. Although much of the literature seems to support both open and arthroscopic techniques, interpretation is difficult because not all patients begin with the same level of soft tissue involvement.

46. Should a patient with a confirmed rotator cuff tear undergo physical therapy? Can physical therapy make a rotator cuff tear worse?

Recent evidence supports the value of a supervised nonoperative strengthening program for chronic, full-thickness rotator cuff tears, although the range in improvement and overall satisfaction varies from 33% to 90%. However, an acute partial-thickness tear may progress if rehabilitation programs address rotator cuff strengthening too aggressively and in isolation.

47. What are the options for management of an irreparable rotator cuff tear secondary to arthropathy?

Because each patient has different levels of pain and functional disability, options for the management of arthropathy vary. Patients with mild degrees of pain usually are treated with analgesics and exercise programs to maintain levels of ADL function. Shoulder arthrodesis and total shoulder arthroplasty are options in severe cases.

48. When developing an outcome measure for shoulder function, is the evaluation of strength of the opposite shoulder important to measure?

Yes; the use of the contralateral limb as an internal control eliminates confounding variables such as age. Thus shoulder outcome tools should measure involved and uninvolved shoulder strength.

49. What are some of the common physical therapy interventions for shoulder (rotator cuff) pain, and are they effective?

According to a Cochrane Database Systematic Review, the following statements can be made regarding common physical therapy interventions for shoulder (rotator cuff) pain:
- Exercise (rotator cuff) is effective in the short-term recovery in rotator cuff disease.
- Exercise (rotator cuff) has long-term benefits with respect to function.
- Exercise and nonthrust mobilization (posterior/inferior glide of glenohumeral joint) are more effective than exercise alone.
- Laser is not any more effective than placebo for rotator cuff tendinitis.
- Ultrasound is of no additional benefit than exercise (rotator cuff) alone.

50. If a patient cannot attend formal physical therapy programs after surgical repair of the rotator cuff, is a standardized home program effective?

The literature has indicated that a standardized home program (to include written and video instructions) for patients following rotator cuff repair resulted in favorable outcomes in regards to range of motion, strength, and patient-reported outcomes.

Bibliography

Bartolozzi A, Andreychik D, Ahmad S: Determinants of outcome in the treatment of rotator cuff disease, *Clin Orthop Rel Res* 308:90-97,1994.

Blanchard T et al: Diagnostic and therapeutic impact of MRI and arthrography in the investigation of full-thickness rotator cuff tears, *Eur Radiol* 9:638-642, 1999.

Brotzman SB: Rehabilitation of the shoulder. In Jobe FW et al, editors: *Clinical orthopaedic rehabilitation,* St Louis, 1996, pp 91-141, Mosby.
Brems JJ: Digital muscle strength measurement in rotator cuff. *Am J Sports Med* 7:102-110, 1979.
Cofield RH: Current concepts review: rotator cuff disease of the shoulder, *J Bone Joint Surg* 67A:974-979, 1985.
Gore DR et al: Shoulder-muscle strength and range of motion following surgical repair of full-thickness rotator cuff tears, *J Bone Joint Surg* 68:266-272, 1986.
Green S, Buchbinder R, Hetrick S: Physiotherapy interventions for shoulder pain, *Cochrane Database Syst Rev* (2):CD004258, 2003.
Hawkins RJ et al: Surgery of full thickness rotator cuff tears, *J Bone Joint Surg* 67A:1349-1355, 1985.
Hawkins RJ et al: *Arthroscopic subacromial decompression: a two to four year follow-up*, Annual Meeting of Arthroscopy Association of North America, 1992.
Hertel R et al: Lag signs in the diagnosis of rotator cuff rupture, *J Shoulder Elbow Surg* 5:307-313, 1996.
Holtby R, Razmjou H: Validity of the supraspinatus test as a single clinical test in diagnosing patients with rotator cuff pathology, *J Orthop Sports Phys Ther* 32:194-200, 2002.
Jost B et al: Clinical outcome after structural failure of rotator cuff repairs, *J Bone Joint Surg* 82A:304-314, 2000.
Lashgari C, Yamaguchi K: Natural history and nonsurgical treatment of rotator cuff disorders. In Norris T, editor: *OKU shoulder and elbow 2,* Rosemont, Calif, 2002, pp 155-162, AAOS.
Matsen FA et al: *Practical evaluation and management of the shoulder,* Philadelphia, 1994, WB Saunders.
Murrell GAC, Walton JR: Diagnosis of rotator cuff tears, *Lancet: Res Lett* 357:769-770, 2001.
Neer CS II et al: *Tears of the rotator cuff: long-term results of anterior acromioplasty and repair,* ASES 4th Meeting, Atlanta, 1988.
Pearsall AW et al: Radiographic findings associated with symptomatic rotator cuff tears, *J Shoulder Elbow Surg* 12:122-127, 2003.
Reinhold MM et al: Electromyographic analysis of the rotator cuff and deltoid musculature during common shoulder external rotation exercises, *J Orthop Sports Phys Ther* 34:385-394, 2004.
Rockwood CA, Matsen FA: Rotator cuff. In *The shoulder,* ed 2, Philadelphia, 1998, pp 755-839, WB Saunders.
Roddey TS et al: A randomized controlled trial comparing 2 instructional approaches to home exercise instruction following arthroscopic full-thickness rotator cuff repair surgery, *J Orthop Sports Phys Ther* 32:548-559, 2002.
Rokito AS et al: Strength after surgical repair of the rotator cuff, *J Shoulder Elbow Surg* 5:12-17, 1996.
Rokito AS et al: Long-term functional outcome of repair of large and massive chronic tears of the rotator cuff, *J Bone Joint Surg Am* 81:991-997, 1999.
Smidt GL, editor: *J Orthop Sports Phys Ther (Special Issue)* 18(1), July 1993.
Wilk KW, editor: *J Orthop Sports Phys Ther (Special Issue)* 18(2), August 1993.
van Holsbeeck E et al: Subacromial impingement: open versus arthroscopic decompression, *Arthroscopy* 8:173-178, 1992.
Walker SW et al: Isokinetic strength of the shoulder after repair of a torn rotator cuff, *J Bone Joint Surg* 69:1041-1044, 1987.

Chapter 39

Shoulder Instability

Michael L. Voight, PT, DHSc, OCS

1. How do the size, shape, and orientation of the glenoid fossa affect glenohumeral joint stability?

The glenoid cavity can be described as an irregularly shaped oval, much like an inverted comma. On the basis of studies conducted by Saha, the average height is 35 mm and the average width is 25 mm. Saha also demonstrated that in 75% of the specimens examined, the glenoid fossa was retroverted approximately 7 degrees. In the remaining 25%, the glenoid was anteverted from 2 to 10 degrees. The glenoid is also tilted from superomedial to inferolateral an average of 15 degrees. The depth of the fossa is enhanced by the glenoid labrum, which can contribute up to 50% of the fossa's depth.

2. Describe the passive stabilizing mechanisms for the glenohumeral joint.

Passive stability is provided by the bony geometry, glenoid labrum, limited joint volume, negative intra-articular pressure, adhesion and cohesion, and capsuloligamentous structures. The glenohumeral joint has a slightly negative pressure of −4.0 mm Hg, which creates a relative vacuum. As long as the relative vacuum effect is maintained, limited joint volume does not allow the joint surfaces to be easily distracted or subluxated.

The close match of the articular surfaces produces intermolecular forces of surface tension, cohesion, and adhesion, which provide continued coupling of the humerus to the glenoid. Adhesion refers to the attraction of unlike substances (joint fluid to bone), whereas cohesion refers to the attraction of like substances (joint fluid to joint fluid). In addition, the glenoid labrum deepens the fossa by 5 mm in an anteroposterior direction and by 9 mm in the superior and inferior direction.

3. What are the primary static stabilizers of the glenohumeral joint?

The superior, middle, and inferior glenohumeral ligaments provide anterior stability. With the arm in the adducted position, the superior glenohumeral and coracohumeral ligaments act in a suspensory role to resist inferior translation of the humeral head. As the arm is brought up into the mid range of abduction, the middle glenohumeral ligament provides more of a stabilizing role. In addition, as the arm is abducted to 45 degrees and beyond, the anterior and posterior portions of the inferior glenohumeral ligament complex become the stabilizers to resist inferior translation. Above 90 degrees of abduction, the inferior glenohumeral ligament becomes the primary stabilizing function. The anterior band of the inferior glenohumeral ligament complex is the primary restraint to anterior translation at 90 degrees of abduction. Posterior stabilization of the glenohumeral joint with the arm at 90 degrees of abduction is provided primarily by the posterior band of the inferior glenohumeral ligament complex.

4. Describe the mechanisms for achieving dynamic stability at the glenohumeral joint.

Stability is achieved through three mechanisms: (1) joint compression of matching concave-convex surfaces as the muscles press the humeral head into the fossa; (2) synergistic, coordinated contraction of the rotator cuff muscles, acting to steer the humeral head into the glenoid in different positions of arm rotation; and (3) dynamization or tensioning of the glenohumeral ligaments through the direct attachment or blending of the rotator cuff tendons into the glenohumeral capsule and ligaments. In addition, the glenoid fossa has an upward, lateral, and forward orientation that serves as a shelf for the humeral head. This source of stability is provided by the normal muscle control of the scapular protractors. When these muscles (serratus anterior, upper trapezius) become weakened, dynamic stability may be lost and the humeral head may simply slide down and off the near vertical glenoid fossa.

5. What is the most common direction and mechanism of injury causing shoulder instability?

Subcoracoid anterior dislocation is the most common direction of dislocation. The most common mechanism of injury for anterior shoulder dislocation is an indirect force with the arm in an abducted, extended, and externally rotated position. The majority of dislocations result from trauma.

6. What is the most common nerve injury after anterior shoulder dislocation?

Injury to the axillary nerve has an overall incidence of approximately 30%. The risk of axillary nerve injury increases with age, duration of dislocation, and force of trauma. The most common type of axillary nerve injury is traction neurapraxia. Because the axillary nerve originates at the posterior cord of the brachial plexus and its anterior branch (humeral circumflex) wraps directly around the humeral wall in the area of the surgical neck, the nerve can be exposed to trauma. Anterior dislocation may cause traction to the portion of the axillary nerve lying in close relation to the capsular structures. Most patients respond to conservative treatment over 10 weeks.

7. Describe the most common mechanism of posterior shoulder dislocation.

A posterior dislocation results most commonly from axial loading of the arm in an adducted, flexed, and internally rotated position. The classic mechanism of injury is either a blow to the front of the shoulder or a fall onto the outstretched arm. Lesser tuberosity fractures are common and often cause the humeral head to become locked in the dislocated position. Posterior dislocations are less common than anterior and account for only 2% to 4% of all dislocations.

8. Why is posterior shoulder dislocation more likely than anterior dislocation after electric shock or convulsive seizures?

Electric shock and convulsive seizures can result in violent contracture of all muscle groups surrounding the shoulder girdle. The combined strength of the latissimus dorsi, pectoralis major, and subscapularis overwhelms the infraspinatus and teres minor muscles by virtue of greater muscle bulk. As a result, the stronger internal rotators simply overpower the relatively weaker external rotators, resulting in a posterior dislocation.

9. What is multidirectional instability with atraumatic onset?

Multidirectional instability is a symptomatic glenohumeral subluxation or dislocation in more than one direction. The basic pathologic changes of multidirectional instability include (1) a loose, redundant, or torn joint capsule; (2) a lax ligamentous mechanism; and (3) a weakened musculotendinous system.

10. In describing shoulder instability, what is meant by the acronym TUBS?

- **T**—Traumatic onset
- **U**—Unidirectional (anterior)
- **B**—Bankart lesion (usually present)
- **S**—Surgery (success rate with nonoperative treatment is >20%)

11. What is meant by the acronym AMBRI in describing shoulder instability?

- **A**—Atraumatic onset
- **M**—Multidirectional in nature
- **B**—Bilateral (usually)
- **R**—Rehabilitation (success with conservative treatment is usually >80%)
- **I**—Inferior capsular shift (procedure of choice if conservative treatment fails)

12. What type of lesion is characterized by the by the acronym ALPSA?

The ALPSA lesion as originally described by Neviaser stands for **A**nterior **L**abroligamentous **P**eriosteal **S**leeve **A**vulsion. This will often accompany a traumatic anterior dislocation and is characterized by the labrum and periosteal sleeve of the anterior glenoid being avulsed and displaced medially.

13. What type of lesion is characterized by the acronym HAGL?

The HAGL lesion occurs with traumatic dislocation when the arm is forced into a hyperabducted position. The acronym stands for **H**umeral **A**vulsion of the **G**lenohumeral **L**igament.

14. Describe the load-shift test.

The load-shift test allows evaluation of glenohumeral translation. A compressive axial load is applied to the humeral head to reduce it into the glenoid. This reduction is important because the humeral head may be resting in a subluxated position, which may give a false sense of the direction of the instability. Anterior and posterior forces then are placed on the proximal humerus, and the direction and degree of translation are determined.

15. Describe the anterior release test.

The patient is supine and the shoulder is placed in 90-degree abduction and 90-degree external rotation (apprehension position) while a posterior-directed force is applied to the humeral head (anterior surface of shoulder). The posterior force is then released; if the patient experiences pain and apprehension, then the test is considered positive.

16. What are the sensitivity and specificity of commonly performed shoulder instability tests?

Test	Sensitivity (%)	Specificity (%)
Load-shift (under anesthesia)	83*	100
Sulcus sign	Not reported	Not reported
Apprehension	57	100
Relocation	30	50
Anterior release	92	89
M&IGHL/PC tests	Not reported	Not reported

*Hawkins suggests it may be overly sensitive.

17. What type of grading scheme is used to assess increased glenohumeral translation?

Anterior translation of 25% or less of the humeral head diameter is considered normal. Hawkins suggested a grading system that may be more appropriate for reporting the test result than distance or percentages:

- Grade I—The humeral head can be felt to ride up the face of the glenoid to the glenoid rim but cannot be felt to move over the rim edge. Grade I corresponds to approximately up to 50% of humeral head translation.
- Grade II—The humeral head can be felt to move over the glenoid rim but reduces with release of pressure, corresponding to clinical subluxation. For grade II the humeral head has more than 50% translation.
- Grade III—The head remains dislocated on release, corresponding to clinical dislocation.

18. Describe the clinical tests for posterior shoulder instability.

In addition to the load-shift test, posterior instability can be assessed with the jerk test. The arm is flexed to 90 degrees with internal rotation, and an axial load is delivered to the shoulder in a posterior direction. The arm is brought into a horizontally adducted position, and posterior slippage is noted. The arm then is brought back into a horizontally abducted position. A jerk may be experienced when the humeral head relocates onto the glenoid fossa.

19. What radiologic studies and views are best suited for confirming or evaluating shoulder instability?

The recommended views in a trauma series include a true anteroposterior (AP) view, a true scapular lateral view, and an axillary view. The most commonly obtained views of the shoulder include the AP view of the shoulder with the humerus in both internal and external rotation, a true AP of the glenoid view, a scapulolateral (Y) view, an axillary view, a West Point projection, and a Stryker notch view.

20. Describe the Hill-Sachs and reverse Hill-Sachs lesions.

The Hill-Sachs lesion is a compression fracture of the posterolateral aspect of the humeral head. It results from impact on the anteroinferior rim of the glenoid during an anterior dislocation of the shoulder. A reverse Hill-Sachs lesion involves a compression fracture of the anteromedial humeral head as the result of a posterior dislocation.

21. What is the suggested radiologic view to visualize a Hill-Sachs lesion?

The Hill-Sachs lesion is demonstrated best by either the internal rotation or the Stryker notch views; each has a sensitivity of 92%. The detection of a Hill-Sachs lesion is prognostically important because patients with a Hill-Sachs lesion may be prone to redislocation.

22. What is a Bankart lesion? What is its significance?

A Bankart lesion is an avulsion or detachment of the anterior portion of the inferior glenohumeral ligament complex and glenoid labrum off the anterior rim of the glenoid. Although a Bankart lesion can contribute to increased translation of the humeral head, complete dislocation requires associated capsular injury. Bankart lesions can contribute to recurrent instability.

23. Describe the clinical presentation of a posterior shoulder dislocation.

Observation is often difficult because most patients hold the shoulder in the traditional sling position of adduction and internal rotation. External rotation usually is limited, and it is not uncommon to find the posteriorly dislocated shoulder locked into internal rotation secondary to a fracture of the lesser tuberosity. Observation usually reveals a prominent coracoid process and a flattening of the anterior aspect of the shoulder.

24. What is the suggested initial medical treatment for anterior shoulder dislocation? Why is early relocation important?

Initial treatment includes application of ice and use of a sling. Acute glenohumeral dislocations should be reduced as quickly and gently as possible because early relocation quickly reduces stretch and compression of neurovascular structures, minimizes the degree of muscle spasm that must be overcome to reduce the joint, and prevents progressive enlargement of the humeral head defect in the locked dislocation.

25. Following reduction for an anterior dislocation, should the arm be immobilized in internal or external rotation?

Postreduction management after traumatic anterior shoulder dislocation is controversial. A 10-year prospective study by Hovelius comparing immobilization with no immobilization found no difference in recurrence rates. The position of immobilization is also controversial. Itoi investigated immobilizing the arm in internal rotation (IR) or external rotation (ER) after initial traumatic anterior dislocation. The recurrence rate was approximately 30% in the IR group and 0% in the ER group at a mean follow-up time of 15.5 months, suggesting external rotation as the position of immobilization. However, it is still more customary to immobilize the arm in IR at this time.

26. What is the most common complication in managing a traumatic anterior dislocation?

Recurrence is the most common complication. Other complications include fractures of the humerus, vascular injuries, neural injuries, and rotator cuff tears (more common in patients >40 years).

27. What accounts for the high incidence of recurrent dislocation?

Several factors have been identified as contributing to recurrence and instability. Age at the time of onset correlates most closely to recurrence. Patients under the age of 20 years may have a recurrence rate up to 80%, whereas after the age of 40 the rate drops to under 10%. Males have a higher recurrence rate than females, and most recurrences are seen within 2 years of the initial traumatic dislocation. The recurrence rate varies inversely with the severity of the initial trauma. If dislocation occurs a second time in younger patients, the chance of frequent recurrence is almost 100%.

28. What is the incidence of associated rotator cuff tears in patients older than 40 years? Why is the rate increased?

The incidence of rotator cuff tears after acute dislocation in patients older than 40 years ranges from 35% to 86%. The reason for the variability in numbers is the unknown amount of rotator cuff pathology before the initial dislocation. With dislocation of the humeral head anteriorly, the anterior and/or posterior structures are disrupted. With dislocations in younger patients, the anterior capsuloligamentous complex tends to disrupt because it is less strong than other tissues in the shoulder. In older patients, the posterior structures (rotator cuff and greater tuberosity complex) are weaker by attrition and tend to disrupt, leaving the anterior capsuloligamentous complex intact.

29. What nonoperative management is appropriate after anterior shoulder dislocation?

After an initial period of immobilization, a regimen of shoulder rehabilitation should be implemented. Initially, range of motion exercises are instituted to help prevent stiffness. Positions of abduction and external rotation should be avoided to prevent excessive stress on the anterior capsule. Strengthening of the shoulder musculature is of paramount importance to improve dynamic stability. Because the capsular stabilizing structures are compromised, the shoulder has a greater dependence on dynamic stabilizing mechanisms. Early focus is placed on the stabilizers of the scapula. The scapula must provide a stable base on which the humerus can rotate and maintain the glenoid in a position that provides maximal congruence with the humeral head. The core scapular exercises are scaption, protraction, retraction, and seated press-up.

Once scapular stability is addressed, emphasis is placed on reestablishing the strength of the rotator cuff musculature, which is the main dynamic stabilizer of the glenohumeral joint. Exercises should be performed in the scapular plane, which provides the greatest congruence between the humeral head and glenoid and minimizes the stress placed on the anterior capsule. The supraspinatus can be isolated with prone horizontal abduction and external rotation. Activation of the teres minor and infraspinatus draws the humeral head posteriorly and thus unloads the stress on the damaged anterior structures. These two muscles are best isolated with prone external rotation with the arm positioned in 90-degree abduction. In addition to strengthening exercises, proprioception exercises should be used to enhance the patient's sense of position.

30. What nonoperative management is appropriate after posterior shoulder dislocation?

Reduction is accomplished by longitudinal forward traction on the arm with the elbow bent, accompanied by anterior pressure on the humeral head. The arm then is brought into an adducted, externally rotated, and internally rotated position to reduce the humeral head back into the glenoid fossa.

Principles of nonoperative treatment include pain management, activity modification, and a shoulder strengthening program involving the scapular and rotator cuff musculature. Nonoperative treatment produces superior results in posterior instability compared with anterior instability. The joint is immobilized for only 2 to 3 weeks in a handshake cast. Integral to the strengthening program is the periscapular and rotator cuff musculature. External rotation and posterior deltoid strengthening are emphasized during rehabilitation. Push-ups and bench press activities should be avoided. The patient must be instructed to avoid activities that place the shoulder at the limits of flexion, internal rotation, or horizontal adduction. Otherwise the shoulder may redislocate.

31. What nonoperative management is appropriate for multidirectional instability?

Overall, patients tend to respond well to rehabilitation. Aggressive physical therapy with strengthening of the scapular stabilizers and rotator cuff musculature frequently provides sufficient dynamic stability. If the patient does not respond to conservative treatment, an inferior capsular shift should be included as part of the surgical procedure.

32. Describe the modern surgical management of patients for whom operative treatment is advisable.

Several different surgical procedures are used to control shoulder instability. The success and/or failure rate for each is quite variable and highly dependent on the skill of the surgeon. Currently, the gold standard is some variation of capsulorrhaphy, which directly affects the size and/or orientation of the glenohumeral capsule:

- Bankart repair—suturing of the anterior capsule and labrum to the anterior glenoid rim
- Capsular shift—tightening of the joint capsule, depending on the precise amount and location of laxity
- Staple capsulorrhaphy—securing the detached anterior capsule and labrum onto the glenoid
- Thermal capsulorrhaphy—thermal shrinkage of the capsular collagen tissue to restore normal stability
- Putti-Platt procedure—subscapularis and capsular shortening

33. How does the outcome of immediate surgical stabilization compare to the nonoperative management of shoulder instability in the young, healthy adult?

Kirkley conducted a prospective randomized clinical trial comparing the effectiveness of immediate arthroscopic stabilization versus immobilization and rehabilitation in first time, traumatic anterior shoulder dislocations. At an average of 32 months' follow-up, a significant reduction in redislocation and an improvement in disease-specific quality of life were afforded by early arthroscopic stabilization in patients less than 30 years of age with a first-time, traumatic anterior dislocation of the shoulder.

The Bankart lesion was noted in a very high percentage of traumatic first-time dislocations—97% in one series of patients who underwent arthroscopic evaluation soon after their injury. The standard of care in the overhead athlete is early repair of the capsular structures. With the Bankart lesion, the capsulolabral complex avulses from the glenoid. If the anteroinferior labrum and capsule do not heal in their anatomic position, the depth of the concavity will be lost in that isolated area, thereby contributing to an increased recurrence rate, especially when the arm is placed in a position of abduction and external rotation. Early stabilization in athletic high risk patients should diminish progressive soft tissue and bony damage.

34. How does surgical repair of shoulder instability affect proprioceptive ability?

Potzl et al. examined the proprioceptive ability (joint repositioning) of patients with recurrent anterior shoulder instability preoperatively and at at least 5 years postoperatively. At 5 years postoperatively, the joint position sense improved significantly, to the level of normal, healthy shoulders.

35. What are SLAP lesions?

Superior labrum anterior and posterior (SLAP) lesions most often result from a sudden downward force on a supinated outstretched upper extremity or from a fall on the lateral shoulder. Patients complain of popping and sliding of the shoulder, especially with overhead activities. The average time to diagnosis from onset of symptoms is about 2.5 years.

36. What are the types of a SLAP lesion?

In 1990 Stephen Snyder coined the name SLAP lesion to describe a more extensive injury pattern involving the superior labrum. Snyder further classified superior labrum disorders into four types:

- Type I—degenerative fraying of the labrum
- Type II—avulsion of the superior labrum and biceps tendon
- Type III—bucket-handle tears of the superior labrum
- Type IV—same as grade II or III with extension into the biceps tendon

Maffet and co-workers described additional types of SLAP lesions:

- Type V—an anterior-inferior Bankart lesion that propagates superiorly to the biceps tendon
- Type VI—an unstable flap tear of the labrum with separation of the biceps anchor
- Type VII—a superior biceps-labral detachment that extends anteriorly beneath the middle glenohumeral ligament

37. Describe the special tests used to evaluate SLAP lesions.

- **O'Brien test**—The patient's arm is placed in flexion to 90 degrees with full internal rotation and horizontal adduction. The patient then attempts to resist a forward (extension) force at the wrist. Pain indicates a positive test.
- **SLAP test**—The patient's extended/supinated arm is abducted to 90 degrees. The examiner pushes down at the wrist while using the thumb of the opposite hand to shift the humeral head in a superior direction. Crepitus and pain are considered positive findings.
- **Load-shift test**—The examiner's thumb is used to push the humeral head superiorly and anteriorly while the arm is held in abduction and external rotation with the elbow flexed.

- **Kibler test**—The patient places the hand on the hip. The examiner pushes anteriorly on the humeral head while an anterior superior force is applied to the humerus through the elbow.

38. What are the sensitivity and specificity of commonly performed tests to determine the presence of a SLAP or Bankart lesion?

Test	Sensitivity (%)	Specificity (%)
Active compression	54-100	11-98.5
Anterior slide	8-78	84-91
Crank test	35-91	56-93
Clunk test	Not reported	Not reported
MRI	42-89	88-92

In general the physical tests appear to be more specific than sensitive.

39. Describe the treatment for SLAP lesions.

Many patients respond well to nonsteroidal antiinflammatory drugs, cortisone injection, or rehabilitation of the rotator cuff and periscapular stabilizers, limiting strengthening to <90 degrees. Patients failing nonoperative management are candidates for arthroscopic debridement (types I and III) and repair (types II and IV) using suture anchors, absorbable tacks, or transglenoid fixation (Caspari technique).

Bibliography

Bahr R, Craig EV, Engebretson L: The clinical presentation of shoulder instability including on field management, *Clin Sports Med* 14:761-776, 1995.

Bigliani LU, editor: *The unstable shoulder,* Chicago, 1996, American Academy of Orthopedic Surgeons.

Bottoni CR et al: A prospective, randomized evaluation of arthroscopic stabilization versus nonoperative treatment in patients with acute, traumatic, first-time shoulder dislocations, *Am J Sports Med* 30:576-580, 2002.

Burkhead WZ, Rockwood CA: Treatment of instability of the shoulder with an exercise program, *J Bone Joint Surg* 74A:890-896, 1992.

Cleeman E, Flatow EL: Shoulder dislocations in the young patient, *Orthop Clin North Am* 31:217-229, 2000.

Dines DM, Levinson M: The conservative management of the unstable shoulder including rehabilitation, *Clin Sports Med* 14:797-816, 1995.

Hawkins RJ, Misamore GW: *Shoulder injuries in the athlete,* New York, 1996, Churchill Livingstone.

Hovelius L: Primary anterior dislocation of the shoulder in young patients: a ten year prospective study, *J Bone Joint Surg* 78A:1677-1684, 1996.

Itoi E et al: A new method of immobilization after traumatic anterior dislocation of the shoulder: a preliminary study, *J Shoulder Elbow Surg* 12:413-415, 2003.

Kirkley A et al: Prospective randomized clinical trial comparing the effectiveness of immediate arthroscopic stabilization versus immobilization and rehabilitation in first traumatic anterior dislocations of the shoulder, *Arthroscopy* 15:507-514, 1999.

Maffet MW, Gartsman GM, Moseley B: Superior labrum-biceps tendon complex lesions of the shoulder, *Am J Sports Med* 23:93-98, 1995.

Matsen FA et al: Glenohumeral instability. In Rockwood MA, Matsen FA, editors: *The shoulder,* Philadelphia, 1998, WB Saunders.

Mosely JB et al: EMG analysis of the scapular muscles during a shoulder rehabilitation program, *Am J Sports Med* 20:128-134, 1992.

Neer CS: Involuntary inferior and multidirectional instability of the shoulder: etiology, recognition, and treatment, *Instr Course Lect* 34:232-238, 1985.

Nord KD, Masterson JP, Mauck BM: Superior labrum anterior posterior (SLAP) repair using the Neviaser portal, *Arthroscopy* 20(suppl 2):129-133, 2004.
Petersen SA: Posterior shoulder instability, *Orthop Clin North Am* 31:263-274, 2000.
Potzl W et al: Proprioception of the shoulder joint after surgical repair for instability: a long-term follow-up study, *Am J Sports Med* 32:425-430, 2004.
Saha AK: Dynamic stability of the glenohumeral joint, *Acta Orthop Scand* 42:491-505, 1971.
Saha AK: Mechanism of shoulder movements and a plea for the recognition of the "zero" position of the glenohumeral joint, *Clin Orthop Scand* 173:11, 1983.
Snyder SJ et al: SLAP lesions of the shoulder, *Arthroscopy* 6:274-279, 1990.
Speer KP: Anatomy and pathomechanics of shoulder instability, *Clin Sports Med* 14:751-760, 1995.
Stayner LR et al: Shoulder dislocations in patients older than 40 years of age, *Orthop Clin North Am* 31:231-239, 2000.
Taylor D, Arciero R: Pathologic changes associated with shoulder dislocations, *Am J Sports Med* 25:306-311, 1997.
Tzannes A et al: An assessment of the interrater reliability of tests for shoulder instability, *J Shoulder Elbow Surg* 13:18-23, 2004.
Yuehuei H, Friedman RJ: Multidirectional instability of the glenohumeral joint, *Orthop Clin North Am* 31:275-283, 2000.

Chapter 40

Adhesive Capsulitis

Jeffrey D. Placzek, MD, PT

1. Describe the epidemiology of adhesive capsulitis.

Adhesive capsulitis, or "frozen shoulder," is more common in females than males and occurs most often in the age range of 40 to 60 years. Bilateral involvement is seen in about 12% of patients. The incidence is 2% in the general population and 10% to 35% in diabetic patients.

2. What are the predominant cell types in adhesive capsulitis? What growth factors are present?

Fibroblasts and myofibroblasts are the predominant cell types. The presence of type III collagen in those with adhesive capsulitis indicates new deposition of collagen within the capsule. The frequency of staining for transforming growth factor β, platelet-derived growth factor, and hepatocyte growth factor is greater in adhesive capsulitis tissue than in tissue from patients with nonspecific synovitis.

3. Define primary and secondary adhesive capsulitis.

Lundberg described stiff shoulder with insidious onset as **primary adhesive capsulitis.** Frozen shoulder after some type of trauma or inciting event is classified as **secondary adhesive capsulitis.**

4. What imaging techniques are useful for the diagnosis of adhesive capsulitis?

Plain films are useful in excluding other pathology, but no pathognomonic changes are associated with capsulitis. Arthrography is the gold standard for diagnosis. The normal capsular volume decreases from 25 ml to about 6 ml with obliteration of the biceps sheath, axillary fold, and subscapular bursa. Dynamic ultrasonography is 91% sensitive and 100% specific for the detection of capsulitis.

5. What MRI findings are associated with adhesive capsulitis?

Thickening of the coracohumeral ligament (CHL) to >4 mm is 95% specific and 59% sensitive for the diagnosis of adhesive capsulitis. Thickening of the capsule in the rotator interval to >7 mm has a specificity of 86% and sensitivity of 64%. Obliteration of the fat triangle between the CHL and the coracoid process was 100% specific but 32% sensitive.

6. Describe the natural resolution of adhesive capsulitis.

Reeves described the three classic stages of adhesive capsulitis:

- The early painful stage (freezing) lasts 2 to 9 months. Patients have diffuse pain and difficulty sleeping on the affected side. Patients begin to have restricted movement secondary to pain.
- The stiffening stage (freezing) lasts 4 to 12 months. Progressive loss of ROM and decreased function are noted.
- The recovery stage (thawing) lasts 5 to 24 months, with gradual increases in ROM and decreased pain.

7. What outcomes are associated with the natural resolution of adhesive capsulitis?

The time to resolution is quite variable, averaging 12 to 36 months. Approximately 20% to 60% of patients have some limitation in ROM and residual pain for up to 10 years.

8. What are the outcomes associated with a home stretching program for adhesive capsulitis?

Griggs et al. found that 90% of patients reported a satisfactory outcome. However, after 22 months, patients still had restricted range of motion as compared to the contralateral side. Abduction was 145 degrees, flexion was 155 degrees, passive internal rotation at 90 degrees of abduction was 29 degrees, and external rotation was 60 degrees.

9. What factors have been proposed in the pathogenesis of adhesive capsulitis?

Cervical spine disorders, autoimmune disorders, tendonitis, hypothyroidism, diabetes, hormonal disorders, and poor posture have been postulated as predisposing factors for capsulitis.

10. What is the role of physical therapy for the treatment of capsulitis?

Exercise has been found to be more effective than modalities, nonsteroidal antiinflammatory drugs, or steroid injections. Nicholson found that mobilization significantly improved ROM into abduction. However, mobilization offered no significant advantage over exercise alone in other motions. One study found mobilization to be more effective than manipulation for increasing ROM. Numerous case studies have found mobilization to be effective in treating adhesive capsulitis.

11. Do end range mobilization techniques improve range of motion in patients with adhesive capsulitis?

Vermeulen et al. found that passive abduction increased from 96 to 159 degrees, flexion increased from 122 to 154 degrees, external rotation increased from 21 to 41 degrees, and the mean glenohumeral capsular volume increased from 10 to 15 cc.

12. Does translational mobilization increase glenohumeral abduction?

In a cadaver model, Hsu et al. found increases in glenohumeral abduction after both ventral and dorsal translational mobilization. Small improvements in external rotation were found after ventral translational mobilization.

13. What outcomes are associated with steroid injections for capsulitis?

Although steroid injections may provide transient relief of pain, no studies show conclusive evidence that they increase ROM or function. This may be due to the fact that few studies differentiate between injections given at different stages of the disease.

14. How does translational manipulation differ from traditional long lever manipulation?

Translational manipulation uses linear forces applied at the humeral head to restore normal kinematic gliding associated with glenohumeral movements. By avoiding long lever forces, translational manipulation minimizes the stress applied to the brachial plexus as well as the glenohumeral, acromioclavicular, scapuloclavicular, and scapulothoracic joints.

15. What outcomes are associated with traditional long lever manipulation under anesthesia for capsulitis?

Despite reported complications of dislocation, fracture, brachial plexus injury, rotator cuff tearing, and failure to regain ROM secondary to pain, manipulation under anesthesia remains a proven treatment technique with a low incidence of the above complications. Hill and Bogumill reported significant increases in ROM immediately and in the long term (flexion = 139 degrees, abduction = 143 degrees, external rotation = 54 degrees, and internal rotation = 63 degrees) after manipulation.

16. What outcomes are associated with translational manipulation under anesthesia for capsulitis?

Placzek et al. reported significant increases in ROM immediately and in the long term (flexion = 163 degrees, abduction = 163 degrees, external rotation = 84 degrees, and internal rotation = 69 degrees) after manipulation. Furthermore, pain was significantly reduced (7.6/10 down to 1.5/10), and function was significantly increased (Wolfgang score of 5.5/16 increased to 14.1/16).

17. What outcomes are associated with the brisement technique (arthrographic distention)?

Distention arthrography in general provides minimal immediate increases in ROM. However, it speeds improvement in ROM over the next several weeks to months. The steroids and local anesthetics used usually provide some pain relief.

18. What outcomes are associated with arthroscopic release for capsulitis?

In general, ROM gains have been somewhat less than with manipulation under anesthesia. The best results have been published by Jerosch et al., where abduction improved from 75 to 165 degrees, external rotation improved from 3 to 75 degrees, external rotation and abduction improved from 4 to 81 degrees, and internal rotation improved from 17 to 59 degrees. Arthroscopic capsular release may be particularly helpful in recalcitrant cases in which therapy and manipulation have failed.

19. Is traditional long lever manipulation under anesthesia associated with intra-articular lesions?

Loew et al. found that in a group of 30 patients 22 had localized synovitis in the rotator interval and 8 had disseminated synovitis. After manipulation, the capsule was ruptured superiorly in 11 patients, anteriorly in 24, and posteriorly in 16. In 4 patients an iatrogenic SLAP lesion was found, 3 had partial tearing of the subscapularis, and 4 had anterior labral detachments. Two patients had tears of the middle glenohumeral ligament. Although manipulation is effective for increasing range of motion, certain iatrogenic intra-articular damage can occur.

Bibliography

Griggs SM, Ahn A, Green A: Idiopathic adhesive capsulitis. A prospective functional outcome study of nonoperative treatment, *J Bone Joint Surg* 82A:1398-1407, 2000.

Harryman DT, Lazarus MD, Rozencwaig R: The stiff shoulder. In Rockwood CA, Matsen FA, editors: *The shoulder,* ed 2, Philadelphia, 1998, pp 1064-1112, WB Saunders.

Hill JJ Jr, Bogumill H: Manipulation in the treatment of frozen shoulder, *Orthopedics* 11:1255-1260, 1988.

Hsu AT et al: Changes and abduction and rotation range of motion in response to simulated dorsal and ventral translational mobilization of the glenohumeral joint, *Phys Ther* 82:544-556, 2002.

Jerosch J: 360 degree arthroscopic capsular release in patients with adhesive capsulitis of the glenohumeral joint—indication, surgical technique, results, *Knee Surg Sports Traumatol Arthrosc* 9:178-186, 2001.

Loew M, Heichel TO, Lehner B: Intra-articular lesions in primary frozen shoulder after manipulation under general anesthesia, *J Shoulder Elbow Surg* 14:16-21, 2005.

Mengiardi B et al: Frozen shoulder: MR arthrographic findings, *Radiology* 233:486-492, 2004.

Placzek JD, Kulig K: Translational manipulation under anesthesia: new concepts in adhesive capsulitis management, *Orthop Phys Ther Clin North Am* 7:1-23, 1998.

Placzek JD et al: Long term effects of translational manipulation for adhesive capsulitis, *Clin Orthop* 356:181-191, 1998.

Placzek JD et al: Theory and technique of translational manipulation for adhesive capsulitis, *Am J Orthop* 4:173-179, 2004.

Vermeulen HM et al: End range mobilization techniques and adhesive capsulitis of the shoulder joint: a multiple subject case report, *Phys Ther* 80:1204-1213, 2000.

Chapter 41

Total Shoulder Arthroplasty

Tim L. Uhl, PT, PhD, ATC

1. Describe the typical patient who might undergo total shoulder arthroplasty (TSA).

Traditionally the age of the patient who undergoes TSA is 55 to 70 years. However, in cases of arthritis resulting from previous dislocation and avascular necrosis, the patient's age may be in the range of 40 to 50 years. Approximately equal numbers of males and females undergo TSA.

2. How many TSAs and hemiarthroplasties are performed each year?

Approximately 15,000 TSAs and hemiarthroplasties were performed in 1998 in the United States.

3. What are the typical indications for TSA?

Medical indications for TSA include osteoarthritis, osteoarthritis secondary to previous trauma such as shoulder instability or surgery, rheumatoid and other inflammatory arthritis, avascular necrosis of the humeral head, and rotator cuff tear arthropathy. Patients' symptoms often include shoulder pain, functional limitations in motion, and radiographic deterioration of the glenohumeral joint. Primary glenohumeral degenerative joint disease presents with central wearing of the humeral head, known as the "Friar Tuck" pattern of central baldness. The glenoid surface wears out primarily on the posterior margin, predisposing the joint to posterior subluxation.

4. What are the typical contraindications for TSA?

- Active infection
- Neurologic compromise of either deltoid or rotator cuff musculature
- Neurotrophic shoulder
- Unrealistic expectation of shoulder function after surgery
- Lack of appropriate motivation to perform rehabilitation program after surgery

5. What is the difference between unconstrained, constrained, and reverse TSA?

Unconstrained TSA more closely resembles normal anatomic configuration of the glenohumeral joint and allows more humeral motion (see figure). Constrained TSA uses a ball-and-socket design that makes the glenoid function more like a true ball-and-socket but reduces humeral motion.

A third type of prosthesis, called a reverse prosthesis, has been developed to place the ball component on the glenoid side and the socket on the humeral side (see figure). This design is advantageous for patients with a deficient cuff because it places the deltoid in a better biomechanical position by medializing the center of rotation so more fibers assist in elevation. The prosthesis can also be placed to lengthen the fibers of the deltoid to take advantage of the length-tension relationship, thereby improving function.

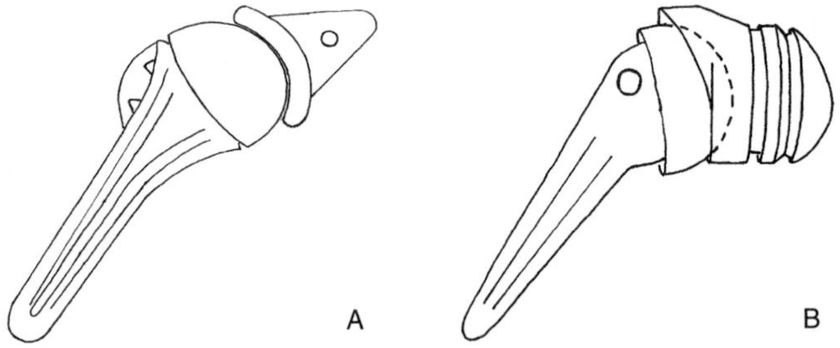

(A) Unconstrained total shoulder arthroplasty with standard polyethylene glenoid component. **(B)** Semiconstrained total shoulder arthroplasty with superior hooded glenoid component.

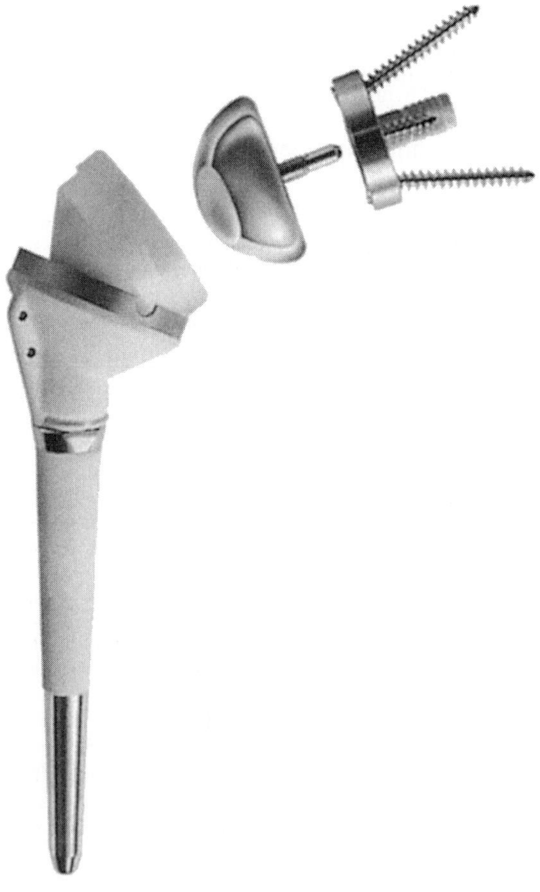

Reverse prosthesis total shoulder arthroplasty using the Delta III (Depuy International Ltd). *(From Boileau P et al: Grammont reverse prosthesis: design, rationale and biomechanics,* J Shoulder Elbow Surg *14(1, supplement):151s, 2005.)*

6. What is the difference between hemiarthroplasty and TSA?

Hemiarthroplasty is the replacement of the humeral component and is also known as humeral head replacement (HHR). A hemiarthroplasty is indicated when the humeral head is deteriorated or fractured but the glenoid surface is intact. Hemiarthroplasty is the surgery of choice if the patient has insufficient glenoid bone to support a glenoid component. When the physical demands are heavy after surgery, a hemiarthroplasty is indicated. Hemiarthroplasty is indicated when arthritis and rotator cuff deficiencies coexist. A badly eroded glenoid cannot stabilize a glenoid component securely, and a nonfunctional rotator cuff produces unbalanced muscular forces on the glenoid, leading to loosening. Hemiarthoplasty can replace the entire humeral head or be a resurfacing prosthesis.

TSA is the replacement of both humeral head and glenoid. This procedure is undertaken when both joint surfaces are damaged and both are reconstructable. TSA is recommended in patients with osteoarthritis and rheumatoid arthritis.

7. Is there a benefit in choosing hemiarthroplasty versus TSA?

It appears that TSA is the best option for treatment of patients with glenohumeral arthritis. Multiple studies showing consistent relief of pain and improved function support this statement. There are times, however, when the deteriorated bone of the glenoid cannot support the prosthesis or the deficiency of the rotator cuff requires the use of hemiarthroplasty.

8. What factors and conditions should be present for a person to consider undergoing a TSA or hemiarthroplasty?

Patients who have failed conservative management but have functioning deltoid and rotator cuff musculature, demonstrate appropriate motivation toward rehabilitation, and are in sufficient health are candidates for a TSA or hemiarthroplasty. Patients without erosion of the glenoid have been found to have improved function following a hemiarthroplasty. Patients suffering from osteoarthritis or osteonecrosis tend to have higher levels of function following surgery than patients with rheumatoid arthritis and cuff tear arthropathy.

9. Can a hemiarthroplasty be converted to a TSA if the hemiarthroplasty fails?

Yes, but it should be considered as a salvage procedure because a recent report determined that nearly 50% of patients who had undergone this procedure were unsatisfied with the outcome at 2 years. The advent of the modular components could lead one to believe that converting to a total shoulder replacement would be a good choice; however, recent evidence suggests that this is not the case.

10. What postoperative complications are associated with TSA?

The incidence of complications in a constrained TSA is about 25%. Most complications are due to mechanical loosening, instability, and implant failure. The incidence of complications in an unconstrained TSA is 14%. Instability accounts for approximately 38% of the postoperative complications. Tearing of the rotator cuff accounts for approximately 13% of postoperative complications. Heterotopic ossification has been reported in up to 40% of patients with TSA but is often minimal and not limiting unless it bridges the glenohumeral joint, restricting forward elevation. Glenoid component loosening occurs in approximately 2% to 4% of patients. Superior humeral migration occurs at the same incidence; it often is associated with glenoid component loosening but is usually not as painful. Intraoperative fractures of the glenoid and humerus occur in <2% of cases. Operative complications are slightly higher in patients with rheumatoid arthritis because of poor tissue quality. Nerve injuries and infections have been reported in less than 1% of patients.

11. What causes components to loosen?

Symptomatic loosening of glenoid and humerus components occurs in 3.5% of patients with TSA. The many contributing factors include glenoid preparation, soft tissue balancing, wear debris, bone reabsorption, prosthetic design, component geometry, and biomaterials. One major concern is the eccentric load placed on the glenoid component by the humeral component, particularly if the humerus has migrated superiorly. The humerus can migrate superiorly because of rotator cuff tear, poor humeral fixation, and soft tissue imbalance. During arm elevation the eccentric load of a proximal migrated humeral component can produce a "rocking horse" effect on the glenoid component that loosens the glenoid component.

12. What are the postoperative goals after TSA?

The primary goal is to relieve pain. Approximately 90% of patients report no pain or slight pain after hemiarthroplasty or TSA. The secondary goal is to restore normal function, specifically shoulder range of motion. Regaining upper extremity strength and ensuring stability of the components are additional postoperative goals.

13. How long will a TSA remain functional?

In a multicenter study of 470 cases of TSA, failure of prosthesis was defined as need for reoperation or patient dissatisfaction. This study reported that at 5-year follow-up 3% of the procedures had failed. A smaller study of 53 operations, using similar criteria, reported that at 11-year follow-up 27% had failed. A study of 29 patients that had surgery at age 50 or younger revealed that 84% of the TSA prostheses were still intact 20 years postoperatively with approximately 50% of these patients reporting satisfactory or better results

14. How much active motion and function are expected after hemiarthroplasty or TSA?

A recent publication by Orfaly has demonstrated that in the hands of outstanding surgeons both procedures can provide excellent improvement in function, decrease pain, and improve range of motion. At an average of 4 years' follow-up, 37 TSAs and 28 hemiarthroplasties were found to have an average pain reduction from 64 to 12 preoperatively to postoperatively. The ASES functional score improved from 39 to 88 out of 100 in the TSA group and from 42 to 84 out of 100 in the hemiarthroplasty group. Both groups' active elevation improved approximately 50 degrees, and external rotation improved 30 degrees.

15. Can a patient participate in sports after TSA?

Yes. The patient should be counseled by the physician and therapist that activities that expose the patient to high-impact events are not recommended because of the potential trauma to the prosthesis. However, sports such as swimming, bowling, dancing, and bicycling can be resumed when appropriate healing has occurred.

16. What is meant by limited-goal rehabilitation? To what type of patient is this applied?

Limited-goal rehabilitation is meant for patients who have deficient rotator cuff and deltoid musculature and significant bony deficiency that does not tolerate the typical rehabilitation program. Patients who have long-standing rheumatoid arthritis and rotator cuff arthropathy as well as some revision arthroplasties may fall into this category. The focus of limited-goal rehabilitation is pain relief and stability. The shoulder functions primarily at the side with elevation restricted at or below 100 degrees and external rotation of 20 degrees.

17. When should postoperative rehabilitation begin for TSA and hemiarthroplasty?

Ideally rehabilitation begins preoperatively. Education about postoperative exercise regimens and typical postoperative symptoms alleviates the patient's apprehension. Early passive motion should be initiated on day 1 or 2 after surgery to prevent intra-articular adhesions and soft tissue contractures. However, the surgeon may modify this procedure, depending on bony or soft tissue quality and fixation during surgery. The most common reason for TSA and hemiarthroplasty revision surgery is contracture between the deltoid and rotator cuff because of prolonged immobilization.

18. Describe the technique of early passive motion (EPM).

EPM, as described by Neer, begins on the second day postoperatively. The patient takes an appropriate pain medication 45 minutes before EPM and applies dry or moist heat to relax the muscles. The patient first performs pendulum exercises. The patient sits or lies in a recumbent position while the therapist slowly elevates the relaxed arm in the scapular plane, applying slight traction. This maneuver is repeated 3 to 5 times twice daily. The point of maximal elevation, based on the surgical procedure, should be determined by the surgeon and communicated to the therapist. Typically, passive external rotation is also started with the arm at the side.

19. Is all passive elevation the same?

No. Passive elevation in the supine position produces less electromyographic (EMG) activity in shoulder musculature than passive elevation in the upright position. Minimal EMG activity has been recorded in the supraspinatus, infraspinatus, and anterior deltoid during supine self-assisted and helper-assisted elevation. However, more EMG activity is noted in the supraspinatus, infraspinatus, and anterior deltoid during passive elevation in an upright position using a pulley or a stick.

20. What is the Neer-phased rehabilitation program?

Charles Neer popularized three phases of shoulder rehabilitation for TSA, hemiarthroplasty, and rotator cuff repairs.

- **Phase I** consists primarily of passive motion exercises, including passive movement of the involved arm by a therapist or family member. Phase I also incorporates the use of assist devices such as rope and pulley, stick, or tabletop to aid the patient in performing passive and active assisted exercises independently.
- **Phase II** consists primarily of active motion exercises. The patient progresses from active assisted to active exercises without assistive devices. The treating clinician must respect healing time frames and incorporate creative techniques to regain coordinated active range of motion.
- **Phase III** consists of resistive exercises. Use of resistive devices, such as light weights and rubber tubing, is incorporated to regain shoulder strength.

21. Why do some patients need abduction pillows?

The surgical repair and the status of the rotator cuff musculature dictate the necessity of an abduction pillow or splint postoperatively. The surgeon examines the quality of the soft tissues during the operation and at closure decides whether excessive tension is placed on the rotator cuff tendons with the arm at the side. Patients with undue tension with the arm at the side or poor tissue may be placed in an abduction splint to reduce stress on the compromised structures and allow healing.

22. What are the standard precautions after TSA?

Each surgery is different, and communication with the surgeon is critical. Events during surgery must be communicated to the therapist to ensure postoperative rehabilitation enhances rather than damages the repair. However, some standard precautions are recommended. Self-transfers and ambulation with crutches should be avoided until adequate strength is regained (often about 6 months). If the patient is suffering from osteoarthritis, therapists are urged to avoid cardinal plane flexion activities because posterior glenoid wear is common and may predispose the patient to posterior subluxation. Patients undergoing TSA because of arthritis from previous dislocations may have weak deltoid and/or unstable joints, which may delay the resistive exercise phase. Patients with rheumatoid arthritis often have weak or torn rotator cuff tissues and proceed slowly through rehabilitation; they need frequent verbal reinforcement. Patients undergoing TSA because of rotator cuff tear arthropathy, congenital defects, neoplasm, and Erb's palsy deformity most commonly fall into the limited-goal rehabilitation program.

23. What are typical outcomes for a reverse total shoulder prosthesis?

Pain predictably improves although may not be completely eliminated, elevation typically reaches 90 to 100 degrees, and function improves when measured by ASES or Constant score to 60% to 70% of a maximum score. Complications range from 10% to 20%.

Bibliography

Bishop JY, Flatow EL: Humeral head replacement versus total shoulder arthroplasty: clinical outcomes—a review, *J Shoulder Elbow Surg* 14(1, suppl):s141-s146, 2005.

Boileau P et al: Grammont reverse prosthesis: design, rationale, and biomechanics, *J Shoulder Elbow Surg* 14(1, suppl):s147-s161, 2005.

Brems JJ: Rehabilitation following total shoulder arthroplasty, *Clin Orthop* 307:70-85, 1994.

Carroll RM et al: Conversion of painful hemiarthroplasty to total shoulder arthroplasty: long-term results, *J Shoulder Elbow Surg* 13:599-603, 2004.

Cuomo F, Checroun A: Avoiding pitfalls and complications in total shoulder arthroplasty, *Orthop Clin North Am* 29:507-518, 1998.

Healy WL, Iorio R, Lemos MJ: Athletic activity after joint replacement, *Am J Sports Med* 29:377-388, 2001.

Hettrich CM et al: Preoperative factors associated with improvements in shoulder function after humeral hemiarthroplasty, *J Bone Joint Surg* 86-A:1446-1451, 2004.

Kelley MJ, Ramsey MJ: Osteoarthritis and traumatic arthritis of the shoulder, *J Hand Ther* 13:148-162, 2000.

Matsen FA et al: Glenohumeral arthritis and its management. In Rockwood CA, Matsen FA, editors: *The shoulder*, ed 2, Philadelphia, 1998, pp 840-964, WB Saunders.

McCann PD et al: A kinematic and electromyographic study of shoulder rehabilitation exercises, *Clin Orthop Rel Res* 288:179-188, 1993.

Neer CS: *Shoulder reconstruction*, Philadelphia, 1990, WB Saunders.

Orfaly RM et al: A prospective functional outcome study of shoulder arthroplasty for osteoarthritis with an intact rotator cuff, *J Shoulder Elbow Surg* 12:214-221, 2003.

Smith KL, Matsen FA III: Total shoulder arthroplasty versus hemiarthroplasty: current trends, *Orthop Clin North Am* 29:491-506, 1998.

Sperling JW, Cofield RH, Rowland CM: Minimum fifteen-year follow-up of Neer hemiarthroplasty and total shoulder arthroplasty in patients aged fifty years or younger, *J Shoulder Elbow Surg* 13:604-613, 2004.

Chapter 42

Acromioclavicular and Sternoclavicular Injuries

Terry R. Malone, PT, EdD, ATC, and
Andrea Lynn Milam, PT, MSEd

ACROMIOCLAVICULAR INJURIES

1. What are the typical mechanisms of acromioclavicular (AC) injury?

The most common mechanism of AC injury is direct force to the tip of the shoulder with the arm adducted against the body. As a result, the acromion is driven downward or inferiorly, with resultant ligament disruption. The location and number of ligaments affected are directly related to the level of force; both AC and coracoclavicular (CC) ligament complexes are at risk for injury.

A secondary mechanism of AC injury is indirect force, as when a person falls on an outstretched hand, generating an impact load at the acromion through the humeral head. This injury typically involves only the AC capsule and ligaments.

2. Who is at risk for AC injury?

AC injury most commonly occurs in men rather than women and in relatively young, as opposed to older, people. AC injuries are approximately 4 or 5 times more prevalent than sternoclavicular injuries.

3. What is the common name for AC joint injury?

The layman's term for AC joint injury is *shoulder separation.*

4. Describe the structure and function of the AC joint.

The AC joint is a diarthrodial plane joint, connecting the outer end of the clavicle with the anterior medial portion of the acromial process. It has fibrocartilage surfaces. The facet (surface) joint shapes include a convex clavicle and a concave acromion. An interesting component of the joint is the intra-articular fibrocartilaginous meniscus-like disk that is interposed between the joint surfaces. This disk typically begins to degenerate during the third and fourth decades of life. The AC joint, in concert with the sternoclavicular joint, allows the clavicle to serve as a crankshaft, keeping the arm in a functional position in relationship to the body. The clavicle rotates early and late during abduction and elevation of the humerus.

5. What are the ligaments of the AC joint?

The three major supporting ligaments to the AC joint are the conoid, trapezoid, and acromioclavicular ligaments. The conoid and trapezoid ligaments are collectively referred to as the coracoclavicular ligament.

The (superior and inferior) AC ligaments reinforce the joint capsule. Their primary role is to control **horizontal movements** of the clavicle. The superior portion is reinforced by the insertional fibers of the deltoid and trapezius muscles.

Vertical stability of the clavicle (AC joint) is controlled by the coracoclavicular ligaments (conoid and trapezoid). The conoid lies medial to the joint, runs posteriorly, and is triangular in shape, whereas the trapezoid is positioned laterally, in the sagittal plane, and is quadrilateral in shape. The orientation of the coracoclavicular ligaments is critical to controlling the rotation of the clavicle, enabling full elevation of the arm. This dual pattern of fiber orientation is particularly significant in that it is also the feature that makes a "simple surgical procedure" unlikely and unsuccessful.

6. Describe the acute presentation of a patient with an AC injury.

The patient with an AC injury often cradles the involved arm by grasping and supporting the elbow with the uninvolved hand. This position reduces the gravitational pull of the weight of the arm inferiorly and also provides some stabilization of the arm next to the trunk.

7. What radiographs are taken to diagnose AC injuries?

Patients sometimes receive x-ray examinations in both loaded (weighted) and unloaded patterns to determine the level of clavicle displacement. The key to this technique is that the weight must be freely suspended from the arm, using no muscular action to hold it in space. A second key to obtaining appropriate diagnostic information via radiograph views of the AC joint is to decrease the intensity of exposure, because overexposure of the joint typically occurs with normal intensities.

Special radiographic angles have been used to delineate the AC joint space more accurately. The usual (normal) anteroposterior view superimposes the joint space onto the spine of the scapula. To correct for this, Zanca recommends a 10- to 15-degree superior angulation view. The visualization of the coracoid is best provided by a supine notch view. Other possible modifications include a scapulolateral view.

8. How are AC injuries classified?

Because AC injury may include two ligament complexes, the classification scheme is somewhat complex. Rather than the simpler first-, second-, and third-degree pattern typically used with specific ligamentous implications, the AC scheme incorporates modifications reflecting horizontal and vertical motions. It also adds descriptors of the rare extreme vertical displacement injuries, classified as types IV to VI.

Acromioclavicular Classification Scheme

Type	Clinical Findings	Instability	Radiographs
Type I: sprain of AC ligaments; AC and CC ligaments are intact	Mild to moderate pain at AC joint General movement is pain-free Tender to palpation	None; minimal ligament damage	Normal
Type II: complete disruption of AC ligaments; sprain of CC ligaments	Moderate to severe pain at both AC joint and CC interspace Limited function	Definite horizontal instability; possible slight change in vertical stability	Slight elevation of clavicle
Type III: complete disruption of AC and CC ligaments	High-riding clavicle Exquisite pain Inability to use UE Affected arm often	AC (horizontal) and CC (vertical) instability	25%-100% increase in CC space

Acromioclavicular Classification Scheme *continued*

Type	Clinical Findings	Instability	Radiographs
	cradled with unaffected extremity		
Types IV, V, and VI	Severe pain and limited function Extreme drooping of involved upper extremity	Horizontal and vertical (surgical intervention directed at restoration of ligamentous complexes and muscular insertions)	Severe displacement of CC follows Type IV: superior and posterior displacement of clavicle Type V: 100%-300% increase of CC interspace compared with normal Type VI: clavicle displaced inferior to coracoid (subcoracoid dislocation)

9. How are type I AC injuries treated?

Treatment of type I AC injuries does not require immobilization. Ice is recommended for pain modulation and the patient may return to activity as comfortably tolerated. If activity exposes the patient to contact or impact forces, a donut pad placed over the shoulder helps to protect the joint. The pad is designed to allow distribution of impact around the AC joint rather than onto it; it is an oblong, dense foam base with the center removed (area of the AC) and is covered by thermoplastic material (taped in place). If used during an athletic event, the thermoplastic surface is covered with temper-foam to protect others.

10. Describe the treatment for type II AC injuries.

Patients who have sustained a type II AC injury typically use a sling as needed, and apply ice as a pain modulator. Range of motion (ROM) exercises are initiated on an as-tolerated basis, often beginning in a passive form to minimize muscle activation of the trapezius and deltoid groups. An exercise program designed to fit the patient's needs generally includes functional progression. If the shoulder is exposed to impact forces, the donut pad should be used as the patient returns to function. Specific strengthening exercises may be required, depending on patient activities. The anatomic presence and positions of the deltoid and trapezius fibers act as reinforcement to the AC joint capsule and thus are often part of the considerations for the long-term rehabilitation program. Usually the athlete can return to full function within 2 to 3 weeks after injury.

11. Describe the operative and nonoperative approaches to type III AC injuries.

The most appropriate treatment for type III AC injuries is somewhat controversial.

OPERATIVE MANAGEMENT

Surgical techniques have been used to address the instability created by the disrupted ligaments. Surgeons generally attempt to pull or stabilize the clavicle downward, often to the coracoid, via a metal screw, Dacron tape, wire, or pins. Complications of such procedures can include infection, pin breakage, pin/wire migration, and resection of the clavicle or coracoid as the wire cuts through the bone. Even after surgery, residual AC joint deformity or discomfort may occur, complicating rehabilitation and ultimate function. Early postoperative management often includes 4 to 6 weeks of immobilization after surgical intervention and a rehabilitation program thereafter. Functional outcomes following this procedure appear to be quite similar to those obtained through nonsurgical management. Hence current treatment is more often directed toward conservative, nonsurgical management.

NONOPERATIVE MANAGEMENT

Conservative management is much like that for a second-degree acromioclavicular injury, but with a greater reliance on an immobilizing support device because of the vertical instability typically associated with a type II AC injury. Also because of associated vertical instability, a residual step deformity remains at the distal clavicle, even after healing is complete. Fortunately, this deformity rarely becomes a disability, and functional outcomes are equal in patients managed with or without surgery. Because disability is most likely a problem in patients who regularly expose the arm to high-intensity demands, surgeons may consider surgical treatment under such conditions. However, it is becoming relatively rare for surgical interventions to be used as part of the management of an acute type II AC injury.

12. Describe the initial treatment for significant (type III or greater) AC injuries.

Reduction and maintenance for comfort is the rule. Because type IV, V, and VI injuries may be corrected surgically, physician follow-up is important. Although the stated treatment is reduction, in reality the arm is immobilized or supported in a sling, but true reduction is not maintained. Devices have been designed to pull the humerus superiorly and the clavicle inferiorly, but their success is minimal because they are frequently associated with a lack of patient compliance. The most commonly used device is the Kenny-Howard harness, which incorporates this combination. In reality, the outcomes of treatment with a harness or benign neglect are quite similar.

13. What can be done to minimize or prevent AC injuries?

In sports where tackling is the rule, shoulder pads are frequently worn. If you place a donut pad under one side, it is important also to pad the uninjured side to avoid alteration of shoulder pad alignment. Shoulder pads work via a cantilever design that enables forces to be placed onto the anterior and posterior thorax rather than the underlying area. Pads must be fitted properly and stabilized to the thorax. A good rule is that the proper fit of the shoulder pad is more important than its size or "model."

14. What are the long-term consequences of AC injury?

Patients often develop a step deformity at the AC joint, where the clavicle appears to sit higher on the affected side than on the normal side. In addition, the patient may experience some pain with high-demand activity. Of interest, significant disability is relatively rare, even with an obvious deformity. Patients experience long-term arthritis of the joint but again with limited symptoms. In fact, postsurgical patients have similar long-term outcomes.

15. What can be done for the patient whose pain is associated with weight lifting?

Pain with weight lifting is a common complaint in athletes with a previous AC injury. The wide-grip bench press is the primary culprit for such pain. The anterior fly-type maneuver, which replicates the cross-arm adduction test for AC pain and provocation, should also be avoided.

Although it might be helpful to do so, athletes usually hesitate to use a narrower grip during weight lifting because it decreases the maximal load that can be handled during bench press. Antiinflammatories, local ice application before and after exercise, and exercise modification can be used successfully in select patients. Other patients will not have a successful outcome because of established osteolysis of the distal clavicle.

16. What other athletes are prone to AC problems?

Racquet-using athletes or throwing athletes may develop AC symptoms related to sport activities. They may exhibit symptoms on follow-through (cross-arm motions) as well as during weight training with wide-grip bench press, dips, or cross-arm fly maneuvers. Partial ROM (restricted ranges) during weight training and decreased maximal effort and repetitions of throwing can be helpful in alleviating pain or minimizing AC problems.

17. What is the natural history of conservatively treated type III AC separations?

Interestingly, most surgeons today do not recommend surgical intervention for these patients, as the residual deformity potentially associated with nonoperative management does not seem to be a significant problem and very limited functional differences in outcomes are seen. In fact, a study of 25 non–operatively managed type III AC separations showed very minimal changes at 1 year with the vast majority having no significant deficits, as evidenced through full ROM, nearly normal strength in most groups, and a minimal deficit in bench press at 1 year.

18. What is the surgical procedure of choice for arthritic AC disability?

Physicians often excise the distal clavicle of patients with recalcitrant pain and disability of the AC joint. The Mumford procedure is designed to remove approximately 0.5 to 2 cm of the distal clavicle, which prevents impingement with crossed-arm movements. Rehabilitation after the procedure is directed toward pain modulation and support for the first 10 to 14 days, followed by functional progression related to the specific needs of the patient.

19. Discuss briefly the role of AC joint mobilization.

AC mobilization can be successfully used in patients presenting with decreased elevation and limited cross-arm motion (horizontal adduction). Mobilization exercises are usually performed from behind, using the horizontally placed thumb to move the clavicle forward. The therapist should maintain as much contact with the distal clavicle as possible to minimize the point of pressure. The arm is supported on a plinth or tabletop as mobilization is performed. Improvements in ROM may follow this procedure.

STERNOCLAVICULAR INJURIES

20. What is the typical mechanism of sternoclavicular (SC) injury?

SC injury is relatively rare but may result from direct trauma, as in an athlete who sustains direct force to the clavicle via impact collision with another player or a hard surface, such as a goal post or equipment. The more common method of SC injury is indirect, as when someone lying on their side receives an external load that causes a rolling of the body over the shoulder, thus combining compression and twisting. Anterior injuries are more common than posterior injuries; posterior dislocation is quite rare but may have serious implications.

21. Who is at risk for SC injuries?

SC injuries are far more common in men than in women and are more prevalent in relatively young, rather than older, people, but they are much less common than AC injuries. Acromioclavicular injuries occur 4 or 5 times more frequently than sternoclavicular injuries.

22. Describe the structure and function of the SC joint.

The SC joint, like the AC joint, contains a meniscus-like disk. Because the articulating surfaces of the sternum and clavicle are typically incongruent, the disk becomes the contact surface of the joint. The actual joint surfaces are saddle-shaped, using the disk independently to enable the unique actions of the clavicle in relation to the sternum (i.e., the disk works or stays with either the sternum or the clavicle during specific actions). The movements allowed by the joint are elevation and depression, protraction and retraction, and rotation.

23. What ligaments support and control the SC joint?

The SC ligament complex includes the capsule itself, which is directly reinforced by the anterior and posterior SC ligaments. The costoclavicular ligament is quite strong and assists with the pivoting action of the clavicle in relation to the anchored, underlying first rib. The interclavicular ligament supports the superior aspect, reinforcing the position of the clavicle to minimize inferior displacement, which endangers the underlying brachial plexus and subclavian artery.

24. Which radiographic views are used to assess SC injuries?

Special radiographic views can be used to assess the SC joint. These views minimize superimposed structures. Hobbs recommends that patients be x-rayed in a sitting position, leaning forward with elbows supported on the x-ray table. In this position a vertical (superior) radiograph is taken. Rockwood uses a "serendipity" view in which the patient is positioned supine with the x-ray tube angled approximately 40 degrees from the vertical and directed toward the clavicle.

25. How are SC injuries classified?

Sternoclavicular Injury Classification

Type	Description
Mild sprain	Ligaments intact
Moderate sprain (subluxation)	Ligaments partially disrupted
Severe sprain (dislocation)	Total disruption of ligaments Two subtypes: 1. anterior dislocation 2. posterior dislocation

26. Describe the treatment for a mild sprain of the SC joint.

No instability is present with a mild sprain. Ice can be used for pain modulation; in addition a sling can be worn for protection from additional trauma for 2 to 4 days or until the patient is pain-free. A gradual return to activities should follow, as tolerated, through a functional progression.

27. Describe the treatment for a moderate sprain (subluxation) of the SC joint.

This type of injury requires immobilization and protection. Most patients wear a clavicle strap to maintain proper clavicular orientation and a sling to support the weight of the arm. Both devices are used for 2 to 4 weeks, followed by rehabilitation progression dictated by need and symptoms.

28. What is the initial treatment for an anterior severe sprain (dislocation) of the SC joint?

The first approach to treating an SC injury is to ensure that reduction is maintained. The majority of sternoclavicular dislocations occur anteriorly, and can be reduced with firm digital pressure. The decision to reduce and immobilize SC dislocations, however, is somewhat controversial. Many SC dislocations are stable after reduction, and patients often do well with brief immobilization and progression of activities, as tolerated. To reduce the dislocation, the patient is positioned supine and a pad is placed posteriorly, allowing shoulder extension. A posterior force applied to the proximal (displaced) clavicle completes the reduction. A sling is typically worn for 3 to 6 weeks.

29. What is the initial treatment for a posterior severe sprain (dislocation) of the SC joint?

The rare posterior sternoclavicular dislocation occurs with abrupt and extreme shoulder extension while the trunk position is maintained, thus permitting a fulcrum/lever sequence. In such cases, reduction may occur via an open procedure in the operating room (as above), particularly because a closed technique may not be successful. An open procedure uses forceps to pull the clavicle into the correct position. The patient with a posterior SC dislocation may present as a medical emergency because of the potential for significant injury to underlying organs and structures.

Typically, a figure-of-eight harness is used for posterior dislocations after reduction is achieved for a minimum of 4 weeks. Some physicians combine the clavicle harness with the arm sling.

For both anterior and posterior injuries, use of ice is followed by gentle, controlled movements after immobilization, leading to progressive functional rehabilitation.

30. What are the long-term consequences of SC injuries?

After reduction of a SC injury, most patients have no significant long-term disability. If chronic joint instability develops, corrective surgery can be performed, but the results are not uniformly positive. Potential adverse outcomes following such a procedure include arthritis and pain, particularly in high-demand patients.

31. What type of surgical procedures are performed on patients with SC instability and disability?

Although relatively rare, some patients experience recurrent dislocations and demonstrate instability, leading to chronic disability and pain. Surgical intervention results are inconsistent, and the surgery is difficult to perform. Most procedures use some type of graft material (subclavius tendon, palmaris longus muscle, or toe extensor muscle) to redevelop proximal stability of the SC pivot joint. Unfortunately, mixed, rather than consistent, postsurgical results are typical.

Bibliography

Branch TP et al: The role of the acromioclavicular ligaments and the effect of distal clavicle resection, *Am J Sports Med* 24:293-297, 1996.

Cook FF, Tibone JE: The Mumford procedure in athletes: an objective analysis of function, *Am J Sports Med* 16:97-100, 1988.

Cox JS: The fate of the acromioclavicular joint in athletic injuries, *Am J Sports Med* 9:50-53, 1981.

Donatelli RA, editor: *Physical therapy of the shoulder,* ed 3, New York, 1997, Churchill Livingstone.

Galpin RD, Hawkins RJ, Grainger RW: A comparative analysis of operative versus nonoperative treatment of grade III acromioclavicular separations, *Clin Orthop* 193:150-155, 1985.

Kelley MJ, Clark WA, editors: *Orthopedic therapy of the shoulder,* Philadelphia, 1995, JB Lippincott.

Morrison DS, Lemos MJ: Acromioclavicular separation: reconstruction using synthetic loop augmentation, *Am J Sports Med* 23:105-110, 1995.

Rockwood CA, Matsen FA, editors: *The shoulder,* ed 2, Philadelphia, 1998, WB Saunders.

Schlegel TF et al: A prospective evaluation of untreated acute grade III acromioclavicular separations, *Am J Sports Med* 29:699-703, 2001.

Snyder SJ, Banas MP, Karzel RP: The arthroscopic Mumford procedure: an analysis of results, *Arthroscopy* 11:157-164, 1995.

Walsh WM et al: Shoulder strength following acromioclavicular injury, *Am J Sports Med* 13:153-158, 1985.

Weaver JK, Dunn HK: Treatment of acromioclavicular injuries: especially complete acromioclavicular separation, *J Bone Joint Surg* 54A:1187-1194, 1972.

Wojtys EM, Nelson G: Conservative treatment of grade III acromioclavicular dislocations, *Clin Orthop* 268:112-119, 1991.

Yap JJL et al: The value of weighted views of the acromioclavicular joint: results of a survey, *Am J Sports Med* 27:806-809, 1999.

Zanca P: Shoulder pain: involvement of the acromioclavicular joint (Analysis of 1,000 cases), *Am J Roentgenol Radium Ther Nucl Med* 112:493-506, 1971.

Chapter 43

Scapulothoracic Pathology

Tim L. Uhl, PT, PhD, ATC, and Tracy Spigelman, MEd, ATC

1. What is the role of the scapula in glenohumeral movement?

The scapula provides a mobile base for humeral motions in all directions; assists in providing an appropriate muscle length-to-tension ratio for rotator cuff and deltoid musculature throughout arm elevation; and serves as a bony attachment for most of the upper quarter proximal musculature. The scapula and surrounding musculature are critical in force transmission from the lower extremities and trunk to the arm in throwing activities.

2. What are the 3-D kinematics of the scapula with respect to the humerus and trunk in arm elevation?

Scapular motion occurs in three cardinal planes during arm elevation: upward rotation, external rotation, and posterior tilt. In a healthy person as the arm is elevated in the scapular plane, the scapula rotates upwardly $\approx 50 \pm 4.8$ degrees, externally rotates about a vertical axis $\approx 24 \pm 12.8$ degrees, and tilts posteriorly about a horizontal axis $\approx 30 \pm 13.0$ degrees.

3. What muscular force couples act on the scapula during arm elevation?

A force couple is two or more lines of force acting on different points of the same structure to produce rotation. The upper trapezius, lower trapezius, and serratus anterior are involved in scapular upward rotation. The posterior tilting and external rotation of the scapula are thought to result from action of the lower serratus anterior musculature and lower trapezius.

4. Does the scapular musculature activation pattern change when the glenohumeral joint is injured?

Yes. Several different studies have demonstrated that motor activity level or onset of motor activity is altered in patients with impingement or glenohumeral instability. Diminished serratus anterior activity has been documented in throwers with unstable shoulders and swimmers with impingement. Delayed onset of serratus anterior activity in overhead reaching has been demonstrated in swimmers with impingement.

5. Can abnormal scapular movement be associated with rotator cuff impingement?

Yes. Diminished scapular movement, particularly in posterior tilting and superior translation, has been associated with rotator cuff impingement symptoms.

6. Define scapular dyskinesia.

Scapular dyskinesia describes abnormal or atypical movement of the scapula during normal active motion tasks, such as reaching overhead. Similar terms used in the literature include abnormal scapulohumeral rhythm, scapular winging, and scapular dysrhythmia.

7. How common is scapular dyskinesia?

It is very common. According to Warner, 64% of patients diagnosed with an unstable glenohumeral joint present with some form of scapular dyskinesia, while all patients with impingement demonstrated some degree of scapular dyskinesia.

8. What populations need to be suspected for scapula pathology?

Scapular pathology should be suspected of any overhead athlete or patient who presents with pain in the shoulder region, regardless of the patient's age. Current research suggests little league baseball players as young as 10 years old present with increased upward scapular rotation compared with nonathletic children of the same age.

9. What causes scapular dyskinesis?

It is not clear whether the scapula dyskinesis is primary or secondary to shoulder pathology. The general consensus is that deficiency of the scapular musculature, particularly the serratus anterior and trapezius, is often involved. The deficiency may be simple weakness, tightness, or a compensatory motor pattern developed in response to pain. Congenital deformities such as scoliosis or Sprengel's deformity may cause scapular dyskinesis.

10. What is Sprengel's deformity?

Also called Eulenburg's deformity, Sprengel's deformity is failure of the scapula to descend during normal development. Typically it is seen in infancy or early childhood as a prominent lump in the web of the neck. The scapula often is hypoplastic, abnormally shaped, and malrotated so that the superomedial angle is curved anteriorly into the supraclavicular region and the inferior angle abuts the thoracic spine. Arm abduction may be limited. Associated musculoskeletal deformities such as scoliosis, rib abnormalities, Klippel-Feil syndrome, and spina bifida are common.

11. What is "SICK" scapula syndrome?

SICK scapula stands for **s**capular malposition, **i**nferior medial border prominence, **c**oracoid pain, and dys**k**inesis. It is a severe form of scapular dyskinesis associated with overuse syndrome and fatigue. The SICK scapula is commonly found in overhead athletes and can be noted by a unilateral drop in the affected shoulder.

12. How is abnormal scapular movement assessed?

Abnormal scapular movement or scapular dyskinesis can be observed during static or dynamic activities. Three-dimensional analysis allows precise measurements of the scapula. Several clinical methods of measurement exist; one of the most common is the lateral scapular slide test, which measures the distance between T8 and the inferior angle of the scapula in three positions: (1) arm at side, (2) hands on waist, and (3) arms abducted to 90 degrees with maximal internal rotation. A lateral displacement >1.5 cm between the involved and uninvolved side is considered an indication of scapular muscle dysfunction. Intra-tester and inter-tester reliability measurements of this test have been reported at 0.84 to 0.88 and 0.65 to 0.88, respectively.

Differences in vertical height between the affected and unaffected scapula should also be assessed to determine abnormal tilting or protraction. Burkhart, Morgan, and Kibler describe this as the "infera." The infera is measured with the athlete standing with arms at the side. A bubble goniometer is used to determine vertical height differences between superomedial borders of the affected and unaffected scapula in centimeters. A large height difference is considered to be 2 to 3 cm or more.

13. How is scapular dyskinesis treated?

The first step is to perform a complete neuromuscular examination of the shoulder girdle and cervical region. Based on the findings, tight structures need to be stretched and weak structures need to be strengthened. Strengthen the scapular protractors with resistance exercises that emphasize scapular protraction that activates the serratus anterior without overactivating the upper trapezius. One of the most important treatments is education about proper posture and typical movement of the scapula. Biofeedback techniques, such as mirrors, verbal cueing, tactile cueing, and video monitoring during exercises, are helpful for the patient to visualize the trunk and scapula. The patient benefits by observing the trunk and scapula during exercises in order to learn how to voluntarily control scapular musculature.

14. Which scapular muscles should be targeted for rehabilitation?

There are approximately 20 muscles attached to the scapula; however, those most involved in stabilization of the scapula against the thoracic wall are the rhomboids major and minor; upper, middle, and lower trapezius muscles; serratus anterior; and the rotator cuff musculature. The muscular force couples mentioned previously should be the focus for rehabilitation. Strengthening and stabilization of these muscles will help reestablish neuromuscular pathways and aid in prevention of instability and secondary impingement, labral pathology, and certain overuse pathologies by maintaining glenohumeral joint congruency.

15. Which exercises target the scapula muscles?

Current EMG research on scapular rehabilitation suggests the following exercises most effectively target the scapular stabilizers. The push-up–plus elicits 80% maximum voluntary contraction (MVC) of serratus anterior activity, prone flexion overhead for lower trapezius elicits 95%, and rows elicit 112% MVC for upper trapezius and middle trapezius muscles. In addition, forces generated from the lower extremity during throwing are transferred through the scapula to achieve increased power; thus the scapula is considered an integral part of the kinetic chain. All scapular rehabilitation should include a strong lower extremity and core strengthening program.

16. How does dyskinesis differ from scapular winging?

Scapular winging typically is associated with long thoracic nerve palsy. Scapular winging is noted when the patient leans into a wall, supporting his or her weight with the arms, or when resistance is applied to outstretched arms as the patient attempts to forward flex. The entire medial and inferior border of the scapula lifts off the thoracic wall because of serratus anterior deficiency.

17. List the muscles that attach to the scapula, the peripheral nerves innervating each muscle, and the corresponding root levels.

- Biceps; musculocutaneous; C5, C6
- Triceps; radial; C6-C8, T1
- Supraspinatus; suprascapular; C4-C6
- Deltoid, all components; axillary; C5, C6
- Teres major; lower subscapular; C5-C7
- Pectoralis minor; medial pectoral with communicating branch of lateral pectoral; C6-C8, T1
- Latissimus dorsi; thoracodorsal; C6-C8
- Subscapularis; upper and lower subscapular; C5-C7
- Infraspinatus; suprascapular; C4-C6
- Teres minor; axillary; C5, C6
- Rhomboids major and minor; dorsal scapular; C4, C5
- Levator scapulae; dorsal scapular; C4, C5, and cervical 3 and 4
- Trapezius, all portions; spinal accessory (cranial nerve XI) and ventral ramus; C2-C4
- Serratus anterior; long thoracic; C5-C8

18. What causes long thoracic nerve palsy?

Long thoracic nerve palsy typically presents idiopathically without a history of macrotrauma. Several mechanisms have been described, such as surgical complications, viral illnesses, immunizations, and trauma (often a traction mechanism).

19. What is the standard treatment for long thoracic nerve palsy?

The palsy usually resolves gradually over time. An electromyographic (EMG) study confirms the diagnosis and can be used to track progress. Strengthening exercises for the weak serratus anterior should be delayed until EMG indicates regeneration. The patient should restrict heavy pushing and overhead lifting activities. Some patients have benefited from a shoulder orthotic that keeps the scapula pressed against the thoracic wall to relieve pain.

Rehabilitation exercises should focus on maintaining range of motion during nerve recovery to prevent joint stiffness. Frequently long thoracic nerve palsy requires 1 year or longer for return to normal function. Long-term follow-up (6 years; range: 2 to 11 years) of iatrogenic long thoracic palsy reported residual symptoms in 25 of 26 patients. Eighty-one percent could not lift or pull heavy objects, 54% could not work with hands above shoulder level, and 58% could not participate in sports such as tennis and golf.

20. What is scapulothoracic dissociation?

Scapulothoracic dissociation results from severe trauma involving lateral displacement of the scapula. It has been described as closed, traumatic forequarter amputation. This injury typically is associated with motorcycle, motor vehicle, or farm implement accidents. The lateral displacement of the scapula ruptures surrounding soft tissue. Typical associated injuries are clavicle fracture, significant neurovascular damage, and major trauma.

21. A patient's symptoms include severe shoulder and neck pain and a drooped shoulder after cervical lymph node resection. What do you suspect is the cause?

One complication of a lymph node or benign tumor removal is iatrogenic injury to the spinal accessory nerve. The injury typically involves the trapezius but often spares the sternocleidomastoid muscle. Trapezius weakness is often noted with the inability to lift the arm above horizontal, and the involved side presents with drooped posture. Patients describe significant shoulder pain, with a sensation of heaviness or the feeling that the shoulder is being pulled out of socket on the involved side.

22. Define snapping scapula.

Snapping scapula is attributed to friction between the mobile scapula with its attached soft tissues and the relatively stable thorax wall. The noise or grating sound may be audible or sensed by the patient. The incidence of grating in the general population has been reported to be as high as 70%. A general friction sound is typically nonpathologic. Grating, loud snapping, or popping sounds associated with pain are thought to be pathologic. Anatomic explanations for snapping scapula include thickened bursa, bone spurs on the scapula or a rib, Luschka's tubercle (an exostosis at the superomedial angle of the scapula), and osteochondroma (a common scapular tumor). A tangential scapulolateral view or computed tomographic scan is more helpful in identifying anatomic anomalies associated with snapping scapula than standard anteroposterior scapular radiographs.

23. What is the differential diagnosis of snapping scapula?

Pain may be referred from the glenohumeral joint; cervical nerve root compression or cervical joint disease may also be present. Thoracic disk disease should be ruled out, along with thoracic outlet syndrome. Tumors also must be considered and evaluated with appropriate imaging studies.

24. How is snapping scapula treated?

Conservative management with antiinflammatory medication, physical therapy modalities, and exercise to strengthen the lower trapezius and serratus anterior musculature often is prescribed. Supportive strapping or bracing may be beneficial. Injection of bupivacaine (Marcaine) may be helpful. Surgical treatment is rare and should be considered only if diagnostic imaging demonstrates the presence of an exostosis or a space-occupying lesion in the scapulothoracic space.

25. What does wasting in the infraspinatus fossa with sparing of the supraspinatus fossa suggest?

This suggests suprascapular nerve compression along its course through the spine of the scapula. A ganglion cyst may be present, or the spinoglenoid ligament may compress the suprascapular nerve to the infraspinatus, sparing the supraspinatus. This disorder presents as weakness in external rotation and wasting in the infraspinatus fossa. A surgical release of the compressing tissues may be necessary if magnetic resonance imaging, EMG, and nerve conduction studies indicate compression and slowing of nerve conduction.

Bibliography

Burkhart SS, Morgan CD, Kibler WB: The disabled throwing shoulder: spectrum of pathology part III: the SICK scapula, scapular dyskinesis, the kinetic chain, and rehabilitation, *Arthroscopy* 19:641-661, 2003.

Butters KP: The scapula. In Rockwood CA, Matsen FA, editors: *The shoulder,* ed 2, Philadelphia, 1998, pp 391-427, WB Saunders.

Donner TR, Kline DG: Extracranial spinal accessory nerve injury, *Neurosurgery* 32:907-910, 1993.

Glousman R et al: Dynamic electromyographic analysis of the throwing shoulder with glenohumeral instability, *J Bone Joint Surg* 70A:220-226, 1988.

Hawkins RJ, Bokor DJ: Clinical evaluation of shoulder problems. In Rockwood CA, Matsen FA, editors: *The shoulder,* ed 2, Philadelphia, 1998, pp 164-197, WB Saunders.

Inman VT, Saunders M, Abbott LC: Observations of the function of the shoulder joint, *J Bone Joint Surg* 26A:1-31, 1944.

Kauppila LI, Vastamaki M: Iatrogenic serratus anterior paralysis: long-term outcome in 26 patients, *Chest* 109:31-34, 1996.

Kendall FP et al: *Muscles: testing and function, with posture and pain,* ed 5, Baltimore, 2005, Williams & Wilkins.

Kibler WB: The role of the scapula in athletic shoulder function, *Am J Sports Med* 26:325-337, 1998.

Ludewig PM, Cook TM, Nawoczenski DA: Three-dimensional scapular orientation and muscle activity at selected positions of humeral elevation, *J Orthop Sports Phys Ther* 24:57-65, 1996.

Lukasiewicz AC et al: Comparison of 3-dimensional scapular position and orientation between subjects with and without shoulder impingement, *J Orthop Sports Phys Ther* 29:574-586, 1999.

Manske RC, Reiman MP, Stovak ML: Nonoperative and operative management of snapping scapula, *Am J Sports Med* 32:1554-1565, 2004.

Marin R: Scapular winger's brace: a case series on the management of long thoracic nerve palsy, *Arch Phys Med Rehabil* 79:1226-1230, 1998.

McClure PW et al: Direct 3-dimensional measurement of scapular kinematics during dynamic movements in vivo, *J Shoulder Elbow Surg* 10:269-277, 2001.

Mourtacos SL, Sauers EL, Downar JM: Adolescent baseball players exhibit differences in shoulder mobility between the throwing and nonthrowing shoulder and between divisions of play [abstract], *J Athletic Training* 38:S-72, 2003.

Myers JB et al: Scapular position and orientation in throwing athletes, *Am J Sports Med* 33:263-271, 2005.

Plafcan DM et al: An objective measurement technique for posterior scapular displacement, *J Orthop Sports Phys Ther* 25:336-341, 1997.

Scovazzo ML et al: The painful shoulder during freestyle swimming: an electromyographic cinematographic analysis of twelve muscles, *Am J Sports Med* 19:577-582, 1991.

Wadsworth DJ, Bullock-Saxton JE: Recruitment patterns of the scapular rotator muscles in freestyle swimmers with subacromial impingement, *Int J Sports Med* 18:618-624, 1997.

Warner JJP et al: Scapulothoracic motion in normal shoulders and shoulders with glenohumeral instability and impingement syndrome, *Clin Orthop* 285:199, 1992.

Woo VE, Marchinksi L: Congenital anomalies of the shoulder. In Rockwood CA, Matsen FA, editors: *The shoulder,* ed 2, Philadelphia, 1998, pp 99-163, WB Saunders.

Chapter 44

Fractures of the Proximal Humerus and Humeral Shaft

Jay D. Keener, MD, PT

1. How are clavicle fractures classified?

Clavicle fractures are classified according to their location. Middle-third fractures are the most prevalent, occurring in about 80% of clavicle fractures. Proximal-third and distal-third fractures occur in 5% and 15%, respectively, of clavicle fractures.

2. Describe the subclass of distal-third clavicle fractures.

Distal-third fractures of the clavicle are subclassified into three groups. Type I fractures are nondisplaced because the coracoclavicular ligaments remain attached to the medial fragment. Type II fractures result in detachment of the coracoclavicular ligaments from the medial fragment and displacement of the fracture. Type III fractures involve the articular surface of the acromioclavicular joint without detachment of the coracoclavicular ligaments. Type III fractures lead to joint degeneration rather than displacement.

3. What nerve is most frequently injured with a fracture of the clavicle?

The most frequently injured nerve is the ulnar nerve, as it passes between the first rib and the fractured clavicle.

4. How are middle-third clavicle fractures usually treated?

Closed treatment is used for middle-third clavicle fractures. The most common methods of closed immobilization include casting, sling and swathe, or figure-of-eight dressings. No closed method can maintain a reduction; therefore a sling and swathe is most commonly used to maintain patient comfort while the fracture heals.

5. What are the indications for operative treatment of clavicle fractures?

- Open fracture
- Impending open fracture
- Interposition of soft tissues
- Nerve or vascular injury requiring repair
- Displaced type II distal clavicle fractures
- Severe deformity in young women (relative indication)

6. When should shoulder motion be initiated in closed treatment of clavicle fractures?

Most middle-third clavicle fractures require 6 weeks of immobilization for union to occur. The elbow, wrist, and forearm should be used immediately after the fracture to prevent atrophy and stiffness.

7. What is the incidence of proximal humerus fractures?

Proximal humerus fractures are common injuries, representing 4% to 5% of all extremity fractures. The majority of proximal humerus fractures occur in patients over 65 to 70 years of age. Several studies have shown that the incidence of proximal humerus fractures is increasing. The explanation for the rising incidence is believed to be related to the high prevalence of osteoporosis in the aging population.

8. Describe the Neer classification of proximal humerus fractures.

Fractures of the proximal humerus can occur in several patterns. Fractures typically propagate through the greater tuberosity, lesser tuberosity, surgical neck, and/or anatomic neck. Fractures are classified according to the number of displaced fracture fragments and dislocation of the humeral head. The number of fragments can vary from 1 to 4. Fracture fragments are considered to be present only when displaced 1 cm or more or angulated a minimum of 45 degrees.

9. What are the deforming muscular forces responsible for the pattern of fracture displacement encountered with proximal humerus fractures?

The greater tuberosity is displaced in a posterior and superior direction from the pull of the supraspinatus and infraspinatus muscles. Displaced greater tuberosity fractures also create a tear in the rotator cuff in the region of the rotator interval. The subscapularis will pull displaced lesser tuberosity fractures medially. The humerus displaces medially and internally rotates from the pull of the pectoralis major with displaced surgical neck fractures. In addition, varus angulation and shortening are common because of the pull of the deltoid muscle on the humeral shaft. Often the humeral head will abduct because of the unopposed force of the rotator cuff, further contributing to the varus alignment of the humeral head. The biceps tendon frequently will become trapped within the fracture fragments with displaced surgical neck fractures.

10. How often do nerve injuries accompany proximal humerus fractures?

Nerve injury following proximal humerus fractures is common, especially with displaced fractures. Clinically detectable nerve injuries following proximal humerus fractures have been reported in up to 45% of cases. The axillary and suprascapular nerves are most commonly involved. Often these injuries are incomplete and may manifest as temporary weakness that recovers along the same course of time as fracture healing. One author reported a 6.1% incidence of brachial plexus injuries following displaced proximal humerus fractures. EMG studies have revealed a very high incidence of occult nerve injury following both nondisplaced (52%) and displaced (82%) fractures. The risk of neurovascular injury following fractures of the proximal humerus is greater in high-energy injuries, fracture-dislocations, and penetrating trauma.

11. What percentage of proximal humerus fractures can be treated nonoperatively?

The majority of proximal humerus fractures are minimally displaced (considered one-part fractures) and can be treated successfully with conservative measures. Approximately 80% of proximal humerus fractures meet the criteria for conservative treatment. Fractures of the surgical neck are often accompanied by a moderate degree of displacement and angulation. Because of the high degree of mobility available at the glenohumeral joint, angulation of 30 to 45 degrees and translation of up to 75% of the width of the humeral shaft can be tolerated as long as there is good apposition of the fracture fragments.

12. When is the treatment of conservatively managed proximal humerus fractures initiated?

Numerous authors have noted that early range of motion is critical for successful outcomes following proximal humerus fractures. The shoulder is immobilized in a sling or cuff and collar for comfort and to facilitate fracture reduction afforded by the weight of the arm. Elbow, wrist, and hand range of motion exercises are initiated immediately. Pendulum exercises are initiated as soon as tolerable for most stable one-part fractures. The shoulder is evaluated clinically at 1-week intervals to assess for clinical signs of early union. Once the humerus and the proximal fragments move as one unit with gentle shoulder range of motion exercises, formal range of motion exercises are initiated. Early fracture stability is usually noted at 2 to 3 weeks from the time of injury.

13. What are the outcomes of conservatively treated proximal humerus fractures?

The outcomes of conservatively treated proximal humerus fractures are generally good. Fracture union rates are greater than 90% in those patients with minimally displaced fractures. Early range of motion of the shoulder has been shown to improve the functional outcome following proximal humerus fractures. Most patients will regain near normal function of the shoulder following these injuries and experience minimal residual pain. A patient can expect 130- to 150-degree elevation, near symmetric external rotation range of motion, and only mild weakness and functional limitations compared with the opposite shoulder.

14. What are the indications for surgical management of proximal humerus fractures?

The decision to operatively stabilize proximal humerus fractures is primarily related to the severity of displacement of the fracture fragments and the risk of avascular necrosis and dislocation of the humeral head. There is some debate about the degree of deformity that is tolerable at the surgical neck. Fracture angulation at the surgical neck greater than 45 degrees or translation of the humeral shaft leading to minimal contact of the bony fragments is best treated surgically. Displacement of the greater tuberosity is not tolerated well because of the risk of fragment impingement within the subacromial space. Therefore greater tuberosity displacement greater than 5 mm is another indication for surgery. Lesser tuberosity displacement greater than 1 cm is best treated operatively. Anatomic neck and head split fractures generally require operative treatment in the form of hemiarthroplasty. Fractures associated with humeral head dislocations require open reduction followed by fracture stabilization or hemiarthroplasty.

15. When is proximal humeral replacement (hemiarthroplasty) preferred over fracture fixation for the management of proximal humerus fractures?

The decision to replace the proximal humerus in order to provide fracture stabilization is based on several factors including the risk of avascular necrosis of the humeral head, the quality of bone, and the age and functional demands of the patient. Displaced four-part fractures, head split fractures, anatomic neck fractures, and three- and four-part fracture dislocations are best treated with hemiarthroplasty. Displaced three-part fractures in older patients or those with poor bone quality is another indication for hemiarthroplasty.

16. What are the final outcomes of surgical fixation of proximal humerus fractures?

The outcomes of surgically managed proximal humerus fractures are variable. Factors related to outcome include the type of fracture, the preoperative function of the patient, and the development of a complication related to the injury or surgery itself. Both percutaneous pinning and open reduction and internal fixation provide reliable results as long as bony union occurs and avascular necrosis of the humeral head does not develop. Patients undergoing a structured exercise program do better than those who do not. Most patients will regain functional range of motion of the shoulder. Most will attain active shoulder elevation to 120 to 150 degrees, external rotation to 30 to 45 degrees, and internal rotation to the lumbar spine. Studies using validated outcome scales note mild residual functional problems such as occasional pain, slight weakness, and limited function following three- and four-part fractures of the proximal humerus. These studies also note poor function or a significant complication in 10% to 40% of patients with displaced three- and four-part fractures.

17. What are the outcomes of hemiarthroplasty for the treatment of proximal humerus fractures?

Most studies of displaced proximal humerus fractures report inferior results from hemiarthroplasty as compared to fracture fixation. However, hemiarthroplasty remains the treatment of choice in many complex fracture patterns. Complications such as malunion and nonunion of the tuberosity fragments and humeral component malposition are thought to be related to poor outcomes. Most patients experience reliable pain relief following hemiarthroplasty for proximal humerus fractures; however, functional outcomes can be quite variable. The majority of patients can use the involved extremity well for activities of daily living below shoulder height, but overhead function is variable. A good outcome following hemiarthroplasty for humerus fracture is elevation to 110 to 130 degrees, external rotation to 30 degrees, minimal to no pain, and only a modest functional limit. These goals are generally achieved in between 60% and 70% of patients.

18. How often do nerve injuries accompany humeral shaft fractures?

Radial nerve injuries complicate between 6% and 18% of humeral shaft fractures. Other nerve injuries are rare, although brachial plexus injuries have been reported in higher energy trauma. Risk factors for radial nerve injuries include high-energy fractures, open fractures, and distal-third humeral shaft fractures. Over 90% of radial nerve injuries will recover spontaneously over a 4-month period.

19. What is the usual treatment for fracture of the humeral shaft?

The majority of humeral fractures can be treated conservatively. Most fractures are treated for a short period of time in a plaster or fiberglass coaptation splint. Within 1 to 2 weeks, the arm is placed in a prefabricated functional brace.

20. How do functional braces facilitate reduction of humeral shaft fractures?

Functional braces work in conjunction with the muscles of the upper arm. Compression of the soft tissue of the upper arm by the brace combined with gravity helps to align the fracture fragments. The elbow is left free for range of motion facilitating muscle activity, further enhancing muscle support around the fracture fragments.

21. What are the outcomes of conservative management of humeral shaft fractures?

Most patients with humeral shaft fractures do well with conservative measures. Conservative treatment generally shows fracture union rates greater than 90% to 95% for those injuries that meet the criteria for surgical management. Fracture union is usually obtained between 8 and 12 weeks. Between 80% and 98% of patients will obtain full range of motion and function of the shoulder and elbow joints.

22. What are the indications for surgical management of humeral shaft fractures?

There are several well-recognized indications for surgical management of humeral shaft fractures. These include pathologic fractures, associated brachial plexus injuries, associated forearm fractures (floating elbow), open fractures with high-grade soft tissue injury, vascular repair, bilateral humerus fractures, multiple trauma, and inability to maintain adequate alignment (varus angulation of 20 degrees, sagittal plane angulation of 30 degrees, or shortening of 3 cm).

23. What is the recommended treatment for radial nerve palsies associated with humeral shaft fractures?

Radial nerve palsy occurs in 6% to 18% of humeral shaft fractures. The majority of radial nerve palsies represent neurapraxic injuries and will improve with observation alone (>90%). Splinting and range of motion exercises of the hand are encouraged to prevent contracture formation. Electromyography and nerve conduction tests are performed after 3 months if failure of improvement of the palsy is noted clinically. Exploration and neurolysis or repair of the nerve is performed if no signs of recovery are seen after 3 to 4 months. Indications for acute nerve exploration include penetrating open fractures, high-grade soft tissue injuries, or secondary nerve palsies (in some cases).

24. What are the outcomes of surgical management of humeral shaft fractures?

Both open reduction and internal fixation (ORIF) and intramedullary fixation (IMF) produce reliable clinical results. The rate of fracture union following ORIF generally ranges from 94% to 98% whereas union rates following IMF range from 87% to 94%.

Both types of surgery are associated with low but significant rates of complications. Residual elbow pain is more common following ORIF. Shoulder pain and the need for repeat surgery are more common following IMF. Direct comparisons between the two surgical techniques show trends toward slightly better outcomes following ORIF.

Bibliography

Bigliani LU, Flatow EL, Pollock RG: Fractures of the proximal humerus. In Rockwood CA et al, editors: *Fractures in adults*, Philadelphia, 1996, pp 1055-1107, Lippincott-Raven.

Boileau P et al: Shoulder arthroplasty for the treatment of the sequelae of fractures of the proximal humerus, *J Shoulder Elbow Surg* 10:299-308, 2001.

Brumback RJ et al: Intramedullary stabilization of humeral shaft fractures in patients with multiple trauma, *J Bone Joint Surg* 68:960-970, 1986.

Chapman JR et al: Randomized prospective study of humeral shaft fracture fixation: intramedullary nails versus plates, *J Orthop Trauma* 14:162-166, 2000.

Darder A et al: Four-part displaced proximal humeral fractures: operative treatment using Kirschner wires and a tension band, *J Orthop Trauma* 7:497-505, 1993.

de Laat EA et al: Nerve lesions in primary shoulder dislocations and humeral neck fractures. A prospective clinical and EMG study, *J Bone Joint Surg Br* 76:381-383, 1994.

Hawkins RJ, Switlyk P: Acute prosthetic replacement for severe fractures of the proximal humerus, *Clin Orthop* 289:156-160, 1993.

Hintermann B, Trouillier HH, Schafer D: Rigid internal fixation of fractures of the proximal humerus in older patients, *J Bone Joint Surg Br* 82:1107-1112, 2000.

Jakob RP et al: Four-part valgus impacted fractures of the proximal humerus, *J Bone Joint Surg Br* 73:295-298, 1991.

Lind T, Kroner K, Jensen J: The epidemiology of fractures of the proximal humerus, *Arch Orthop Trauma Surg* 108:285-287, 1989.

McCormack RG et al: Fixation of fractures of the shaft of the humerus by dynamic compression plate or intramedullary nail. A prospective randomized trial, *J Bone Joint Surg Br* 82:336-339, 2000.

Pollock FH et al: Treatment of radial nerve palsy associated with fractures of the humerus, *J Bone Joint Surg* 63:239-243, 1981.

Rose SH et al: Epidemiologic features of humeral fractures, *Clin Orthop* 168:24-30, 1982.

Sarmiento A et al: Functional bracing of fractures of the shaft of the humerus, *J Bone Joint Surg* 59:596-601, 1977.

Sarmiento A et al: Functional bracing for comminuted extra-articular fractures of the distal third of the humerus, *J Bone Joint Surg Br* 72:283-287, 1990.

Stableforth PG: Four-part fractures of the neck of the humerus, *J Bone Joint Surg Br* 66:104-108, 1984.

Visser CP et al: Nerve lesions in proximal humeral fractures, *J Shoulder Elbow Surg* 10:421-427, 2001.

Wijgman AJ et al: Open reduction and internal fixation of three- and four-part fractures of the proximal part of the humerus, *J Bone Joint Surg Am* 84:1919-1925, 2002.

Zagorski JB et al: Diaphyseal fractures of the humerus. Treatment with prefabricated braces, *J Bone Joint Surg* 70:607-610, 1988.

Chapter 45

Nerve Entrapments of the Shoulder Region

Robert A. Sellin, PT, DSc, ECS, and
Edward Schrank, MPT, DSc, ECS

1. How is the spinal accessory nerve usually injured?

The spinal accessory nerve (cranial nerve XI) is a purely motor nerve and supplies motor fibers to the upper, middle, and lower trapezius muscles as well as the sternocleidomastoid. Mechanisms of injury include tumor, surgical procedures to the posterior triangle, and stretch and whiplash injuries.

2. Describe the typical presentation of a patient with a spinal accessory nerve injury.

The patient's symptoms may include a drooping shoulder girdle and/or flat upper trapezius muscle on the involved side. Shoulder pain is a major disabling factor, often attributed to traction at the brachial plexus. Winging of the scapula caused by trapezius weakness increases with abduction, whereas winging caused by serratus anterior weakness increases with forward elevation. If the level of injury is above the innervation of the sternocleidomastoid, the patient also may demonstrate weakness in rotating the face toward the opposite shoulder. Symptoms may seem to mimic shoulder dysfunction, with pseudoweakness of the rotator cuff secondary to decreased stability of the scapula, which in turn can contribute to rotator cuff pathology.

3. What surgery is performed for spinal accessory nerve palsy?

The Eden-Lange procedure is used for correction of spinal accessory nerve palsy; in this procedure the levator scapulae are transferred to the acromion and the rhomboids are transferred to the infraspinatus fossa. Excellent outcomes are expected in 75% of patients.

4. What are the common sites of entrapment of the suprascapular nerve?

The suprascapular nerve courses from nerve roots C5 and C6 and runs posterolaterally to the suprascapular notch beneath the transverse scapular ligament. The nerve is commonly injured at the suprascapular notch by ganglia or tumor. Injury at the suprascapular notch affects both the supraspinatus and the infraspinatus muscles and mimics rotator cuff pathology. The presenting symptoms include shoulder joint pain, weakness in external rotation, and, to a lesser degree, weakness in abduction.

The suprascapular nerve is also susceptible to traction and compression injuries as it travels around the spine of the scapula through the fibro-osseous tunnel formed by the spinoglenoid ligament and the spine of the scapula. Injury at this level results in strength changes in the infraspinatus muscle and shoulder pain, with sparing of the supraspinatus muscle. There may be wasting in the infraspinatus fossa. Overhead athletes are prone to suprascapular nerve injury at the spine of the scapula.

5. What diagnostic tests are available to help confirm suprascapular nerve injury?

Electromyography and nerve conduction studies are usually considered the criterion standard for diagnostic testing for suprascapular nerve injury, although when each test is used alone, it is not directly diagnostic. In patients with weakness, electrodiagnostic testing has shown a diagnostic accuracy of 91% in leading to a single, correct diagnosis. Diagnostic nerve blocks of the suprascapular nerve at the suprascapular notch have been used with a positive result—defined as temporary relief of the pain being experienced by the patient. Sensitivity and specificity studies are lacking with regard to the value of diagnostic nerve blocks for this problem. Magnetic resonance imaging has been shown to have a sensitivity and specificity of 94.5% and 100%, respectively, in detecting muscular edema associated with nerve injury, using electromyography and nerve conduction studies as the reference standard.

6. What nerve is most commonly injured after anterior shoulder dislocation?

The axillary nerve is most vulnerable to injury in anterior shoulder dislocations as it travels from the quadrilateral space, passing anteriorly and lying against the surgical neck of the humerus. The incidence of axillary nerve injury has been reported to be between 19% and 55% following anterior shoulder dislocations and up to 58% of proximal humeral fractures. Full recovery of axillary nerve injury resulting from dislocation or fracture occurs 85% to 100% of the time with nonoperative management within 6 to 12 months from the time of injury.

7. Describe the motor and sensory distributions of the musculocutaneous nerve.

The musculocutaneous nerve, which arises from the roots of C5, C6, and sometimes C7, is the terminal branch of the lateral cord of the brachial plexus. It innervates and penetrates the coracobrachialis muscle and travels between and innervates the biceps brachii and brachialis muscles. The musculocutaneous nerve emerges lateral to the biceps tendon as the lateral antebrachial cutaneous nerve, providing sensory innervation to the lateral forearm. Damage to this nerve causes weakness in elbow flexion and supination and numbness or paresthesias in the lateral forearm.

8. What are the common mechanisms of injury to the musculocutaneous nerve?

Injuries result from fractures or dislocations of the humerus, fracture of the clavicle, gunshot or stab wounds, entrapment by the coracobrachialis muscle, heavy exercise, and complications from anterior shoulder surgery. Musculocutaneous nerve injury attributable to a shoulder harness in a motor vehicle accident also has been reported.

9. What is rucksack palsy?

Rucksack palsy is an injury to the upper trunk of the brachial plexus or long thoracic nerve. The problem was described in soldiers serving in Vietnam, who carried their packs or "rucksack" with heavy loads of ammunition (60 to 80 lb). The rucksack usually compromised the upper trunk or long thoracic nerve, which arises from the C5-C7 nerve roots. Patients' symptoms may include shoulder pain and isolated scapular winging, or global symptoms of upper trunk involvement. Electromyographic testing is helpful in differentiating the location and severity of the lesion. Return of function is generally good, and recovery is proportional to the severity and chronicity of the lesion. The injury is more likely to occur on the nondominant side.

10. What surgical interventions are available for long thoracic nerve palsy?

- Transfer of the sternal head of the pectoralis major to the inferior angle of the scapula (91% satisfactory results)
- Thoracodorsal or medial pectoral nerve to long thoracic nerve transfer

11. What are the common causes of brachial plexus injuries?

Gunshot wounds, traction to arm or neck, fractures of the humerus, dislocations of the shoulder, primary nerve tumors, metastatic breast cancer, and radiation therapy can cause brachial plexus injuries. Closed injuries account for the majority of brachial plexus injuries, and 75% of injuries occur at the root level.

12. What are the clinical signs and symptoms of typical brachial plexus injuries?

- **Upper trunk** lesions affect the suprascapular, musculocutaneous, and axillary nerves as well as parts of the median and radial nerves. Patients' symptoms include weakness in shoulder flexion, abduction, and extension as well as marked weakness in elbow flexion, supination, and pronation and in wrist flexion. Areas of numbness and paresthesia may include the lateral forearm and hands as well as the thumb and index fingers.
- The **middle trunk** is rarely injured in isolation. Lesions produce weakness in the general distribution of the radial nerve, partially involving the triceps and sparing the brachioradialis.
- **Lower trunk** lesions cause motor weakness in muscles innervated by the ulnar nerve, the C8 components of the radial nerve, and muscles innervated by the distal median nerve, including the thenar muscles and the lumbricales. Patients have profound weakness of hand intrinsic muscles and sensory changes in the medial forearm (medial antebrachial cutaneous nerve), the medial hand, and the entire ring and little fingers.
- Lesions of either the **posterior or the anterior division** are rare in isolation, although a posterior division lesion has been reported. Posterior division lesions are similar in presentation to posterior cord lesions.
- **Lateral cord** lesions are similar to upper trunk lesions with sparing of the suprascapular nerve and upper trunk contributions to the axillary and radial nerves. Normal shoulder strength in flexion, extension, abduction, and external rotation; weakness in elbow flexion, supination, and pronation and wrist flexion; and numbness in the lateral forearm implicate the lateral cord.
- **Medial cord** lesions are similar to lower trunk lesions with sparing of C8 contributions to the radial nerve. Finger extension has normal strength.
- **Posterior cord** lesions are rare in isolation.

13. What key muscle tests help to differentiate a C5-C6 root injury from a lateral cord lesion?

A C5-C6 root lesion affects all C5-C6 muscles, whereas an upper trunk lesion spares the dorsal scapular nerve to the rhomboids and the long thoracic nerve to the serratus muscles. A lateral cord lesion spares the suprascapular nerve (shoulder external rotation and abduction) as well as contributions to the posterior cord.

14. What is thoracic outlet syndrome?

Thoracic outlet syndrome (TOS) refers to the compression of the neurovascular structures (roots or trunks of the brachial plexus and axillary or subclavian arteries) between the neck and axilla. TOS can be subdivided into vascular or neural compression symptoms, or both, depending on which specific structures within the cervicoaxillary canal are compromised. True neurologic TOS manifests as a chronic lower trunk brachial plexopathy caused by anatomic anomalies. The anomalies include a taut band extending from near the tubercle of the first thoracic rib to the tip of either the C7 transverse process or a rudimentary cervical rib. The C8 and T1 anterior primary rami can be stretched around this band either before or after forming the lower trunk. Electromyography may show evidence of denervation in the intrinsic hand muscles, but this is not common. Neural compression symptoms occur more commonly than vascular symptoms. The cause of TOS also can be traumatic. A midshaft fracture of the clavicle occasionally results in injury to the blood vessels or brachial plexus situated between the clavicle and first thoracic rib. With this type of injury, the terminal portion of the subclavian artery, the initial portion of the subclavian vein, and the proximal aspects of the cords of the brachial plexus may be damaged.

15. Describe the various tests used to evaluate a patient suspected of having TOS.

- The **Adson maneuver** is performed in the sitting or standing position with the examiner palpating the radial pulse in the patient's abducted and extended arm. The examiner extends and externally rotates the arm as the patient rotates his or her head toward the examiner and takes a deep breath. A diminished or absent radial pulse suggests compression of the subclavian artery by the scalene muscles. Specificity has been reported from 32% to 87%.
- The **Allen test** is similar to Adson's test except the arm is abducted 90 degrees and the elbow is flexed 90 degrees. The patient turns his or her head away from the examiner and holds the breath. A diminished or absent radial pulse is a positive finding. Specificity has been reported from 18% to 43%.
- In the **Roos test** the patient holds both arms in the 90/90 position of the Allen test and then rapidly opens and closes the fingers for 3 minutes. Inability to maintain the test position, diminished motor function of the hands, or decreased sensation or paresthesia are suggestive of TOS secondary to neurovascular compromise.
- In the **Wright test** the arm is hyperabducted so that the hand is brought over the head with the elbow and arm in the coronal plane. Wright advocated performing the test in the sitting and then supine positions. Taking a breath or rotating or extending the head and neck may have an additional effect. The pulse is palpated for differences. This test is used to detect compression in the costoclavicular space.
- The **costoclavicular syndrome test or military brace** is accomplished by palpating the radial pulse and drawing the patient's shoulder down and back. A positive test is indicated by the absence of the pulse. Sensitivity has been reported at 95%, with specificity from 53% to 85%.
- In the **provocation elevation test** the patient elevates both arms above the horizontal and rapidly opens and closes the hands 15 times. If fatigue, cramping, or tingling occurs, the test is positive for vascular insufficiency and TOS.
- In the **shoulder girdle passive elevation test** the patient crosses one arm on the chest. The examiner stands behind the patient and passively elevates the shoulder girdle upward and forward (passive shoulder shrug). The position is held for 30 seconds. A positive test is reported if the pulse becomes stronger, skin color improves, or hand temperature increases. The patient also may report a "relief phenomenon," which can range from numbness, pins and needles, or pain as the ischemia to the nerve is released.
- In the **Halstead maneuver,** the radial pulse is palpated and the examiner applies a downward traction on the arm while the patient's neck is hyperextended and the head is rotated to the opposite side. Absence or decreased pulse indicates a positive test for TOS.

16. How many TOS tests should be performed in a clinical exam?

The false-positive rate for all of the TOS tests is relatively high. Many of them test only the vascular component of TOS. One way to decrease the chance of a false-positive test is to perform at least three different tests. The literature reports a false-positive rate of 12% when two TOS tests are performed. If three or more are performed, the false-positive rate can be reduced to 2% or less. Gillard reports a mean sensitivity and specificity of 72% and 53%, respectively, when the Adson, hyperabduction, and Wright tests are used in a cluster.

17. What outcomes are associated with physical therapy treatment of TOS?

Physical therapy treatment of TOS shows the following typical outcomes: 60% will have symptomatic improvement, 24% will not change, and 16% continue to worsen.

18. What outcomes are associated with surgical treatment of TOS?

The frequency of good to excellent results varies widely, ranging from 24% to 90%. Abnormal SSEPs and arterial photoplethysmography correlate with improved results.

19. What causes "dead arm syndrome"?

Dead arm syndrome historically has been attributed to various causes, including recurrent transient anterior shoulder subluxation, rotator cuff tear, labral tears, and psychological disorders. Often radiographs and electromyograms are normal, and the young athlete is frustrated. The mechanism of injury in overhead-throwing athletes appears to be related to acceleration in the late cocking phase of throwing. The injury also can be caused by direct trauma to the arm. Some believe a type 2 **s**uperior **l**abral **a**nterior to **p**osterior (SLAP) lesion, with or without rotator cuff involvement, is the underlying cause. Although many symptoms described by patients suggest possible neural compromise, true neurologic changes are rarely, if ever, present.

20. What is a "burner"?

A "burner" or "stinger" is a nerve injury that often occurs during sporting activities, most frequently football. It is generally thought to be a traction or compression injury of the upper trunk of the brachial plexus or the fifth or sixth cervical roots. The disorder usually produces transient pain, numbness, and paresthesia. Chronic burner syndrome may result from nerve root compression in the intervertebral foramina secondary to disk disease in older collegiate and professional athletes.

21. Describe the clinical findings of a patient with Pancoast's tumor.

Pancoast's tumor can compromise the C8-T1 roots of the brachial plexus via compression from the apex of the lung. The presenting symptoms of the patient are sensory changes in the medial forearm and hand, including the fourth and fifth digits. Other signs may include intrinsic muscle wasting, Horner syndrome, and a history of night pain. Clinicians should be especially suspicious of a Pancoast tumor in smokers who have these symptoms and no history of trauma or neurologic disease.

22. What is Horner syndrome?

Horner syndrome consists of unilateral enophthalmos (sunken eyeball), ptosis (drooping eyelid), miosis (contraction of the pupil), and flushing of the face caused by ipsilateral involvement of the sympathetic chain fibers in the cervical sympathetic chain or upper thoracic cord.

23. What are the most common peripheral nerve injuries that affect the shoulder region?

The most common peripheral nerve injury involving the shoulder region is the "burner" followed by injuries involving the cervical root, axillary nerve, suprascapular nerve, and long thoracic nerve. Football players have the greatest number of peripheral nerve injuries.

24. Are cowboy collars effective in preventing burners and stingers in football players?

No. Research does not show that cowboy collars significantly prevent burners and stingers. However, they are better than shoulder pads alone in the prevention of cervical hyperextension injuries.

25. What does reduce the occurrence of burners and stingers in football players?

Strength training to the cervical spine and shoulder girdle musculature is an effective way to reduce the occurrence of burners and stingers in football players.

Bibliography

Bartosh RA, Dugdale TW, Nielsen R: Isolated musculocutaneous nerve injury complicating closed fracture of the clavicle, *Am J Sports Med* 20:356-359, 1992.

Black KP, Lombardo JA: Suprascapular nerve injuries with isolated paralysis of the infraspinatus, *Am J Sports Med* 18:225-228, 1990.

Burkhard SS, Morgan CD, Kibler BW: Shoulder injuries in overhead athletes: the "dead arm" revisited, *Clin Sports Med* 19:125-159, 2000.

Cummins CA et al: Suprascapular nerve entrapment at the spinoglenoid notch in a professional baseball pitcher, *Am J Sports Med* 27:810-812, 1999.

Cummins CA, Messer TM, Schafer MF: Infraspinatus muscle atrophy in professional baseball players, *Am J Sports Med* 32:116-120, 2004.

Daube JR: Rucksack paralysis, *JAMA* 208:2447-2452, 1969.

Dubuisson AS, Kline DG: Brachial plexus injury: a survey of 100 consecutive cases from a single service, *Neurosurgery* 51:673-682 (discussion 682-683), 2005.

Gillard J et al: Diagnosing thoracic outlet syndrome: contribution of provocative tests, ultrasonography, electrophysiology, and helical computed tomography in 48 patients, *Joint Bone Spine* 68:416-424, 2001.

Kuhlman GS, McKeag DB: The "burner": a common nerve injury in contact sports, *Am Fam Physician* 60:2035-2042, 1999.

Levitz CL, Reilly PJ, Torg JS: The pathomechanics of chronic, recurrent cervical nerve root neuropraxia. The chronic burner syndrome, *Am J Sports Med* 25:73-76, 1997.

Logigian EL et al: Stretch induced spinal accessory nerve palsy, *Muscle Nerve* 11:146-150, 1988.

Markey KL, Di Benedetto M, Curl WW: Upper trunk brachial plexopathy. The stinger syndrome, *Am J Sports Med* 21:650-655, 1993.

Marx RG, Bombardier C, Wright JG: What do we know about the reliability and validity of physical examination tests used to examine the upper extremity? *J Hand Surg [Am]* 24:185-193, 1999.

McIlveen SJ et al: Isolated nerve injuries about the shoulder, *Clin Orthop Rel Res* 306:54-63, 1994.

Nardin RA, Rutkove SB, Raynor EM: Diagnostic accuracy of electrodiagnostic testing in the evaluation of weakness, *Muscle Nerve* 26:201-205, 2002.

Novak CB, Collins ED, Mackinnon SE: Outcomes following the conservative management of thoracic outlet syndrome, *J Hand Surg* 20:542-548, 1995.

Perlmutter GS, Leffert RD, Zarins B: Direct injury to the axillary nerve in athletes playing contact sports, *Am J Sports Med* 25:65-68, 1997.

Rankine JJ: Adult traumatic brachial plexus injury, *Clin Radiol* 59(9):767-774, 2004.

Rowe CR: Recurrent transient anterior subluxation of the shoulder: the "dead arm" syndrome, *Clin Orthop Rel Res* 223:11-19, 1987.

Safran MR: Nerve injury about the shoulder in athletes, part 1: suprascapular nerve and axillary nerve, *Am J Sports Med* 32:803-819, 2004.

Safran MR: Nerve injury about the shoulder in athletes, part 2: long thoracic nerve, spinal accessory nerve, burners/stingers, thoracic outlet syndrome, *Am J Sports Med* 32(4):1063-1076, 2004.

Tirman PF et al: Association of glenoid labral cysts with labral tears and glenohumeral instability: radiologic findings and clinical significance, *Radiology* 190:653-658, 1994.

Warrens AN, Heaton JM: Thoracic outlet compression syndrome: the lack of reliability of its clinical assessment, *Ann R Coll Surg Engl* 69:203-204, 1987.

Section VI

The Elbow and Forearm

Chapter 46

Functional Anatomy of the Elbow

Jeffrey D. Placzek, MD, PT

1. Describe the joints of the elbow.

The elbow consists of three joints: the ulnohumeral, radiocapitellar, and proximal radioulnar joints. The olecranon forms the greater sigmoid notch of the ulna, which articulates with the trochlea to form a uniaxial ginglymoid joint. The radiocapitellar and proximal radioulnar joints form a trochoid or pivoted joint. The thin elbow capsule and synovial membrane define the confines of the joint, beginning proximal to the coronoid and olecranon fossae and ending beyond the tips of the coronoid and olecranon processes. Because the maximal volume of the capsule is 15 to 30 ml at 80-degree flexion, the elbow often is held in this position to minimize pain from capsular distention secondary to acute hemiarthrosis.

2. What is the normal carrying angle of the elbow?

The carrying angle of the elbow varies with flexion and extension, ranging from 6 degrees of varus with full flexion to 11 degrees of valgus in full extension. In men the mean value is between 11 and 14 degrees (full extension). Some studies show that women tend to have larger carrying angles than men, with an average value between 13 and 16 degrees.

3. Describe the articular geometry of the distal humerus.

The articular surface has a 30-degree anterior angulation, 5 to 7 degrees of internal rotation, and 6 to 8 degrees of valgus tilt.

4. Describe the interosseous membrane (IOM) of the forearm.

The interosseous membrane is composed of the central band, the proximal band, several accessory bands, and the membranous portion. The most important structure is the central band, which originates from the radius and is angled distally to attach to the ulna at a 21-degree angle. The central band is 1.5 to 2 cm wide and is responsible for 71% of the IOM stiffness after excision of the radial head.

5. What portion of the longitudinal growth of the upper arm does the elbow contribute?

The elbow accounts for only 20% of the total longitudinal growth of the humerus. The proximal humerus accounts for the remaining 80%.

6. What structures contribute to elbow stability?

Elbow stability is maintained by a combination of bony and soft tissue components. Primary stabilizers include the coronoid (ulnohumeral joint), lateral ulnar collateral ligament, and anterior band of the medial collateral ligament. Secondary stabilizers include the radial head, extensor and flexor muscle masses, and joint capsule.

7. Describe the medial ligamentous complex.

The main constraint to elbow valgus instability is the medial collateral ligament (MCL). The MCL originates on the central two thirds of the anteroinferior medial condyle and inserts onto the anteromedial coronoid. It has three distinct bundles. The anterior bundle, which is the strongest, inserts on the anterior coronoid and greater sigmoid notch. The thin posterior bundle attaches to the posterior greater sigmoid notch. The oblique bundle is variable in its attachments. The anterior bundle is divided into anterior and posterior bands. The anterior band is the primary restraint to valgus stress from 30 to 90 degrees while the posterior band tensions from 90 to 120 degrees.

8. Describe the lateral ligamentous complex.

The lateral collateral ligament (LCL) complex consists of the radial collateral ligament (lateral epicondyle to annular ligament), the annular ligament (anterior to posterior edge of sigmoid notch), the accessory collateral ligament (variable, posterior annular ligament to supinator crest), and the lateral ulnar collateral ligaments (LUCLs, lateral epicondyle to supinator crest), which blend intimately with the underlying joint capsule and more superficial extensor tendons. The LUCL insertion may be broad-based or bilobed and is the primary constraint to posterolateral rotatory instability.

9. Describe the most important varus and valgus stabilizers of the elbow at 0 and 90 degrees of flexion.

Varus stress at the elbow is resisted by the LCL, anconeus muscle, and joint capsule. With full extension, the LCL contributes 14% of the restraint to varus stress; 54% is provided by the joint surface and 32% by the capsule. With 90 degrees of flexion, restraint to varus stress provided by the LCL, joint articulation, and capsule changes to 9%, 78%, and 13%, respectively.

Valgus stress is resisted mainly by the fan-shaped MCL complex, which consists of anterior, intermediate, and posterior fibers. The anterior oblique fibers are taut throughout flexion-extension and are the most important valgus stabilizers. The posterior oblique ligaments are taut only during flexion. At full extension, contributions from the MCL, joint surface, and anterior capsule to resisting valgus stress are equal. At 90 degrees of flexion, the MCL contributes 54% of the resistance, the radial head contributes 30%, and the remainder is supplied by articular congruity and the anterior capsule.

10. Describe posterolateral rotatory instability.

Posterolateral rotatory instability (PLRI) is a common pattern of acute elbow instability caused by a fall onto an outstretched arm. The humerus rotates internally on the elbow, which undergoes external rotation and valgus loading as the elbow flexes. Specifically, the ulnar rotates externally while the radiohumeral joint subluxates posterolaterally, allowing the coronoid to pass under the trochlea as the ulna swings into a valgus position.

11. What is the Morrey elbow instability scale?

Morrey described five elbow instability types based on damage to particular structures about the elbow:

- Type 0—elbow reduced and stable when stressed
- Type I—PLRI with a positive shift test; torn LUCL
- Type II—perched condyles, unstable elbow with varus stress; torn LUCL and anterior and posterior capsules
- Type IIIa—posterior dislocation of the elbow with valgus instability; torn LUCL, posterior MCL, and anterior and posterior capsules
- Type IIIb—posterior dislocation of the elbow with gross instability; torn LUCL, anterior MCL, posterior MCL, and anterior and posterior capsules

12. During closed-chain upper extremity exercise, how much weight is transmitted through the radiocapitellar and ulnohumeral joints?

Approximately 60% of the force is transferred through the radiocapitellar joint and 40% through the ulnohumeral joint. The greatest amount of force is transmitted between 0 and 30 degrees of flexion.

13. Describe normal arthrokinematics at the elbow.

Motion at the elbow is primarily gliding for both flexion and extension. Rolling occurs in the final 5 to 10 degrees of range of motion (ROM) for both flexion and extension. Minimal adduction may occur with flexion and minimal abduction with extension, although the magnitude of these movements is debated.

14. Differentiate "normal" from "functional" elbow ROM.

The normal average ROM of the elbow is from 0 degrees (full extension) to 150 degrees (full flexion), with 85 degrees of supination and 80 degrees of pronation. However, activities of daily living usually can be accomplished with a ROM of 30 to 130 degrees of flexion, 50 degrees of supination, and 50 degrees of pronation. If pronation and supination are normal with good motion of the wrist and shoulder, functional mobility may occur with as little as 75 to 120 degrees of motion.

15. Where is the axis of flexion and extension in the elbow? Where is the axis during pronation and supination?

The axis of flexion of the elbow is a line through the center of the capitellum and the center of curvature of the trochlear groove, colinear with the distal anterior humeral cortex. Motion resembles a "loose hinge," with 3 to 5 degrees of rotation and varus/valgus motion during the flexion arc. During pronation and supination, the radius rotates along an axis passing through the center of the radial head and the distal ulnar fovea. The radial head translates 1 to 2 mm proximally during pronation.

16. Which muscle is considered the "workhorse" of elbow flexion?

The brachialis muscle is the primary flexor of the elbow, inserting approximately 1 cm distal to the coronoid onto both the ulna and the capsule. The brachioradialis has the longest lever arm.

17. Describe the effect of speed on muscle recruitment during supination.

During slow, unresisted supination activity, the supinator may act independently. However, all rapid and resisted movements are assisted by the biceps. This holds true regardless of elbow position.

18. Describe the effects of speed and joint angle on pronation activity.

The pronator quadratus is the primary pronator of the forearm, regardless of elbow position. With increasing speeds or resistance, activity of the pronator teres increases.

19. What is the effect of changing forearm position on muscle testing of elbow flexion strength?

Resisting elbow flexion with the forearm in neutral position places maximal stress on the brachioradialis muscle. Testing the elbow with the forearm pronated minimizes biceps activity. Forearm position does not affect activity of the brachialis.

20. At what position are elbow flexion strength and supination strength maximal?

Elbow flexion strength is maximal at 90 to 110 degrees of flexion. The biceps acts most strongly as a supinator at 90 degrees of flexion. Pronation strength is 15% to 20% less than supination strength in the normal elbow.

21. Describe the innervation of the various muscles controlling movement at the elbow.

Action	Muscles	Nerve Root	Nerve
Flexion	Brachialis	C5, C6	Musculocutaneous
	Biceps brachii		—
	Brachioradialis		Radial
Extension	Triceps	C7	Radial
	Anconeus		
Pronation	Pronator teres	C6, C7	Median
	Pronator quadratus		
Supination	Biceps	C5, C6	Musculocutaneous
	Supinator	C5, C6, C7	Deep branch of radial

22. Which arteries supply blood to the elbow?

Three arcades surround the elbow joint. The medial arcade is formed by the superior and inferior ulnar collateral arteries and the posterior ulnar recurrent artery. The posterior arcade is formed by the medial and lateral arcades and the middle collateral artery. The lateral arcade is formed from the radial and middle collateral, radial recurrent, and interosseous recurrent arteries.

23. What is the order (and approximate age) of ossification of structures around the elbow?

Ossification follows the acronym CRMTOL: **c**apitellum (6 months to 2 years), which includes the lateral crista of the trochlea; **r**adial head (4 years); **m**edial epicondyle (6 to 7 years); **t**rochlea (8 years); **o**lecranon (8 to 10 years); and **l**ateral epicondyle (12 years).

24. Describe the anatomy of the ulnar nerve at the elbow.

The ligament of Osborne is present in all elbows, and two thirds of elbows will also display a discrete arcade of ligament of Struthers. An average of one capsular branch diverges from the ulnar nerve 7 mm proximal to the medial epicondyle. An average of three motor branches to the flexor carpi ulnaris (FCU) is typical. Approximately 45% of elbows will have an aponeurosis distal to Osborne's ligament that runs between the FCU and medial epicondylar muscles.

25. The medial antebrachial cutaneous nerve is subject to painful neuromas if disrupted during surgery. Where do branches of this nerve typically cross the medial elbow?

Approximately 61% of the time a branch is noted an average of 1.8 cm above the medial epicondyle; 100% of the time branches cross distal to the medial epicondyle at an average distance of 3.1 cm.

26. What is the blood supply to the extensor carpi radialis brevis (ECRB) tendon?

The radial recurrent artery supplies the tendon through branches on its medial and lateral borders. Important contributions are given from the posterior branch of the radial collateral artery and more minor contributions from the interosseous recurrent artery. These arteries form a superficial network with the deep portion of the tendon being nearly avascular.

27. What is the relationship of the posterior interosseous nerve (PIN) near the lateral elbow?

Pronation of the forearm increases the distance from the capitellum to the PIN to an average of 52 mm. Supination draws the nerve proximal with an average distance of 33 mm from the capitellum.

Bibliography

Degeorges R, Masquelet AC: The cubital tunnel: an anatomical part of its distal part, *Surg Radiol Anat* 24:169-176, 2002.

Diliberti T, Botte M, Abrams R: Anatomical considerations regarding the posterior interosseous nerve during posterolateral approaches to the proximal part of the radius, *J Bone Joint Surg* 82A:809-813, 2000.

Gonzalez MH et al: The ulnar nerve at the elbow and its local branching: an anatomic study, *J Hand Surg Br* 26:142-144, 2001.

Hollinshead WH: *Anatomy for surgeons,* Vol 3, New York, 1969, Harper & Row.

Lowe JB, Maggi SP, Mackinnon SE: The position of crossing branches of the medial antebrachial cutaneous nerve during cubital tunnel surgery in humans, *Plast Reconstr Surg* 114:692-696, 2004.

O'Driscoll SW, Morrey BF, Korinek S: Elbow subluxation and dislocation: a spectrum of instability, *Clin Orthop Rel Res* 280:186-197, 1992.

Schneeberger AG, Masquelet AC: Arterial vascularization of the proximal extensor carpi radialis brevis tendon, *Clin Orthop* 398:239-244, 2002.

Simon SR, editor: *Orthopaedic basic science,* Rosemont, Ill, 1994, American Academy of Orthopaedic Surgeons.

Yamaguchi K et al: The extraosseous and intraosseous arterial anatomy of the adult elbow, *J Bone Joint Surg* 79A:1653-1662, 1997.

Chapter 47

Common Orthopaedic Elbow Dysfunction

T. Kevin Robinson, PT, DSc, OCS

1. Describe an elbow with joint effusion.

All three joints of the elbow complex are affected because they have a common joint capsule. The joint swelling is most evident in the triangular space between the radial head, tip of the olecranon, and lateral epicondyle. The elbow is held in the loose packed position of about 70 degrees of flexion, because in this position the joints have maximal volume.

2. What is "little league elbow"?

Little league elbow is a generic term referring to several overuse injuries in young throwers. Examples include osteochondritis dissecans of the capitellum with or without loose bodies, injury and premature closure of the proximal radial epiphysis, overgrowth of the radial head, and medially stressed valgus overuse. The repetitive valgus stress of throwing results in microtrauma of the medial anterior oblique ligament and compression of the radiocapitellar joint. Repeated traction on the olecranon at the site of the triceps brachii insertion may produce olecranon apophysitis or an olecranon stress fracture. Excessive repeated traction through the medial elbow may result in enlargement of the medial humeral epicondyle as well as inflammation of the medial humeral apophysis. Osteochondrosis dissecans of the radial head and/or capitellum or osteochondrosis of the capitellum (Panner's disease) may result from compressive forces through the lateral elbow during the throwing motion. These same forces can result in injury to the proximal radial epiphysis and early closure of its growth center.

3. How is little league elbow treated?

In general, little league elbow is treated with relative rest and absolutely no throwing for up to 1 year. If significant fragmentation or separation of the medial humeral apophysis is seen on plain radiographs, surgery may be indicated.

4. Describe the recommended sequence of pitches for adolescent athletes.

One of the main causes of elbow injury in adolescent athletes is throwing pitches that they are not physically prepared to perform. Baseball's Medical and Safety Advisory Committee has recommended when various pitches should be introduced. The first pitch introduced is the fast ball at 8 years, followed by the change-up at 10 years, the curve ball at 14 years, the knuckle ball at 15 years, and the slider and fork ball at 16 years.

5. What functional tests help to confirm the diagnosis of little league elbow?

Flexing and extending the elbow with maintenance of valgus stress should elicit elbow pain. Valgus stress testing may reveal pain and increased range. Loss of passive elbow extension may result from early flexion contracture, which is common in professional pitchers and may represent serious damage in children or adolescents.

6. What is lateral epicondylitis?

The term "tendonitis" has been used to describe a hypothetical chronic inflammatory process in the overused tendon. However, histologic examinations of excised pathologic tendons have consistently failed to display the presence of inflammatory cells. Instead, the tissue is characterized by the presence of dense populations of fibroblasts, vascular hyperplasia, and disorganized collagen, termed by Nirschl as angiofibroblastic hyperplasia. Angiofibroblastic hyperplasia appears to be the result of a failed healing response to microtears, combined with vascular deprivation in the tendon's origin, preventing healing to occur.

7. Which structure is most commonly involved in lateral epicondylitis (tennis elbow)?

The most commonly involved structure is the extensor carpi radialis brevis (ECRB) tendon followed by the extensor digitorum communis (EDC) tendon. These tendons may be histologically indistinguishable at the common origin. The ECRB tendon has the greatest EMG activity of the forearm muscles, especially in the acceleration and early follow-through phases of the tennis swing. Tendon fibers attaching to the periosteum are relatively avascular and tend to heal very slowly. Immature granulation tissue is present at the injury repair site.

8. What are the differential diagnoses for lateral epicondylitis?

- Entrapment of the radial nerve
- Degenerative changes of the radiocapitellar joint
- Posterolateral rotatory instability
- Occult fractures of the radial head or lateral humeral epicondyle
- Posterior epicondylitis at the triceps attachment to the olecranon
- Panner's disease
- Tumor of the capitellum or in the supinator muscle
- Rheumatoid arthritis
- Tendinitis of the long head of the biceps (caused by insertion on the radius)
- Cervical spinal problems

9. Are forearm support bands (counterforce braces) an effective orthosis for lateral epicondylitis?

Counterforce braces consist of a flexible band that fits around the proximal forearm and applies pressure to the underlying tissues during activity. These braces may reduce acceleration forces by 46%. While one study showed that they increase the rate of fatigue in unimpaired people, other studies have shown decreased pain threshold with no changes in isokinetic strength.

10. Describe the incidence and demographics of lateral epicondylitis.

Lateral epicondylitis most commonly occurs in patients between 35 and 50 years of age. The incidence varies in different populations. In studies performed at industrial health clinics, epicondylitis was most commonly associated with work-related activities (35% to 64% of all reported cases). Tennis players also are at high risk; 10% to 50% will have symptoms at some time in their career. Risk increases with poor stroke mechanics, striking the ball off center, improper grip size, and harder court surfaces. Amateurs tend to have lateral epicondylitis secondary to the backhand whereas professionals usually have medial epicondylitis because of forceful serving.

11. What is the best treatment for lateral epicondylitis?

Corticosteroid injections have shown short-term improvement (6 weeks) with this condition; however, the few long-term follow-up studies for this intervention show success rates at 60% or lower. There has been one study that has compared both corticosteroid injection and physical therapy. Hart found that at 6 weeks, 92% of patients receiving corticosteroid injection reported improvement in symptoms compared to 47% of patients receiving physical therapy. However, at 52 weeks only 69% of patients receiving corticosteroid injections had positive outcome measurements (self-reported and blinded assessments) compared to 91% for the physical therapy interventions. The physical therapy intervention used was nine treatments of pulsed ultrasound, deep friction massage, and an exercise program. Studies comparing the effects of phonophoresis versus ultrasound have shown that both treatment options result in decreased pain and increased pressure tolerance in selected soft tissue injuries, but the addition of phonophoresis does not augment the benefits of ultrasound alone.

12. What is the Mills maneuver? Is it an effective treatment for lateral epicondylitis?

Numerous studies have reported that about 10% of patients with lateral epicondylitis are unresponsive to conservative treatment. A final option before surgery is the Mills maneuver, which is intended to pull apart the two surfaces joined by a painful scar. Once separation is attained, permanent lengthening of the common extensor tendon results. In one study of over 100 resistant cases, repeat manipulation was needed in only six patients and surgical intervention was needed in only one patient over a 20-year period. The maneuver is performed with the patient in supine position, the wrist in full flexion, and the forearm fully pronated. The elbow is moved suddenly from a flexed position to full extension. This maneuver is painful because it places maximal stretch on the scar. Wadsworth recommends performing the maneuver only after the site is injected with 0.5 ml of methylprednisolone and 0.5 ml of 2% lidocaine.

13. What are the common surgical treatments of lateral epicondylitis?

Nirschl and Pettrone recommend a procedure in which the degenerated extensor carpi radialis brevis origin is resected and the lateral epicondyle is decorticated. In a 10-year follow-up study, pain relief was noted in over 90% of patients. Spencer and Herndon recommend simple fasciotomy of the extensor origin. They reported "excellent" or "good" results in 96% of 23 patients. Other studies have reported "excellent" or "good" results in 31 of 35 patients at long-term follow-up. This technique is recommended because of its simplicity, minimal complications, and recovery time of 3 to 4 weeks. Arthroscopic release of the ECRB tendon has excellent results in 80% to 95% of the cases with early return to work (approximately 2 weeks).

14. What other treatments are available for lateral epicondylitis?

Autologous blood injections demonstrate ~79% pain relief in those who have failed steroid injection and exercise. Platelet-derived growth factor is thought to stimulate a healing response. Lithotripsy studies have shown mixed reviews with little benefit shown over placebo in the blinded studies.

15. What is radial tunnel syndrome? Why is it confused with lateral epicondylitis?

The radial tunnel is about 2 inches in length, extending proximally from the capitellum of the humerus, between the brachioradialis and brachialis, and distally through the supinator muscle. The radial nerve may become entrapped in this tunnel, resulting in persistent pain around the lateral epicondyle and an aching sensation in the extensor and/or supinator muscle mass distal to the lateral epicondyle. Tennis elbow straps may increase symptoms because of increased pressure compression over the radial tunnel.

16. What is "nursemaid's elbow"?

Nursemaid's elbow ("pulled elbow") is subluxation of the radial head, usually in children younger than 5 years. It usually occurs when a child is forcefully pulled or jerked by the arm with the arm in extension. Radiographs are of little benefit, even with comparison views of the uninvolved elbow. The combination of patient history and limitation of motion, especially absence of supination of the elbow, usually makes the diagnosis. A sudden pull on the extended elbow while the forearm is pronated may produce a tear in the distal attachment of the annular ligament to the radial neck. The radial head penetrates partially through the tear as it is distracted from the capitellum. Then the proximal part of the annular ligament slips into the radiohumeral joint, where it becomes trapped between the joint surfaces once the pull is released. The source of pain is the trapped annular ligament. The entrapped ligament can be freed by suddenly supinating the forearm while the elbow is flexed.

17. Describe medial epicondylitis.

Medial epicondylitis has been called golfer's elbow, medial tennis elbow, and even swimmer's elbow. It is an overuse injury that results from repetitive valgus stress on the medial elbow combined with wrist flexion and pronation. The patient with medial epicondylitis usually presents with pain, inflammation, and point tenderness at the medial epicondyle where the flexor/pronator group originates.

18. What are the differential diagnoses for medial epicondylitis? How are they ruled out?

The differential diagnoses for medial epicondylitis are medial collateral ligament (MCL) injuries, ulnar nerve injuries, and degenerative changes of the medial elbow joint. Both medial epicondylitis and MCL injury can create pain on valgus stress testing. It is possible to differentiate the two injuries by applying valgus stress to a slightly flexed elbow while the wrist is flexed and the forearm pronated. This arm position eliminates the symptoms attributed to medial epicondylitis and results in a painless valgus stress test, provided that the ulnar collateral ligament (UCL) is uninjured. Passive wrist extension and active resisted wrist flexion and pronation can further distinguish medial epicondylitis from UCL injury. A positive Tinel's sign, tenderness of the ulnar nerve to palpation, and paresthesia and numbness in the fourth and fifth fingers confirm ulnar nerve injuries. According to Nirschl, 60% of patients with medial epicondylitis have ulnar nerve symptoms. Radiographic changes include bone spurs and degenerative disease.

19. What is olecranon bursitis?

The olecranon bursa is located between the skin and tip of the olecranon process. Bursitis is caused by trauma because of chronic overuse (e.g., leaning on the elbow ["student's elbow"]) or by direct impact that results in inflammation or infection. The differential diagnoses include fracture of the olecranon process of the ulna, gout, rheumatoid arthritis, and synovial cyst of the elbow joint. Usually the elbow joint is not involved because the bursa and joint do not communicate unless rheumatoid arthritis is present. If the joint is infected, all motion is resisted.

20. Describe the management of olecranon bursitis.

Traumatic bursitis is managed symptomatically with immobilization in a splint, compressive dressings, and contrast baths. Aspiration of the bursa usually does not prevent recurrence of swelling because of continued flexion and extension activities. If the bursa is painful and prevents activity, aspiration is indicated and may be both diagnostic and therapeutic.

Bibliography

Bennett JB, Tullos HS: Acute injuries to the elbow. In Nicholos JA, Hershman EB, editors: *Upper extremity in sports medicine,* St Louis, 1990, pp 319-334, Mosby.

Brody LT: The elbow, forearm, wrist and hand. In Hall CM, Brody LT, editors: *Therapeutic exercise: moving toward function,* Philadelphia, 1999, pp 626-663, Lippincott Williams & Wilkins.

Buettner CM, Leaver-Dunn D: *Prevention and treatment of elbow injuries in adolescent pitchers,* Champaign, Ill, 2000, Athletic Therapy Today.
Dimberg L: The prevalence and causation of tennis elbow (lateral humeral epicondylitis) in a population of workers in an engineering industry, *Ergonomics* 30:573-580, 1987.
Hart LE: Corticosteroid injections, physiotherapy, or a wait-and-see policy for lateral epicondylitis? *Clin J Sports Med* 12:403-404, 2002.
Klaiman MD et al: Phonophoresis versus ultrasound in the treatment of common musculoskeletal conditions, *Med Sci Sports Exercise* 30:1349-1355, 1998.
Knebel PT et al: Effects of the forearm support band on wrist extensor muscle fatigue, *J Orthop Sci Phys Ther* 29:677-685, 1999.
Nirschl RP, Pettrone F: Tennis elbow. The surgical treatment of lateral epicondylitis, *J Bone Joint Surg* 61A:832-839, 1979.
Noteboom T et al: Tennis elbow: a review, *J Orthop Sci Phys Ther* 25:357-366, 1994.
Spencer GE, Herndon CH: Surgical treatment of epicondylitis, *J Bone Joint Surg* 35A:421-424, 1953.

Chapter 48

Elbow Fractures and Dislocations: Patterns, Classifications, and Management

Jeffrey D. Placzek, MD, PT

1. How are fractures of the distal humerus classified?

Distal humeral fractures historically have been divided into extra-articular and intra-articular, with the following subdivisions: supracondylar, epicondylar, transcondylar, condylar, intercondylar, capitellar, and trochlear fractures. In an attempt to develop a universal system, the AO/ASIF classification encompasses all periarticular distal humeral fractures.

AO/ASIF Class	Description	Treatment
Type A: Extra-articular Fractures		
A1	Avulsion fractures with no loss of column support to articular surface	Brief immobilization with early ROM
A2	Metaphyseal fractures with limited comminution	Nondisplaced: cast/brace <3 weeks Displaced: ORIF

continued

AO/ASIF Class	Description	Treatment
A3	Significant metaphyseal comminution	ORIF with 4.5 DC plates
Type B: Partial Articular Fractures		
B1	Lateral column disruption	ORIF with plates and/or screws
B2	Medial column disruption	ORIF with plates and/or screws
B3	Disruption of capitellum or trochlea	ORIF with or without primary fragment excision
Type C: Entire Articular Fractures		
C1	Intercondylar split without comminution	ORIF
C2	C1 with metaphyseal comminution	ORIF with or without bone graft
C3	C2 with articular surface comminution	ORIF with or without excision and with or without bone graft

AO/ASIF, Arbeitsgemeinschaf fur Osteosynthesefragen/Association for the Study of Internal Fixation; *ORIF,* open reduction and internal fixation.

2. Define Malgaigne (supracondylar) fractures.

Most commonly seen in children, Malgaigne fractures occur above the olecranon fossa and are characterized by dissociation of the humeral diaphysis from the condyles of the distal humerus. Fracture lines may extend distally to involve the articular surface. In adults intercondylar fractures are much more common and must be suspected.

3. Describe two classification systems for Malgaigne fractures.

The simpler system, based on the mechanism of injury, includes either extension-type or flexion-type supracondylar fractures. Falls onto an outstretched hand can produce the more common extension-type supracondylar fracture (80%), in which the fracture line passes from anterodistal to posteroproximal on lateral radiographs. Flexion-type supracondylar fractures result from force directed against the posterior aspect of a flexed elbow. The fracture line passes obliquely from anteroproximal to posterodistal on lateral radiographs. When displaced, the sharp proximal bone fragment often pierces the triceps and overlying skin, creating an open fracture.

A more comprehensive classification system, based on the presence of intercondylar extension and fracture comminution, is used more commonly in adults. Four types of supracondylar fractures are recognized:

- Type I—fractures without intercondylar extension
- Type II—fractures with intercondylar extension but without comminution
- Type III—fractures with intercondylar extension and supracondylar comminution
- Type IV—fractures with intercondylar extension and intercondylar comminution

4. How are supracondylar fractures managed in adults?

Anatomic reduction with stable fixation in adults is best achieved with plate-and-screw fixation (see table). External fixators are used when rapid stabilization of the elbow is required (e.g., vascular disruption), when an open wound is associated with significant soft tissue injury or loss, or when plate-and-screw fixation is precluded by extensive bone loss or comminution. External fixator pins are placed laterally into the distal humerus and dorsally into the ulna. Skin incisions followed by blunt dissection to bone under direct visualization help to prevent injury to the radial nerve. Ulnar pins are inserted with the forearm in 30 degrees of supination to permit forearm rotation.

Treatment of Supracondylar Fractures in Adults

Fracture Type	Operative Treatment
Type I	Medial, lateral, or triceps splitting with application of medial- and lateral-column 3.5-mm reconstruction plates Orthogonal configuration preferred over parallel placement Medial-column plate applied to medial ridge; lateral-column plate placed on posterior column surface
Types II and III	Transolecranon exposure followed by reduction and lag-screw fixation of intercondylar fracture Reduce and stabilize supracondylar component with medial and lateral plates Use bone graft in regions of supracondylar comminution (autogenous graft)
Type IV	Same as type III, but do not use lag-screw construct to fix intercondylar component because mediolateral condylar distance will decrease, creating joint incongruity

5. Describe the classification and management of supracondylar fractures in children.

The Gartland classification of supracondylar humerus fractures in children is based on the degree of displacement. Treatment ranges from percutaneous pin placement to formal open reduction and internal fixation (ORIF). Short-term immobilization in a bivalved cast is common to all treatments.

Treatment of Supracondylar Fractures in Children

Class	Description	Extension-Type	Flexion-Type
Type I	Undisplaced fracture	Immobilization at 90° of flexion	Immobilization in near-extension
Type II	Displaced with one intact cortex	Closed reduction and percutaneous pin placement (two lateral)	Closed reduction and percutaneous pin placement (two lateral)
Type III	Complete displacement	Closed reduction and crossed-pin placement (two lateral, one medial); ORIF if unstable	Closed reduction and crossed-pin placement (two lateral, one medial); ORIF if unstable

6. How are Granger (epicondylar) fractures classified and managed?

Lateral epicondylar fractures are extremely rare and usually are managed symptomatically with brief splinting followed by early ROM exercises. The medial epicondyle—a traction apophysis for the wrist flexors and medial collateral ligament—is the last ossification center to fuse with the humeral metaphysis (age 15 to 20 years). Fractures are classified as undisplaced, minimally displaced, displaced >5 mm but proximal to the elbow joint, and entrapped (usually between the olecranon and trochlea). Acute fractures are differentiated from chronic tension stress injuries (little league elbow). Treatment of nonincarcerated fragments involves closed manipulation with short-term immobilization (10 to 14 days) with the forearm pronated and the elbow and wrist flexed. ORIF is indicated for incarcerated fractures causing ulnar neuropathy. Chronic stress fractures are treated conservatively with brief immobilization and activity modification.

7. Which age-group is most susceptible to transcondylar humerus fractures?

Transcondylar fractures usually are seen in older adult patients as a consequence of osteoporotic bone. The fracture line passes between the articular surface and the old epiphyseal line, traversing the coronoid and olecranon fossae. Treatment ranges from closed reduction and splinting to percutaneous pinning or ORIF. Excessive callus formation in the coronoid or olecranon fossa may result in loss of motion.

8. How are condylar fractures classified in adults?

Condylar fractures are rare in adults, representing <5% of all distal humerus fractures. Lateral condylar fractures, which include the capitellum and lateral epicondyle, are more common than medial condylar fractures. In *Rockwood's Handbook of Fractures*, Milch describes two types of fractures based on the presence of the lateral trochlear ridge: type I fractures leave the lateral trochlear ridge intact, whereas type II fractures, which are less stable, include the lateral trochlear ridge as part of the fracture fragment. Jupiter describes Milch fractures as high or low, based on extension of the fracture line into the supracondylar region. Low Jupiter fractures are equivalent to Milch type I fractures and high Jupiter fractures to Milch type II fractures. Preferred treatment in adults is ORIF with early ROM exercises.

9. How are condylar fractures classified in children?

In children, both Milch and Jacob systems are used. The Jacob system accounts for fracture displacement:

- Stage I fractures are undisplaced with an intact articular surface.
- Stage II fractures have moderate displacement.
- Stage III fractures are unstable elbow injuries with fragment displacement and rotation.

Closed treatment of initially nondisplaced fractures in a long-arm cast is associated with a loss of reduction. Frequent serial radiographs are recommended to detect fracture displacement. ORIF is recommended for stage II fractures and for failed closed treatment.

10. Define intercondylar fractures.

Intercondylar fractures are the most common distal humerus fractures in adults. Usually they result from forces directed against the posterior aspect of a flexed elbow that cause the ulna to impact the trochlea. The resultant force splits the condyles, which are pulled apart by the flexor (medial) and extensor (lateral) muscle masses.

11. Describe three classification systems for intercondylar fractures in adults.

The universal AO/ASIF classification of intercondylar fractures includes subtypes C1, C2, and C3. The Jupiter classification describes the shape and direction of the fracture as high T, low T, Y, H, medial lambda, or lateral lambda. Riseborough and Radin describe four types: type I (undisplaced), type II (slight displacement with no condylar fragment rotation in the frontal plane), type III (displacement of the condylar fragments with rotation), and type IV (type III fracture with severe comminution of the articular surface).

12. How are intercondylar fractures managed?

Treatment of intercondylar fractures must be individualized according to the patient's age, medical status, bone quality, and fracture pattern. Older adult patients with osteoporotic bone and comminuted articular fractures may be managed with either closed treatment (cast/traction) or total elbow arthroplasty using a semiconstrained device. In general, ORIF with plates and screws is the preferred treatment for intercondylar fractures.

13. What are typical functional outcomes after an intra-articular distal humerus fracture?

Approximately 70% of patients have a good or excellent outcome; 25% have fair and 5% have poor outcomes. Other typical outcomes are the following: mean flexion arc, ≈112 degrees; pronation and supination, ≈75 degrees each; grip strength, ≈80% of the contralateral side. About 75% of patients return to their previous occupation.

14. Describe the three types of capitellar fractures.

Capitellar fractures are rare, representing <1% of all elbow fractures. Shear stress in the coronal plane may produce three types of fracture patterns:

- Type I fractures involve both osseous and cartilaginous portions of the capitellum, producing a Han-Steinthal fragment.
- Type II fractures of the capitellum shear off the articular cartilage with little underlying subchondral bone. This "uncapped condyle" is called a Kocher-Lorenz fragment.
- Type III fractures are markedly comminuted compression fractures of the capitellum.

15. How are capitellar fractures managed?

Treatment of nondisplaced fractures involves placing the elbow in maximal flexion and forearm pronation to allow the radial head to act as an internal splint. However, extreme flexion in the face of soft tissue edema can cause vascular compromise and subsequent compartment syndrome. Immobilization at 90 degrees of flexion in a long-arm cast decreases the risk of compartment syndrome but is associated with loss of fracture reduction. Displaced fractures are treated with ORIF or fragment excision. Type I fractures are exposed through the anconeus surgical approach. Provisional fixation with Kirschner wires simplifies placement of small-fragment cancellous bone screws (directed posterior to anterior) or Herbert screws (placed anterior to posterior and buried below the articular surface). Excision of fracture fragments is indicated for most displaced type II fractures and for severely comminuted type III fractures.

16. Define Laugier (trochlear) fractures.

Trochlear fractures are rare injuries produced by coronal shear forces directed against the trochlea by the coronoid process. Often associated with capitellar fractures, trochlear fractures are distinguished by a double-arc sign on lateral distal humerus radiographs. One arc represents the lateral ridge of the trochlea, and the other arc represents capitellar subchondral bone.

17. How are trochlear fractures managed?

Trochlear fractures are managed much like capitellar fractures. Nondisplaced fractures are managed by splinting and casting with early ROM exercises. Displaced fractures with significant osseous fragments are exposed through an extended lateral Kocher approach and stabilized via cancellous or Herbert screws. Severely comminuted or extensive articular injuries are managed via excision followed by early ROM exercises.

18. Describe the Colton classification of olecranon fractures.

Colton modified the original Schatzker classification system of olecranon fractures to include the following classes: undisplaced, displaced, oblique, and transverse fractures; comminuted fractures; and fracture-dislocations.

19. How are undisplaced olecranon fractures treated?

Treatment of undisplaced fractures involves immobilization in a long-arm cast with the elbow in 45 to 90 degrees of flexion for approximately 3 weeks. Radiographic evaluation 5 to 7 days after cast application is needed to rule out fracture displacement. Protected ROM in a hinged brace with 90 degrees of maximal flexion is initiated at 3 weeks. Fracture union is not expected until 6 to 8 weeks after injury. Joint stiffness and loss of motion are common, particularly in older adult patients who undergo prolonged immobilization.

20. How are displaced olecranon fractures treated?

Displaced fractures or fractures associated with a loss of active elbow extension are commonly treated with tension band wiring, 3.5-mm DC/reconstruction plates, or excision of up to 50% of the olecranon fragment and reattachment of the triceps. The coronoid must be intact.

21. What outcomes are associated with olecranon fractures?

Decreased ROM is noted in 50% of patients. Deficits usually are minimal, and patients maintain a functional ROM. Paresthesias, usually transient, are noted in 10% of patients. Nonunion occurs in about 5% of olecranon fractures. Approximately 85% of patients have no complaints at long-term follow-up; 50% will show arthritic changes as compared to 11% in the uninjured extremity. Approximately 22% of plates used for fixation require removal, and up to 50% of tension band wires will need to be removed.

Treatment of Displaced Olecranon Fractures

Modified Colton Type	Treatment
Avulsion fracture	Tension band wiring or excision of small fragment
Oblique fracture	Bicortical screws/plates to prevent shortening
Transverse fracture	Tension band wiring
Comminuted fracture	
Coronoid intact	Excision (up to 50%) with triceps reattachment
Coronoid fracture	Plate/screw fixation
Fracture dislocation	Reduce dislocation; ORIF of radial head (no early excision); ORIF of olecranon as above

22. Describe the Regan and Morrey classification of coronoid fractures.

Three types of coronoid fractures, based on fragment size, were described by Regan and Morrey. Type I is a tip avulsion fracture, type II involves <50% of the coronoid, and type III involves >50% of the coronoid and is associated with recurrent elbow dislocations. Management of type I and type II fractures is short-term immobilization in flexion, followed by early ROM exercises. Type III fractures with associated elbow instability are best managed with ORIF.

23. Do type I fractures represent true avulsions of the coronoid?

No. The brachialis inserts an average of 11 mm distal to the tip of the coronoid. Therefore most type I fractures represent shear fractures of the tip of the coronoid.

24. Summarize the mechanisms of injury and general management of radial head fractures.

Radial head fractures result from indirect trauma (e.g., fall onto an outstretched hand) when longitudinal forces drive the radial head into the capitellum. Because of the mechanism of injury, concomitant Essex-Lopresti injury to the distal radioulnar joint (DRUJ), capitellum, and medial collateral ligament must be ruled out. A mechanical block to motion or elbow instability is an indication for operative intervention. Aspiration of an elbow hemarthrosis with injection of lidocaine through a direct lateral approach can decrease pain and allow evaluation of passive ROM. ORIF is accomplished by placing cortical screws, Herbert screws, or miniplates in the anterolateral quadrant of the radial head (nonarticulating surface).

25. How are radial head fractures classified in adults?

Mason's classification of radial head fractures in adults was modified by Johnston. Recommended treatment is listed in the following table.

Fracture	Description	Management
Type I	Undisplaced fracture involving <25% of head	Splint and ROM as pain subsides
Type II	Marginal fracture with displacement of head	Excision or ORIF if angulation >30°, more than one third of head is fractured, or displacement >3 mm Otherwise treat conservatively with splinting and early ROM
Type III	Entire head comminuted	Early vs late radial head excision; repair DRUJ; repair/reconstruct MCL
Type IV	Associated elbow dislocation or Monteggia fracture	Reduce elbow; assess Monteggia or Essex-Lopresti injury; repair DRUJ; reconstruct MCL

ROM, Range of motion; *ORIF,* open reduction and internal fixation; *DRUJ,* distal radioulnar joint; *MCL,* medial collateral ligament.

26. How are radial head fractures classified in children?

In children, 90% of proximal radial fractures involve either the physis or the radial neck and are associated with fractures of the olecranon, coronoid, and medial epicondyle. The O'Brien classification is based on the degree of angulation of the radial neck. ORIF is indicated with angulation >60 degrees, failed closed reduction, complete displacement of the radial head, or >4 mm of radial head translocation. Radial head excision in children is associated with a high incidence of overgrowth and poor outcome.

O'Brien Type	Angulation	Treatment
Type I	<30°	Simple immobilization
Type II	30-60°	Closed reduction and immobilization
Type III	>60°	ORIF with Kirschner wires

27. How are elbow dislocations classified?

Elbow dislocations are classified based on the position of the ulna and radius relative to the distal humerus. Several types of elbow dislocation are recognized: posterior, posterolateral, posteromedial, medial, lateral, anterior, and divergent.

28. What are the most and least common types of elbow dislocations?

Posterolateral elbow dislocations account for 11% to 28% of injuries to the elbow and are more common than other types of elbow dislocation. The incidence of posterolateral dislocations is highest in the 10- to 20-year-old age-group and frequently is associated with sports-related injuries.

Divergent elbow dislocations are rare and consist of two types: anteroposterior and mediolateral (divergent).

29. Which fractures are commonly associated with elbow dislocations?

Medial or lateral epicondyle fractures (12% to 34%) can become entrapped in the joint, causing a mechanical block to motion. They are seen more commonly in children. ORIF is occasionally necessary.

Coronoid process fractures (5% to 10%) are seen most commonly with posterior dislocations. Fragments are graded as type I, II, or III as size increases. Type III fractures are associated with recurrent dislocations, and ORIF is recommended.

Radial head fractures involving the proximal intra-articular portion of the radius are managed nonoperatively in the absence of a bony mechanical block to motion. ORIF is indicated with concomitant radial head dislocation.

30. What complications are associated with elbow dislocations?

- Loss of motion (average of 10- to 15-degree loss of extension with simple dislocations)
- Loss of strength (15% average)
- Chronic instability
- Redislocation
- Posttraumatic arthritis
- Neurologic or vascular injury
- Compartment syndrome (Volkmann's ischemic contracture)
- Ectopic calcification of the capsule or collateral ligaments (75% of cases)
- Heterotopic ossification of the capsule (5%), collateral ligaments, or brachialis

31. What are typical outcomes for triad injuries of the elbow (radial head fracture, coronoid fracture, and ligament instability)?

Typical outcomes include the following: flexion arc, ≈112 degrees; pronation/supination arc, ≈136 degrees; complications resulting in reoperation, ≈20%. Approximately 78% of patients have a good to excellent result.

Bibliography

Aslam N, Willett K: Functional outcome following interim fixation of intra-articular fractures of the distal humerus (AO type C), *Acta Orthop Belg* 70:118-122, 2004.
Bailey CS et al: Outcome of plate fixation of olecranon fractures, *J Orthop Trauma* 15:542-548, 2001.
Bucholz RW: *Orthopedic decision making,* ed 2, St Louis, 1996, Mosby.
Canale ST, editor: *Operative orthopaedics,* ed 9, St Louis, 1998, Mosby.
Colton CL: Fractures of the olecranon in adults: classification and management, *Injury* 5:121-129, 1973.
Hotchkiss RN: Displaced fractures of the radial head: internal fixation or excision?, *J Am Assoc Orthop Surg* 5:1-10, 1997.
Ikeda M et al: Comminuted fractures of the radial head. Comparison of resection and internal fixation, *J Bone Joint Surg* 87:76-84, 2005.
Jupiter JB et al: Intercondylar fracture of the humerus, *J Bone Joint Surg* 67A:226-239, 1985.
Karlssson MK et al: Fractures of the olecranon: a 15 to 25 year follow-up of 73 patients, *Clin Orthop* 403:205-212, 2002.
Koval KJ, Zuckerman JD, editors: *Rockwood's handbook of fractures*, Philadelphia, 2002, Lippincott Williams and Wilkins.
Levine AM, editor: *Orthopaedic knowledge update: trauma,* Rosemont, Ill, 1998, American Academy of Orthopaedic Surgeons.
Pugh DM et al: Standard surgical protocol to treat elbow dislocations with radial head and coronoid fractures, *J Bone Joint Surg* 86A:1122-1130, 2004.
Regan W, Morrey B: Fractures of the coronoid process of the ulna, *J Bone Joint Surg* 71A:1348-1354, 1989.
Riseborough EJ, Radin EL: Intercondylar "T"-fractures of the humerus in the adult, *J Bone Joint Surg* 51A:130-141, 1969.
Webb LX: Distal humerus fractures in adults, *J Am Assoc Orthop Surg* 4:336-344, 1996.

Chapter 49

Nerve Entrapments of the Elbow and Forearm

John L. Echternach, PT, DPT, EdD

1. How are nerve compressions of the ulnar nerve classified?

McGowan's classification consists of three classes:

- Class 1—The patient has symptoms only.
- Class 2—The patient has both signs and symptoms, including dysesthesia and mild weakness in the ulnar nerve distribution.
- Class 3—The patient has primarily objective signs, such as objective loss of sensation, weakness, and atrophy (at least in the beginning stage) of muscles in the ulnar nerve distribution, most notably the intrinsic muscles in the hand.

The McGowan classification has proved useful to hand surgeons for determining which patients may need decompression of the ulnar nerve at the elbow.

2. What are the common sites of compression of the ulnar nerve at the elbow?

From proximal to distal, the first compression site is the ligament of Struthers, which may cause either ulnar or median nerve symptoms. The ulnar nerve also can be compressed above the elbow by the fascia that enshrouds the upper arm and at the point where it leaves the fascia, known as the medial intermuscular septum or arcade of Struthers. The ulnar nerve is compressed most often at the level of the medial condyle or just below as it enters the cubital tunnel between the two heads of the flexor carpi ulnaris muscle.

3. What are the sensitivity or provocation tests for cubital tunnel syndrome?

Test results for cubital tunnel syndrome include the following: Tinel's sign = 0.70, elbow flexion = 0.32, pressure provocation = 0.55, pressure-flexion test = 0.91.

4. What percentage of asymptomatic people have a positive elbow flexion test?

Approximately 10% will have a positive elbow flexion test.

5. What is a Martin-Gruber anastomosis? Explain its clinical significance.

A Martin-Gruber anastomosis is an anastomosis from the median nerve to the ulnar nerve in the forearm before the median nerve crosses the wrist. The Martin-Gruber anastomosis may confuse understanding of symptoms in patients with compressions of either the ulnar or the median nerve. It is found in approximately 8% to 54% of the population, according to various studies. Leibovic and Hastings described four types of this anastomosis: type I (60%)—motor branches sent from the median to the ulnar nerve to innervate "median" muscles; type II (35%)—motor branches sent from the median to the ulnar nerve to innervate "ulnar" muscles; type III (3%)—motor fibers sent from the ulnar to the median nerve to innervate "median" muscles; type IV (1%)—motor fibers sent from the ulnar to the median nerve to innervate "ulnar" muscles.

6. What other types of communication between the ulnar and median nerves occur in the forearm other than the Martin-Gruber anastomosis?

There is a communication referred to by some as the Marinacci communication or the reverse Martin-Gruber anastomosis, which is an ulnar to median communication. This communication often is unrecognized. In a recent study of 100 patients (200 arms), researchers reported that they found the Marinacci communication in 7 arms. Their conclusion was that the Marinacci communication is more common than usually suspected in the general population. However, in another study of ulnar to median nerve anastomosis in the forearm, the authors did not find the ulnar to median anastomosis or the Marinacci anastomosis in any of the 50 subjects they examined. The ulnar to median anastomosis in the forearm, or the Marinacci communication, is still considered rare enough that individual cases are reported.

7. At what site above the elbow may the median nerve be compressed?

The ligament of Struthers runs from a bony projection toward the medial epicondyle. The median nerve, along with the ulnar nerve in some instances, passes below this bony projection. The ligament may be a site of compression of both nerves, but more typically only the median nerve is involved.

8. Define radial tunnel syndrome.

In radial tunnel syndrome, the deep branch of the radial nerve is compressed in the forearm, causing pain and occasionally weakness in the most distally supplied muscles of the radial nerve. There is no sensory loss because the compression occurs below the level of the superficial radial nerve. Signs and symptoms include deep, aching pain in the upper dorsal forearm without tenderness over the lateral epicondyle or radial head. The tenderness is located just below the radial head in the groove formed between the brachioradialis muscle and the extensor carpi radialis. Patients also may have a positive long-finger sign—when the patient extends the wrist and fingers and pressure is applied to the third digit to resist extension, the extensor fascia tightens in the area of the radial tunnel, increasing symptoms. Weakness may be found in the extensors of the thumb, the abductor pollicis longus, and the extensor indicis.

9. What five tests are commonly used for the diagnosis of radial tunnel syndrome?

1. Compression over the radial tunnel
2. Long-finger test
3. Wrist extension
4. Resisted supination
5. Cuff test—a blood pressure cuff is applied above the source of pain in a peripheral nerve distribution, and by decreasing vascularity to the compression site reproduces the pain syndrome

10. Which test for radial tunnel syndrome has the highest sensitivity?

The differential motor latency test conducted in pronation and supination has the highest sensitivity for radial tunnel syndrome, >0.3 ms difference between positions being sensitive for the detection of radial tunnel syndrome. Clinically, palpation for pain over the radial tunnel area has the greatest sensitivity, followed by resisted supination and the long-finger test.

11. What are the possible sites of compression in radial tunnel syndrome?

The fibrous edge of the proximal portion of the supinator muscle (arcade of Frohse), tendinous origins of the extensor carpi radialis brevis, the distal edge of the supinator, and the vascular leash of Henry are all possible compression sites.

12. Which nerve is compressed in pronator teres syndrome?

Pronator teres syndrome refers to compression of the median nerve as it passes through the pronator teres muscle in the forearm. Other sites of compression in the proximal forearm are the bicipital aponeurosis and the fascia (arch) of the flexor digitorum superficialis.

13. Define anterior interosseous syndrome.

The anterior interosseous nerve is compressed below the level of the pronator teres muscle as it becomes an independent branch of the median nerve.

14. How can pronator teres syndrome be clinically differentiated from anterior interosseous syndrome?

In patients with pronator teres syndrome, forearm pain is increased by resisted pronation. Patients also may have pain on palpation in the pronator teres area; weakness in muscles supplied by the median nerve; feeling of numbness in the hand, especially the second and third digits; and, occasionally, complaints of easy fatigue with the use of the hand muscles.

Patients with anterior interosseous syndrome show weakness only in the muscles supplied by the anterior interosseus nerve. Some clinicians suggest testing the pronator quadratus with the elbow flexed; resisting pronation puts the pronator teres at a disadvantage and demonstrates weakness in the pronator quadratus. Patients complain of aching in the forearm but no sensory changes. They are unable to make an OK sign by pinching the thumb and index finger together because of weakness of the flexor pollicis longus.

15. What are the common signs, symptoms, and EMG/NSC changes noted in carpal tunnel syndrome, anterior interosseous syndrome, and pronator teres syndrome?

	Symptoms	Signs	EMG/NCS Findings
Carpal tunnel syndrome	Numbness and tingling in digits 1-3½ Weak grip Hand weakness Wrist and hand pain (especially at night)	Decreased sensation of digits 1-3½ Weakness of thenar muscles	Distal latency prolongation of median nerve (motor and sensory) across wrist Possible denervation of thenar muscles and lateral lumbricals
Anterior interosseous syndrome	Weakness of pinch Denies numbness and tingling May have anterior forearm pain	Weakness of FPL, PQ, and FDP (lateral) Normal sensation	Denervation of FPL, PQ, and FDP (lateral) Normal median motor and sensory nerve distal latencies at wrist and normal forearm conduction velocity
Pronator teres syndrome	Numbness and tingling in digits 1-3½ Deep anterior forearm pain Increased symptoms with forceful pronation activities (e.g., twisting off lids) Hand weakness	Weakness of thenar muscles Questionable weakness of FPL, PQ, and FDP (lateral) Decreased sensation of digits 1-3½	Decreased forearm conduction velocity (may have conduction block across elbow) Possible median motor and sensory distal latency prolongation at wrist May have denervation in thenar muscles, lateral lumbricals, FPL, PQ, and FDP (lateral) Pronator teres is spared

16. At what sites may the superficial radial nerve be compressed?

Occasionally patients have symptoms of sensory loss in the distribution of the superficial radial nerve without other evident problems with the radial nerve. Compression may occur when the superficial radial nerve emerges from beneath the brachioradialis muscle and enters the fascia, investing the extensor muscles of the forearm. Some dog handlers loop the leash of a dog that they are training over their forearm and hold the leash below the loop. When the dog pulls on the leash, the loop tightens around the distal aspect of the forearm, compressing the radial nerve under the loop (dog handler's syndrome). Other names for this syndrome are Cheralgia paresthetica and handcuff palsy.

17. What is Saturday night palsy?

Saturday night palsy is a compression injury in the portion of the radial nerve between the radiospiral groove and lateral intermuscular septum. Typical causes are periods of relatively severe compression of the radial nerve in the region of the posterior aspect of the humerus. The typical patient is an inebriated person on Saturday evening who loses consciousness with the arm slung over the back of a chair, hence the name Saturday night palsy.

18. Describe the symptoms and signs of Saturday night palsy.

Patients typically have weakness of the triceps and loss of function of the wrist extensors as well as the finger and thumb extensors. Sensory loss varies, depending on the level of the lesion. If the compression site is above the branches for the superficial radial nerve, the patient has sensory loss in the radial nerve distribution. If the compression is below the site of the superficial radial nerve branches and above the site for innervation to the brachioradialis and wrist extensors, the patient reports loss of wrist extension but no loss of sensation. Saturday night palsy is considered a high radial nerve palsy because it occurs in the upper arm, not in the forearm. This distinction is important in differentiating Saturday night palsy from radial nerve compressions of the forearm described previously.

19. Can the radial nerve be compressed by fibrous bands at the level of the radial head?

Yes. The most proximal site of compression of the deep branch of the radial nerve is the point where it crosses close to the radial head. Compressions of the deep branch of the radial nerve may be confused with tennis elbow or lateral epicondylitis. The surgical literature reports no differentiation in terms of clinical symptoms. Neural tension testing (provocative tests for neural tension) is a relatively recent concept. No research relates compression of the deep branch of the radial nerve at the level of the radial head to a positive test for neural tension.

20. Discuss the relative frequency of the various limb injuries and nerve compressions.

Injuries to the median nerve are much more common at the wrist; carpal tunnel syndrome accounts for over 90% of median nerve problems in the upper extremity. Pronator teres syndrome and anterior interosseous nerve syndrome are much less common. Pronator teres syndrome is the most difficult of the disorders of the median nerve to diagnose definitively. For every 100 carpal tunnel syndromes diagnosed, one pronator teres syndrome is diagnosed. Anterior interosseous nerve syndrome is also relatively rare but may be distinguished more easily than pronator teres syndrome and therefore may be diagnosed more frequently with certainty. Lesions of the ulnar nerve around the elbow are the most common problem encountered on examining the ulnar nerve and in the upper extremity are second only to carpal tunnel syndrome in incidence. Compression of the ulnar nerve at the level of the wrist is the second most common site for localized lesions of the ulnar nerve. Compressions of the median nerve at the ligament of Struthers, the ulnar nerve at the arcade of Struthers, and the radial nerve in the arm are much less frequent.

21. What are the surgical options and outcomes for cubital tunnel syndrome?

Surgical options include decompression alone, subcutaneous transposition, intramuscular transposition, submuscular transposition, medial epicondylectomy, and arthroscopic epicondylectomy. Positive results vary from 70% to 95% with few differences between procedures other than minor benefits from submuscular transfer with advanced-staged ulnar nerve compression.

22. How frequently is there loss of ulnar nerve function following a total elbow joint arthroplasty?

The incidence of ulnar nerve complications following total joint arthroplasty varies considerably. Some reports carry no information about ulnar neuropathy following this procedure. Others have reported an incidence of up to 26%. Most of the literature seems to indicate a 6% to 10% complication rate of ulnar nerve problems following total joint arthroplasty, with most of these resolving over time. Many patients have subclinical nerve changes before their surgery secondary to arthritis, synovitis, and swelling.

Bibliography

Amoiridus A, Vladronikolis IG: Verification of the median-to-ulnar and ulnar-to-median nerve motor fiber anastomosis in the forearm: an electrophysiological study, *Clin Neurophysiol* 114:94-98, 2003.

Dawson DM, Hallett M, Welbourn AJ: *Entrapment neuropathies,* ed 3, Philadelphia, 1999, Lippincott-Raven.

Dumitru D: *Electrodiagnostic medicine,* Philadelphia, 2002, vol 1 and 2, Hanley & Belfus.

Echternach JL: Loss of ulnar nerve function following a total elbow joint arthroplasty, *Clinical Electrophysiology Newsletter* 14:11-14, 2000.

Hildebrand KA et al: Functional outcome of semiconstrained total elbow arthroplasty, *J Bone Joint Surg Am* 82A:1379-1386, 2000.

Kelly EW, Coghlan J, Bill S: Five- to thirteen-year follow up of the GSB III total elbow arthroplasty, *J Shoulder Elbow Surg* 13:434-440, 2000.

Kimura J: *Electrodiagnosis in diseases of muscle and nerve,* ed 2, Philadelphia, 1989, FA Davis.

Konin JG et al: *Special tests for orthopedic examination,* ed 2, Thorofare, NJ, 2002, Slack.

Kupfer DM et al: Differential latency testing: a more sensitive test for radial tunnel syndrome, *J Hand Surg* 23:859-864, 1998.

Leibovic SJ, Hastings H: Martin-Gruber revisited, *J Hand Surg* 17:47-53, 1992.

Liveson JA: *Peripheral neurology: case studies in electrodiagnosis,* Philadelphia, 1991, FA Davis.

Mansat P, Morrey BF: Semiconstrained total elbow arthroplasty for ankylosed and stiff elbows, *J Bone Joint Surg Am* 82A:1260-1268, 2000.

Meenakshu-Sundaram S, Sundar B, Arunkumar MJ: Marinacci communication: an electrophysiological study, *Clin Neurophysiol* 114:233-247, 2003.

Millender LH, Louis DS, Simmons BP: *Occupational disorders of the upper extremities,* New York, 1992, Churchill Livingstone.

Moro JK, King GJ: Total elbow arthroplasty in the treatment of posttraumatic conditions of the elbow, *Clin Orthop Relat Res* 370:102-114, 2000.

Novak CB et al: Provocation testing for cubital tunnel syndrome, *J Hand Surg* 19:817-820, 1994.

Omer GE, Spinner M, VanBeele AL: *Management of peripheral nerve problems,* ed 2, Philadelphia, 1998, W.B. Saunders.

Resende LA et al: Ulnar-to-median nerve anastomosis in the forearm. Review and report of 2 new cases, *Electromyogr Clin Neurophysiol* 40:253-255, 2000.

Spinner M: *Injuries to the major branches of the peripheral nerves of the forearm,* ed 2, Philadelphia, 1978, W.B. Saunders.

Spinner RJ, Morganlander JC, Nunley JA: Ulnar nerve function following total elbow arthroplasty: a prospective study comparing preoperative and postoperative clinical and electrophysiological evaluation in patients with rhuematoid arthritis, *J Hand Surg (Am)* 25:360-364, 2000.

Stancic MF, Burgic N, Micovic V: Marinacci communication. Case report, *J Neurosurg* 92:860-862, 2000.

Sunderland S: *Nerve and nerve injuries,* ed 2, New York, 1990, Churchill Livingstone.

van der Lugt JC, Geskus RB, Rozing PM: Primary Souter-Srathclyde total elbow prosthesis in rheumatoid arthritis, *J Bone Joint Surg Am* 86A:434-440, 2004.

Section VII

The Wrist and Hand

Chapter 50

Functional Anatomy of the Wrist and Hand

Paul Simic, MD, and Amanda L. Simic, MS, OTR, CHT

1. What areas of the hand typically have autonomous innervation?

Normally, the dorsal thumb-index web space is innervated by the radial nerve. The tip of the little finger is innervated by the ulnar nerve. The median nerve provides sensation to the volar tip of the index finger.

2. Name the tendons in the six dorsal compartments of the hand.

The first compartment consists of the abductor pollicis longus and extensor pollicis brevis. The extensor carpi radialis brevis and extensor carpi radialis longus are in the second compartment. In the third compartment the extensor pollicis longus passes radially to Lister's tubercle to insert on the thumb. The fourth compartment contains the four tendons of the extensor digitorum and the "fellow traveler" extensor indicis proprius. In the fifth compartment is the tendon for the fifth digit—the extensor digiti minimi. Finally, the extensor carpi ulnaris passes through the sixth compartment.

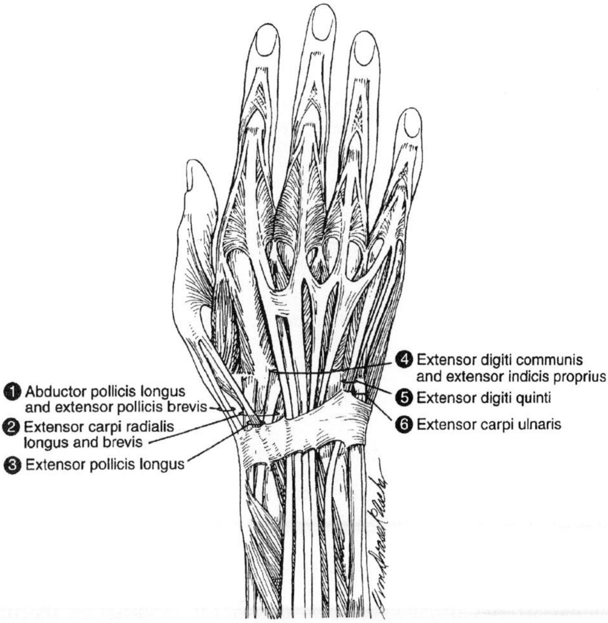

Wrist extensor compartments. (*From Watson N, Smith RJ, editors:* Methods and concepts in hand surgery, *Stoneham, Mass, 1986, Butterworth, with permission.*)

3. What deeper structures do the palmar creases identify?

The distal palmar crease is generally at the level of the necks of the metacarpals. The proximal palmar crease serves as a landmark for the superficial palmar arterial arch. The intersection of cardinal line and ulnar ring is the hook of the hamate. The intersection of the cardinal line and thenar crease is the origin of the motor branch of the median nerve. The intersection of the cardinal line and radial long finger is where the motor branch inserts into the thenar muscles.

4. Name the 10 structures that pass through the carpal tunnel.

The eight tendons of the flexor digitorum superficialis (FDS) and flexor digitorum profundus (FDP) pass through the carpal tunnel. The FDS tendons to the long and ring fingers are superficial to the FDS tendons to the index and little fingers. The flexor pollicis longus and, of course, the median nerve also pass through the tunnel. The flexor carpi radialis tendon is not considered to be an occupant of the carpal tunnel because it passes through its own compartment.

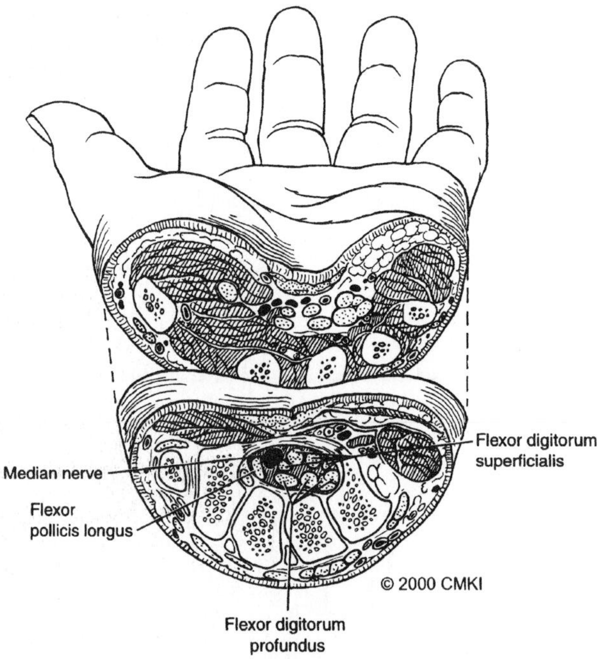

Ten structures that travel through the carpal tunnel. (*From the Christine M. Kleinert Institute for Hand and Microsurgery, Inc., with permission.*)

5. Describe the relationship of the contents of Guyon's canal.

From radial to ulnar, the ulnar artery and ulnar nerve pass through the canal. The flexor carpi ulnaris tendon is most ulnar but lies outside Guyon's canal.

6. What is the relationship between the digital nerves and arteries?

The common digital arteries usually bifurcate 0.5 to 1.0 cm distal to the bifurcation of the common digital nerves in the palm. They are contiguous in the distal half of the fingers. The arteries are deep to the nerves. In general, if the artery is lacerated, so is the nerve.

7. Describe the anatomy of the flexor sheath.

The pulleys are called annular (A) and cruciate (C), names derived from their respective configurations. They prevent the tendons from bowstringing when the fingers are flexed.

- A1 pulley—on the volar plate of the metacarpal phalangeal joint
- A2 pulley—over the proximal portion of the proximal phalanx
- C1 pulley—over the mid-portion of the proximal phalanx
- A3 pulley—on the volar plate of the proximal interphalangeal (PIP) joint
- C2 pulley—over the proximal middle phalanx
- A4 pulley—at the mid-portion of the middle phalanx
- C3 pulley—on the distal aspect of the middle phalanx
- A5 pulley—attached to the volar plate of the distal interphalangeal (DIP) joint

The odd-numbered annular pulleys (A1, A3, A5) are located at the joints, and even-numbered pulleys (A2 and A4) are located over bone. After the two initial annular pulleys, the cruciate and annular pulleys alternate. The A2 and A4 pulleys are considered the most crucial.

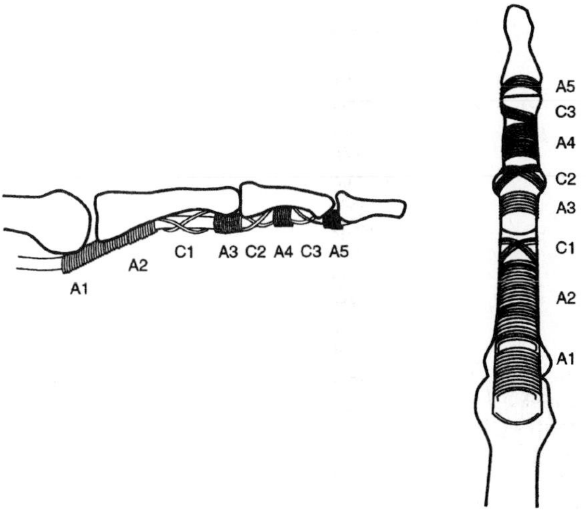

Anatomy of the flexor sheath.

8. What are the anatomic landmarks for the zones of flexor tendon injury in the hand?

- Zone 1—distal to the insertion of the FDS
- Zone 2—distal palmar crease, formerly called "no man's land"
- Zone 3—distal to the distal edge of the transverse carpal ligament
- Zone 4—carpal tunnel
- Zone 5—distal portion of the forearm

9. What are the zones of injury of the extensor tendon?

1. DIP
2. Middle phalanx
3. PIP
4. Proximal phalanx
5. Metacarpophalangeal (MCP)
6. Metacarpal
7. Dorsal retinaculum
8. Distal forearm

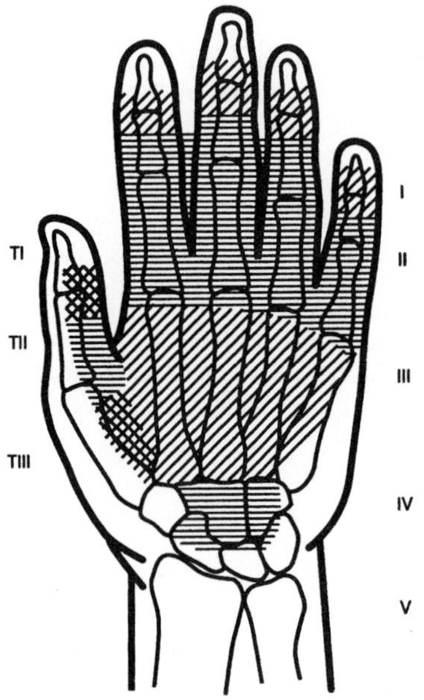

Zones of flexor tendon injury.

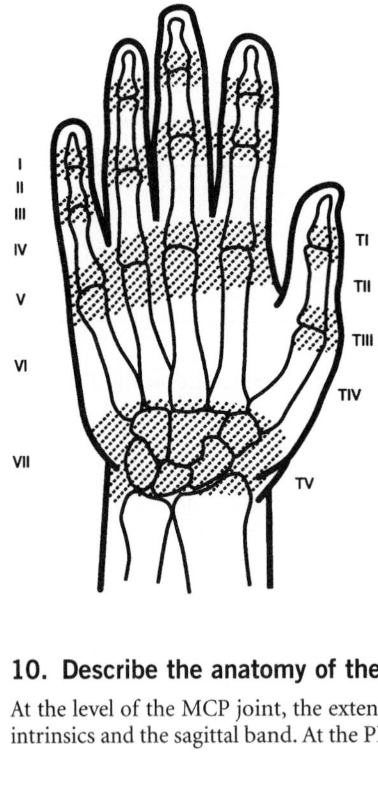

Zones of extensor tendon injury.

10. Describe the anatomy of the extensor mechanism of the fingers.

At the level of the MCP joint, the extensor tendon is centralized by the conjoined tendons of the intrinsics and the sagittal band. At the PIP level, the extensor tendon essentially trifurcates into the central slip and the two lateral bands. The central slip inserts on the base of the middle phalanx. The lateral bands insert on the base of the distal phalanx. The lateral bands displace volarly with flexion and dorsally with extension.

11. What is the function of the retinacular ligaments?

The transverse retinacular ligaments attach from the flexor sheath to the conjoined lateral bands, thus stabilizing the lateral bands. Lateral displacement of the bands may lead to a boutonnière deformity, whereas contracture and dorsal displacement may lead to swan neck deformity. The oblique retinacular ligament runs from the proximal volar aspect of the PIP to the dorsal terminal extensor tendon. This ligament links the movement of the DIP and PIP joints. PIP flexion allows DIP flexion, whereas PIP extension promotes DIP extension.

12. Name the eight carpal bones.

Starting radially and proximally, they are the scaphoid (Sc), lunate (Lu), triquetral (Tri), and pisiform (Pi). Starting distally and radially, they are the trapezium (Tm), trapezoid (Td), capitate (Ca), and hamate (Ha).

13. Describe the structure of the carpal ligaments.

The majority of the carpal ligaments are intracapsular. They can be categorized into two groups: intrinsic and extrinsic. The intrinsic ligaments begin and end on the carpal bones, while the extrinsic ligaments connect the radius and ulna to the carpus. The names of the carpal ligaments describe their origins and insertions. The volar ligaments are believed to be the strongest and most important. The major extrinsic ligaments are the radioscaphoid, radiocapitate, long radiolunate, ulnocapitate, short radiolunate, ulnotriquetral, and ulnolunate. Among the major intrinsic ligaments are the scapholunate interosseous, lunotriquetral, triquetral-hamate-capitate complex, and the numerous distal carpal row interosseous ligaments.

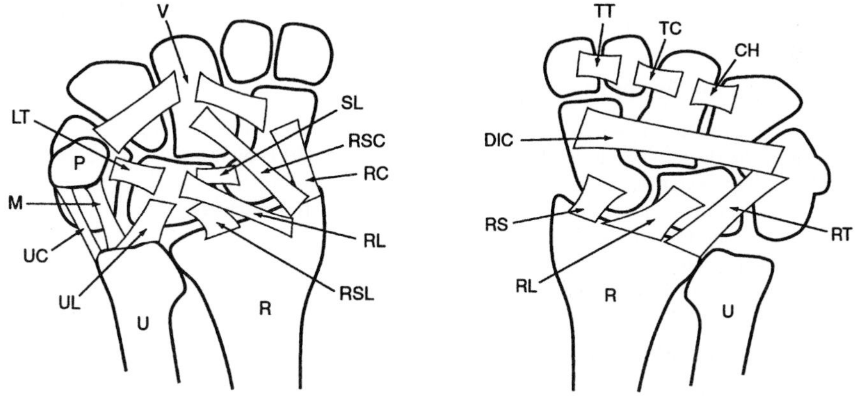

Volar carpal ligaments. Dorsal carpal ligaments.

14. Where is the space of Poirier?

The ulnocapitate and radiocapitate ligaments attach to the palmar aspect of the capitate, forming an inverted V. The triangular-shaped area at the base of this V is called the space of Poirier. This area of relative weakness is frequently the location of perilunate dislocations.

15. What is the normal range of motion of the wrist?

- Flexion—0 to 80 degrees (60% from midcarpal joint, 40% from radiocarpal joint)
- Extension—0 to 70 degrees (33% from midcarpal joint, 66% from radiocarpal joint)
  Flexion is dominated by midcarpal joint motion and extension by radiocarpal motion.
- Radial deviation—0 to 20 degrees (scaphoid volar flexion, lunate volar flexion)
- Ulnar deviation—0 to 30 degrees (scaphoid dorsiflexion, lunate dorsiflexion)
- Total radial/ulnar deviation arc—50 degrees (60% from midcarpal joint, 40% from radiocarpal joint)
- Pronation and supination—0 to 80 degrees, 160 degrees total arc of motion

16. What is the functional range of motion of the wrist?

Opinions vary; one study suggests 10 degrees of flexion, 30 degrees of extension, 10 degrees of radial deviation, and 15 degrees of ulnar deviation. Others suggest 40 degrees of flexion, 40 degrees of extension, and a combined 40-degree radial/ulnar deviation arc.

17. Describe the kinematics of the wrist.

The distal carpal row interosseous ligaments are multiple and strong. Hence the distal row moves as a unit. Excluding the pisiform, the proximal row has no tendinous attachments. Thus the distal row moves first, and the proximal row follows its lead. With wrist flexion the distal row flexes and ulnar-deviates. Extension causes the distal row to extend and deviate radially. With radial deviation, the distal row deviates radially, extends, and supinates. The exact opposite occurs with ulnar deviation. The proximal carpal row extends with ulnar deviation and flexes with radial deviation.

18. Describe the main area of motion during wrist flexion and extension.

Both the radiocarpal and midcarpal joints contribute to flexion and extension at all ranges of motion. However, two thirds of flexion occurs at the radiocarpal joint, whereas slightly more extension occurs at the midcarpal joint.

19. Describe the motion of the fingers and thumb.

- MCP joint of the thumb—0 to 90 degrees of flexion-extension with an average of 55 degrees
- IP joint of the thumb—85 to 90 degrees of flexion with slight pronation; usually allows 0 to 20 degrees of hyperextension
- Finger MCP joints—30 to 45 degrees of extension, 85 to 100 degrees of flexion, and 20 to 60 degrees of abduction/adduction
- PIP joints—no extension and 100 to 115 degrees of flexion
- DIP joints—10 to 20 degrees of extension and 80 to 90 degrees of flexion

20. Describe the blood supply of the scaphoid.

The scaphoid receives its blood supply through its ligaments. The main arterial supply enters around the midpoint (waist) of the scaphoid; additional vessels enter distally. The more proximal portion of the scaphoid receives nutrients in a retrograde fashion. This precarious situation can be disrupted by fractures and explains the relatively high incidence of avascular necrosis.

21. Describe the normal anatomy of the distal radius.

The distal radius tilts in two planes. It normally has approximately 11 degrees of volar tilt and 23 degrees of ulnar inclination. It consists of two facets—the lunate and scaphoid fossae.

22. What position of the wrist allows maximal grip strength?

Maximal power grip is achieved with 35 degrees of extension and 7 degrees of ulnar deviation. In full flexion only 25 percent of grip strength can be achieved.

23. Describe the musculature of the hand.

Musculature of the Hand

Muscle	Origin	Insertion	Action	Innervation
Abductor pollicis brevis	Fr, Tm, Sc	Lateral base of proximal phalanx of thumb	Abduction of thumb	RBMN
Flexor pollicis brevis	Superficial head: Fr, Tm Deep head: Ca, Td	Lateral base of proximal phalanx of thumb	Flexion of thumb MCP	Superficial: RBMN Deep: deep ulnar
Opponens pollicis	Fr, Tm	Lateral/anterior shaft of 1st MC	Medial rotation during opposition	RBMN
Adductor pollicis	Oblique head: Ca, Td, base of 2nd MC Transverse head: shaft of 3rd MC	Medial base of proximal phalanx of thumb	Adduction of thumb	Deep ulnar
Abductor digiti minimi	Pisiform	Medial base of 5th proximal phalanx	Abduction of 5th at MCP	Deep ulnar
Flexor digiti minimi	Hook of hamate	Medial base of 5th proximal phalanx	Flexion of 5th at MCP	Deep ulnar
Opponens digiti minimi	Hook of hamate	Anterior shaft of 5th MC	Opposition of 5th	Deep ulnar
Palmaris brevis	Medial palmar aponeurosis	Skin	Deepens palm	Superficial ulnar
Lumbricals	1 and 2: single heads from lateral FDP 3 and 4: double heads from medial 3rd FDP	Lateral sides of extensor expansions of 2-5	Flexion of MCPs and extension of PIPs and DIPs	1 and 2: median 3 and 4: ulnar
Dorsal interossei	Double heads from adjacent MCs	Extensor expansions of fingers 2, 3, and 4 on side	Abduction of 2nd and 4th MCPs, medial/lateral deviation of 3rd	Deep ulnar

continued

Musculature of the Hand *continued*

Muscle	Origin	Insertion	Action	Innervation
		allowing abduction	MCP	
Palmar interossei	Single heads from MCs 1, 2, 4, and 5	1 to medial thumb proximal phalanx 2, 4, and 5 to side of extensor expansions of 2, 4, and 5 for adduction	Adduction of fingers 1, 2, 4, and 5	Deep ulnar

Fr, Flexor retinaculum; *Tm,* trapezium; *Sc,* scaphoid; *Ca,* capitate; *Td,* trapezoid; *MC,* metacarpal; *FDP,* flexor digitorum profundus; *MCP,* metacarpophalangeal; *PIP,* proximal interphalangeal; *DIP,* distal interphalangeal; *RBMN,* recurrent branch of medial nerve.

24. Describe the anatomy of the carpal tunnel.

TRANSVERSE CARPAL LIGAMENT

- Extends from proximal carpal row (pisiform and scaphoid tubercle) to distal row (hook of hamate and trapezial ridge) through proximal aspect of second through fifth metacarpals.
- Width = 22 mm
- Length = 26 mm
- Thickness:
  1. Proximal = 0.6 mm
  2. Mid-portion = 1.6 mm
  3. Distal = 0.6 mm

CARPAL CANAL

- Depth
  1. Entrance to canal = 12 mm
  2. Mid-portion = 10 mm
  3. Distal end = 13 mm
- Average cross-sectional area = 17 mm^2
- Smallest cross-sectional area = 16 mm^2 (at distal carpal row)
- Volume = 5.84 ml
- Carpal tunnel release increases canal volume by 25% and changes the shape from oval to round. This is associated with a concomitant change in the shape of Guyon's canal from triangular to a vertical oval.

25. What is the average pressure (in mm Hg) in the carpal tunnel at different wrist positions?

	Normal	With Carpal Tunnel Syndrome
Neutral position:	2	32
Full flexion:	31	94
Full extension:	35	110
After carpal tunnel release:	5	—

26. Describe the force transmission across the radiocarpal joint with axial wrist loading.

With the wrist in neutral position during axial carpal loading:

- 80% across distal radius (60% through scaphoid facet, 40% lunate facet)
- 20% across distal ulna

27. What are the two possible communications (anastomosis or interconnection) between the median and ulnar nerves?

- Martin-Gruber anastomosis—In this anomaly, nerve fibers that were destined to be with the ulnar nerve when the median nerve was formed (by contributions from the lateral and medial cords of the brachial plexus) have stayed with the median nerve until the proximal forearm, where they finally join the ulnar nerve. This nerve interconnection explains why some patients with high ulnar nerve lesion have retained function in an area that typically is innervated by the ulnar nerve.
- Riche-Cannieu interconnection—This less common anomaly occurs with a pattern similar to the Martin-Gruber anastomosis. In this case, however, motor nerves to intrinsic muscles have stayed with the median nerve rather than the ulnar nerve at the level of the brachial plexus and rejoin the ulnar nerve in the hand.

28. Describe the bony anatomy of the metacarpophalangeal joint.

It is a condyloid (triaxial) joint with a trapezoidal shaped metacarpal head on axial cross-section. This results in a more narrow width dorsally. In flexion, the wider head has greater bony contact with the proximal phalanx, resulting in greater stability. The metacarpal head is a near perfect circle in the sagittal plane. For 10% of patients, the thumb metacarpal head is flat, in which case the joint acts more like a hinge with mobility relying upon capsular laxity.

29. Explain the cam effect of the metacarpophalangeal joint.

The cam effect at this joint is due to the eccentric origin of the collateral ligaments, dorsal to the axis of rotation. Additionally, prominences are found volarly over which the collateral ligaments pass, increasing the tension from 60 to 90 degrees of flexion. Thus, the collateral ligaments tighten in flexion, giving stability to the MCP joint when gripping. In extension, the collateral ligaments relax, allowing abduction-adduction motion, thus improving fine motor movements.

30. Describe the anatomy of the proximal interphalangeal joint (PIP).

It is a single-axis hinge joint with a bicondylar proximal phalanx head and intercondylar groove that articulates with the saddle-shaped median ridge of the middle phalanx base. This provides significant lateral stability. The PIP joint does not have a cam effect; thus the collateral ligaments have equal tension in flexion and extension.

31. What is the clinical and anatomic significance of thumb interphalangeal joint active extension versus hyperextension?

All thenar muscles (except opponens pollicis) insert at least partially into the dorsal apparatus of the thumb, and therefore act to extend the IP joint. They cannot, however, hyperextend the IP joint, which requires intact function of the extensor pollicis longus (EPL) muscle and tendon. Thus a patient with either radial nerve palsy or EPL tendon laceration may still exhibit thumb IP active extension, but not hyperextension.

32. Where is the EIP tendon in relation to the EDC tendon?

The extensor indicis proprius (EIP) tendon almost always is ulnar to the extensor digitorum communis EDC tendon.

33. Describe the insertion of the dorsal interossei (DI) tendons.

The superficial belly inserts through the medial tendon to the lateral tubercle at the base of the proximal phalanx and acts as an abductor. The deep belly continues as the lateral tendon to the transverse fibers of the dorsal apparatus, acting to flex the MCPs and extend the IPs. The first DI tendon inserts 100% medial, the second DI tendon inserts 60% medial and 40% lateral, the third DI tendon inserts 6% medial and 94% lateral, and the fourth DI tendon inserts 40% medial and 60% lateral.

34. Describe the cross-section of the median and ulnar nerves.

- Median—6% motor, 94% sensory; motor branch may arise radial (60%), central (22%), or volar/radial (18%)
- Ulnar—45% motor, 55% sensory; motor branch arises dorsal ulnar

35. Describe the anatomy of the superficial branch of the radial nerve (SBRN).

The SBRN exits between the brachioradialis (BR) and the extensor carpi radialis longus (ECRL) at approximately 9 cm proximal to the radial styloid. It bifurcates 5.1 cm proximal to the styloid and develops into five dorsal digital nerves.

Bibliography

Bednar JM, Osterman AL: Carpal instability: evaluation and treatment, *J Am Acad Orthop Surg* 1:10-17, 1993.

Gellman H et al: An in vitro analysis of wrist motion: the effect of limited intercarpal arthrodesis and the contributions of the radiocarpal and midcarpal joints, *J Hand Surg* 13A:378-383, 1988.

Ruby LK: Carpal instability, *J Bone Joint Surg* 77A:476-487, 1995.

Simon SR et al: Kinesiology. In Simon SR, editor: *Orthopaedic basic science,* Rosemont, Ill, 1994, pp 519-623, American Academy of Orthopaedic Surgeons.

Strickland JW: Flexor tendons: acute injuries. In Green DP, editor: *Operative hand surgery,* ed 4, New York, 1999, pp 1851-1897, Churchill Livingstone.

Chapter 51

Common Orthopaedic Dysfunction of the Wrist and Hand

Darren Gustitus, OTR, CHT

1. Describe clinical assessment of contracture of the oblique retinacular ligament.

Measure distal interphalangeal (DIP) flexion with the proximal interphalangeal (PIP) joint both extended and flexed. An increase in DIP motion with the finger flexed indicates contracture of the oblique retinacular ligament (ORL). If DIP motion is unchanged, range of motion probably is limited by joint contracture. If DIP motion is worse with flexion, the contracture is probably in the lateral bands.

2. How is the flexor digitorum superficialis clinically isolated when testing flexion at the PIP joint?

Passively extend all the fingers except the test finger. This maneuver prevents individual flexion of the flexor digitorum profundus (FDP) but allows function of the flexor digitorum superficialis (FDS).

3. What occurs anatomically during a positive scaphoid shift test?

The scaphoid shift test assesses the integrity of the scaphoid-lunate ligament. The evaluator applies pressure to the volar surface of the scaphoid with their thumb while passively holding the wrist in ulnar deviation. The evaluator maintains pressure over the scaphoid with the thumb while passively moving the wrist into radial deviation and slight flexion. At this time the evaluator releases pressure from the scaphoid. A positive test is indicated if the patient feels a painful "clunk" of the scaphoid. The scaphoid normally flexes with radial deviation of the wrist. If the integrity of the scaphoid-lunate (SL) ligament is adequately disrupted, pressure from the evaluator's thumb will cause the scaphoid to glide onto the dorsal rim of the radius. Release of the thumb from the scaphoid causes the scaphoid to fall back into volar flexion, sometimes eliciting an audible, painful "clunk."

4. Describe the Bunnell-Littler test.

Measure PIP range of motion (ROM) with the metacarpophalangeal (MCP) joint flexed and extended. If the PIP has more ROM with the MCP flexed, the test is positive and indicative of intrinsic muscle tightness.

5. How can the intrinsics be clinically isolated when testing extension at the PIP joint?

The patient is asked to extend the interphalangeal (IP) joints while the examiner holds the metaphalangeal (MP) joint flexed.

6. Describe the test for vascular integrity of the radial and ulnar arteries.

The Allen test is used to evaluate vascular integrity. The examiner compresses the patient's ulnar and radial arteries at the wrist and instructs the patient to open and close the hand several times so that the hand appears pale. The examiner then releases one artery and notes how long it takes for the fingers to recover their normal color (usually <5 seconds). The test is performed for each artery and is useful in evaluating patency.

7. Describe splinting techniques for various upper extremity nerve injuries.

- Median nerve—Must maintain thumb abduction.
- Radial nerve—Must maintain wrist extension; may use outrigger for passive finger extension.
- Ulnar nerve—Must attempt to avoid claw deformity; use a splint that keeps the MCP joints flexed and the IP joints extended.

8. In general, what is the appropriate position of the MCP joints in splinting? Why?

The MCP joints should be splinted in some degree of flexion and not in an extended position. In the extended position, the collateral ligaments are shortened, whereas in the flexed position they are stretched. Consequently, it is easier to regain full flexion when the MCP joints are splinted in the flexed position. Because of the cam effect of the metacarpal head, the collateral ligaments are lengthened and therefore stretched in flexion.

9. What is the best position to splint the hand after injury or surgery to prevent ligament shortening and possible fixed deformity?

The hand should be positioned with the wrist in extension, the MCP joint flexed, the IP joint extended, and the thumb palmarly abducted. Rehabilitation can be achieved more quickly and easily from this so-called safe position.

10. Define the syndrome of the quadriga.

If a surgical procedure or injury prevents the proximal excursion of a single flexor profundus tendon, the full flexion of the adjacent profundus tendon may be impaired. This phenomenon can occur only in the long, ring, and small fingers because of the anatomic arrangement of the flexor profundus tendons and their origin from a common muscle belly. If the excursion of one profundus tendon is limited, the muscle cannot move the other tendons to their full extent. Verdan coined the term quadriga from the Roman chariot in which the reins to four horses were controlled and operated by a single rider.

11. Explain extrinsic tightness with respect to the extensor tendons.

If the extrinsic (long) extensor tendon or tendons are adherent (for example, to the metacarpal after a fracture has healed), excursion distal to this point is limited. Adherence limits simultaneous flexion of the MCP and PIP joints. If the MCP joint is flexed, the PIP joint is pulled in extension by the adhered tendon, and if the PIP joint is flexed, the MCP joint is pulled into extension. The test for extrinsic extensor tightness is exactly opposite to the test for intrinsic tightness.

12. What is a mallet finger? How does it develop?

A mallet finger may develop after an injury to the extensor mechanism at the DIP joint, resulting in "droop" of the finger into flexion at the DIP joint. Such injuries include tendon rupture at the distal phalanx, laceration at or proximal to the DIP joint, avulsion fracture of the extensor tendon, or any injury that results in the loss of integrity of the extensor tendon insertion at the base of the distal phalanx. Loss of integrity usually is caused by a force applied to the tip of an actively extended finger, which forces the DIP joint into flexion.

13. What is a trigger finger?

A trigger finger is "locked" or attempts to lock in a position of flexion. If the flexor tendon cannot reenter the fibro-osseous canal at the level of the A1 pulley because of thickening of the A1 pulley and reactive inflammation of the synovium of the flexor tendon, it assumes a flexed or "locked" position. Treatment is injection of corticosteroids into the tendon sheath or release of the A1 pulley.

14. What is Dupuytren's contracture? Which structures in the hand usually are involved?

Dupuytren's contracture is a familial disease characterized by the development of new fibrous tissue in the form of nodules and cords in the palmar and digital fascia of the hand. The fibrous tissue leads to flexion contractures of the digits. Dupuytren's contracture is more common in Northern Europeans, diabetic patients, alcoholic patients, patients with liver disease, and patients who smoke. Men outnumber women by about 9 to 1. Dupuytren's contracture involves certain components of the palmar fascia, the pretendinous bands, the superficial transverse ligament, the spiral band, the natatory ligament, the lateral digital sheet, and Grayson's ligament. Treatment is usually surgical. Active splinting improves ROM in 59% of patients who comply with the program.

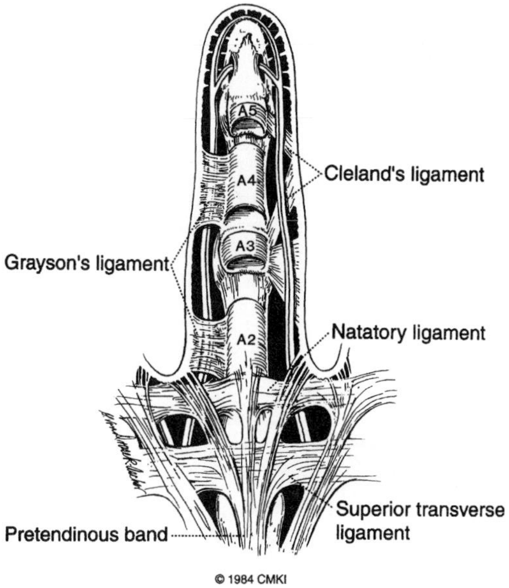

Structures involved in Dupuytren's contracture. (*From the Christine M. Kleinert Institute for Hand and Microsurgery, Inc., with permission.*)

15. What is Kienböck's disease?

It is avascular necrosis of the lunate, usually as a result of distant trauma. Treatment is radial shortening or ulnar lengthening.

16. What is a ganglion cyst?

Ganglion is a Greek word meaning "cystic tumor." Ganglions are mucus-filled cysts that account for 50% to 70% of all soft tissue tumors of the hand and wrist; they are more prevalent in women (female to male ratio of 3:1). There is no occupational proclivity, although the tendency to develop ganglions is seen with repetitive wrist activity. Dorsal wrist ganglions are the most common and account for 60% to 70% of all ganglions. The next most common site is the radial volar wrist (20%), followed by the flexor sheath of the fingers and the DIP joint. When ganglions become painful or noticeably enlarged, aspiration and cortisone injection may be indicated. Surgical removal of the cyst, in most cases, provides reliable definitive treatment.

17. Define swan neck deformity.

Swan neck deformity describes the posture of a finger in which the DIP joint is flexed and the PIP joint is hyperextended, giving the overall appearance of a swan neck. This deformity can be flexible or fixed. The many causes of swan neck deformity include volar plate deficiency at the PIP joint, FDS tendon incompetence, intrinsic muscle contracture, chronic mallet finger, and excessive traction by the extensor apparatus. This deformity usually does not respond to conservative splinting or an exercise program and requires operative management.

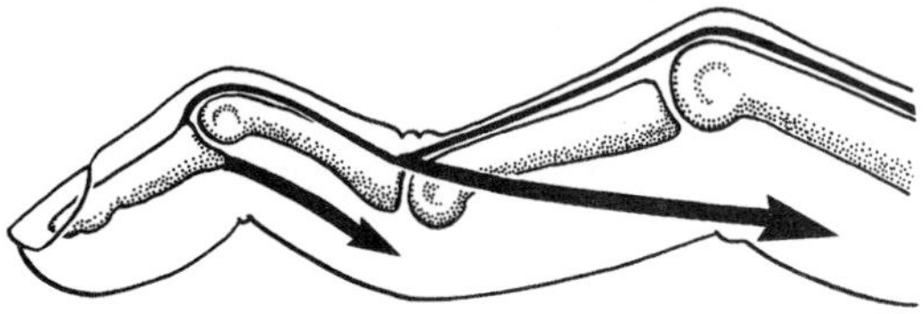

18. What is a boutonnière deformity?

A boutonnière (buttonhole) deformity is opposite in appearance to the swan neck deformity; it describes the posture of a finger in which the DIP joint is hyperextended and the PIP joint is flexed. It is caused by "buttonholing" of the head of the proximal phalanx through the extensor mechanism at the PIP joint (central slip injury), which allows the lateral bands of the extensor mechanism to move volarly. The result is extension of the DIP joint with flexion of the PIP joint. In contrast to swan neck deformity, boutonnière deformity responds to a specific and conventional splinting and exercise program.

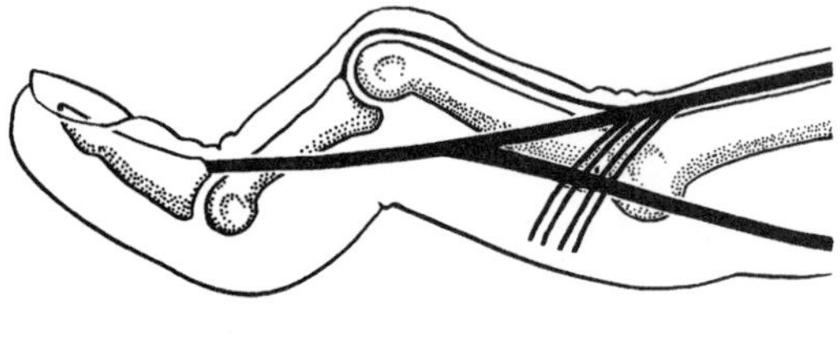

19. What is a pseudo-boutonnière deformity?

A pseudo-boutonnière deformity presents similar to a boutonnière deformity in that the patient has a digit with a PIP joint flexion contracture. With a pseudo-boutonnière deformity, there has been an injury to the volar plate of the digit, resulting in scarring of the digit into a flexed posture at the PIP joint. The pseudo-boutonnière deformity does not result in tightness, as evidenced by passive mobility of the DIP joint with the PIP joint held in extension.

20. What is de Quervain's disease? How is it treated?

de Quervain's disease is the inflammation of tendons and synovium, specifically the abductor pollicis longus and extensor pollicis brevis tendons and their surrounding synovium. It is also called stenosing tenosynovitis of the first dorsal compartment of the wrist. Finkelstein's test may help to diagnose de Quervain's disease by eliciting pain over the radial side of the wrist. The test is performed by ulnar deviation of the hand after a fist is made over the flexed thumb. Caution should be taken in interpreting a positive Finkelstein test. Many causes other than de Quervain's disease can generate pain with this maneuver, including first carpometacarpal arthritis, Wartenberg's disease, and arthrosis of the radiocarpal and intercarpal joints. Anomalous tendons, multiple slips of the abductor pollicis longus tendon, and multiple subcompartments within the first compartment have been implicated as the cause for failure of nonoperative treatments, such as use of nonsteroidal antiinflammatory drugs, local steroid injection, and thumb and wrist immobilization. If nonoperative treatment fails, surgical release of the first dorsal compartment provides the best result.

21. What is the most common type of injury in the upper extremity?

Fingertip injuries are the most common type, and their treatment is perhaps the most controversial. Treatment may include healing by secondary intent, skeletal shortening and closure, skin grafting, and flap coverage (especially with bone exposure and skin loss).

22. What types of flaps are used for closure of fingertip defects?

- V-Y advancement (triangular volar)
- Double V-Y (Kutler)
- Moberg volar vascularized advancement
- Neurovascular island (Cook procedure)
- Cross-finger flap (tissue is obtained from the dorsum of one finger to cover the volar aspect of an adjacent finger)
- Thenar and hypothenar flaps (for defects of the volar aspect of digital fingertips)

23. What is the most common joint disease in the upper extremity?

Osteoarthritis or degenerative joint disease is caused by cartilage deterioration and new bone formation at the joint surface. The carpometacarpal joint of the thumb and the DIP joints are the most commonly involved joints in the hand. Pain relief, function maintenance, prevention of associated deformities, and patient education are the hallmarks of management.

24. What nerve is implicated by dysesthesia or numbness in the palmar triangle? Discuss its clinical relevance.

The palmar cutaneous branch of the median nerve, which arises from the median nerve approximately 5 to 6 cm proximal to the wrist and does not pass through the carpal tunnel, is the nerve implicated in numbness of the palmar triangle. This knowledge may assist the clinician in diagnosing a nerve compression more proximal than the carpal tunnel. In addition, neuroma formation is an especially difficult problem to solve after inadvertent transection of the palmar cutaneous branch during carpal tunnel release and may cause "scar tenderness" after surgery.

25. What long-standing rehabilitation problem may occur when proximal phalanx fractures do not allow rigid fixation and early motion?

When range of motion exercises must be delayed to await fracture healing, adhesion of the flexor and extensor tendons to the fracture callus site is common. Adhesion can prevent tendon excursion and sometimes leads to either flexion contracture or extensor lag at the PIP joint, depending on postfracture position and healing pattern.

26. Describe the "lumbrical plus" finger. What causes it?

A lumbrical plus finger results in paradoxical extension of the PIP joint during attempted flexion of the finger. It occurs when the FDP is ineffective because of laceration, scarring, or amputation. "Pull" of the FDP through the lumbrical attachment to the finger causes extension of the PIP joint, which may occur when a flexor tendon graft is "too long."

27. What is the most common infection in the finger?

Paronychia, or infection of the nailfold, is the most common finger infection. It is treated by incision and drainage, and administration of antibiotics.

28. What is a felon?

A felon is an infection of the finger pulp. It is treated with lateral incision and drainage.

29. What changes in the hand are commonly associated with rheumatoid arthritis?

- Extensor tendon rupture (usually in the ring and small fingers)
- Rupture of the flexor pollicis longus tendon (Mannerfelt syndrome)
- Synovitis and degeneration of the radioulnar and radiocarpal joints (with sparing of the midcarpal)
- Palmar and ulnar dislocation of the MCPs
- Swan neck deformities of the fingers
- Boutonnière deformity of the thumb

30. Define focal dystonia.

Focal dystonia (writer's cramp) is characterized by excessive agonist and antagonist muscle activity. Treatment involves changing pen sizes, using biofeedback, administering β-blockers, or injecting botulinum toxin.

31. What structures compose the triangular fibrocartilage complex (TFCC)?

The TFCC consists of the articular disk, the meniscal homolog, the tendon sheath of the extensor carpi ulnaris, the disk-lunate and disk-triquetral ligaments, and the disk-carpal and ulnocapitate ligaments. The TFCC distributes force and stabilizes the ulnar wrist.

32. How are TFCC tears diagnosed?

Diagnoses are made by clinical exam and imaging studies. Ulnar-sided wrist pain may indicate TFCC. Arthrography has a 27% false-positive rate, and false positives may be as high as 50% with MRI. The sensitivity of both modalities is about 85%.

33. What is the total excursion of normal flexor and extensor tendons?

- EDC—about 50 mm
- FDP—about 70 mm

34. What extensor tendon injuries should be repaired?

Injuries in which >50% of the tendon is lacerated should be repaired.

35. When are extensor tendon repairs weakest?

Extensor tendons lose 10% to 50% of their strength between postoperative days 5 and 21.

36. How long should extensor tendon repairs be protected?

- Zones I and II—6 to 8 weeks
- Zones III and IV—6 weeks
- Zones V to VII—4 to 6 weeks

37. Describe the rehabilitation of an extensor tendon injury.

For zones V to VII, dynamic splinting is begun at postoperative day 3. The wrist is held at about 40 degrees of extension, with the MCPs and IPs at 0 degrees in an elastic outrigger. Active flexion with passive extension is done 10 times/hour. Dynamic splinting is discontinued by the third or fourth week, and active ROM is started. Finger extension exercises are started at week 4, finger flexion strengthening at week 6, and resistive exercises at week 7.

38. How are flexor tendons nourished in the synovial sheaths of the fingers?

They are nourished in two ways—through the vincula, which are small blood vessel networks, and by synovial fluid diffusion.

39. When should a flexor tendon be repaired?

When >60% of the tendon is lacerated, it should be repaired.

40. When are flexor tendon repairs weakest?

Flexor tendons are weakest between postoperative days 6 and 12.

41. How much gliding of flexor tendons does joint motion produce?

Each 10 degrees of DIP motion produces 1 to 2 mm of FDP gliding, whereas each 10 degrees of PIP motion produces about 1.5 mm of FDP and FDS gliding.

42. List and briefly describe the three rehabilitative approaches to the treatment of flexor tendons.

- Immobilization—a conservative treatment approach, immobilizing the patient for a duration of 3 to 4 weeks in a dorsal blocking splint with the wrist in 10 to 30 degrees of flexion, 40 to 60 degrees of MCP flexion, and full IP extension. This treatment approach is primarily used with children and other individuals who are unable to adhere to more complex protocols.
- Early passive mobilization—a treatment approach having various subprotocols including, but not limited to, Kleinert, modified Duran, and Washington. These protocols exist on the theory that passive mobilization of the tendon will result in increased tendon excursion with fewer adhesions and increased healing of the tendon. The modified Duran protocol uses a DBS with a strap to maintain the hand against the back of the splint. PROM is performed to the digits in flexion. The IP joints are actively extended while holding the MPs in full passive flexion. The Kleinert and Washington protocols also use a DBS; however, they use rubber band traction with a palmar pulley providing passive flexion to the digit(s). The patient performs hourly active extension within the brace. The splints are worn for 3 to 6 weeks as appropriate with treatment progressing according to the patient's progress.
- Early active mobilization—another treatment approach having various subprotocols; developed for the treatment of zone II tendon repairs. Early active mobilization protocols apply a controlled amount of stress to the repaired tendons, encouraging increased tendon glide with fewer adhesions. Various subprotocols use varying techniques for applying the controlled stress, including, but not limited to, active contraction while using rubber band traction and active contraction in a tenodesis splint.

43. What pulleys are essential for flexor tendon function?

Absence of an A4 pulley results in loss of 85% of work and excursion. Absence of A2 results in loss of excursion but no loss in work. An intact A2 and A4 are essential, but the addition of A3 significantly improves function, especially of the FDS.

44. In general, what are the expected outcomes after flexor tendon repair?

On average, patients regain 75% of grip strength, 77% of finger pressure, 75% of pinch strength, 76% of PIP motion, and 75% of DIP motion.

45. Describe the difference between the congenital anomalies camptodactyly and clinodactyly.

- Camptodactyly is a flexion deformity of a digit in the anteroposterior plane. It more commonly occurs bilaterally at the PIP joint of the small finger. However, other joints and digits can be affected. This flexion deformity is caused by tightening of the skin, ligaments, and tendons; abnormal musculature; and irregularly shaped bones.
- Clinodactyly is a curving of a digit in the coronal plane. It commonly occurs bilaterally at the middle phalanx of the small finger into radial deviation. However, other phalanges and digits can be affected. The deformity is caused by shortening of the phalanx on most often the radial side of the digit.

46. Describe the benefits of pressure therapy in the therapeutic management of a burned hand.

Pressure therapy is an essential key to preventing or controlling hypertrophic scarring after a burn. Pressure garments applying approximately 25 mm Hg pressure will help control scarring by decreasing circulation to the maturing scar tissue, thereby preventing excessive growth of the scar tissue. This will help the scar to mature into a flat, soft, and pliable scar. Pressure garments are typically elastic customized garments worn over the affected area 24 hours a day.

47. What scar contractures can potentially occur after a burn to the dorsum of the hand? What scar contractures can occur after a burn to the palmar surface of the hand?

Burns to the dorsum of the hand can potentially result in the following contractures of the hand: MP joint hyperextension, IP joint flexion or hyperextension, flattening of the transverse arch, ulnar rotation of the fifth digit, thumb extension and adduction, thenar contractions, and interdigital web space contractions. Burns to the palmar surface of the hand can potentially result in the loss of thumb and finger extension and abduction.

48. Transfer of a muscle-tendon unit will result in what change in muscle grade using a 0 to 5 muscle grading scale?

Tendon transfers do not automatically result in any loss of muscle grade. Other variables can affect and decrease the muscle grade of a transfer; however, loss is not automatic.

49. How does systemic lupus erythematosus (SLE) differ from rheumatoid arthritis (RA) with regard to arthritis and pathodynamics?

SLE and RA are both autoimmune disorders that result in chronic inflammation of the body's tissues. SLE attacks and breaks down the joint capsule, causing ligament and volar plate laxity, and tendon subluxation. Subsequent deformities, including joint instabilities and subluxations, occur because of the lost integrity of ligaments and tendons. RA, however, causes inflammation of the synovium, resulting in erosion of cartilage and bone. RA can develop into a multitude of joint deformities, and loss of motion.

50. What are common wrist and hand deformities developed by patients with a diagnosis of systemic lupus erythematosus?

Common wrist and hand deformities include MP joint ulnar drift, MP volar subluxation, swan neck deformities, boutonnière deformities, lateral IP deformities, inability to extend the MP joint, thumb MP flexion posture, type 1 thumb deformity (thumb flexion and IP joint hyperextension), radiocarpal and intercarpal subluxation or dislocation, and dorsal subluxation of the distal ulna.

51. Define Raynaud's phenomenon and discuss its etiology, clinical presentation, and treatment.

Raynaud's phenomenon is a vasospastic disorder of unknown origin. It is often experienced by individuals with vascular disorders, including systemic lupus erythematosus and atherosclerosis, as well as with rheumatoid arthritis. It is also commonly seen in response to repeated digital trauma, vibration, and prolonged cold exposure. The presenting symptoms of Raynaud's phenomenon often include a "triple response" of vascular changes, although not all individuals experience three color changes and the order of the color changes varies. Typically the digit(s) will assume a blanched appearance (lack of blood flow because of vasospasm), followed by cyanosis (venous pooling), and then followed by reddening of the digit(s) as arterial blood flow returns to the digit(s). Raynaud's phenomenon can also occur in the feet, nose, ears, and tongue. Only two color changes have to occur for Raynaud's phenomenon to be diagnosed. Treatment for this disorder consists of surgical removal of the proximal obstruction; patient education on the effects of smoking and caffeine, avoidance of cold and vibration, and avoidance of vasoconstrictive medications; biofeedback; and use of oral vasodilatory medications.

Bibliography

Brand PW: *Mechanics of tendon transfers. Rehabilitation of the hand and upper extremity,* ed 5, St Louis, 2002, Vol 46, p 779, Mosby.

Cannon N et al: *Diagnosis and treatment manual for physicians and therapists,* ed 4, Indianapolis, 2001, Hand Rehabilitation Center of Indiana.

Dobyns J: *Management of congenital hand anomalies. Rehabilitation of the hand and upper extremity,* ed 5, St Louis, 2002, Vol 118, p 1902, Mosby.

Green DP, Hotchkiss RN, Pederson WC: *Green's operative hand surgery,* New York, 1998, Churchill Livingstone.

Grigsby deLinde L, Knothe B: *Therapist's management of the burned hand. Rehabilitation of the hand and upper extremity,* ed 5, St Louis, 2002, Vol 90, p 1494, Mosby.

Kleinert HE, Cash SL: Management of acute flexor tendon injuries in the hand, *Instr Course Lect* 34:361-372, 1985.

Kleinert HE, Meares A: In quest of the solution to severed flexor tendons, *Clin Orthop* 104:23-29, 1974.

Kleinert HE et al: Primary repair of flexor tendons, *Orthop Clin North Am* 4:865-876, 1973.

Light TR: *Hand surgery update 2,* Rosemont, Ill, 1999, American Academy of Orthopaedic Surgeons.

Littler JW: The finger extensor mechanism, *Surg Clin North Am* 47:415-432, 1967.

Melvin J: *Systemic lupus erythematosus of the hand. Rehabilitation of the hand and upper extremity,* ed 5, St Louis, 2002, Vol 102, pp 1667-1674, Mosby.

Pettengill KS, van Strien G: *Postoperative management of flexor tendon injuries. Rehabilitation of the hand and upper extremity,* ed 5, St Louis, 2002, Vol 27, pp 439-452, Mosby.

Skirven T: Clinical examination of the wrist, *J Hand Ther* 9:99-100, 1996.

Taras J, Lemel MS, Ross N: *Vascular disorders of the upper extremity. Rehabilitation of the hand and upper extremity,* ed 5, St Louis, 2002, Vol 52, pp 892-893, Mosby.

Verdan C: Syndrome of the quadriga, *Surg Clin North Am* 40:425-426, 1960.

Witt J, Pess G, Gelberman RH: Treatment of deQuervain's tenosynovitis: A prospective study of the results of injection of steroids and immobilization in a splint, *J Bone Joint Surg* 73A:219-222, 1991.

Young L, Bartell T, Logan SE: Ganglions of the hand and wrist, *South Med J* 81:751-760, 1988.

Chapter 52

Fractures and Dislocations of the Wrist and Hand

Paul Simic, MD, and Amanda L. Simic, MS, OTR, CHT

1. Define boxer's fracture.

Typically, fractures of the metacarpal necks of the ring and small fingers are called boxer's fractures. The name is derived from the mechanism of injury. The fracture usually occurs when a person strikes or punches. The fracture usually angulates the apex dorsally, because the volar cortex comminutes and the intrinsic muscles cause a flexed position secondary to crossing the metaphalangeal (MP) joints volar to their axis of motion. Usually boxer's fractures can be treated nonoperatively with closed reduction and casting. The acceptable degree of angulation is undecided, but most surgeons accept up to 10 to 15 degrees in the second and third digits, 30 to 35 degrees in the fourth, and 50 degrees in the fifth.

2. What is a baseball finger?

Baseball finger, another name for mallet or drop finger, is typically a flexion deformity of the distal interphalangeal (DIP) joint resulting from injury of the extensor tendon to the base of the distal phalanx. This injury usually occurs during catching a ball (hence the name) or striking something with the finger extended and the tendon tight. The usual treatment is splinting of the DIP joint for 4 to 6 weeks. Average extensor lag after stack splinting is 8 degrees. Late management includes tenodermodesis, Fowler's tenotomy, or oblique retinacular ligament (ORL) reconstruction.

3. What is a jersey finger?

A jersey finger is avulsion of the flexor digitorum profundus (FDP) tendon from the distal phalanx. The result is inability to flex the DIP. Treatment is surgical reattachment. Some loss of extension is common. Surgery should be performed soon after injury especially if the tendon is completely retracted to the palm.

4. Describe the usual angulation of proximal phalanx fractures.

The angulation of proximal phalanx fractures, like that of most fractures, depends on two factors: the mechanism of injury and the muscles acting as a deforming force on the fractured bone. Typically, proximal phalanx fractures present with apex volar angulation. The proximal fragment is flexed by the interossei, which insert into its base, and the distal fragment is pulled into hyperextension by the central slip, which inserts into the base of the middle phalanx.

5. What is the usual or ideal position of immobilization of phalanx fractures?

Stable fractures often can be treated with buddy taping and early movement. If a fracture requires reduction and immobilization, the best position is the position of function, with the MP joints in almost full flexion and the interphalangeal (IP) joints in full extension. The MP joints rarely become stiff in full flexion because of the cam effect of the metacarpal hands on the collateral ligaments. The proximal interphalangeal (PIP) joints are least likely to become stiff in full extension.

6. Describe Bennett's fracture and Rolando's fracture.

Both are fractures of the base of the thumb metacarpal. Bennett's fracture typically results from an axial force directed against a partially flexed metacarpal (often in a fight). The smaller of the two fracture fragments stays in place, attached to the anterior oblique ligament. The rest of the digit is pulled dorsally and radially by the abductor pollicis longus, whereas the more distal attachment of the adductor pollicis contributes additional dorsal displacement. Rolando's fracture involves more comminution with the two fragments; usually a third large dorsal fragment in a Y- or T-shaped pattern is also present.

7. Describe the diagnosis and treatment of lateral collateral ligament injuries of the PIP joint.

Lateral dislocations are caused by an abduction or adduction force across the extended finger, usually in such sports as basketball, football, and wrestling. The radial collateral ligament (RCL) is injured more often than the ulnar collateral ligament (UCL). The PIP joint is stressed radially and ulnarly between 0 and 20 degrees. Angulation >20 degrees is an indication of collateral injury. The injury is treated with buddy taping and motion. The length of treatment depends on the degree of injury (complete or incomplete).

8. What are the differences between a dorsal and a volar PIP dislocation?

Dorsal dislocation is more common and results from hyperextension of the joint. The volar plate usually is injured at its attachment to the distal phalanx. Such injuries usually are treated with buddy taping for 3 to 6 weeks. Volar PIP dislocations are much less common. The injured tissue is the central slip. If the dislocation is treated with buddy taping, a boutonnière deformity probably will result. Hence volar dislocation should be treated with immobilization of the PIP joint in full extension.

9. Define gamekeeper's thumb.

An injury to the UCL of the thumb MP joint is called a gamekeeper's thumb because British gamekeepers often developed UCL laxity resulting from their method of putting down wounded rabbits. Today, however, it is seen most commonly in skiers. On exam the thumb is most tender over the ulnar aspect of the MP joint. The MP joint is stressed in both flexion and extension and in comparison with the other side. Often radiographic stress views confirm the diagnosis.

10. What is a Stener lesion?

With a complete tear of the UCL, the adductor aponeurosis often will be found between the torn UCL. This is called a Stener lesion and can prevent the ligament from healing. For this reason, most physicians recommend surgical treatment of complete UCL ruptures.

11. How is gamekeeper's thumb treated?

Acute partial ruptures can be treated with a thumb spica cast for 4 weeks. The treatment of complete ruptures is controversial. Most believe that is should be treated surgically. Tears in the middle of the ligament can be repaired directly. If the ligament is avulsed, it is reattached with a bone anchor or tied over a button.

12. Describe the radiographic evaluation of the wrist.

1. Anteroposterior (AP): three smooth arcs should be visible on the normal AP radiograph—across the distal radius; across the distal scaphoid, lunate, and triquetral; and across the proximal capitate and hamate.
2. Lateral: the radiolunatocapitate should form a straight line with the third metacarpal joint.

- Normal scapholunate (SL) angle—30 to 60 degrees
- Normal capitolunate (CL) angle—0 to 30 degrees

3. Flexion, extension, radial deviation, and ulnar deviation views, along with above, are enough to diagnose 90% of wrist injuries.
4. Special views
   - Scaphoid-radial oblique (supinated posteroanterior view)—with the forearm pronated 45 degrees from neutral, a full profile view of the scaphoid is obtained.
   - AP with fist compression or passive longitudinal compression may accentuate scapholunate dissociation and widening of the scapulolunate interval.
   - Carpal tunnel view—for this view, the wrist is in maximal dorsiflexion with the beam directed 15 degrees toward the carpus.

13. Describe Colles', Barton's, and Smith's fractures.

The most common of the three is Colles' fracture, which is extra-articular with dorsal angulation, displacement, and shortening. Barton's fracture is an intra-articular shear fracture that may be dorsal or volar. A Smith's fracture is often called a reverse Colles' fracture. It is an extra-articular fracture with volar displacement and angulation.

14. What are chauffeur's and die-punch fractures?

A chauffeur's fracture is an intra-articular, triangular-shaped fracture involving the radial styloid. A die-punch fracture describes a depressed fracture of the lunate fossa.

15. When is surgery indicated for distal radius fractures?

An unstable fracture (one that cannot be held in position with a splint or cast) is an indication for surgery. Radial shortening >5 mm, dorsal angulation >20 degrees, and articular step-off >1 to 2 mm are also reasons to consider surgery.

16. Name the five factors that may contribute to instability of a distal radius fracture after closed reduction.

- Initial angulation >20 degrees
- Dorsal metaphyseal comminution >50% of the width of the radius
- Intra-articular fracture
- Age >60 years
- Considerable osteoporosis

17. What are the outcomes from volar plating of distal radius fractures?

Flexion and extension average 55 to 60 degrees, pronation/supination averages 75 degrees, and grip is approximately 75% to 80% of the contralateral side.

18. What is the second most common fracture of the wrist?

Scaphoid fractures are the second most common wrist fracture after distal radius fractures. They usually result from a fall on a dorsiflexed wrist. The diagnosis is made from the patient's history and from exam findings of pain and swelling in the anatomic snuff box. Of course, radiographs are taken, but pain and tenderness justify initiation of treatment.

19. Where is the scaphoid most commonly fractured?

Around 65% of scaphoid fractures occur at the waist, while 10% occur at the distal body, 15% through the proximal pole, and 8% at the tuberosity. Because of differences in blood supply, fracture location can determine healing rates and times to union. The average time to union for waist fractures is 10 to 12 weeks, and 90% heal. It takes 12 to 20 weeks for proximal pole fractures to heal, and only 60% to 70% heal with cast treatment. Tuberosity and more distal fractures almost always heal in 4 to 6 weeks.

20. What are the treatment guidelines for scaphoid fractures?

1. Nondisplaced fractures: long-arm thumb spica for 6 weeks, then short-arm cast until the fracture is radiographically healed
2. Displaced fractures (i.e., 1-mm step-off, >60-degree scapulolunate angulation, or >15-degree lunatocapitate angulation):
   - With acceptable reduction (i.e., <1-mm step-off, <25-degree lateral intrascaphoid angulation, or <35-degree anteroposterior angulation), use a long-arm spica cast.
   - With unacceptable reduction, use open reduction with Herbert or compression screw or staple fixation; cast for 2 to 3 weeks, then encourage early movement.

21. Define Kienböck's disease.

Kienböck's disease is defined by the radiographic finding of avascular necrosis of the lunate. The exact etiology is uncertain, but the probable cause is some combination of a traumatic event, repeated microtrauma, and/or injury to the ligaments carrying blood supply to the lunate. It also has been associated with relative shortening of the ulna compared with the radius (ulnar negative variance).

22. What are the four stages of Kienböck's disease?

- Stage 1—sclerosis
- Stage 2—fragmentation
- Stage 3—collapse
- Stage 4—arthritis

23. Describe the classification of carpal instabilities.

The loss of the normal carpal ligaments and/or normal bony anatomy can lead to wrist instability. Wrist instability is classified as dissociative (CID) or nondissociative (CIND).

- CID—Carpal instability dissociative results from loss of the intrinsic ligaments. There are two types of CID:
  1. Dorsal intercalated segment instability (DISI) results from disruption between the scaphoid and lunate, allowing the scaphoid to rotate into volar flexion. The remaining components of the proximal row, the lunate and triangular muscles, rotate into dorsiflexion because of loss of connection to the scaphoid. DISI is the most common clinical pattern of carpal instability The SL angle is >60 degrees, and the CL angle is >30 degrees.
  2. Volar intercalated segment instability (VISI) results from disruption of the ligamentous support to the triangular and lunate and leads to volar rotation of the lunate and extension of the triangular. It is the second most common instability. The SL angle is <30 degrees, and the CL angle is >30 degrees.
- CIND—A tear of the extrinsic ligaments can cause midcarpal or radiocarpal instability and is called carpal instability nondissociative.
- CIC—Carpal instability combined is caused by disruption both within and between rows, as seen in a transscaphoid perilunate fracture dislocation.
- Axial carpal instability—This is usually caused by violent trauma that results in longitudinal disruption.

24. What is scapholunate dissociation?

A complete tear of the scapholunate ligaments may result from a hyperextension injury and can lead to scapholunate dissociation, which disrupts normal proximal row kinematics. The lunate and triquetrum extend abnormally, supinate, and deviate radially. The scaphoid tilts into flexion, pronation, and ulnar deviation. This abnormal positioning affects how the wrist bears loads and can lead to pain, weakness, and arthritis.

25. Describe Watson's test.

Watson's test is used to discern scapholunate dissociation. The wrist is moved from ulnar to radial deviation while pressure is applied over the volar tuberosity of the scaphoid. A positive test results when a painful clunk is felt from the proximal pole of the scaphoid as it subluxates over the rim of the radius.

26. What is the Terry Thomas sign?

A posteroanterior radiograph of the wrist that shows a gap >3 to 5 mm between the scaphoid and lunate, especially in comparison with the other side, suggests scapholunate dissociation (SLD). It is named after the English comedian who had a space between his front teeth. A more familiar eponym might be the Alfred E. Newman sign.

27. How is SLD treated?

Acute SLD can be treated with closed reduction and percutaneous pinning or open reduction, internal fixation, and repair of the ligament. Less than acute injuries can be treated with repair or reconstruction of the ligament and reinforcement of the capsule. Chronic injuries can be treated with limited or complete fusion, proximal row carpectomy, styloidectomy, or total wrist arthroplasty.

28. Define lunotriquetral dissociation.

A complete tear of the lunotriquetral ligament (possibly from a fall on a pronated, radially deviated, outstretched hand) may result in lunotriquetral dissociation, which disrupts the normal proximal row kinematics. The scaphoid and lunate tilt into flexion, and the untethered triquetrum moves proximally. This arrangement can lead to pain, weakness, and arthritis.

29. What is the ballottement test?

The lunate is held in place with one hand, and the pisotriquetral joint is displaced anteriorly and posteriorly with the other hand. Pain, crepitus, a click, or gross displacement suggests lunotriquetral dissociation.

30. How is lunotriquetral dissociation treated?

Acute lunotriquetral dissociation usually is treated with a cast or splint. The treatment of chronic injuries is unclear. Some recommend ligament repair or reconstruction, whereas others recommend limited arthrodesis.

31. How are thumb UCL avulsion fractures best treated?

Small avulsion fractures of the thumb ulnar collateral ligament with minimal (<2.0 mm) displacement are best treated with open reduction and internal fixation. Minimally displaced UCL avulsion fractures frequently have significant rotation that prevents successful fracture healing even with prompt cast immobilization.

32. Describe the Galeazzi fracture-dislocation.

In the Galeazzi fracture-dislocation of the forearm, fracture of the radial shaft includes a distal ulna dislocation. This injury was termed a "fracture of necessity," stemming from the inherent instability of the fracture-dislocation and the need for surgical intervention. A key element of treatment is to stabilize the radius with internal fixation and restore the length of the radius. The stability of the distal radioulna joint (DRUJ) is assessed, and if unstable, repair of the triangular fibrocartilage complex (TFCC) and/or the capsule of the DRUJ is recommended.

33. Describe the Essex-Lopresti injury.

Essex-Lopresti injuries are a variant of Galeazzi fractures, except that the radial head has an intra-articular fracture combined with a dislocation of the distal ulna, tearing the capsule of the DRUJ and/or the TFCC. Injuries that have less than 1 to 2 mm of articular step-off, have less than 30% of the radial head joint surface involved, and that are angled less than 30 degrees can be treated nonoperatively by immobilizing the forearm in supination to help reduce the DRUJ for 3 weeks before starting range of motion exercises. Fractures not within these criteria are best treated with open reduction and internal fixation.

34. Describe the evaluation and treatment of acute, unstable DRUJ injuries.

In the case of Galeazzi fracture-dislocations or Essex-Lopresti injuries, once the fractures have been reduced and stabilized, the DRUJ is reduced with the forearm in full supination. If the distal ulna redislocates when the forearm is brought to neutral forearm rotation, a repair of the TFCC and/or DRUJ capsule and ligaments is indicated. In these injuries, the TFCC and the entire DRUJ capsule detach peripherally from the ulna with or without a fracture of the ulna styloid.

35. Describe the evaluation and treatment of late subluxation or dislocation of the DRUJ.

Late subluxation or dislocation of the DRUJ is often due to attritional injuries secondary to a malunion of the distal radius, with shortening, loss of radial inclination, or radial translation of the distal fracture fragment. Definitive treatment may require reconstruction of the DRUJ with or without corrective osteotomy of the distal radius. Persistent subluxation of the DRUJ should be evaluated following corrective osteotomy. Patients with persistent dorsal ulna subluxation relative to the radius may require reconstruction of the volar ligaments, whereas persistent volar subluxation may require reconstruction of the dorsal ligaments.

Bibliography

Cooney WP, Linscheid RL, Dobyns JH: Fractures and dislocations of the wrist. In Bucholz RW et al, editors: *Fractures in adults,* ed 4, New York, 1996, pp 745-867, Lippincott-Raven.

Dinowitz M et al: Failure of cast immobilization for thumb ulna collateral ligament avulsion fractures, *J Hand Surg* 22:1057-1063, 1997.

Fernandez DL, Palmer AK: Fractures of the distal radius. In Green DP, editor: *Operative hand surgery,* ed 4, New York, 1999, pp 929-985, Churchill Livingstone.

Glickel SZ et al: Ligament replacement for chronic instability of the ulnar collateral ligament of the metacarpophalangeal joint of the thumb, *J Hand Surg,* 18A:930-941, 1993.

Green DP, Butler TE: Fractures and dislocations in the hand. In Bucholz RW et al, editors: *Fractures in adults,* ed 4, New York, 1996, pp 607-745, Lippincott-Raven.

Heyman P et al: Injuries of the ulnar collateral ligament of the thumb metacarpophalangeal, *Clin Orthop Rel Res* 292:165-171, 1993.

Kozin SH, Thoder JJ, Lieberman G: Operative treatment of metacarpal and phalangeal shaft fractures, *J Am Acad Orthop Surg* 8:111-121, 2000.

Orbay JL, Fernandez DL: Volar fixed-angle plate fixation for unstable distal radius fractures in the elderly patient, *J Hand Surg* 29:96-102, 2004.

Ruby L: Carpal fractures and dislocations. In Browner BD et al, editors: *Skeletal trauma: fractures, dislocations, and ligamentous injuries,* Philadelphia, 1992, pp 1025-1059, WB Saunders.
Ruby LK: Carpal instability, *J Bone Joint Surg* 77A:476-487, 1995.
Wright TW, Horodyski M, Smith DW: Function outcome of unstable distal radius fractures: ORIF with a volar fixed-angle tine plate versus external fixation, *J Hand Surg* 30:289-299, 2005.

Chapter 53

Nerve Entrapments of the Wrist and Hand

John J. Palazzo, PT, DSc, ECS, and Kathleen Galloway, PT, MPT, DSc

1. What is Wartenberg's disease?

Wartenberg's disease, also known as superficial radial nerve entrapment and cheiralgia paresthetica, occurs infrequently and is often confused with de Quervain's disease. Because of its superficial location along the distal radius, the nerve is easily compressed between the brachioradialis and extensor carpi radialis longus tendons with pronation and ulnar deviation. Superficial radial nerve entrapment creates a pattern of pain, numbness, and tingling over the dorsal lateral aspect of the hand. Wrist movement or blunt trauma aggravates the symptoms.

2. How is de Quervain's disease clinically differentiated from superficial radial nerve entrapment?

Finkelstein's test may be positive for both disorders. They can be differentiated by percussion along the anatomic course of the nerve, visual inspection for the presence or absence of edema along the dorsal lateral aspect of the hand, and sensory testing. Dellon described a nerve traction test for the superficial radial nerve. The patient is asked to pronate the forearm for up to 1 minute. If numbness and tingling are elicited or exacerbated over the superficial radial nerve field, entrapment is suspected. In addition, a positive Tinel's sign on resisted pronation is confirmative. Electrodiagnostic tests can confirm the abnormality by demonstrating an absent superficial radial sensory response when the median and dorsal ulnar cutaneous responses are normal.

3. How is median nerve entrapment at the wrist clinically differentiated from a C8 root level compromise?

Symptoms of median nerve entrapment at the wrist include daytime and nocturnal pain, reduced perceptions of sensation in the radial three and one-half digits, and intrinsic muscle weakness. Nontraumatic cervical root lesions have symptoms including vague neck complaints, digital numbness and tingling, fine motor skill limitations, and muscle weakness. Median nerve entrapments are made worse with repetitive use and prolonged wrist flexion. Median nerve sensibility is limited to its nerve field, whereas sensory changes associated with a cervical root level lesion are dermatomal. Manual muscle testing of C8 ulnar- and radial-innervated muscles compared with median nerve–innervated muscles may indicate global C8 muscle weakness, whereas isolated median muscle weakness localizes the level of pathology.

4. Describe the clinical manifestations of compression of the deep motor branch of the ulnar nerve.

The second, third, and fourth digits are unable to abduct because of deep motor branch nerve pathology. The fifth digit should abduct because the intact abductor digiti minimi is innervated by the superficial ulnar motor branch. Sensation in the ulnar nerve field should be intact. Visual inspection may reveal ulnar guttering of the deep motor branch intrinsic muscles rather than the hypothenar musculature. Lastly, manual compression applied by the examiner's thumb and index finger to the first web space (first dorsal interosseous/adductor pollicis muscle group) elicits pain compared with the same test applied to the abductor digiti minimi or the opposite side. This simple provocative pinch test appears to be a sensitive but nonspecific test; it is often present with ulnar neuropathy at the elbow and other sites as well. The mechanism of injury is associated with long-standing pressure in the palm, often an occupational hazard associated with pipe cutters, mechanics, and cyclists.

5. A complete ulnar nerve lesion at the wrist may produce motor paralysis of which muscles in the hand?

The majority of the intrinsic hand muscles receive their motor innervation from the ulnar nerve. A complete lesion of the ulnar nerve at the wrist causes extreme motor weakness or atrophy of up to 14½ muscles, listed below in the order of innervation sequence:

- One subcutaneous muscle (the palmaris brevis, which puckers the skin over the hypothenar muscle group)
- Three hypothenar muscles (abductor digiti minimi, flexor digiti minimi, and opponens digiti minimi)
- Two medial lumbricals (numbers 3 and 4, which are in the palm, just radial to and originating from the third and fourth flexor digitorum profundus tendons)
- Three palmar interosseous muscles that adduct the fingers
- Four dorsal interosseous muscles that abduct the fingers
- One and one-half thenar muscles (adductor pollicis, both oblique and transverse heads, and the deep half of the flexor pollicis brevis muscle)
- Total hand muscle/nerve scores: ulnar = 14½, median = 4½, radial = 0

6. What is the significance of a positive Froment's sign?

Ulnar nerve lesions result in a significant loss in hand grip strength. Weakness of the adductor pollicis, flexor pollicis brevis, and first dorsal interosseous muscles sharply impairs the pinching power of the thumb against the index finger. A simple test is to ask the patient to pinch a piece of stiff paper between the thumb and index finger while the examiner attempts to pull it away. The patient with an ulnar-deficient hand substitutes the flexor pollicis longus, causing hyperflexion of the thumb DIP joint to hold the thumb opposed to the radial side of the index finger. As the patient tries harder, the thumb flexes more and the pinch becomes weaker and fails.

7. Describe the tunnel of Guyon and a related nerve entrapment.

The lateral border of the tunnel of Guyon is the hook of the hamate, and the medial border is the pisiform bone. The floor is the joining of the ulnar extension of the transverse carpal ligament and pisohamate ligament. The overlying palmar fascia and palmaris brevis form the roof. The principal contents of the tunnel include the ulnar nerve and ulnar artery. The flexor carpi ulnaris inserts on the pisiform, but no tendons are contained within the tunnel of Guyon. Ganglia, fracture of the hamate hook, displacement of the pisiform bone, anomalous muscles, repetitive trauma, hypothenar hammer syndrome, arthritis, ulnar artery thrombosis, or aneurysm can cause various patterns of ulnar nerve involvement, ranging from complete motor and sensory to partial motor or sensory-only symptoms.

8. What is the significance of the palmaris brevis sign?

The palmaris brevis muscle is located on the ulnar aspect of the hand, superficial to the hypothenar muscle mass. When it contracts, it causes puckering of the skin on the ulnar border of the hand. To contract the muscle, ask the patient to abduct the small finger, which should cause a wrinkle over the proximal hypothenar region. The muscle receives innervation by the only motor twig of the superficial branch of the ulnar nerve as it passes immediately out of the tunnel of Guyon. The presence or absence of this muscle is usually detected by side-to-side comparison. The muscle is absent in complete ulnar neuropathies at the wrist. Ulnar nerve lesions at the wrist, affecting only the deep motor branch, spare the muscle.

9. Name underlying systemic pathologies that may present with carpal tunnel syndrome.

- Kidney disease
- Thyroid disease
- Liver disease
- Diabetes, both NIDDM and IDDM

10. What is the mechanism for production of carpal tunnel syndrome in repetitive and factory workers?

There does appear to be evidence, in an animal model, that repetitive use induces nerve pathology. Clark et al. studied rats that were trained to perform a repetitive task with a 60% maximum force level 4 times per minute, 2 hours per day, and 3 days per week for a total of 12 weeks. After 6 weeks there was an increase in the threshold for limb withdrawal to a painful stimulus. Histochemical analysis of the median nerves at the wrist, at 12 weeks, demonstrated increases in macrophages, collagen, and connective tissue. Grip strength and median nerve conduction were significantly decreased relative to the prestudy values.

Dias et al. evaluated 327 women of working age with carpal tunnel syndrome (CTS) to identify prevalence. Dias found that women who did repetitive work, however, did not have a higher incidence of CTS as compared to women who performed nonrepetitive work or to nonworking women.

11. What are important factors to consider when reading an electromyograph (EMG) and nerve conduction velocity (NCV) report for a patient with suspected carpal tunnel syndrome?

Median motor studies include stimulation of the median nerve proximal to the carpal tunnel with recording over the abductor pollicis brevis muscle. Median sensory studies can be antidromic, which means that the stimulus is opposite of the physiologic direction of response transmission. In a sensory antidromic study, the nerve is stimulated proximally with a recording over that same nerve distally. For the median nerve, a typical antidromic sensory study involves stimulation proximal to the wrist and recording 14 cm distally in either digit I or digit II, or possibly digit III. A palmar segment can be studied to more closely analyze the carpal tunnel involvement by performing the same antidromic study with digital recording and stimulation in the palm. The distal portion (from the palm to the fingers) is subtracted from the entire 14-cm distance to calculate the nerve conduction velocity across the carpal tunnel. Another method of evaluating the median sensory nerve involves stimulation of the nerve distally in the hand or palm and recording over the median nerve at the wrist. A focal conduction can be calculated directly when the median nerve is stimulated in the palm and the recording is made at the wrist. The NCV component of the report should contain latency, distance, amplitude, nerve conduction values, and temperature values.

12. Describe the classic findings of median nerve compression at the wrist.

Median nerve compromise at the wrist results in numbness or pain in the radial three and one-half digits. These complaints are noted particularly at night. Patients also may complain of referred pain in the forearm or as proximal as the shoulder. Patients note an increased frequency of dropping items, apparently attributable to sensory loss. Such symptoms are more common in women than men. Symptoms are exacerbated with sustained activity, such as cumulative trauma disorders or repetitive wrist flexion associated with assembly occupations. Objective features of median nerve compromise vary with acuity of the lesion. In the early stages of median nerve compromise, sensory changes are negative. Two-point discrimination may be reduced along the second and third digits and the radial aspect of the fourth digit. Tapping over the median nerve at the wrist crease may produce an electric shock sensation to the median-innervated digits. Tinel's sign (the presence of electric shock) provides clarification of pathology when it is positive and generally is detected only with moderate-to-severe cases of median nerve entrapment. Phalen's test (wrist flexion test) is conducted with the wrists in complete volar flexion for up to 60 seconds. It is positive with aggravation of median nerve signs and symptoms. Thenar eminence manual muscle testing reveals reduced strength in the abductor pollicis brevis in long-standing cases of median nerve entrapment with muscle atrophy. Long-standing cases also are associated with deterioration of manual dexterity as sensorium and muscle atrophy persist.

13. Are clinical examination tests valid for evaluating carpal tunnel syndrome?

Tinel's sign is used clinically to evaluate the status of peripheral nerve function. A tingling sensation, paresthesia, or electrical shock felt distal to the tapping site in the median nerve distribution to the thumb, index, middle, or ring fingers is considered a positive Tinel's sign. Reported values of specificity range from 55% to 95%, and sensitivity ranges from 45% to 75%. Tinel's sign may be present in normal people and is not descriptive of abnormality; therefore it may be more useful to rule out carpal tunnel syndrome when it is negative.

Diagnostic Tests for Carpal Tunnel Syndrome

Author (Year)	CTS Hands	Control Hands	Edx+	Sensitivity (%)	Specificity (%)	PPV (%)	NPV (%)
Provocative Tests							
Phalen's Test (Wrist Flexion Test)							
DeKrom (1990)	44	49	Yes	48*	53*	49*	52*
Gonzalez del Pino (1997)	200	200	No	87	90	90*	87*
Williams (1992)	30	30	No	87	100	100	88
Golding (1986)	39	71	Yes	10*	86*	29*	64*
Gellman (1986)	67	50	Yes	71	80	82*	69*
Phalen (1972)	598	†	No	81*	NR	NR	NR
Kuhlman (1997)	142	86	Yes	51	76	78	49

continued

Diagnostic Tests for Carpal Tunnel Syndrome ***continued***

Author (Year)	CTS Hands	Control Hands	Edx+	Sensitivity (%)	Specificity (%)	PPV (%)	NPV (%)
Gerr (1998)	57	181	Yes	53*	58*	25*	83*
Tetro (1998)	95	96	No	61	83	79‡	68‡
Tinel's Sign							
DeKrom (1990)	44	49	Yes	25*	59*	35*	47*
Gonzalez del Pino (1997)	200	200	No	33	97	88*	69*
Williams (1992)	30	30	No	67	100	100	75
Golding (1986)	39	71	Yes	26*	80*	42*	66*
Gellman (1986)	67	50	Yes	44	94	91*	56*
Phalen (1972)	598	†	No	70	NR	NR	NR
Kuhlman (1997)	142	86	Yes	23	87	75	41
Gerr (1998)	57	181	Yes	14*	79*	17*	74*
Tetro (1998)	95	96	No	74	91	89‡	78‡
Wrist Extension Test							
DeKrom (1990)	44	49	Yes	41*	55*	45*	51*
Median Nerve Compression Test							
DeKrom (1990)	44	49	Yes	5*	94*	40*	52*
Gonzalez del Pino (1997)	200	200	No	87	95	95*	88*
Williams (1992)	30	30	No	100	97	97	100
Kuhlman (1997)	142	86	Yes	28	74	65	39
Durkan (1991)				87	90		
Tetro (1998)	95	96	No	75	93	91‡	79‡
Tourniquet Test (Blood Pressure Cuff Test)							
DeKrom (1990)	44	49	Yes	70*	20*	44*	43*
Golding (1986)	39	71	Yes	21*	87*	47*	67*
Gellman (1986)	67	50	Yes	65	60	68*	57*
Physical and Sensory Exam							
Thenar Atrophy							
DeKrom (1990)	44	49	Yes	16*	94*	70*	55*
Golding (1986)	39	71	Yes	3*	100*	100*	65*
Phalen	598	†	No	36*	NR	NR	NR
Gerr (1988)	57	181	Yes	16*	90*	33*	77*
Abductor Pollicis Brevis Weakness							
DeKrom (1990)	44	49	Yes	39	80	63	59
Kuhlman (1997)	142	86	Yes	66	66	76	54
Gerr (1998)	57	181	Yes	37*	76*	33*	79*
Sharp Pinwheel Test Hyperesthesia							
DeKrom (1990)	44	49	Yes	25	90	69	57
Sharp Pinwheel Test Hypoesthesia							
DeKrom (1990)	44	49	Yes	39	66	46	59

Diagnostic Tests for Carpal Tunnel Syndrome ***continued***

Author (Year)	CTS Hands	Control Hands	Edx+	Sensitivity (%)	Specificity (%)	PPV (%)	NPV (%)
Golding (1986)	39	71	Yes	15*	93*	55*	67*
Kuhlman (1997)	142	86	Yes	51	85	85	51
Two-Point Discrimination							
Gellman (1986)	67	50	Yes	33	100	100*	53*
Gerr (1998)	57	181	Yes	16*	78*	18*	75*

From Wiederien et al: *Carpal tunnel syndrome: a literature review for the effect of the median nerve compression test on median nerve conduction across the carpal tunnel,* 1999, U.S. Army–Baylor University.
Edx+, Use of electrodiagnosis as gold standard for diagnosis; *PPV,* positive predictive value; *NPV,* negative predictive value; *NR,* not reported.
*Indicates values that were not presented but calculated from published data.
†Negative hands of same 50 subjects served as the controls.
‡Hypothetical population incidence rate of 0.50.

14. What are the most sensitive electromyographic indicators for carpal tunnel syndrome when reading an EMG report?

Median sensory studies typically show the earliest abnormalities in carpal tunnel syndrome. Reports can be interpreted more easily when there is an indication both of the site of median sensory nerve stimulation and recording and of the distance traveled by the stimulus between onset and recording.

Lew et al. examined the sensitivity and specificity for several median sensory conductions in determining carpal tunnel syndrome. They examined the wrist to digit, palm to digit (subtracted from the wrist to digit), and palm to wrist median sensory studies in 44 normal and 136 symptomatic hands. They found that the short segment from the palm to wrist was the most sensitive (75%) for carpal tunnel syndrome.

15. What is the clinical difference between an anterior interosseous nerve injury and median nerve injury at the wrist?

The anterior interosseous nerve, which innervates the flexor pollicis longus, pronator quadratus, and flexor digitorum profundus to the index and long fingers, may be injured traumatically or become inflamed spontaneously. Pain along the volar surface of the forearm may be associated with local trauma or heavy muscle exertion. As weakness develops, fine motor control suffers and pinching motion is reduced. Physical examination reveals absent or reduced flexion of the IP joint of the thumb and DIP joint of the index finger caused by weakness of the flexor pollicis longus and flexor digitorum profundus muscles. Sensation to the volar surface of the forearm and median-innervated digits is intact. Percussion over the nerve may produce radiating pain along the path of the nerve distally to the pronator quadratus.

16. What are the outcomes for steroid injection versus splinting for CTS?

Graham et al. followed 73 patients (99 hands) presenting with a diagnosis of CTS. All subjects were given a neutral wrist splint to wear for 9 weeks and underwent up to three steroid injections. Following the 9-week conservative treatment trial, subjects with persistent symptoms were scheduled for a carpal tunnel release, while those with symptom resolution were followed for up to 1 year. Ten percent of the limbs with initial resolution of symptoms following the 9- week splint/injection intervention remained symptom-free at the 1-year follow-up visit. The researchers noted that those who maintained long-term benefits with splinting and steroid injection interventions had a shorter duration of symptoms (less than 3 months) and had fewer sensory complaints when conservative measures were initiated.

17. What are the differences in risks and outcomes between open and endoscopic CTR procedures?

A meta-analysis of studies evaluating the differences between endoscopic and open carpal tunnel release surgical procedures identified three quality studies on the subject. All three revealed no difference between open and endoscopic surgery in symptom relief, and there was no difference in the risk of permanent median nerve injury. There was a conflict in outcomes of return to work and function between the two types of surgery. Endoscopic carpal tunnel release surgery seems to be more likely to produce reversible nerve injury although endoscopic surgery produces a better grip strength outcome with less scar tenderness.

18. What are the normative EMG and nerve conduction values used to define pathology in carpal tunnel syndrome and how are they applied in a patient case setting?

To control for the effects of temperature, some examiners use comparisons between nerves in the same limb. The following are some guidelines:

- Perform a median/ulnar sensory orthodromic study.
- Difference greater than 10 m/sec in velocity or 0.5 msec in latency between median and ulnar sensory studies in the palm to wrist segment is considered abnormal.
- Difference greater than 0.5 msec between radial and median sensory studies (stimulate at wrist and record from thumb) over a 10-cm distance is considered abnormal.
- Absence of median sensory response is abnormal.

Bibliography

Clark BD et al: Performance of a high-repetition, high-force task induces carpal tunnel syndrome in rats, *J Orthop Sports Phys Ther* 34:244-253, 2004.

Dawson DM, Hallett M, Millender LH: Digital nerve entrapment in the hand. In *Entrapment neuropathies,* ed 2, Boston, 1990, pp 254-255, Little Brown.

Dellon AL, Mackinnon SE: Radial sensory nerve entrapment in the forearm, *J Hand Surg* 11A:199-205, 1986.

Dias JJ et al: Carpal tunnel syndrome and work, *J Hand Surg (Br)* 4:329-333, 2004.

Durkan J: A new diagnostic test for carpal tunnel syndrome, *J Bone Joint Surg* 73A:535-538, 1991.

Finkelstein H: Stenosing tendovaginitis at the radial styloid process, *J Bone Joint Surg* 12A:509-539, 1930.

Graham RG et al: A prospective study to assess the outcomes of steroid injections and wrist splinting for the treatment of carpal tunnel syndrome, *Plast Reconst Surg* 113:550-556, 2004.

Lew HL et al: Sensitivity, specificity, and variability of nerve conduction velocity measurements in carpal tunnel syndrome, *Arch Phys Med Rehabil* 86:12-16, 2005.

Nora DB et al: What symptoms are truly caused by median nerve compression in carpal tunnel syndrome? *Clin Neurophysiol* 116:275-283, 2005.

Seror P: Tinel's sign in the diagnosis of carpal tunnel syndrome, *J Hand Surg* 12B:364-365, 1987.

Stewart JD: *Focal peripheral neuropathies,* New York, 1987, Elsevier.

Szabo RM: Superficial radial nerve compression syndrome. In Szabo RM, editor: *Nerve compression syndromes diagnosis and treatment,* Thorofare, NJ, 1989, pp 194-195, Slack.

Thoma A et al: A Systematic Review of reviews comparing the effectiveness of endoscopic and open carpal tunnel decompression, *Plast Reconst Surg* 113:1184-1191, 2004.

Wiederien R et al: *Carpal tunnel syndrome: a literature review for the effect of the median nerve compression test on median nerve conduction across the carpal tunnel,* unpublished manuscript prepared by United States Army-Baylor University Graduate Program in Physical Therapy, 1999.

Wilbourn AJ: *Ulnar neuropathy,* Rochester, Minn, 1985, p 27, American Association of Electromyography and Electrodiagnosis.

Section VIII

The Spine

Chapter 54

Functional Anatomy of the Spine

Brady Vibert, MD, and Harry N. Herkowitz, MD

1. How many degrees of freedom are available in the spine?

The vertebrae are capable of performing all six motions in space: flexion and extension, right and left rotation, right and left bending, superior and inferior translation, anterior and posterior translation, and right and left lateral translation.

2. Describe Fryette's laws of spinal biomechanics.

1. In the cervical spine, side-bending and rotation occur to the same side.
2. When the lumbar and thoracic areas of the spine are in neutral position, side-bending and rotation occur to the opposite side.
3. When the lumbar and thoracic areas of the spine are in extreme flexion, side-bending and rotation occur to the same side.
4. In actuality, spinal movement is highly variable among different people and even in the same person in different regions of the thoracolumbar spine.

3. Describe the normal ranges of motion of each section of the spine.

- C0-C1—10 to 15 degrees of flexion/extension, 8 degrees of lateral flexion, minimal rotation
- C1-C2—10 degrees of flexion/extension, 45 degrees of rotation, little or no lateral flexion
- C3-C7—64 degrees of flexion, 24 degrees of extension, 40 degrees of lateral flexion, 40 degrees of rotation
- T1-S1—80 degrees of flexion, 25 degrees of extension, 45 degrees of rotation, 35 degrees of lateral flexion

In general flexion/extension and lateral flexion increase from cranial to caudal. Rotation decreases from cranial to caudal.

4. How many natural curves are contained in the spine? Describe their orientations.

There are four curves in the sagittal plane of the spine, and they alternate lordosis and kyphosis:

Curve	Defined By	Curve Orientation	Normal Saggital Plane	Weight-Bearing Axis
Cervical	C1-C7	Lordosis		C1, C7
Thoracic	T1-T12	Kyphosis	30-40°	T10
Lumbar	L1-L5	Lordosis	55-65°	
Sacral	S1-S5	Kyphosis		S2

5. Define scoliosis.

Scoliosis can be defined broadly as any abnormal curvature of the spine in the coronal plane. A more specific definition is any abnormal curvature in the coronal plan >10 degrees. Any variant curve <10 degrees is considered spinal asymmetry.

6. List the important ligaments of the cervical and the lumbar spine. Specify their origin, insertion, attachment, and function.

Name	Origin	Insertion	Attachment	Function	Upper Cervical Name Change
Anterior longitudinal ligament	Skull	Sacrum	Anterior surface of vertebral bodies	Limits extension	Atlantoaxial and anterior atlanto-occipital membrane
Posterior longitudinal ligament	Skull	Sacrum	Posterior surface of vertebral bodies	Resists hyperflexion, posterior disk protrusion	Tectoral ligament
Ligamentum flavum	Anterior surface of lamina above	Superior margin of lamina below		Prestresses disk Helps extend flexed spine	Posterior atlanto-occipital membrane
Interspinous ligament	Posterior aspect of superior spinous process	Anterior/inferior aspect of interior spinous process		Limits flexion	
Supraspinous ligament	Occipital protuberance to upper lumbar spine	Across tips of spinous processes		Limits flexion	Ligamentum nuchae
Transverse ligament	Body of C1	Body of C1	Across posterior dens	Retains odontoid process of C2 in place against anterior arch of atlas	
Alar ligament	Bilateral extension from sides of dens	Occipital condyles		Secondary stabilizer C1-C2	
Apical ligament	Tip of dens	Foramen magnum		Secondary stabilizer C1-C2	

7. Describe the anatomy of the intervertebral disk.

Each motion segment has one disk, with the exception of C1-C2. The disk is an avascular structure composed of an outer annulus fibrosus, an inner nucleus pulposus, and a cartilaginous end-plate interface superior and inferior to the vertebral body. The jelly-like nucleus pulposus acts as a shock absorber, and the annulus helps to stabilize and transmit the loads transmitted to the nucleus pulposus by axial loading. The biomechanical vertical compression forces to which the nucleus is exposed are converted into horizontally directed forces that the tough outer annulus helps to absorb and distribute to the motion segment. The fibers of the annulus are arranged in alternating perpendicular lamellar fibers, arranged at a 45-degree angle to the vertebral end plates. Disk height is larger anteriorly in the cervical and lumbar spine and shorter anteriorly in the thoracic spine, which accounts for the cervical and lumbar lordosis and thoracic kyphosis.

8. How does the disk obtain its nutrition?

Because the disk is avascular, the disk cells must obtain their nutrition through local diffusion. Diffusion of uncharged solutes, such as glucose, occurs primarily through the end plates. Negatively charged solutes diffuse through the annulus.

9. What is the effect of exercise on disk nutrition?

Exercise provides nutrition through pumping of the disk, which aids in solute transport and possibly promotes nutrition through increasing external local vascularity.

10. What changes occur in the disk with aging?

As the spine ages, degenerative changes occur, and the chemical composition of the nucleus pulposus changes. In the nucleus pulposus of a youth, type II collagen, proteoglycans, and water are abundant. Over time, the nucleus decreases proteoglycan production, loses water, and produces less type II collagen. It begins to resemble the annulus, which consists mostly of type I collagen. Whereas young disks maintain height, aging disks lose height with degeneration and water loss.

11. Describe the facet articulations of the spine.

- Occiput anterior (OA)—At the atlanto-occipital joint is an articulation between the condyles of the occipital bone and superior facets of the atlas (C1). The anterior and posterior occipital membranes and joint capsule support this articulation.
- Atlantoaxial (AA)—Great mobility is needed at C1-C2, where 50% of cervical rotation occurs. As a result of the strong coupling pattern at this joint, axial rotation is associated with vertical translation and contralateral side-bending. The facets of C1-C2 are horizontally aligned but biconvex in design. As a result, C1 is vertically at its highest position in neutral rotation and in its lowest position in full left or right lateral rotation.
- Cervical—The facet joints are angulated at 45 degrees to the vertical in the sagittal plane at C2-C7. This orientation allows increased mobility compared with the thoracic and lumbar portions of the spine, including the coupled axial rotation observed with lateral bending.
- Thoracic—In the thoracic spine, the facet joints are oriented at 60 degrees to the vertical in the sagittal plane. This orientation leads to increased rigidity in the thoracic spine, with decreased axial rotation in the lower thoracic spine compared with the upper thoracic spine. This decrease is secondary to transitioning of the facets to a more lumbar-type facet.
- Lumbar—In the lumbar spine, the facet joints are vertically oriented, and their configuration allows little rotation and flexion. The superior facets are oriented dorsomedially, almost facing each other. The inferior facet processes face ventrolaterally. This configuration allows a locking-in of each articulation of the superior facets from the lower vertebrae with the inferior processes of the upper vertebrae.

12. How does the spine receive loads in different postures? What is the effect of a backrest or lumbar support?

Nachemson measured intradiskal pressure with pressure transducers placed at L3-L4 in normal patients at different postures. His research showed that the least loaded condition is lying supine. In vivo loads increase sequentially with lying on the side, standing, sitting in a chair, standing with flexed spine, sitting in a chair with flexed spine, standing with flexed spine carrying a weight, and sitting in a chair with flexed spine carrying a weight. The relative loads are as follows:

- Lying on the side—25%
- Standing—100%
- Seated—145%
- Standing with forward bend—150%
- Seated with forward bend—180%

The loads on the lumbar spine are lower during supported sitting than during unsupported sitting because part of the weight of the upper body is supported by the backrest. Backward inclination and use of a lumbar support further reduce the loads.

13. What are the dimensions of the spinal canal? How does the canal size change in different areas of the spine?

The space available for the cord (SAC) is defined as the area posterior to the posterior longitudinal ligament and anterior to the ligamentum flavum. The normal canal opening is about 17 to 20 mm in the cervical spine. Stenotic symptoms often occur when this space decreases to <14 mm. The SAC is narrowest at T5. The spinal cord is approximately 42 cm long in women, 45 cm long in men, and 10 mm in diameter. Two levels of enlargement correlate with the levels of upper and lower extremity innervation: the C4-T1 level and the L2-S3 level. The end of the cord, the conus medullaris, starts at the T10-T11 disk level. The L1-L2 disk level marks the end of the conus medullaris and the start of the cauda equina.

14. How are the facet joints innervated?

The spinal nerve divides into ventral and dorsal rami. The dorsal primary ramus gives medial, lateral, and intermediate branches to the facet joints and paraspinal muscles. The medial branches are especially important in facet joint innervation. Two branches—superior and inferior—innervate the facet joint above and below the level of the nerve root. For example, the descending medial branch of L1 and the ascending medial branch of L3 innervate the L2-L3 facet.

15. Where is the nerve root in relation to the pedicle and disk in the cervical and lumbar portions of the spine?

In the cervical spine, the spinal nerve roots exit directly lateral from the spinal canal adjacent to the corresponding disk and superior to the inferior pedicle. The nerve roots are numbered for the cervical vertebra above which they pass. For example, the C4 nerve root exits beneath the C3 pedicle and above C4. Because there are eight cervical nerve roots but only seven cervical vertebrae, the numbering changes at C7-T1. Here the eighth cervical root passes. Thus, the nerve root passing under the pedicle of T1 is the T1 nerve root.

In the lumbar spine, the nerve root passes directly under the pedicle for which it is named. For example, the L4 nerve root passes beneath the pedicle of L4 at the L4-L5 intervertebral level. The nerve root is usually superior to the disk at that level, whereas the cervical nerve roots exit at the level of the disk.

16. How does spinal movement affect the size of the intervertebral foramen?

Cadaver studies indicate that foramen size increases in flexion by 24% and decreases in extension by 20%. Changes caused by lateral bending and axial rotation are not as impressive.

17. Describe the function of the facet joints and their role in load-bearing.

The facets are thought to protect the lumbar spine against torsional disk damage. They decrease the allowable rotation to which an intervertebral disk is exposed and share spinal load with the disk. Investigators debate the exact amount of load that the facets bear, but estimates range from 9% to 25%, depending on whether the spine is flexed or extended. If the spine is arthritic, the facets may bear almost 50% of the load.

18. Describe the form and function of the uncinate processes.

The uncinate processes, which are fully developed by age 18, are thought to prevent posterior translation as well as some degree of lateral bending. They are also thought to be a guiding mechanism for flexion and extension in the cervical spine.

19. What happens during the straight-leg raise test?

Investigators have shown that the L4, L5, S2, and S3 nerve roots run in a sigmoid course through the foramina, with slack that can be taken up. The S1 nerve root runs a relatively straight course through the foramen. During a straight-leg raise (SLR) test, the sciatic nerve trunk is drawn downward through the greater sciatic notch, pressing tightly against the anterior bony structures. From 0 to 30 degrees, at 5 cm above the horizontal position, movement of the nerve at the greater sciatic notch already has begun. After a bit more elevation, the lumbosacral plexus is moving against the sacral ala, without root movement. From 35 to 70 degrees, the nerve roots begin moving. At 70 to 90 degrees, the nerve roots no longer move, but more tension is placed on all of the neural structures. The seated SLR has been shown in some studies to be more sensitive than the supine SLR.

20. Which muscles are recruited to initiate and complete lumbar flexion and extension?

Flexion is initiated by the abdominal muscles and the vertebral portion of the psoas. With further flexion, the erector spinae muscles are recruited as the forward moment acting on the spine increases. As the spine is further flexed, the posterior hip muscles are activated. At full flexion the erector spinae muscles become inactive and are at full stretch. These muscles and the posterior ligaments supply passive restriction to further forward flexion. To extend from this position, the pelvis tilts backward and the spine extends backward, using the above muscles in reverse sequence.

21. How effective are lumbosacral corsets for relief of spinal disk pressure?

Maximal disk load reduction with tight corsets is approximately 20% to 30%. The use of an abdominal corset with a chair back brace also may be helpful in diminishing loads applied to the lumbar spine.

22. What changes in lumbar spine intervertebral flexion and extension can be expected following lumbar disk replacement surgery?

A recent study has shown that at a mean follow-up of 8.7 years, at least 2 degrees of intervertebral motion are maintained in 66% of patients. The study found the mean range of motion for all disks to be 3.8 degrees.

23. List the ratios of disk height to vertebral body height in the cervical, lumbar, and thoracic areas of the spine.

- Cervical—1:4
- Thoracic—1:7
- Lumbar—1:3

24. What active range of motion in the cervical spine is required to perform activities of daily living?

In order to perform activities of daily living, 65 to 70 degrees both of rotation and of flexion and extension are needed. In a recent study, shoe-tying required the greatest amount of flexion and extension (66.7 degrees), while driving a car in reverse (67.6 degrees) and crossing the street (≈85 degrees) necessitated the greatest rotation.

25. Describe the effect on spinal loading of the double SLR, supine sit-up, trunk curl, and reverse curl.

- A double SLR involves mostly the psoas muscle; little abdominal muscle function can be measured.
- A supine sit-up with the knees and hips bent eliminates psoas recruitment and actively strengthens the abdominal muscles; however, because of greatly increased disk pressure, these exercises should be avoided.
- A trunk curl or half sit-up, in which only the shoulder blades clear the floor, lessens lumbar motion, recruits abdominal muscle function, and lessens the load on the disks.
- A reverse curl, in which the knees are brought to the chest and the buttocks are raised from the floor, activates the internal and external obliques as well as the rectus abdominus but with less disk pressure than sit-ups.

26. What lumbar pressures are involved in commonly used exercises and postures?

Standing—100%	Sit-up—210%
Fowler's position—35%	Reverse curl—140%
Bilateral SLR—150%	Prone extension—130%

27. What are the differences in lumbar spine muscle kinematics between patients with chronic low back pain and normal subjects?

Chronic low back pain patients have been found to have earlier activation and significantly longer activation of their erector spinae musculature as compared to normal controls during a lifting exercise. Longer contraction may suggest that chronic low back pain patients have changed their motor program from an open to a closed loop system.

28. What is the effect of age on cervical spine range of motion?

Average adolescent flexion-extension measures approximately 130 degrees whereas adult men (average age 37) have only 117 degrees of flexion-extension. Similarly, rotation decreased from 160 to 153 degrees for these same age-groups. This exemplifies the importance of cervical spine range of motion exercises beginning in young adulthood.

29. What are the effects of lumbar diskectomy on trunk musculature?

At 2 months after surgery, patients undergoing lumbar spine diskectomy were found to have 44% decreased trunk flexion strength and 36% decreased trunk extension strength when compared to controls. This may indicate a need for formal trunk strengthening following lumbar spine surgery.

30. What is the effect of leg length discrepancy on spinal motion during gait?

There is a significant asymmetrical lateral bending motion in the lumbar spine during gait in patients with leg length discrepancies of 3 cm. This may lead to accelerated degenerative changes in the lumbar spine.

31. How much nerve root movement occurs in the lumbar spine with SLR?

- L4—1.5 mm
- L5—3.0 mm
- S1—4.0 mm
- Sacral ala—4.5 mm
- Sciatic notch—6.5 mm

32. How much nerve root movement occurs in the lumbar spine with forward flexion while standing?

- L1-L2—2 to 5 mm
- L3—2.0 mm
- L4—0 mm

33. How much dural movement occurs in the cervical spine with flexion and extension?

- C5—Approximately 3 mm
- C8—Approximately 9 mm
- T1—Approximately 13 mm
- T5—Approximately 7 mm
- T10—Approximately 2 mm

34. Describe key vertebral landmarks.

- L5—Smallest lumbar spinous process
- L3—Largest lumbar transverse process
- C7—Most prominent cervical spinous process
- C6—Most inferior bifid cervical spinous process

Bibliography

Alderink GJ: Three-dimensional analysis of active head and cervical spine range of motion: effect of age in healthy male subjects, *Clin Biomechanics* 17:611-614, 2002.

Bennett SE, Schenk RJ, Simmons ED: Active range of motion utilized in the cervical spine to perform daily functional tasks, *J Spinal Disorders Techniques* 15:307-311, 2002.

Ferguson SA et al: Differences in motor recruitment and resulting kinematics between low back pain patients and asymptomatic participants during lifting exertions, *Clin Biomechanics* 19:992-999, 2004.

Grieve GP: *Common vertebral joint problems,* ed 2, New York, 1988, Churchill Livingstone.

Hakkinen A et al: Trunk muscle strength in flexion, extension, and axial rotation in patients managed with lumbar disc herniation surgery and in healthy control subjects, *Spine* 28:1068-1073, 2004.

Huang RC et al: Long-term flexion-extension range of motion of the Prodisc: total disc replacement, *J Spinal Disorders Techniques* 16:435-440, 2003.

Mitchell FL, Moran PS, Pruzzo MA: *An evaluation and treatment manual of osteopathic muscle energy procedures,* Valley Park, Mo, 1979, p 23, ICEOP.

Mototaka K, Kei M, Katsuji S: The effect of leg length discrepancy on spinal motion during gait, *Spine* 28:2472-2476, 2003.

Nachemson A: Towards a better understanding of back pain: a review of the lumbar disc, *Rheumatol Rehabil* 14:129, 1975.

Panjabi MM, Takata K, Goel VK: Kinematics of lumbar intervertebral foramen, *Spine* 8:348, 1983.

White AA III, Panjabi MM: *Clinical biomechanics of the spine,* ed 2, Philadelphia, 1990, JB Lippincott.

Chapter 55

Mechanical and Diskogenic Back Pain

Stanley V. Paris, PT, PhD, and
M. Elaine Lonnemann, PT, DPT, MSc

1. What is the role of bed rest in acute back pain?

Bed rest has a very limited role. A day or two at the most is recommended, with the possible exception of severe neurologic involvement. "Rest from activity but not from function" is a good adage to follow in this situation.

2. Describe the structure of the intervertebral disk.

Moving centrally from the outer neurovascular capsule are fibrous annular plates, often erroneously called rings (they do not circle the disk). Because the number of anterior and lateral plates is greater than the number of posterior plates, the nucleus in the lumbar spine is positioned slightly posterior within the disk. Between the fibrous outer annulus and the inner fluid nucleus is a transition zone consisting of a loosely arranged collection of fibrous tissue that is highly deformable and acts as a buffer between the nucleus and annulus. The nucleus pulposus is a mucoid protein that binds approximately 3 times its weight in water and allows for distribution of forces.

3. Describe the functions of the intervertebral disk.

Rather surprisingly, because of its extensive water content the disk is not a shock absorber. Instead, the muscles of the spine are responsible for shock absorption. The functions of the intervertebral disk include the following: (1) It provides space and position for the segment to allow the nerve root to pass through the foramen without compromise. (2) It permits, guides, and restrains motion in all directions, with the nucleus acting as an incompressible ball while the ligamentous annulus (90% type I collagen) restrains the nucleus and prevents excessive motion within the segment.

4. What position facilitates disk nutrition?

Side lying or lying on the back with the knees bent and the back flat facilitates nutritional pressure changes. Approximately 80% of the nutrition absorbed within a night's rest occurs within the first hour of rest. Therefore by resting during the lunch hour and again at the end of the workday as well as at night, it is possible to more than double the nutrition to the disk.

Side lying is of value if the knees are drawn up so as to flatten or slightly round the back. However, the moment the back assumes lordosis it loads the posterior disk, restricting its ability to imbibe nutrient fluids through the cartilaginous end plate. Likewise, prone lying is not recommended unless there is a large, firm pillow beneath the abdomen to prevent the formation of lordosis.

5. Describe the innervation of the disk.

The recurrent sinu-vertebral nerve and a gray ramus communicans from the sympathetic chain innervate the disk. They penetrate the outer capsule and may extend as far as the second or third annular lamella.

6. What is the source of diskogenic low back pain?

Peng et al. studied the histologic characteristics of the painful disk. They noted the formation of a zone of vascularized granulation tissue from the nucleus pulposus to the outer part of the annulus fibrosus. Nerve growth was found deep into the annulus fibrosis and nucleus pulposus following the zone of granulation tissue in painful disks. Immunoreactive nerve fibers (such as substance P, neurofilament 2000, and vasoactive intestinal peptide) were more extensive in painful disks than in control disks. Annular tears noted at the periphery of disks were associated with this increased vascular granulation tissue, and nociception from these fibers may be the source of diskogenic low back pain.

7. What are some of the anatomic structures associated with mechanical dysfunction of the facet joint and how might they be a source of mechanical pain?

With regard to the facet joint, there are five common conditions that can lead to pain and disability.

1. **ACUTE SYNOVITIS/HEMARTHROSIS**
   As with any synovial joint, an acute strain to the facet joint may result in effusion and even bleeding into the joint. The strained joint is painful, which causes its muscles to act as involuntary stabilizers, holding the joint against unguarded motion to facilitate initial healing. However, if the joint is held in this position for more than 1 or 2 days, because of pain or the fear of pain, the cross fibers of collagen in the capsule will begin to create capsular stiffness, resulting in a capsular pattern or restriction. Additionally, if their was a hemarthrosis present, adhesion can be expected to form from the fibrinogen in the resolving blood clot.

2. **STIFFNESS**
   As stated previously, stiffness can occur after an acute injury, resulting from collagen cross binding or the deposition of fibrous adhesions following the injury.

3. **MECHANICAL BLOCK**
   Occasionally, most typically at L4/5 in the male, a joint may become painlessly locked in side-bending following stooping to pick up an object. The exact cause of this "locking" can only be speculated, but could be due to a torn or separated meniscoid (all lumbar facets have menisci), a free fragment of articular cartilage, or simply roughness between degenerative joint surfaces.

4. **PAINFUL CAPSULAR ENTRAPMENT**
   On occasion (more commonly in the cervical spine), a sudden awkward movement may result in an acute one-sided pain that prevents the patient from holding the spine erect. In fact any movement towards the pain that slides the superior facet downward seems to cause an acute discomfort. In these circumstances, one can only assume that the facet capsule has become "stuck" between the articular surfaces. The fact that an isometric contraction of the multifidus muscles or a rotation, gapping technique can often produce immediate relief tends to support this hypothesis.

5. **DEGENERATIVE ARTHROSIS**
   Joint degeneration is a fact of age, no doubt hastened by misuse and abuse as well as genetic factors. Arthritic joints are stiff and painful, especially in the early morning.

   It is of interest to note that some spinal segments are hypermobile and perhaps unstable. This should be considered mostly a ligamentous condition, although laxity of the facet capsules may play a small role.

8. Discuss the potential sources of pain associated with dysfunction of the disk.

Several researchers have found nerve endings in the outer two to three layers of the disk. Furthermore when the disk degenerates to the degree that it becomes engorged with blood vessels in an effort to repair the disk, sympathetic nerves accompany the blood vessels. Substance P, a pain facilitator, has also been found in degenerative disks.

Early back pain, particularly that associated with developing instability, is mostly from the disk, is usually felt in the back and buttocks, and is of a deep and vague nature, often poorly localized.

When the disk herniates, one source of pain may be from the mechanical strain on the outer fibers of the annulus. If the prolapse places pressure on a nerve root, a sharper radicular radiating pain may pass from the back into the leg from compression of the dorsal root ganglia. With initial nerve root pressure, there is little pain because it appears that the nerves first have to become engorged and sensitized. Thus nearly 30 minutes may pass from the initial, sharp low back pain (tearing of the annulus) to the onset of radicular leg pain (pressure on the nerve root). Chemical irritation from inflammatory agents of the nociceptive fibers of the outer annulus may also cause pain. Other anatomic structures associated with the disk that are innervated and may cause nociception include the posterior longitudinal ligament (PLL), dural root sleeve, and dural sheath. Diskogenic pain is mediated by the sinu-vertebral nerves; it reaches the rami communicans through the L2 spinal ganglion. The pain may also take another route through the sympathetic nervous system.

9. Describe the articular receptor distribution in the spine.

- Type I—Postural receptors such as Ruffini's corpuscles (greatest in the cervical spine) sense joint position; they have a low threshold and are slow to adapt.
- Type II—Dynamic receptors such as Golgi-Mazzoni fat pads (deep seated in synovium) sense movement; they have a low threshold but adapt rapidly.
- Type III—Inhibitory receptors are found in the outer layers of the facet capsules, in associated ligaments, and in the deep layer of the multifidus.
- Type IV—Nociceptive receptors have a high threshold; they are nonadapting and chemosensitive.

10. Does disk herniation result from weakness and damage to the annulus (outside in) or from pressure pushing the disk outward (inside out)?

The first change noted with diskography is that the nucleus deforms and starts to "leak" or move laterally. The inner annulus has few fibers, like the loose-knit weave of a woolen sweater. It can be stretched considerably without tearing. The fibrous annulus, however, has many fibers. It is more like a cotton shirt, having little elasticity before tearing. Although the inner annulus may degenerate, tears begin at the outer annulus and spread inward, eventually allowing the nucleus to deform. The outer annulus is approximately 3 times as vascular as the capsule of the knee and thus can heal, as postmortem specimens have shown. Therefore determining which patients have an outer annulus injury can aid in selection of the appropriate therapy to promote healing and prevent herniation. Glycosaminoglycan turnover within the annulus requires approximately 500 days; collagen turnover is even slower. Healing, if possible, is still remarkably slow.

11. Which structure is most commonly involved in the patient with low back pain?

Regardless of the primary source of pain—disk, facet, or sacroiliac—the muscles will always be involved, whether voluntarily in a protective manner or involuntarily to guard against low back pain. However, they may also be the primary source of pain following unaccustomed overuse (e.g., the first day of spring gardening). The most common cause of initial low back pain would be injury of the facet joints, followed by ligamentous weakness, sacroiliac strain, and ligamentous pain from the outer annulus. Pain may also develop from ligamentous instability in an unstable segment that is often adjacent to a stiff segment.

12. At what levels does cervical spondylosis most typically occur?

The prevalence of cervical spondylosis is as follows: C5/C6 > C6/C7 > C3/C5 > C7/T1. These changes affect 70% of the population by age 70.

13. At what levels does lumbar disk prolapse most commonly occur?

The prevalence of lumbar disk prolapse usually occurs in the following order: L4/L5 > L5/S1 > L3/L4 > L2/L3 > L1/L2.

14. In the thoracic spine, what are the most common levels of dysfunction that present with clinical symptoms?

The junctional sites T1/2, T12/L1, and T4/5 are the most common levels of dysfunction.

15. Describe a classification of disk herniations.

DISK PROTRUSION (ANNULAR FIBERS INTACT)
- Localized annular bulge (usually laterally)
- Diffuse annular bulge (usually posterior and bilaterally)

DISK HERNIATIONS (ANNULAR FIBERS DISRUPTED)
- Prolapsed (nucleus has migrated through the inner layers but is still contained)
- Extruded (nucleus has broken through the outermost layer)
- Sequestered (nucleus has broken from the disk and is in the spinal or intervertebral canals)

16. Does spontaneous disk resorption occur? What are the proposed mechanisms?

Results reported by Kawaguchi et al. maintain that regression of herniated disks is a process of general tissue repair and remodeling observable in a range of disk herniations rather than a specific autoimmune response.

17. What is the effect of facet angle on disk herniation?

A study by Karacan et al. showed a positive correlation in patients with lumbar disk herniation and asymmetry to sagittalization of facet joints. They noted these alterations were more prominent in the taller patients. Park et al. found that the degree of facet tropism and disk degeneration might be considered a key factor when distinguishing the development of far lateral lumbar disk herniation from posterolateral lumbar disk herniation. A direct relationship between the extent of the degree of facet tropism and the extent of disk herniation was not seen. Other studies by Hagg and Farfan found an unclear relationship between facet tropism and disk degeneration.

18. What is the incidence of disk herniation?

The incidence of disk herniations cannot be answered for the simple reason that it is now believed that most disk herniations do not hurt. Computed tomography (CT) scans of the lumbar spine in asymptomatic subjects with no history of other than minor back discomfort indicate that the rate of disk herniation is 39%. A similar study by Weisel showed 50% abnormalities on CT scans in asymptomatic hospital workers. Disk protrusions are seen in 24% of asymptomatic patients.

19. What are the common causes of radiculopathy?

Neurologic signs arising from the lumbar spine most commonly occur in middle age, are more prevalent in men, and are typically a result of disk herniations, whereas neurologic signs arising from the cervical spine occur later in life, are more prevalent in women, and result from lateral foraminal stenosis caused by osteophytes from the lateral interbody, osteoarthrosis of the facet joints, and perhaps some disk material along with shortening and thickening of the ligamentum flavum.

20. Describe the classic presentation of disk herniations at various spinal levels.

Level	Nerve Root	Dermatome	Myotome	Reflex
C2/C3	C3	Anterior neck and posterior neck	Lateral neck press	None
C3/C4	C4	Nape and anterior shoulder	Shoulder shrug	None
C4/C5	C5	Deltoid anterior arm to base of thumb	Biceps	Biceps
C5/C6	C6	Lateral arm thenar eminence, thumb and index finger	Wrist extensors	Brachioradialis
C6/C7	C7	Posterior arm to index, long, and ring fingers	Triceps	Triceps
C7/C8	C8	Inner aspect of forearm and hand, lateral three fingers	None	
T12/L1	L1	Iliac crest and groin	Psoas	None
L1/L2	L2	Anterior thigh	Psoas	None
L2/L3	L3	Anterior lower thigh and shin	Quadriceps	Knee jerk
L3/L4	L4	Medial calf and big toe	Tibialis anterior	Knee jerk
L4/L5	L5	Lateral leg and anterior foot	Extensor hallucis longus	Extensor digitorum brevis
L5/S1	S1	Lower half of posterior calf, sole of foot, and lateral two toes	Flexor hallucis longus, gastrocnemius	Achilles
L5/S1	S2	Posterior thigh, sole, and plantar aspect of heel	Hamstrings	Lateral, hamstrings

21. Describe the natural history of disk disease.

In 90% to 95% of patients, spinal pain (which often is disk-related) resolves in 3 to 4 months. Lumbar disk herniations are quite common, and most cases have a favorable prognosis. Approximately 45% of patients demonstrate resorption of the herniation over time. In Norway, Weber randomly denied surgery to half of the patients selected for surgery by good and fair criteria (not as liberal as in the United States). At the end of the first year, those who had surgery scored twice as well on assessment as those who did not. By 3 years, however, there was no significant difference between the two groups. Five-year follow-up examination also found no difference.

22. Which is more successful for acute disk herniation—surgery or conservative care?

It has been shown in a summary of the literature that medical management that includes physical therapy is slightly favored over surgery, although both treatment options demonstrate excellent to very good results in 70% of the cases. However, with aggressive medical management that includes manual therapy and stabilization, excellent to good results can be achieved in 90% of the cases, even with paresis.

23. Describe the outcomes of physical therapy for acute low back dysfunction.

Only in the area of acute low back pain (with no specific diagnosis) have satisfactory outcomes been established. The treatments determined to be effective were, in descending order, manipulation, patient instruction, and exercise.

24. Discuss the role of manipulation and manual therapy in the treatment of disk herniation.

Manual therapy has no direct role in the reduction of disk herniations because neither traction nor manipulation has been shown to reduce the disk. However, manual therapy has been demonstrated to be effective, by relaxing the muscles and allowing for movement in the segment.

Manipulation has not been shown to reduce disk herniation. However, Maitland grade I and II oscillations may help to reduce discomfort and pain and thereby promote return to active function. More physical techniques involving stretching and thrust may be of value at the neighboring stiff segments to increase motion and thus improve overall function of the spine, lessening the strain on the level with the disk herniation.

25. What is the effect of rehabilitation after disk surgery?

A systematic review within the framework of the Cochrane Collaboration was performed in 2006; this study reviewed rehabilitation following first-time lumbar disk surgery. Their findings indicated that there is strong evidence (level 1) that intensive exercise programs are more effective on functional status and faster return to work (short-term follow-up) as compared with mild exercise programs. There is no evidence that patients need to have their activities restricted after first-time lumbar disk surgery. There is strong evidence for use of intensive exercise programs (at least if started about 4 to 6 weeks postoperatively), and no evidence that these programs increase the reoperation rate. The preferred method of postsurgical rehabilitation was unclear. It was also noted that there have been no studies investigating whether active rehabilitation programs should start immediately after surgery or at a later time.

26. How does exercise relieve back pain?

1. Repetitive motion gates pain. For example, repetitive motion (e.g., pendulum exercises) centralizes the pain to the shoulder, relaxes spasm, enables more motion, and hastens recovery.
2. If the pain is from an intradiskal source, repetitive motion may alter the chemical balance. T_2-weighted MR studies showed a definite increase in disk water content after repetitive backward bending but no reduction in the size of the protrusion.
3. Extension places a higher stretch on the facet joint capsules than forward bending. Placing the hands in the small of the back and using them as a fulcrum mobilize the facet joints.
4. Repetitive motion enables a patient to get over "fear of movement" and undoubtedly relaxes muscle splinting, thus improving function, decreasing load on the disk, and allowing earlier return to function.
5. Motion performed repetitively may reduce swelling around the nerve and thus the pressure that may cause ischemia.

27. What is the definition of spinal instability?

Spinal instability is a condition in which the osseoligamentous and neuromuscular components of the spine are unable to hold the spine against aberrant motions and slippage, leading to stress on soft tissues and causing pain.

28. Which are more frequently the cause of pain—facet or uncovertebral joints?

Facets are exquisitely innervated, including type IV nociceptors. The innervation of the uncovertebral joints (which exist only in the cervical spine between the second and sixth vertebrae) is similar to that of the disk from the recurrent nerve sinu-vertebral. However, clinically disorders involving the facets or uncovertebral joints cannot be separated in terms of symptoms. Pain from the uncovertebral joints may be similar to that from the disk—deep, vague, and locally appreciated. On the other hand, the facet joints develop superficial and well-localized pain. The uncovertebral joint may produce more serious pain when osteophytes (which commonly develop from these joints) crowd into the intervertebral foramen and entrap a nerve root, producing the more severe radicular pain.

29. Describe the innervation of the facet joints and types of afferent nerve fibers.

The innervation of the facet joints is a branch of the posterior primary ramus, which supplies the skin and muscles to the back. A deep branch arises near the facet joint and innervates that joint, with a larger branch supplying the joint below and another branch traveling to the level above (perhaps only in the lumbar spine). Thus the facet joints on their larger posterior surface have in common with most other joints a triple level of innervation. The anterior innervation is by a branch of the recurrent nerve sinu-vertebral that arches over the intervertebral foramen to supply the ligamentum flava—which are the anterior facet joint capsule!

30. Does leg length difference play a role in back pain and sciatica?

Leg length difference of up to one-half inch is present in 40% of the population and thus seems to be a normal occurrence. In theory, the presence of a short leg causes the back to bend toward the side of the longer leg, placing a greater load on the facet and disk on the longer side and somewhat narrowing the intervertebral foramen. No definitive study, however, has proved that symptomatic dysfunction results.

31. What muscles increase abdominal tone and pressure for stabilization of the lumbar spine?

The oblique and transverse abdominal muscles are important contributors to abdominal tone while the multifidus muscle provides stabilization for the posterior spinal structures.

32. What is the order of soft tissue disruption with forward flexion injury?

Forward flexion injury causes the following order of soft tissue disruption: supraspinous ligament, interspinous ligament, facet capsule, and disk.

33. Discuss the significance of the multifidus muscle.

The multifidus arises from the mamillary process just lateral to the facet joint, and then passes upward and medially, attaching to the adjacent facet joint capsule and to the capsule above before inserting into the spinous process one and two levels above. Acting unilaterally, it tends to bend the spine to the same side and rotate it to the opposite side. Acting bilaterally, it extends the spine. Because the multifidus inserts into the capsules of the facet joints, it tends to pull the capsule out of the way, helping to prevent capsular impingement. As one of the deepest muscles in the back, it is considered to be a primary stabilizer. The multifidus may be damaged during laminectomy or fusion. Even at 5 years after surgery, extensive damage may still be present.

34. What are the effects of dynamic lumbar stabilization exercise programs after diskectomy?

One study demonstrated that following microdiskectomy a 4-week postoperative exercise program can improve pain relief, disability, and spinal function. The exercise program, designed by a physical therapist, concentrated on improving the strength and endurance of the back and abdominal muscles and the mobility of the spine and hips. The program included aerobic exercise and strengthening exercises such as curl-ups and leg lifts to strengthen the erector spinae musculature.

A prospective randomized clinical trial (RCT) by Yilmaz et al. demonstrated with controls that dynamic lumbar stabilization exercises are an efficient and useful technique in the rehabilitation of patients who have undergone microdiskectomy. Outcomes were good for relief of pain and for functional parameters such as strength of the trunk, abdominal, and lumbar spine muscles.

35. What are the effects of disk herniation and surgery on proprioception and postural control?

Leinonen studied proprioception and postural control in patients before and after diskectomy. These variables were found to be diminished when comparing postoperative patients with chronic low back pain caused by disk herniation versus healthy controls.

36. What are the functional results and risk factors for reoperation after disk surgery?

It has been documented that factors including sedentary occupations, exposure to considerable vibration (such as from driving a motor vehicle), cigarette smoking, previous full-term pregnancies, physical inactivity, increased body mass index (BMI), and a tall stature are associated with symptomatic disk herniations. Increased fitness levels and strength have been noted to reduce the risk of disk rupture. Lack of regular physical exercise was a significant predictor for reoperation while gender, age, BMI, occupation, or smoking did not hold as much significance as regular exercise.

37. What are the effects of surgery on pain, spine mobility, and disability?

In a prospective cohort study from the Maine Lumbar Spine Study (Atlas et al.), 400 patients with sciatica caused by lumbar disk herniation were treated either surgically or nonsurgically and then assessed in 10-year follow-up visits. Changes in the modified Roland back-specific functional status scale favored surgical treatment throughout the follow-up period. However, work and disability status at 10 years did not demonstrate a difference between those treated surgically from those treated nonsurgically. A cross-sectional survey by Hakkinen et al. reviewed the results of patients' status post–lumbar disk herniation surgery. They found that 2 months after the operation median leg pain had decreased by 87% and back pain by 81%. However, moderate or severe leg pain was still reported in 25% and back pain in 20% of the patients. Hakkinen noted that pain, decreased trunk muscle strength, and decreased mobility were still present in a considerable proportion of patients 2 months after surgery.

38. What are the effects of low back pain, disk herniation, and surgery on the lumbar multifidus?

In patients with first-episode low back pain, ultrasound measurements indicate that multifidus muscle recovery does not occur spontaneously when the low back pain resolves. Disk herniation has been associated with selective atrophy of type I fibers while the atrophy of type II fibers was more frequent and severe. Findings such as decreased size of type 2 muscle fibers and core/targetoid and/or moth-eaten changes in the type 1 muscle fibers have been noted. Selective type 2 muscle fiber atrophy has been found during intraoperative muscle biopsies. Pathologic changes were present in 88% of patients before surgery. Rantanen et al. reviewed the intraoperative biopsies of patients with disk herniation and 5-year follow-up biopsies. Results showed that patients who have a positive outcome have positive changes in the structure of the multifidus. After a posterior surgical approach, biopsies of the multifidus showed significantly more signs of denervation in the tissue than before surgery.

Bibliography

Atlas SJ et al: Long-term outcomes of surgical and nonsurgical management of sciatica secondary to a lumbar disc herniation: 10 year results from the Maine lumbar spine study, *Spine* 30:927-935, 2005.

Botsford DJ, Esses SI, Ogilvie-Harris DJ: In vivo diurnal variation in intervertebral disc volume and morphology, *Spine* 19:935-940, 1994.

Creighton DS: Positional distraction: a radiological confirmation, *J Manual Manipulative Ther* 1:83-86, 1993.

Dolan P et al: Can exercise therapy improve the outcome of microdiscectomy? *Spine* 25:1523-1532, 2000.

Farfan H, Huberdeau R, Dubow H: Lumbar intervertebral disc degeneration: the influence of geometric features on the pattern of disc degeneration: a post mortem study, *J Bone Joint Surg [Am]* 54:492-510, 1972.

Hagen K et al: The updated Cochrane Review of bed rest for low back pain and sciatica, *Spine* 30:542-546, 2005.

Hagg O, Wallner A: Facet joint asymmetry and protrusion of the intervertebral disc, *Spine* 15:356-359, 1990.

Hakkinen A et al: Pain, trunk muscle strength, spine mobility and disability following lumbar disc surgery, *J Rehabil Med* 35:236-240, 2003.

Hides JA et al: Evidence of lumbar multifidus muscle wasting ipsilateral to symptoms in patients with acute subacute low back pain, *Spine* 19:165-172, 1994.

Kara B et al: Functional results and the risk factors of reoperations after lumbar disc surgery, *Eur Spine J* 14:43-48, 2005.

Karacan I et al: Facet angles in lumbar disc herniation: their relation to anthropometric features, *Spine* 29:1132-1136, 2004.

Kawaguchi S et al: Immunophenotypic analysis of the inflammatory infiltrates in herniated intervertebral discs, *Spine* 26:1209-1214, 2001.

Leinonen V et al: Lumbar paraspinal muscle function, perception of lumbar position and postural control in disc herniation-related back pain, *Spine* 28:842-848, 2003.

Ostelo RW et al: Rehabilitation after lumbar disc surgery, *Cochrane Database Syst Rev* 1, 2006.

Paris SV: Anatomy as related to function and pain, *Orthop Clin North Am* 14:3, 1983.

Paris SV, Nyberg R: Healing of the lumbar intervertebral disc. Presented at the International Society for the Study of the Lumbar Spine, Kyoto, Japan, May 1989.

Park J et al: Facet tropism: a comparison between far lateral and posterolateral lumbar disc herniations, *Spine* 26:677-679, 2001.

Peng B et al: The pathogenesis of discogenic low back pain, *J Bone Joint Surg (Br)* 87B:62, 2005.

Raoul S et al: Role of the sinu-vertebral nerve in low back pain and anatomical basis of therapeutic implications, *Surg Radiol Anat* 24:366-371, 2003.

Rantanen J et al: The lumbar multifidus muscle five years after surgery for a lumbar intervertebral disc herniation, *Spine* 18:568-574, 1993.

Saal JA: Natural history and nonoperative treatment of lumbar disc herniation, *Spine* 21(suppl):2S-9S, 1996.

Weber BR et al: Posterior surgical approach to the lumbar spine and its effect on the multifidus muscle, *Spine* 22:1765-1772, 1997.

Weisel SW et al: A study of computer-assisted tomography. I: The incidence of positive CAT scans in an asymptomatic group of patients, *Spine* 9:549-551, 1984.

Yilmaz F et al: Efficacy of dynamic lumbar stabilization exercise in lumbar microdiscectomy, *J Rehabil Med* 35:163-167, 2003.

Zhao WP et al: Histochemistry and morphology of the multifidus muscle in lumbar disc herniation: comparative study between diseased and normal sides, *Spine* 25:2191-2199, 2000.

Zoidl G et al: Molecular evidence for local denervation of paraspinal muscles in failed-back surgery/postdiscotomy syndrome, *Clin Neuropathol* 22:71-77, 2003.

Chapter 56

Lumbar Spinal Stenosis

Julie M. Fritz, PT, PhD, ATC

1. What is lumbar spinal stenosis?

Lumbar spinal stenosis can be defined as any narrowing of the lumbar spinal canal, nerve root canals, and/or intervertebral foramina that may encroach on the nerve roots of the lumbar spine. Lumbar spinal stenosis can become a painful and potentially disabling condition in affected individuals.

2. How is lumbar spinal stenosis classified?

There are two means of classification commonly used to describe patients with lumbar spinal stenosis; one is based on the anatomic location of the narrowing, the other on the etiology of the narrowing.

ANATOMIC CLASSIFICATION

- Lateral stenosis—narrowing that occurs within the lumbar intervertebral foramina and/or the nerve root canal, causing encroachment around the spinal nerve as it exits
- Central stenosis—narrowing that occurs within the spinal canal, causing encroachment around the nerve roots of the cauda equina housed within the dural sac

ETIOLOGIC CLASSIFICATION

- Primary stenosis—narrowing caused by a congenital malformation or defect in postnatal development. Only about 10% of cases of lumbar stenosis can be considered to be primary stenosis.
- Secondary stenosis—narrowing resulting from acquired conditions such as degenerative changes, spondylolisthesis, fractures, and postsurgical scarring. The most common cause of secondary stenosis is degenerative changes. Secondary stenosis may occur in individuals who already have a degree of primary stenosis.

3. What are the most common structural changes associated with lumbar spinal stenosis?

The majority of cases of lumbar spinal stenosis occur secondary to degenerative changes. Facet joint arthrosis and hypertrophy, bulging and thickening of the ligamentum flavum, loss of disk height and posterior/lateral bulging of the intervertebral disk, and degenerative spondylolisthesis are the most common changes contributing to lumbar spinal stenosis. Other, less common causes of secondary stenosis include fractures, postoperative fibrosis, tumors, and systemic diseases of the bone such as Paget's disease.

4. Is lumbar stenosis a common problem?

Yes; lumbar spinal stenosis is a common cause of low back pain, particularly in older adults. It is the most common reason for undergoing spinal surgery in individuals over the age of 65. Because of increases in life expectancy and improved diagnostic technology, rates of diagnosis of lumbar spinal stenosis and rates of surgery have increased substantially in the past several decades.

5. How will the typical patient with lumbar stenosis present clinically?

Because degenerative changes are the predominant cause leading to lumbar spinal stenosis, affected individuals are generally older than age 50 with a long history of low back pain. Most patients will have symptoms of pain and/or numbness in one or both legs. Chronic nerve compression may lead to diminished lower extremity reflexes and strength or sensation deficits. Lumbar range of motion, particularly in extension, will be limited and painful, often reproducing leg symptoms. Symptoms tend to be posture-dependent, worsening with spinal extension and improving with flexion. Because of this, patients will generally feel better in a sitting position, and worse when standing or walking.

6. Why do patients with lumbar spinal stenosis feel worse when standing than when sitting?

Standing places the lumbar spine in a position close to full extension. Extension of the spine causes further narrowing of the spinal canal. In individuals without stenosis, this narrowing is tolerated without difficulty; however, patients with stenotic narrowing tend to have worse symptoms when standing, or when standing and walking. Sitting causes flexion in the spine and therefore will generally reduce the symptoms of individuals with lumbar spinal stenosis.

7. Are there other factors that exacerbate symptoms for patients with lumbar spinal stenosis?

Axial compression, as is experienced during weight-bearing, also creates increased narrowing of the spinal canal and may exacerbate the symptoms of lumbar spinal stenosis. Research has demonstrated that the narrowing effects of axial compression are similar in magnitude to those of spinal extension. This helps to explain why walking can be difficult for patients with lumbar stenosis. Walking involves extension of the spine and creates increased compressive forces.

8. What is neurogenic claudication?

Neurogenic claudication is defined as poorly localized pain, paresthesias, and cramping of one or both lower extremities of a neurologic origin; symptoms are worsened by walking and relieved by sitting. There can be many causes of claudication; therefore the key distinguishing feature of neurogenic claudication is its neurologic origin—mechanical irritation of the cauda equina. The symptoms of neurogenic claudication are often the reason that an individual with lumbar spinal stenosis is prompted to seek medical treatment.

9. Are there other conditions that might be confused with lumbar stenosis?

Other conditions that have been confused with lumbar spinal stenosis include osteoarthritis of the hip, vascular claudication, unstable spondylolisthesis, and lumbar intervertebral disk herniation.

10. How can lumbar spinal stenosis be differentiated from other conditions with a similar presentation?

The postural-dependency of symptoms (i.e., better with flexion or sitting; worse with extension, standing, and walking) is a unique characteristic of patients with lumbar spinal stenosis. Clinicians have attempted to capitalize on this fact to differentiate spinal stenosis from other conditions with similar symptoms. A "bicycle test" has been described in which the patient first pedals in a upright, seated position with the lumbar spine in extension, and then with the spine in a flexed position. If the individual pedals farther in the spine-flexed position, the test is considered positive for lumbar spinal stenosis. Walking tests have also been described for use in differential diagnosis. The patient walks on a level surface in an upright posture, and also in a slumped or flexed posture. If the patient can walk farther with the spine flexed, the test is considered positive for lumbar spinal stenosis. A variation on this test is to compare walking on a level treadmill versus an inclined treadmill (15-degree incline). The incline of the treadmill causes the patient to flex the spine while walking, and usually will improve walking capacity in patients with lumbar spinal stenosis.

11. How is the diagnosis of lumbar stenosis confirmed?

Diagnostic imaging modalities are generally used to confirm the diagnosis of lumbar spinal stenosis. The most commonly used tests are the following:

- Magnetic resonance imaging—MRI is one of the most commonly used imaging studies to confirm a diagnosis of lumbar spinal stenosis. The anterior-posterior diameter of the spinal canal or the cross-sectional area of the dural sac can be measured to determine the extent of narrowing.
- CT scan—The CT scan is also commonly used to assess the diameter or cross-sectional area in the same manner as described for the MRI.
- Myelography—The anterior-posterior diameter of the spinal canal assessed on a myelogram was one of the first diagnostic imaging tests used to determine the presence of spinal stenosis. The disadvantage of myelography is the potential for adverse reactions to the contrast dye that is required for the test; also, there are reports of reduced diagnostic accuracy as compared with CT scans or MRI.

12. Are plain film x-rays helpful in the diagnosis of lumbar spinal stenosis?

Plain film x-rays can show the degenerative changes such as osteophytes and disk degeneration that are often the cause of lumbar spinal stenosis. Lateral views can demonstrate the diameter of the intervertebral foramina. However, plain film x-rays are limited in their usefulness by their inability to image the central spinal canal and the soft tissue changes that may contribute to lumbar spinal stenosis.

13. What are the most common impairments and functional limitations found in patients with lumbar spinal stenosis?

The most common impairments found during the examination of the patient are restrictions in spinal range of motion. Side-bending is often limited bilaterally; lumbar extension may be quite limited and reproduce or intensify the patient's symptoms. Lumbar flexion is also frequently limited in range, but will often somewhat relieve the symptoms. Deficits in vibratory or pinprick sensation in one or both lower extremities can occur, along with strength or reflex deficits. Many patients will have a positive straight leg raise test. Another common area of impairment is the hip joint. Restricted range of motion, particularly in extension, and weakness of the hip extensors and abductors are common findings. The most widespread functional limitation in patients with lumbar spinal stenosis is diminished walking tolerance.

14. Describe the surgical procedure for a patient with lumbar spinal stenosis.

Surgical treatment of lumbar spinal stenosis is performed to relieve compression on the contents of the central and lateral spinal canals. The most common surgical procedure for patients with lumbar spinal stenosis is a decompression laminectomy in which portions of the vertebral arch are removed to reduce compression of the lumbar spinal nerves. Sometimes a fusion, with or without instrumentation, will also be performed, although this is usually only done if there is evidence of spondylolisthesis along with the spinal stenosis.

15. Should a patient with lumbar spinal stenosis have surgery?

Little is presently known regarding the long-term outcome of surgery for lumbar spinal stenosis, or how these outcomes compare to nonsurgical treatment. Results reported thus far appear to indicate that short-term results are generally good with high percentages of patients expressing satisfaction with their result. The satisfaction tends to deteriorate with time, with only about 60% to 70% of patients satisfied 4 to 7 years after surgery.

16. Will the symptoms of lumbar stenosis continue to worsen over time?

Even less is known about the natural history of lumbar spinal stenosis than is known about surgical results. A few small studies have followed groups of patients who have chosen not to have surgery. The results tend to show that although some patients will deteriorate over time and eventually require surgery, the decline is not inevitable and large percentages of patients can maintain or improve their condition with time. The impact of a structured, nonsurgical treatment intervention on this natural history has not been sufficiently evaluated.

17. Will epidural steroid injections help patients with lumbar stenosis?

Epidural steroid injections are one nonoperative treatment that has been recommended for patients with lumbar spinal stenosis. Some patients will receive short-duration benefits from epidural steroid injections. The effectiveness of injections in reducing symptoms beyond a couple of weeks, however, is less likely.

18. What is the best physical therapy treatment for patients with lumbar stenosis?

Numerous treatment options have been proposed for use by physical therapists in the treatment of patients with lumbar spinal stenosis. Flexion-oriented exercises are advocated in order to capitalize on the postural dependency of symptoms of spinal stenosis. General conditioning activities are useful and may include stationary cycling, aquatic exercise, and walking as tolerated by the patient. Any strength or flexibility deficits identified during the physical examination should be addressed. Mobilization and stretching of the hips may also be helpful.

19. Should traction be used in the treatment of patients with lumbar spinal stenosis?

Pelvic traction has been recommended for the treatment of lumbar spinal stenosis in an attempt to relieve compression that results from the pathology. Although traction may be helpful for pain reduction in some patients, it should be combined with more active forms of therapy in order to improve function.

20. Can deweighted treadmill ambulation help patients with lumbar spinal stenosis?

Deweighted treadmill ambulation uses a harness and traction device to provide a vertical traction force during ambulation on a treadmill. The traction force reduces the axial compression associated with weight-bearing and can permit an individual with lumbar spinal stenosis to walk with reduced symptoms of neurogenic claudication. This treatment technique may hold promise for patients with stenosis because it provides the benefit of traction while keeping the patient active and exercising.

21. Are there published studies documenting patient outcomes with any physical therapy treatment approaches?

Unfortunately there are very few published outcome studies using any of the treatments mentioned above. Simotas et al. reported on the results of 49 patients treated with a program of physical therapy (flexion-oriented exercises) and epidural steroids. After 3 years, 9 patients (18%) had undergone surgery, 12 (24%) reported no change in symptoms, 23 (47%) had some amount of improvement, and 5 (10%) patients experienced worsening of symptoms. Fritz et al. reported the outcomes of two patients undergoing treatment using flexion-oriented exercises and deweighted treadmill ambulation. Both patients showed improved walking tolerance and reduced pain and disability levels with 6 weeks of treatment, and these improvements persisted at the 10-week follow-up visit. Whitman et al. also reported successful outcomes of three patients undergoing treatment involving mobilization of the spine and hips along with flexion-oriented exercises.

22. Should patients with lumbar stenosis wear a brace or corset?

The use of a rigid corset to limit spinal extension or a soft corset for general support has been recommended. A soft corset may provide a measure of relief for patients. A more rigid brace, while effective in limiting or preventing extension, is often cumbersome and restrictive for the patient and should likely be reserved for those individuals not responding to other forms of nonoperative treatment.

23. How should the outcomes of treatment for patients with lumbar stenosis be measured?

Measuring the effectiveness of any treatment for lumbar spinal stenosis is an important consideration. Patient-reported measures such as the Oswestry or Roland Morris disability scales are useful for documenting functional limitations and disability. The measurement of walking tolerance, usually conducted on a treadmill, is an important assessment and monitoring tool because it measures the most common and troublesome functional limitation in these patients.

24. Does stenosis occur in the cervical spine as well?

Yes; stenotic narrowing can and does occur in the cervical spine. Similar to the lumbar spine, the narrowing may occur laterally, in the intervertebral foramen, or centrally, in the spinal canal. The etiology may be primary (i.e., congenital), secondary to degenerative conditions, or a combination of these two factors. The presence of congenital stenosis of the central canal in the cervical spine is a particular concern for participants of collision sports such as football. The normal sagittal plane diameter of the spinal canal in the cervical region is 17 to 18 mm. The diameter of the spinal cord is about 10 mm. If the sagittal plane diameter of the canal is diminished, the safety margin within the canal is compromised, and symptoms of compression of the spinal cord may result.

25. What symptoms will a patient with cervical stenosis exhibit?

The symptoms of lateral and central cervical stenosis differ substantially. Lateral cervical stenosis typically results in compression of the cervical nerve root and produces symptoms of radiculopathy. Central cervical stenosis may compress the spinal cord, resulting in a condition termed cervical myelopathy. Symptoms of radiculopathy include neck and upper extremity pain and paresthesia in a dermatomal pattern. There may also be complaints of upper extremity muscle weakness in the affected arm. Symptoms of myelopathy are often more subtle, particularly in the early stages. Neck pain is not always present. Unsteadiness in gait or clumsiness are often early symptoms. Wasting of the intrinsic hand muscles is common. An extrasegmental distribution of paresthesia in one or both hands and feet may be present, followed by a perception of weakness. Gait disturbances can become severe, significantly interfering with functional activities and safety.

26. What is the typical clinical presentation for patients with cervical stenosis?

The clinical presentation of lateral cervical stenosis (radiculopathy) is typical of lower motor neuron disorders. Signs typically include hyporeflexia of the affected upper extremity accompanied by motor weakness and sensory disturbances consistent with the level of compression of the nerve root. Cervical range of motion is typically limited, and extension and ipsilateral side-bending may exacerbate the upper extremity symptoms. Spurling's test (cervical extension and ipsilateral side-bending with axial compression) is usually positive. Upper extremity symptoms may be reduced or relieved with manual cervical traction.

The signs accompanying central cervical stenosis (myelopathy) are those of upper motor neuron, or long tract, disorders. Weakness with spasticity may be present, along with clonus and positive Hoffmann and Babinski signs. Vibratory sensation is typically diminished in the lower extremities, and both upper and lower extremity reflexes may become hyperactive. Cervical range of motion is typically restricted in all planes. Lhermitte's sign (spinal pain and/or radiating extremity pain and paresthesias with forced cervical flexion or extension) may be present. Spurling's test is expected to be negative, and manual cervical traction will not have any effect on symptoms.

27. Should patients with cervical radiculopathy undergo surgery?

Most cases of cervical radiculopathy can be treated nonsurgically. Only patients with progressive neurologic deterioration are considered surgical candidates, or those who attempt conservative care for at least 3 months with no relief of symptoms. Nonsurgical treatment options include epidural steroid injections and cervical traction. Unfortunately, few controlled studies have been conducted to study the effectiveness of these interventions; however, it appears that they are effective for at least some patients.

28. What is the best treatment for cervical myelopathy?

Surgical management is typically considered once a diagnosis of myelopathy is established because the disorder tends to be progressive and potentially disabling. Performing surgery early in the course of the condition is believed to lead to a better long-term outcome. Laminotomy or laminoplasty are typically performed to increase the dimensions of the central spinal canal, and may be accompanied by cervical fusion.

Bibliography

Atlas SJ et al: The Maine Lumbar Spine Outcome Study, Part III. 1-year outcomes for surgical and non-surgical management of lumbar spinal stenosis, *Spine* 21:1787-1795, 1996.

Bridwell KH: Lumbar spinal stenosis. Diagnosis, management, and treatment, *Clin Geriatr Med* 10:677-701, 1994.

Chang Y et al: The effect of surgical and nonsurgical treatment on longitudinal outcomes of lumbar spinal stenosis over 10 years, *J Am Geriatr Soc (U.S.)* 53:785-792, 2005.

Deyo RA, Cherkin DC, Loeser JD: Morbidity and mortality in association with operations on the lumbar spine. The influence of age, diagnosis, and procedure, *J Bone Joint Surg* 74-A:536-543, 1992.

Dvorak J: Epidemiology, physical examination and neurodiagnostics, *Spine* 23:2663-2673, 1998.

Fritz JM, Erhard RE, Vignovic M: A nonsurgical approach for patients with lumbar spinal stenosis, *Phys Ther* 77:962-973, 1997.

Fritz JM et al: Lumbar spinal stenosis: a review of current concepts in evaluation, management, and outcome measurements, *Arch Phys Med Rehabil* 79:700-708, 1998.

Hurri H et al: Lumbar spinal stenosis: assessment of long-term outcome 12 years after operative and conservative care, *J Spinal Disease* 11:110-115, 1998.

Johnsson KE, Rosen I, Uden A: The natural course of lumbar spinal stenosis, *Clin Orthop* 279:82-86, 1992.

Katz JN et al: Degenerative lumbar spinal stenosis: diagnostic value of the history and physical examination, *Arthritis Rheum* 38:1236-1241, 1995.

Katz JN et al: Seven- to 10-year outcome of decompressive surgery for degenerative lumbar spinal stenosis, *Spine* 21:92-98, 1996.

Penning L: Functional pathology of lumbar spinal stenosis, *Clin Biomech* 7:3-17, 1992.

Porter RW: Spinal stenosis and neurogenic claudication, *Spine* 21:2046-2052, 1996.

Schonstrom N et al: Dynamic changes in the dimensions of the lumbar spinal canal: an experimental study in vitro, *J Orthop Res* 7:115-121, 1989.

Simotas AC et al: Nonoperative treatment for lumbar spinal stenosis: clinical outcome results and a 3-year survivorship analysis, *Spine* 25:197-203, 2000.

Whitman JM, Flynn TW, Fritz JM: Nonsurgical management of patients with lumbar spinal stenosis: a literature review and a case series of three patients managed with physical therapy, *Phys Med Clin N Am* 14:77-103, 2003.

Willen J et al: Dynamic effects on the lumbar spinal canal: axially loaded CT-myelography and MRI in patients with sciatica and/or neurogenic claudication, *Spine* 22:2968-2976, 1997.
Zdeblick TA: The treatment of degenerative lumbar disorders: a critical review of the literature, *Spine* 20(suppl):126s-137s, 1995.

Chapter 57

Spondylolysis and Spondylolisthesis

Matthew G. Roman, PT, OMPT

1. How is spondylolisthesis measured and graded?

Anterior slippage of one vertebral body on an adjacent body is graded I, II, III, and IV according to the percentage of slippage (25, 50, 75, and 100%, respectively). For example, a grade II spondylolisthesis indicates a 25% to 50% subluxation of the vertebral body, a grade III indicates a 50% to 75% translation, etc. Grade V spondylolisthesis indicates the superior vertebral body slips entirely forward on the subjacent body, known as spondyloptosis. These measurements are made on a standing lateral radiograph. Subsequently, Taillard has described a method that expresses the slippage in terms of percentage of the anteroposterior diameter of the distal segment (measurement of forward displacement of the anterior aspect of one vertebral body on the one below divided by the anteroposterior dimension of the distal vertebral body). This method is considered to be more accurate and more reproducible than the Meyerding method. Both methods, however, continue to be commonly used.

2. What is sacral inclination?

Sacral inclination, also known as sacral tilt, is the angle of displacement of the sacrum from the vertical. It is the measurement of the angle between a line drawn along the posterior margin of the first sacral vertebra and its bisection with the true vertical. This angle is measured on a standing lateral radiograph. The sacrum is angled anteriorly in normal upright standing postures, but the angle tends to decrease as the listhesis increases. The sacrum becomes more vertical with progressive listhesis.

3. What is the slip angle?

Also known as sagittal roll, sagittal rotation, and angle of kyphosis, the slip angle is considered to be the most sensitive indication of potential segmental instability. This angle is measured between a line drawn perpendicular to the S1 and S2 vertebral bodies (through the disk space) and a line drawn along the superior end plate of the L5 body. The inferior end plate can also be used; however, the inferior end plate is more commonly deformed with degenerative changes and is

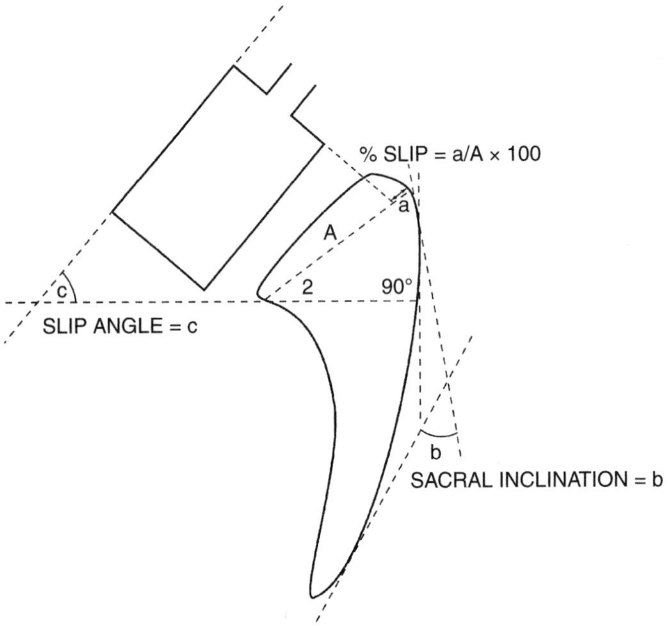

Measurement of sacral inclination, slip angle, and percent slip.

more difficult to consistently identify than the superior end plate. This measurement is critical because it is felt to be the most sensitive measurement to predict progression of the listhesis.

4. What are the types (classifications) of spondylolisthesis and the etiologies of each?

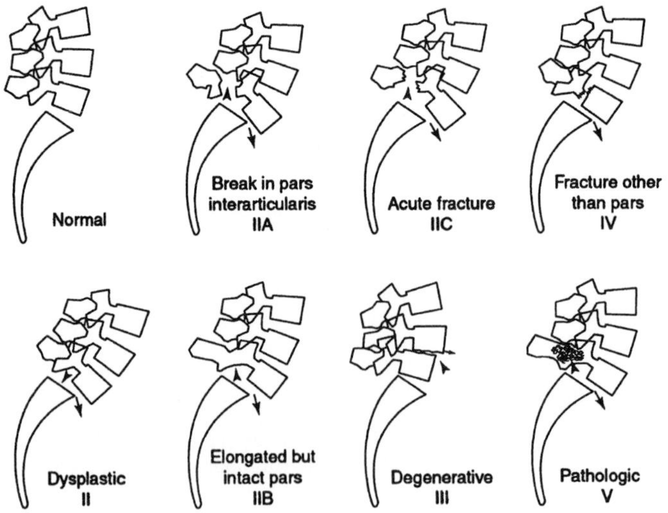

Types of spondylolisthesis.

	Congenital	Isthmic	Degenerative	Traumatic	Pathologic	Iatrogenic
Gender	Females > males, 2:1	Males > females, 2:1	Females > males, 5:1	Seldom seen	Data unavailable	Data unavailable
Age at onset	Congenital	Adolescents	Generally after 40 years	Seldom seen	Data unavailable	Data unavailable
Comorbidities	Questionable accelerated DDD; SBO	Questionable accelerated DDD; SBO		Seldom seen	Local or systemic bone disease	Lumbar stenosis
Most common level	L5-S1	L4-5	L4-5	Seldom seen	Data unavailable	Data unavailable
Progressive or not?	Yes, often caused by attenuation of posterior elements	Uncommon after stress fracture occurs	Gradually, occasionally will autofuse, related to degenerative changes		Data unavailable	Data unavailable
Associated symptoms	Radicular pain is common, associated with nerve root stretch and irritation	LBP, may present with radiculopathy in adulthood; "crisis" LBP at onset possible	Neurogenic claudication associated with stenosis Degenerative LBP		Data unavailable	Data unavailable
Cause	Dysplastic pars interarticularis, dysplastic sacral facets may have sagittal or axial orientation, attenuates with weight-bearing	Stress fracture of pars interarticularis, more common in young gymnasts and football linemen	Degenerative lumbar spine and intervertebral disk changes	Traumatic, producing fracture other than at pars interarticularis that allows listhesis	Tumor, infection, osteoporosis	Excessive decompression of facets at time of surgery

DDD, Degenerative disk disease; *SBO,* spina bifida occulta; *LBP,* low back pain.

5. What is the rate of occurrence of isthmic spondylolisthesis?

The incidence of spondylolysis or spondylolisthesis was found to be 4.4% at age 6. These children were followed into adulthood, where the incidence increased to 6%. The degree of slip was seldom found to progress after adolescence as the listhesis generally occurs concurrently with the fatigue fracture. Interestingly, the spondylolysis was never found to be symptomatic in the population studied by Fredrickson et al. yet was reported by Micheli to be the most common cause of low back pain in adolescents.

6. Does spondylolysis always progress to spondylolisthesis?

No. Nearly 50% of patients who present with isthmic spondylolysis do not progress to spondylolisthesis. Generally speaking, the listhesis occurs at the time of the fatigue fracture. If the anterior translation has not occurred during childhood or adolescence, it seldom occurs in adulthood. In the longitudinal study by Fredrickson et al., progression of the listhesis was found to be unusual after it was initially appreciated in childhood or adolescence. Degenerative spondylolisthesis can occur without isthmic defect because of long-standing segmental instability and/or intervertebral disk degeneration. In a similar fashion, dysplastic spondylolisthesis can occur without a disrupted pars interarticularis. Some cases of dysplastic spondylolisthesis occur with intact, but attenuated posterior elements.

7. Should neurologic compromise be anticipated with spondylolisthesis?

Lower extremity radicular pain in the child is said to be more representative of dysplastic spondylolisthesis, suggesting irritation of the L5 or S1 nerve root, although isthmic spondylolisthesis can present similarly. Isthmic defects are often filled with fibrocartilaginous tissue that is formed in response to the stress fracture and resultant listhesis. The exiting nerve root then is stretched across this fibrous defect, causing nerve root irritation and associated lower extremity radicular signs. Neurologic signs can occur in the form of lower extremity weakness, paresthesia, and occasional bowel or bladder incontinence. Cauda equina symptoms are most commonly associated with dysplastic spondylolisthesis as the nerve roots are stretched across the defect as they exit the sacral foramina. Degenerative spondylolisthesis often results in neurogenic claudication signs indicative of associated spinal stenosis.

8. Does the isthmic pars defect heal when treated?

If diagnosed early and treated with rigid bracing for up to 6 months, the results have been favorable according to radiographic evaluation, clinical improvement in symptoms, and bone scan criteria. Bone scan evaluation is typically used to determine if the fatigue fracture is sufficiently acute to warrant immobilization. Steiner and Micheli describe 78% good or excellent clinical results with the use of a modified Boston brace in grade I spondylolisthesis. The brace was used for 6 months full time, while allowing a flexion exercise program and sports participation within limits of pain complaints. Other reports indicate that the pars defect rarely heals, but clinical results tend to be favorable in response to bracing for the acute spondylolytic crisis. Early in the immobilization period, aggressive abdominal strengthening and stabilization exercises are begun, with return to activity, including sports, as tolerated.

9. What associated morbidity is seen with spondylolisthesis?

When isthmic spondylolisthesis occurs at the L5-S1 level, local instability is rarely seen. However, when it occurs at L4-L5, instability is more common because of the absence of the contribution of the iliolumbar ligament to segmental stability. This level has been shown to be hypermobile or unstable into the third or fourth decade of life. Degenerative changes occurring over the next several years tend to stabilize the progressive isthmic spondylolisthesis, but may lead to degenerative spondylolisthesis later in life.

There is some belief that intervertebral disk degeneration occurs more rapidly in the presence of isthmic spondylolisthesis than in a population without spondylolisthesis. Studies indicate a more rapid rate of degenerative processes after age 25 in patients with isthmic spondylolisthesis than in those without the disorder. Evidence of spina bifida occulta is seen 4 times more often in patients with isthmic and dysplastic spondylolisthesis compared with uninvolved control populations. Reported incidence of spina bifida occulta in dysplastic spondylolisthesis is 40%, with the normal incidence in adults without dysplastic spondylolisthesis being 6%. Spina bifida contributes to the predisposition to isthmic defects in involved patients by the dysplastic posterior elements not forming completely, leaving the posterior ring inherently weak. Transitional anatomy (sacralization of the L5 segment or lumbarization of the S1 segment) is 4 times more likely in those with degenerative spondylolisthesis than in age-matched controls.

10. How is spondylolisthesis diagnosed radiologically?

Standard x-rays are considered to be the gold standard in diagnosis. A lateral lumbar spine film will demonstrate the listhesis of one segment on the distal. Studies have confirmed that the anterior translation is greater in standing, weight-bearing films than in supine, non–weight-bearing films. Therefore some authors suggest both views be taken to demonstrate intersegmental motion. Lumbar spine oblique views are used to evaluate the integrity of the pars interarticularis. The well-described "Scotty Dog" sign shows the presence of the fatigue fracture by a radiolucent area across the "neck" of the "Scotty Dog." Bone scan technology is used to diagnose an acute fatigue fracture of the pars, or to differentiate local tumor or infection as the cause of symptoms. Neuroimaging studies (MRI or CT scan) are used to confirm suspicion of nerve root impingement associated with disk degeneration or the listhesis itself. Serial radiographs are taken to assess for progression of the listhesis. Repeat films are taken at 6- to 12-month intervals when spondylolisthesis is initially diagnosed, and then after a greater interval if no progression is identified.

11. What are the basic principles of conservative management of spondylolisthesis?

Isthmic spondylolisthesis often presents with a spondylolytic crisis in a child or adolescent. When confirmed radiographically, bracing is recommended in the acute case. When worn continuously for 3 to 6 months, the brace provides the pars defect an opportunity to heal. While still in the brace, specific trunk stabilization exercises are performed. The purpose of the exercises is to aggressively and functionally facilitate abdominal muscle contraction without causing segmental lumbar spine movement, which is undesirable during the healing stage as it may disrupt the healing pars. Attempts to restore "normal" lordosis through aggressive repeated extension activities, either standing or prone, are not indicated in treatment. A patient with spondylolisthesis may demonstrate a compensatory reduction in lumbar lordosis as a mechanism to limit the anterior translation stress involved with upright postures. Repeated lumbar extension exercises increase this stress, and have been shown to increase pain complaints in spondylolisthesis patients.

12. What is the role of flexibility exercises in conservative treatment of spondylolisthesis?

Lower extremity flexibility exercises are an integral part of any complete low back rehabilitation program. Hamstring flexibility is often limited in patients with symptomatic spondylolisthesis. Hamstrings become tight subconsciously in order to produce and maintain a posterior pelvic tilt and subsequent reduction in lumbar lordosis, thereby reducing the anterior shear force of the lumbar spine vertebral body. An anterior pelvic tilt may be adopted, allowing the iliopsoas and rectus femoris to adaptively shorten. These opposing forces of reactively shortening lower extremity musculature increase the overall stress and tension within the muscular system of the lumbosacral spine and pelvis, resulting in increased symptoms of pain and dysfunction.

Hamstring spasm that is unresponsive to conservative measures is often relieved by decompression of the L5 or S1 nerve roots at the time of surgery.

13. What are the surgical indications in the child or adolescent with spondylolisthesis?

Surgical indications for children and adolescents with spondylolisthesis are fairly well established. According to Amundson et al., surgical indications include:

- Persistence or recurrence of major symptoms in spite of aggressive conservative management for at least 1 year
- Tight hamstrings, persistently abnormal gait, or postural deformities unrelieved by physical therapy
- Sciatic scoliosis, or lateral shift
- Progressive neurologic deficit
- Progressive slip beyond grade II spondylolisthesis, even when asymptomatic
- A high slip angle (greater than 40 to 50 degrees), because high slip angles are felt to be the most sensitive indicator for progressive listhesis and instability
- Psychological problems associated with postural deformity, or gait deviations associated with a high-grade listhesis

Outcomes from in situ fusion in adolescents with spondylolisthesis have been well documented with very favorable results. Children and adolescents generally fare well following posterolateral fusion procedures, usually returning to unrestricted activity. It is interesting to note that most symptoms associated with spondylolisthesis in the child and adolescent are associated with the segmental instability; therefore in situ fusion can adequately control the symptoms without requiring nerve root decompression. Current recommendations are that decompression without fusion should not be performed "in patients under age 40, and is rarely needed in the child and adolescent years."

14. List the surgical indications for adults with spondylolisthesis.

- Isthmic spondylolisthesis that becomes symptomatic as an adult
- Following trauma
- Associated with progressive degenerative changes
- Degenerative spondylolisthesis associated with progressive symptoms
- Persistent symptoms lasting more than 4 months, interfering with patient's quality of life
- Progressive neurologic deficits
- Progressive weakness
- Bowel/bladder dysfunction
- Sensory loss
- Reflex loss
- Limited walking tolerance (associated with neurologic claudication)
- Associated segmental instability

15. What types of surgical interventions are available for treatment of spondylolisthesis?

In situ fusion has long been the procedure of choice for symptomatic spondylolisthesis, both in adolescent and in adult populations. Commonly, reduction procedures have been complicated by nerve root symptoms, radiculopathy, and occasional motor deficits from disrupting the nerve root during surgery. There is further controversy regarding the need for nerve root decompression accompanying posterolateral fusion in the adult with isthmic spondylolisthesis. Some authors claim decompression is necessary in the presence of any neurologic deficit, while others claim that decompression is effectively accomplished by a successful fusion. Wiltse et al. claim that the fibrocartilage mass decreases in size with successful posterolateral fusion effectively decompressing the nerve root. All authors, however, agree that the presence of bowel or bladder dysfunction and a motor deficit that is significant enough to cause loss of normal ambulation are reasons to decompress the offending nerve root during surgery. Decompression without fusion is often proposed in the treatment of degenerative spondylolisthesis as well. Wide laminectomy and involvement of the facet joints with decompression tend to result in an increased prevalence of associated instability. Substantial debate continues regarding the efficacy of decompression alone versus decompression with fusion in degenerative spondylolisthesis.

Bibliography

Amundson G, Edwards C, Garfin S: Spondylolisthesis. In Rothman RH, Simone FA, editors: *The spine,* ed 3, Vol 1, Philadelphia, 1992, pp 913-969, WB Saunders.

Farfan HF: The pathological anatomy of degenerative spondylolisthesis: a cadaver study, *Spine* 5:412-418, 1980.

Fredrickson BE et al: The natural history of spondylolysis and spondylolisthesis, *J Bone Joint Surg* 66-A: 699-707, 1984.

Gaines RW, Nichols WK: Treatment of spondyloptosis of two-stage L5 and reduction of L4 onto S1, *Spine* 10:680-686, 1985.

Grobler LJ, Wiltse LJ: Classification, non-operative, and operative treatment of spondylolisthesis. In Frymoyer JW, editor-in-chief: *The adult spine: principles and practice,* Vol 2, New York, 1991, Raven Press.

Grobler LJ et al: Etiology of spondylolisthesis. Assessment of the role played by lumber facet joint morphology, *Spine* 18:80-91, 1993.

Hensinger RN: Spondylolysis and spondylolisthesis in children, *Instr Course Lect, Am Acad Orthop Surg* 32:132-151, 1983.

Hodges SD et al: Traumatic L5-S1 spondylolisthesis, *Southern Med J* 92:316-320, 1999.

Ishida Y et al: Delayed vertebral slip and adjacent disc degeneration with an isthmic defect of the fifth lumbar vertebra, *J Bone Joint Surg* 81-B:240-244, 1999.

Love TW, Fagan AB, Fraser RD: Degenerative spondylolisthesis: developmental or acquired? *J Bone Joint Surg* 81-B:670-674, 1999.

Meyerding HW: Spondylolisthesis, *Surg Gynecol Obstet* 54:371-377, 1932.

Micheli LJ, Wood R: Back pain in young athletes: significant differences from adults in causes and patterns, *Arch Pediatr Adolesc Med* 149:15-18, 1995.

Nance DK, Hickey M: Spondylolisthesis in children and adolescents, *Orthop Nurs* 18:21-27, 1999.

Ralston S, Weir M: Suspecting lumbar spondylolysis in adolescent low back pain, *Clin Pediatr* 37:287-293, 1998.

Sanderson PL, Fraser RD: The influence of pregnancy on the development of degenerative spondylolisthesis, *J Bone Joint Surg* 78-B:951-954, 1996.

Shaffer B, Wiesel S, Lauerman W: Spondylolisthesis in the elite football player: an epidemiologic study in the NCAA and NFL, *J Spinal Disord* 10:365-370, 1997.

Steiner ME, Micheli LJ: Treatment of symptomatic spondylolysis and spondylolisthesis with the modified Boston brace, *Spine* 10:937-943, 1985.

Taillard W: Le spondylolisthesis chez l'enfant et l'adolescent, *Acta Orthop Scand* 24:115-144, 1954.

Wiltse LL, Winter RB: Terminology and measurement of spondylolisthesis, *J Bone Joint Surg* 65:768-772, 1983.

Chapter 58

Scoliosis

Paul J. Roubal, PT, PhD

1. What are the major types of scoliosis?

- Functional scoliosis—This may be caused by muscle spasm (secondary to lumbar or thoracic injuries) or leg length discrepancy (which causes a lateral shift in the spine). Functional scoliosis resolves with healing of the lumbar or thoracic injuries or correction of the leg length discrepancy.
- Structural scoliosis—This type of scoliosis is usually idiopathic.
- Congenital scoliosis—This type is caused by vertebral anomalies and is much less common than the other two types of scoliosis.

2. What is the incidence of idiopathic structural scoliosis?

Idiopathic scoliosis affects 1 to 4 people per thousand. Curves >20 degrees are 7 times more common in females than males, and curves >30 degrees have a 10:1 female to male ratio. The incidence drops to about 0.3% overall for curves >20 degrees. Idiopathic scoliosis usually occurs in adolescents between 11 and 14 years of age.

3. What are the possible causes of idiopathic scoliosis?

The role of genetics has been debated. Family history is not helpful in determining curve magnitude. Some form of multifactorial or autosomal dominant inheritance seems to be involved although most recent research suggests a polygenic inheritance pattern. The proprioceptive system and equilibrium imbalances, possibly related to asymmetry in the brain stem, also may be implicated.

4. Describe the clinical presentation of idiopathic scoliosis.

Curves do not straighten when the trunk is flexed forward (Adam's test). Structural curves exhibit rotatory components during forward flexion, and the patient's symptoms usually include rib hump or asymmetry in the trunk, referred to as the angle of trunk rotation (ATR). The ATR is easily measured with the scoliosometer.

5. What types of initial screening processes appear most effective in determining whether aggressive active treatment, such as bracing or surgery, is needed?

The most common method for determining the presence and severity of scoliosis is Adam's test combined with the use of the scoliosometer. Moire photography is moderately effective in screening for scoliosis but is much less cost-effective. Two-tier screening programs, which include both an initial screener and a secondary screener, tend to be the most effective in reducing false-positive diagnoses.

6. When is further evaluation of idiopathic scoliosis advisable?

In general, patients with curves >15 to 20 degrees and a 5- to 7-degree ATR usually are referred for further follow-up by an orthopaedist. Current data, however, recommend at least a 20-degree curve and 7-degree ATR.

7. Describe the Risser classification.

The Risser classification uses ossification of the iliac epiphysis to grade remaining skeletal growth. Ossification starts laterally and runs medially. Ossification of the lateral 25% indicates Risser type 1; of 50%, Risser type 2; of 75%, Risser type 3; complete excursion, Risser type 4; and fusion to the ilium, Risser type 5. Growth in females is usually complete in Risser type 4.

8. Describe the King classification system.

The King classification system describes curve types in idiopathic scoliosis, and the system helps to determine surgical treatment.

- Type I—primary lumbar and secondary thoracic curves
- Type II—primary thoracic and secondary lumbar curves
- Type III—thoracic curves only
- Type IV—large thoracic curves extending into the lumbar spine
- Type V—double thoracic curves

Recent studies have demonstrated some reliability problems with the King classification system. A newer system—the Lenke classification of adolescent idiopathic scoliosis—uses three components: curve type, lumbar spine modifiers, and sagittal thoracic modifiers. It is the most common system in use today for determining surgical intervention treatments. The Lenke system has recently been shown to be much more reliable than the King system.

9. Describe the rate of progression of idiopathic scoliosis.

Curve progression depends on curve size and Risser sign. For curves <20 degrees that are Risser type 0 or 1, progression occurs in 22% versus only 1.6% for curves above Risser type 2. For curves of 20 to 30 degrees and Risser type 0 or 1, progression occurs in 68% versus only 22% for curves above Risser type 2.

10. What treatment options are available for progressive idiopathic scoliosis?

Surgery and bracing have been the gold standard of treatment. There has recently been some research that shows progressive inpatient rehabilitation programs concomitant with development of ongoing home programs derived from this inpatient program have been successful in controlling the progression of scoliotic curves.

11. When should bracing be considered?

Curves <20 degrees generally do not require bracing, particularly when patients are more mature (Risser types 3 to 5). Curves <30 degrees that progress 5 degrees or more over 12 months should be braced. For curves >30 degrees, bracing should be initiated immediately. Bracing is not indicated in skeletally mature patients.

12. Describe the bracing used for scoliosis. How long should the brace be worn?

The first brace, developed immediately after World War II by Blount et al., was named the Milwaukee brace. It was fairly cumbersome, made with stainless-steel bars, and fitted with side straps to reduce lateral deflection and rotation of the spine at the specific points of apexes of curves. Newer, more comfortable braces include the Boston brace (thoracolumbosacral orthosis [TLSO]), which appears to be the most effective; it is made of molded plastic and fitted to the patient. Boston braces enhance adherence to treatment protocols because of ease of use. Generally they must be changed once every 12 to 18 months, depending on the patient's growth and body changes. Braces are most effective when worn 23 hours per day until skeletal maturity is achieved. The effectiveness of bracing is time-dependent: the more the brace is worn, the better the outcome.

13. What forces in braces reduce progression of scoliotic curves?

Computer evaluation of braces determined that the primary correction forces in braces are lateral. Muscle forces and longitudinal traction play minimal roles, if any. Reduction in hyperlordosis also is needed to reduce the curve.

14. What are the outcomes of major brace types in treating idiopathic scoliosis?

The Boston brace, Milwaukee brace, and Charleston bending brace are used most commonly to treat idiopathic scoliosis. Recent studies show that the quality of life scores are higher for Milwaukee and Boston braces than for the Charleston brace. For most curves, the Boston brace appears more effective at preventing curves from progressing, as defined by a lower rate of surgery. Surgical rates for the Charleston brace appear to be approximately 50% higher than for either the Milwaukee or the Boston brace. The greatest difference in outcome is found in King type III curves. King type I and II curves have fairly equal results with Charleston and Boston braces. Boston braces are most appropriate for curves with their apex below T8. Milwaukee braces are best used for curves with the apex above T7. Recent strides have been made in developing strap tension systems with strap transducers instrumented to the Boston brace. These tension systems allow optimal prescribed levels of tensioning so the patient may achieve the best curve correction along with a reduction in curve progression.

15. What curves respond best to bracing?

Curves without severe lumbar hyperlordosis, thoracic lordosis, or hyperkyphosis respond best to bracing. Risser type 0 curves respond best, whereas Risser type 4 or 5 curves rarely respond well. Double major curves respond less favorably to bracing than other curves.

16. How effective is bracing?

Over the years, the efficacy of bracing has been one of the most intensely debated subjects in the treatment of idiopathic scoliosis. Recent reports, however, indicate that the efficacy may be as high as 74% to 81% in halting progression of idiopathic structural scoliosis. In contrast, only 33% of patients do not progress without the use of bracing. Recent studies also show that wearing braces did not affect the quality of life in adolescents compared to observed counterparts. Other recent studies show that brace compliance and a high initial correction are strong indictors for bracing success.

17. What are the indications for surgical intervention?

- Curves >50 degrees in skeletally mature patients
- Curves progressed beyond 40 degrees in skeletally mature patients
- Curves >30 degrees with marked rotation
- Double major curves >30 degrees

18. Define "crankshaft phenomenon."

In a patient with an immature spine, correction of scoliosis with successful posterior fusion may be complicated by continued anterior vertebral body growth, which can increase the curve and vertebral rotation. This problem may be corrected with combined anterior and posterior fusion procedures if a skeletally immature patient must undergo surgery.

19. What type of correction can be expected with surgical intervention?

Surgery in idiopathic scoliosis generally reduces the major coronal curve by approximately 50%, vertebral rotation by approximately 10%, and apical translation by an average of approximately 60%.

20. What is the most common form of surgical intervention in idiopathic scoliosis?

Segmental instrumentation with multihook systems (e.g., Cotrel-Dubousset system) is the most common approach. Fixation is posterior. For more advanced and rigid curves, both anterior and posterior fusions may be incorporated. Patients should be evaluated on an individual basis.

21. List the complications of surgical intervention for idiopathic scoliosis.

- Migration of rods
- Neurologic damage
- Pseudarthrosis
- Renal failure
- Psychological stress
- Blood loss
- Failure of fixation
- Infection
- Respiratory distress

22. What types of treatment other than surgery or bracing have been shown to be effective?

Numerous studies have demonstrated that lateral electrical stimulation (LES) and exercise, either in or out of the bracing, are ineffective. To date, no research has shown that chiropractic care is effective. Physical therapists have recently been used in progressive inpatient and immediate post-inpatient rehabilitation programs for scoliosis.

23. Describe the role of the physical therapist in screening and treating scoliosis.

The physical therapist may train screeners, screen patients, and oversee preoperative and post-operative conditioning programs and progression in patient rehabilitation programs. Pain management, either before or after bracing or surgery, also may be needed.

24. Compare the costs of bracing and surgery.

Most research shows that the costs of bracing and surgery are somewhat comparable. At the start of the new millennium, total surgical costs, which include preoperative and postsurgical care and bracing as well as other medical care, average approximately $50,000. These costs do not include screening. Overall costs would be decreased if screening was used with bracing. Cost estimates do not include loss of income, welfare, social programs, or other direct or indirect medical costs associated with surgical intervention.

25. What are the long-term curve progressions for surgical-treated versus brace-treated curves?

After 22 years, brace-treated curves progressed 7.9 degrees versus 3.5 degrees for surgically treated curves.

26. What are the long-term (20 years or more) quality-of-life outcomes for surgery versus bracing treatment?

No correlation exists between curve size after treatment, curve type, total treatment time, or age at completion of treatment. Approximately 49% of those undergoing surgery, 34% of those treated with braces, and 15% of controls will have some limitation of social activities, mostly because of physical participation in activities or self-consciousness about appearance. Patients treated for scoliosis have about the same health-related quality of life as the general population.

27. What is the natural history of patients with untreated idiopathic scoliosis?

Untreated people with scoliosis are productive and function at a high level at 50-year follow-up. Back pain occurs in 61% as compared to 35% of controls. However, of those with pain 68% describe it as minor or moderate.

Bibliography

Blount WP et al: The Milwaukee brace in the operative treatment of scoliosis, *J Bone Joint Surg Am* 40A:511-525, 1958.

Climent JM, Sanchez J: Impact of the type of brace on the quality of life of adolescents with spine deformities, *Spine* 24:1903-1908, 1999.

Danielsson AJ, Nachemson AL: Radiologic findings and curve progression 22 years after treatment for adolescent idiopathic scoliosis: comparison of brace and surgical treatment with matching control group of straight individuals, *Spine* 26:516-525, 2001.

Danielsson AJ et al: Health related quality of life in patients with adolescent idiopathic scoliosis: a matched follow-up at least 20 years after treatment with brace or surgery, *Eur Spine J* 10:278-288, 2001.

Dubousset J, Herring JA, Shufflebarger H: The crankshaft phenomenon, *J Pediatr Orthop* 9:541-550, 1989.

Fernandez-Feliberti R et al: Effectiveness of TLSO bracing in the conservative treatment of idiopathic scoliosis, *J Pediatr Orthop* 15:176-181, 1995.

Howard A, Wright JG, Hedden D: A comparative study of TLSO, Charleston, and Milwaukee braces for idiopathic scoliosis, *Spine* 23:2404-2411, 1998.

Katz DE, Durrani AA: Factors that influence outcome in bracing large curves in patients with adolescent idiopathic scoliosis, *Spine* 26:2354-2361, 2001.

King HA et al: The selection of fusion levels in thoracic idiopathic scoliosis, *J Bone Joint Surg* 65A:1302-1313, 1983.

Landauer F, Wimmer C, Behensky H: Estimating the final outcome of brace treatment for idiopathic thoracic scoliosis at 6-month follow-up journal, 6:201-207, 2003.

Lenke LG et al: Adolescent idiopathic scoliosis: a new classification to determine extent of spinal arthrodesis, *J Bone Joint Surg* 83A:1169-1181, 2001.

Lenke LG et al: The Lenke classification of adolescent idiopathic scoliosis: how it organizes curve patterns as a template to perform selective fusions of the spine, *Spine* 28:S199-207, 2003.

Lou E et al: Intelligent brace system for the treatment of scoliosis, *Stud Health Technol Inform* 91:397-400, 2002.

Lonstein JE, Winter RB: The Milwaukee Brace for the treatment of adolescent idiopathic scoliosis, *J Bone Joint Surg* 82A:1207-1221, 1994.

Mielke CH et al: Surgical treatment of adolescent idiopathic scoliosis: a comparative analysis, *J Bone Joint Surg* 71A:1170-1177, 1989.

Montgomery F, Willner S: The natural history of idiopathic scoliosis: incidence of treatment in 15 cohorts of children born between 1963 and 1977, *Spine* 22:772-774, 1997.

Nachemson AL, Petersen LE: Effectiveness of treatment with a brace in girls who have adolescent idiopathic scoliosis, *J Bone Joint Surg* 77A:815-822, 1995.

Rigo M, Reiter Ch, Weiss HR: Effect of conservative management on the prevalence of surgery in patients with adolescent idiopathic scoliosis, *Pediatr Rehabil* 6:209-214, 2003.

Roubal PJ, Freeman DC, Placzek JD: Costs and effectiveness of scoliosis screening, *Physiotherapy* 85:259-268, 1999.

Ugwonali OF et al: Effect of bracing on the quality of life of adolescents with idiopathic scoliosis, *Spine J* 4:254-260, 2004.

Weinstein SL et al: Health and function of patients with untreated idiopathic scoliosis: a 50 year natural history study, *JAMA* 5:559-567, 2003.

Weiss HR, Weiss G, Schaar HJ: Incidence of surgery in conservatively treated patients with scoliosis, *Pediatr Rehabil* 6:111-118, 2003.

Willers U et al: Long-term results of Harrington instrumentation in idiopathic scoliosis, *Spine* 18:713-717, 1993.

Chapter 59

Thoracic Spine and Rib Cage Dysfunction

*Timothy W. Flynn, PT, PhD, OCS**

1. What is the incidence of disk disease in the thoracic spine?

The incidence of asymptomatic herniated nucleus pulposus or bulge in the thoracic spine is high. Wood and Garvey reported that the incidence of asymptomatic thoracic disk herniations based on magnetic resonance imaging (MRI) is approximately 37%. On follow-up examination of asymptomatic patients with disk herniation, the authors noted little change in size of the herniation. Symptomatic disks may occur less frequently in the thoracic spine because of the relative limitation of motion in the thoracic region.

2. Describe the normal range of motion (ROM) of the thoracic spine.

The rib cage and sternum attachments limit ROM of the thoracic spine. Inclinometry of T1-T12 indicates that the total range of sagittal plane motion is approximately 36 degrees (16 degrees of flexion and 20 degrees of extension from neutral posture). Frontal plane motion is approximately 44 degrees (24 degrees of right side-bending and 20 degrees of left side-bending from neutral posture).

3. Describe the preferred side-bending and rotation-coupling pattern of the thoracic spine.

In general, when the spine is neither flexed nor extended, side-bending and rotation are coupled to opposite directions (e.g., right side-bending with left rotation). This postulate is based primarily on cadaveric studies without an intact rib cage. According to Lee, clinical observation demonstrates that the coupling pattern is sensitive to which plane of movement is introduced first; she suggests that rotation and side-bending couple to the same side in the thoracic spine when rotation is introduced first. However, in vivo reports have noted a large variation in coupling pattern both within and among individuals. In addition, coupling pattern is sensitive to the plane of reference. Above the apex of the curve, for instance, the opposite coupling pattern appears to predominate, whereas below the apex of the curve coupling patterns to the same side appear to predominate.

4. How many articulations are present on the typical thoracic vertebra?

A typical thoracic vertebra has 12 separate articulations: 4 zygapophyseal articulations, 2 costotransverse articulations, 4 costovertebral articulations, and 2 body-IV disk-body articulations. At present, individual passive assessment of these components is likely to be fraught with difficulty and poor reliability.

---

*The opinions and assertions contained herein are the private views of the author and are not to be construed as official or as reflecting the views of the Department of the Army or the Department of Defense.

5. Describe the typical pattern of rib cage motion.

The typical upper rib motion during respiration is termed pump handle (sagittal plane elevation), whereas lower rib motion is termed bucket handle (frontal plane flaring). Lee's model suggests that during spinal flexion the ribs rotate anteriorly; posterior elements move superiorly and anterior elements move inferiorly. This pattern is termed internal torsional movement. During spinal extension, the opposite movement is proposed, with the ribs rotating posteriorly; posterior elements move inferiorly and anterior elements move superiorly. This pattern is termed external torsional movement. This model has not been validated with in vivo motion studies. Various authors and one case report have outlined the potential clinical presentation and significance of loss of this movement.

6. Describe the cervical rotation lateral flexion (CRLF) test.

The CRLF test determines the presence of first rib hypomobility in patients with brachialgia. The test is performed with the patient in the sitting position. The cervical spine is rotated passively and maximally away from the side being tested (i.e., rotation to the left to test the right side). In this position, the spine is gently flexed as far as possible, moving the ear toward the chest. A test is considered positive when lateral flexion movement is blocked. Lindgren and colleagues reported excellent inter-rater reliability (Kappa value = 1.0) and good agreement with cineradiographic findings (Kappa value = 0.84).

7. Define thoracic outlet syndrome.

Thoracic outlet syndrome (TOS) is perhaps the most controversial symptom complex in surgery. Even the use of established operation criteria before surgery results in relief of symptoms in only 28% of patients undergoing first rib resection. Diagnoses using the traditional positional provocation tests of the upper extremity are unreliable and result in a large number of false positives. Conservative therapy aimed at restoring function to the upper thoracic aperture in patients with TOS decreased symptoms and returned patients to work after intervention and at a 2-year follow-up visit. Therefore conservative management is advocated.

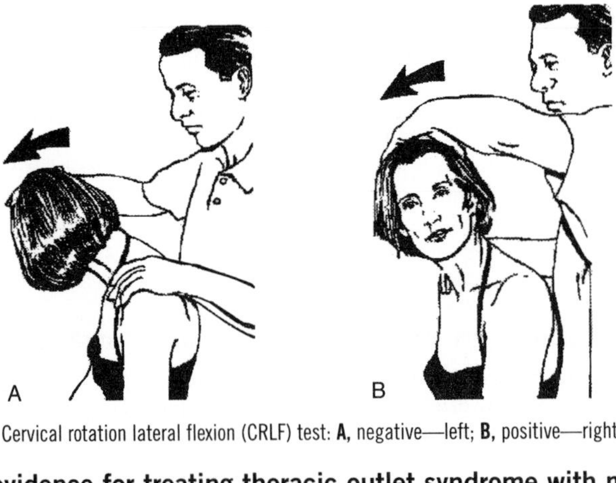

Cervical rotation lateral flexion (CRLF) test: **A,** negative—left; **B,** positive—right.

8. Is there evidence for treating thoracic outlet syndrome with manual therapy procedures?

Lindgren and Leino, in a case series, described treating a subluxation of the first rib with manual therapy procedures (isometric muscle activities) with a subsequent reduction of symptoms attributed to thoracic outlet syndrome.

9. Describe the typical pattern of movement and positional dysfunction of the thoracic spine and rib cage.

In general, the upper two segments of the thoracic spine often have restricted ability to extend fully, resulting in a flexed (kyphotic) posture in this region. The T3-T7 segments often have restricted ability to flex and concurrent external rib torsional dysfunction, resulting in an extended (flat) posture in this region. The T8-T12 segments often have restricted ability to extend, resulting in a flexed (kyphotic) posture in this region.

10. Describe a classification system for thoracic spine and rib cage dysfunction.

Patients in whom specific mobilization is indicated have primary single segmental restriction of either flexion or extension, torsional rib cage dysfunction, and/or first rib restriction. The immobilization category includes patients who require motion restriction. The rib subluxations are the primary candidates for this treatment, which is geared at using the patient's muscle activity to restore normal symmetry and to avoid movement stresses in directions that promote asymmetry. Segmental thoracic hypermobility or instability also is placed in this category.

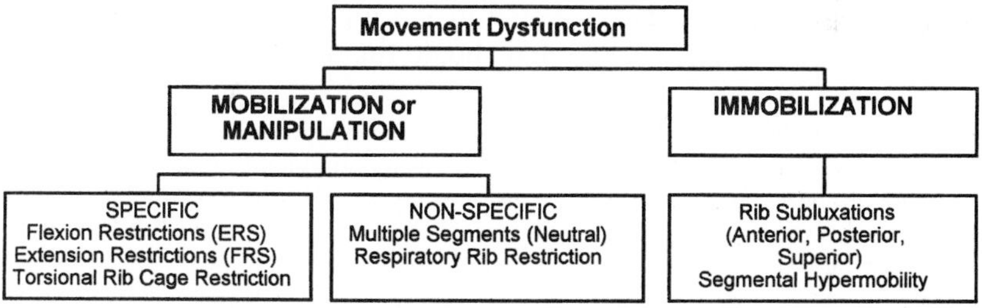

Classification and treatment scheme for thoracic spine and rib dysfunction.

The nonspecific mobilization category does not imply gross mobilization but rather the treatment of multiple segments in the neutral (neither flexed nor extended) spine. Rib cage restrictions in either inhalation or exhalation also fall into this category.

11. Does dysfunction in the thoracic spine contribute to mechanical neck pain?

Cleland and colleagues demonstrated that manipulation of the thoracic spine results in decreased neck pain in individuals with primary cervical complaints. Furthermore, increases in cervical ROM after thoracic manipulation have been observed.

12. Does osteoporosis frequently involve the thoracic spine?

Osteoporosis is associated with loss of bone mass per unit of volume. Loss of bone mass in the axial skeleton predisposes vertebral bodies to fracture, which results in back pain and deformity. An anterior wedge compression fracture is manifested by a decrease in anterior height, usually 4 mm or greater, compared with the vertical height of the posterior body.

13. What are the symptoms of thoracic osteoporosis? How are they treated?

Symptomatic osteoporosis presents as midline back pain localized over the thoracic or lumbar spine, the most common location for fractures. The treatment of osteoporosis is often complex and in severely affected patients should be coordinated with an endocrinologist. Treatment should include exercise, which has been shown to increase bone mass and to slow the decline of skeletal mass. Weight-bearing activities should be emphasized. Men and women over age 60 are at risk for spontaneous osteoporotic fractures of the thoracic spine; the extent of vertebral deformity and multiple fractures appears linked with pain intensity.

14. What is the incidence of musculoskeletal dysfunction mimicking cardiac disease in the emergency department (ED)?

Musculoskeletal chest wall syndromes have been reported in as many as 28% of patients admitted to the ED with acute chest pain but without acute myocardial infarction.

15. Is there a role for thoracic spine manipulation in the treatment of mild compressive cervical myelopathy?

Browder and colleagues described the use of intermittent cervical traction and manipulation of the thoracic spine in a series of patients with mild cervical compressive myelopathy attributed to herniated disk. They noted a substantial reduction of pain and a decreased level of disability following this protocol.

16. The presenting symptoms of a 35-year-old man include pain and stiffness in the thoracic region, which is worse in the morning. On physical exam you note limited chest expansion. What should the differential diagnosis include?

Ankylosing spondylitis (AS) is a chronic inflammatory disease characterized by a variable symptomatic course. Back pain and stiffness are the initial symptoms in 81% of patients. In the thoracic spine, AS causes decreased motion at the costovertebral joints, reduced chest expansion, and impaired pulmonary function. Chest expansion is measured at the fourth intercostal space in men and below the breasts in women. The patient raises both hands over the head and is asked to take a deep inspiration. Normal expansion is ≥2.5 cm.

17. The presenting symptoms of a 44-year-old man include pain in the right T7-T9 region slightly below the inferior lateral angle of the scapula. Further questioning determines that the symptoms are worse 2 to 3 hours after a meal. What should the differential diagnosis include?

Pain from cholecystitis (inflamed gallbladder) typically occurs 1 to 2 hours after ingestion of a heavy meal, with severe pain peaking at 2 to 3 hours. Pain from gallbladder disease is generally transmitted along T8 and T9 nerve segments. Right upper quadrant or epigastric pain is characteristic, but pain often is referred to the angle of the scapula on the right side.

18. Can thoracic spine and rib cage musculoskeletal dysfunction mimic anginal pain?

The T4-T7 thoracic segments frequently have been implicated as the source for initiation of pseudoanginal pain. The primary evidence is in the form of case reports and case series. Hamburg and Lindahl reported six cases of "anginal" pain relieved by manipulation of the midthoracic segments. In many cases, the primary symptoms of diabetic thoracic radiculopathy are severe abdominal and anterior chest pain with minimal back pain.

19. What is Scheuermann's disease? Is it safe to use manual therapy in affected patients?

Scheuermann first described the radiographic changes of anterior wedging and vertebral end-plate irregularity in the thoracic spine associated with kyphosis. The disease also is known as juvenile kyphosis, vertebral osteochondritis, and osteochondritis deformans juvenilis dorsi. Disk material herniated into the vertebral bodies (Schmorl's nodes) is a common associated finding. Patients benefit from even slight increases in motion of the posterior elements at the involved segments. Despite the fact that the basic deformity is not "corrected," maintenance and improvement in range of motion and function may be achieved.

20. Do postural abnormalities of the cervical and thoracic spine contribute to pain?

Poor upper quadrant posture has been implicated as a source of neck and shoulder pain. Patients with more severe postural abnormalities of the thoracic, cervical, and shoulder regions have a significantly increased incidence of pain. In particular, patients with thoracic kyphosis and rounded shoulders reportedly have an increased incidence of cervical, interscapular, and headache pain.

21. Define T4 syndrome.

T4 syndrome describes a group of symptoms including dysfunction within the T2-T7 segments. The clinical presentation includes various combinations of pain in the upper limbs, neck, upper thoracic, and scapular region with cranial headaches. However, the T4 segment is nearly always involved. In addition, patients may report glovelike paresthesias and numbness in one or both hands, often nocturnal in nature. Differential diagnoses include systemic illness, polyneuritis, and nerve root compression. Typical examination findings include tenderness, asymmetry, and limited segmental range of motion and tissue thickening. Furthermore, posteroanterior pressure over the involved thoracic segment reproduces the symptoms. McGuckin (not peer-reviewed) reported 90 cases in which the syndrome occurred more frequently in women (4:1) than men, with a typical presentation between 30 and 50 years. In another case report, two cases of apparent T4 syndrome of 6 to 12 months' duration that were treated successfully by two sessions of T3-T4 manipulation. Treatment includes localized segmental mobilization and/or manipulation.

22. What role can the thoracic spine play in headaches?

Dysfunction of the thoracic spine, in particular the upper five segments, has been implicated as the primary generator of headaches. Examination of the upper thorax spine in patients with headaches is warranted. Treatment using segmental mobilization and/or manipulation has been advocated. The mechanism for the referred pain to the head is unknown.

23. Can low back pain be caused by thoracic dysfunction?

Yes. The lateral branches of the dorsal rami of lower thoracic and upper lumbar segments become cutaneous over the buttocks, and greater trochanter pain in this region can be referred from the thoracic spine.

24. When obtaining a medical history for patients over age 50 who have thoracic spine pain not associated with trauma, why is it important to identify red flags associated with cancer?

Metastatic lesions in the skeleton are much more common than primary tumors of bone (overall ratio = 25:1). The presence of metastases increases with age. Patients age 50 and older are at greatest risk of developing metastatic disease. Metastases occur more commonly in the axial skeleton than in the appendicular skeleton. The thoracic spine is the area of the spine most frequently affected by metastases. Breast cancer is the most common site of tumor origin. In addition, skeletal metastases from tumors of prostate, lung, thyroid, kidney, rectum, and uterine cervix are quite common.

25. Describe the clinical presentation of postherpetic neuralgia.

Postherpetic neuralgia is pain that persists for longer than 1 month after the rash of acute herpes zoster (reactivated chickenpox virus) resolves. The pain can be lancinating or manifest as a steady burning or ache along a thoracic dermatomal pattern. The involved skin area is often hypersensitive to light touch. Postherpetic neuralgia can mimic thoracic radiculopathy or referred pain of thoracic spine origin.

26. Define costochondritis. What treatment can the physical therapist provide?

Costochondritis is an inflammation or irritation of the costochondral junction. Frequently it is referred pain from thoracic or rib dysfunction, probably in the corresponding vertebral level. Examination of the thoracic spine and posterior chest wall is warranted. Treatment using segmental mobilization and/or manipulation has been advocated.

27. If the patient demonstrates inhibition or difficulty in activating the lower trapezius muscle, what should the therapist consider?

The therapist should screen the T8-T12 segments for extension restrictions. Segmental mobilization or manipulation to improve extension may result in immediate improvement of lower trapezius muscle activation. The mechanism is unclear; it could be secondary to localized pain that inhibits maximal muscle firing.

28. If the patient demonstrates inhibition of the serratus anterior muscle or has difficulty in stabilizing the scapula during arm movements, what should the therapist consider?

In the absence of long thoracic neuropathy, the therapist should screen the T3-T7 vertebral segments for flexion restrictions. Segmental mobilization or manipulation to improve flexion often results in immediate improvement of serratus anterior muscle activation. The mechanism is unclear; it may be secondary to localized pain that inhibits maximal muscle firing.

29. What areas of the cervical spine typically refer pain into the thoracic region?

The cervical zygapophyseal joints, especially those at the C5-C6 and C6-C7 spinal levels, and the cervical intervertebral disks and nerve roots, especially at the C5-C6 and C6-C7 spinal levels, commonly refer pain into the middle region of the back.

30. Is thoracic spine dysfunction a contributing factor to complex regional pain syndrome type I (CRPS I)?

CRPS I is a complex and poorly understood syndrome that was previously classified as reflex sympathetic dystrophy. Assessment and treatment of the thoracic spine should be performed in patients presenting with this syndrome. Thoracic spine manipulation has been used in this population with subsequent reduction in pain and dystrophic symptoms.

31. Can treatment of the thoracic spine and rib cage aid in the management of shoulder dysfunction?

Bang and Deyle have demonstrated that manual therapy procedures targeted at impairments of the cervical and thoracic spine result in decreased pain and improved function in patients with shoulder impingement syndrome. In addition, in a small case series Boyle reported that apparent shoulder impingement syndrome was relieved by mobilization of the second rib.

Bibliography

Bang MD, Deyle GD: Comparison of supervised exercise with and without manual physical therapy for patients with shoulder impingement syndrome, *J Orthop Sports Phys Ther* 30:126-137, 2000.

Boyle J: Is the pain and dysfunction of shoulder impingement lesion really second rib syndrome in disguise? Two case reports, *Manual Ther* 4:44-48, 1999.

Browder D, Erhard R, Piva S: Intermittent cervical traction and thoracic manipulation for management of mild cervical compressive myelopathy attributed to cervical herniated disc: a case series, *J Orthop Sports Phys Ther* 34:701-712, 2004.

Cleland J et al: Immediate effects of thoracic manipulation in patients with neck pain: a randomized clinical trial, *Manual Ther* 10:127-135, 2005.

Flynn TW: An evidence-based description of clinical practice: thoracic spine and ribs, *Orthop Phys Ther Clin North Am* 8:1-20, 1999.

Flynn TW, Hall RC: Pseudovisceral symptoms from the costovertebral segments relieved with manual therapy, *J Manual Manipulative Ther* 6:202-203, 1998.

Fruergaard P et al: The diagnoses of patients admitted with acute chest pain but without myocardial infarction, *Eur Heart J* 17:1028-1034, 1996.

Greigel-Morris P et al: Incidence of common postural abnormalities in the cervical, shoulder, and thoracic regions and their association with pain in two age groups of healthy subjects, *Phys Ther* 72:425-431, 1992.

Grieve GP: Thoracic musculoskeletal problems. In Boyling JD, Palastanga N, editors: *Grieve's modern manual therapy,* ed 2, New York, 1994, pp 401-428, Churchill Livingstone.

Hamberg J, Lindahl O: Angina pectoris symptoms caused by thoracic spine disorders: clinical examination and treatment, *Acta Med Scand Suppl* 644:84-86, 1981.

Kikta D, Breder A, Wilbourn A: Thoracic root pain in diabetes: the spectrum of clinical and electromyographical findings, *Ann Neurol* 11:80-85, 1982.

Lee D: Biomechanics of the thorax: a clinical model of in vivo function, *J Manual Manipulative Ther* 1:13-21, 1993.

Lillegard W: Medical causes in the thoracic region. In Flynn T, editor: *The thoracic spine and ribcage: musculoskeletal evaluation and treatment,* Newton, Mass, 1996, pp 107-120, Butterworth-Heinemann.

Lindgren K-A: Conservative treatment of thoracic outlet syndrome: a 2-year follow-up, *Arch Phys Med Rehabil* 78:373-378, 1997.

Lindgren K-A, Leino E: Subluxation of the first rib: a possible thoracic outlet syndrome mechanism, *Arch Phys Med Rehabil* 68:692-695, 1988.

Lindgren K-A, Leino E, Manninen H: Cervical rotation lateral flexion test in brachialgia, *Arch Phys Med Rehabil* 73:735-737, 1989.

Lindgren K-A et al: Cervical spine rotation and lateral flexion combined motion in the examination of the thoracic outlet, *Arch Phys Med Rehabil* 71:343-344, 1990.

Martin GT: First rib resection for the thoracic outlet syndrome, *Br J Neurosurg* 7:35-38, 1993.

McGuckin N: The T4 syndrome. In Grieve G, editor: *Modern manual therapy of the vertebral column,* New York, 1986, pp 370-376, Churchill Livingstone.

Menck J, Requejo S, Kulig K: Thoracic spine dysfunction in upper extremity complex regional pain syndrome type I, *J Orthop Phys Ther* 30:401-409, 2000.

Willems JM, Jull GA, Ng JK-F: An in vivo study of the primary and coupled rotations of the thoracic spine, *Clin Biomechanics* 11:311-316, 1996.

Wood KB et al: Thoracic MRI evaluation of asymptomatic individuals, *J Bone Joint Surg* 77A:1634-1638, 1995.

Wood KB et al: The natural history of asymptomatic thoracic disc herniations, *Spine* 22:525-530, 1997.

Chapter 60

Spine Fractures and Dislocations: Patterns, Classifications, and Management

Eeric Truumees, MD

1. How common is trauma to the spinal column?

There are over 1 million spine injuries per year in the United States alone; 50,000 of these injuries include fractures to the bony spinal column. Males outnumber females 4 to 1 for spinal trauma. Injury is most common at the cervicothoracic and thoracolumbar junctions. The improvement in automobile restraint systems has increased survival rates from major spinal column injury.

2. How many spinal cord injuries occur per year in the United States?

An estimated 16,000 people sustain spinal cord injuries each year, with 11,000 of the injured surviving to reach the hospital. Overall, 10% to 25% of spinal column injuries are associated with at least some neurologic changes. These changes are more common with injuries at the cervical level (40%) than at the lumbar level (20%).

3. What are the most common modes of spinal column injury?

Almost half (45%) are related to motor vehicle accidents (MVAs). Falls account for another 20%. In children falls account for only 9% of significant spine injuries, whereas in older patients they account for 60%. Sports injuries account for another 15%. Of these, diving injuries are the most common. Trampoline, ice hockey, and wrestling are other frequent culprits. Organized football accounts for 42 cervical fractures and 5 cases of quadriplegia per year. This statistic has decreased from 110 and 34, respectively, in 1976 (before the spear tackling rules were enacted). Another 15% of spinal column injuries are related to acts of violence.

4. In what scenarios are spinal column injuries most likely to be missed?

Worsening neurologic deficits occur in only 1.5% of patients diagnosed early but in 10% of patients with missed injuries. Injuries are most commonly missed in patients with a decreased level of consciousness, intoxication, head trauma, or polytrauma. Two, separate noncontiguous spinal injuries occur in as many as 20% of cases. The presence of one obvious spinal injury increases the chance of missing another, more subtle injury. Red flags to alert the practitioner to subtle spine injury are facial trauma, calcaneus fracture, hypotension, and localized tenderness or spasm. Significant injury is also more likely in patients with osteopenia or neuromuscular disease.

5. What is the long-term prognosis of a spinal cord–injured patient?

The average 10-year survival rate in all patients with spinal cord injury is 86%. In patients over 29 years of age, this number drops to 50%. Pneumonia and suicide are the chief causes of death.

6. What are incomplete cord syndromes and how do they affect rehabilitation?

Incomplete cord syndromes reflect injuries in which only part of the cord matter is damaged. While severe, some function below the level of injury is preserved.

Syndrome	MOI/Pathology	Characteristics	Prognosis
Central	Age >50, extension	UE > LE, M + S loss	Fair
Anterior	Flexion-comp (vert art)	Incomplete motor, some sensory	Poor
Brown-Séquard	Penetrating trauma	Ipsilateral motor, contralateral pain/temp	Best
Root	Foraminal comp/disk	Based on level, weakness	Good
Complete	Burst, canal comp	No function below level	Poor

MOI, Method of injury; *UE,* upper extremity; *LE,* lower extremity; *M + S,* motor and sensory; *vert art,* vertebral artery injury; *comp,* compression.

7. How is the pediatric spine differently susceptible to trauma?

For children older than 8 to 10 years, the spine behaves biomechanically like an adult. Younger children have more elastic soft tissues that make multiple, contiguous fractures much more common than in adults. The large size of the child's head relative to the body places the fulcrum for spinal flexion at C2-C3 in children. For children older than 8 years, the fulcrum is at C5-C6. Younger children are therefore far more likely to have upper cervical spine injuries (occiput to C3).

8. What is SCIWORA?

The marked elasticity of the pediatric spinal column is greater than the elastic limit of the cord. Therefore in rare cases, the **S**pinal **C**ord can be **I**njured **W**ithout **O**bvious **R**adiographic **A**bnormality (SCIWORA). More than half of these children will have delayed onset of neurologic symptoms, and therefore close and repeated exams are needed. In recent years, the concept of SCIWORA has been challenged. In any case, the ready availability of MRI makes the concept less critical than in years past.

9. How are gunshot wounds to the spine treated?

Because there is little ligamentous injury associated with civilian weapons, most can be treated closed with external immobilization. As bullet removal often worsens neurologic deficits, surgery is recommended only if the neurologic deficit is progressive, a CSF fistula ensues, or lead poisoning occurs. Surgical indications after colonic perforation are controversial.

10. Describe appropriate steps in the early evaluation of spinal column injury.

In trauma patients, the spine is assumed to be unstable until a secondary survey and radiographs have been performed. Directly examine the back by log-rolling the patient while maintaining in-line traction on the neck. Ecchymosis, lacerations, or abrasions on the skull, spine, thorax, and abdomen suggest that force was imparted to underlying spinal elements. Deformity, localized tenderness, step-off, or interspinous widening warrants further evaluation.

11. Describe appropriate steps in the early management of spinal column injury.

First, immobilize the spine on a backboard with sandbags and a hard collar. After radiographs and a secondary survey have excluded major instability, transfer the patient to a regular bed. Maintain a hard cervical collar until the cervical spine has been formally cleared. Until definitive stabilization can be undertaken, patients with significant thoracolumbar injury should be transferred to a rotating frame or other protective bed. For unstable cervical trauma, traction may be required. High-dose steroid protocols are **no longer considered standard of care** in the acute management of spinal cord injury.

12. How is the level determined in spinal cord injury?

Because the cord ends at the L1-L2 disk space, the level of injury to the spinal column may not match the level of cord injury. The cord level is defined as the lowest *functional* motor level, that is, the lowest level with useful motor function (grade 3 of 5, or antigravity strength). In some cases, a given cord injury will be described as "T_8 motor and T_{12} sensory."

13. Are there any radiographic clues that an injury might be unstable?

The spine is divided into three columns—anterior (the anterior two thirds of the body and disk), middle (the posterior one third of the body and PLL), and posterior (the posterior elements). Injury to two or more columns renders the spine unstable. Other radiographic parameters have also been defined, but vary by spinal level and remain controversial. Clues include significant loss of vertebral height (perhaps >50%), marked or progressive spinal angulation (in some studies, segmental kyphosis >20 degrees), or more than 3 to 4 mm of spondylolisthesis.

14. Why is the level of injury important?

The room available for the cord and the native stability of the spinal column vary significantly from the occiput to the sacrum. In the upper cervical spine, the bony elements are highly mobile and stability comes from the ligaments. Also, the ratio of the size of the canal to that of the cord is large. This extra room allows more displacement before cord injury. In the lower cervical spine, the narrow canal leaves little room for translation before cord compression.

The rib cage and sternum render the thoracic spine inherently more stable than the rest of the spine. Yet, here the canal is narrowest versus cord size. The transition zone between the fixed thoracic and mobile lumbar spine subjects the thoracolumbar junction at higher risk for injury. The mobile lower lumbar spine has a large canal with ample room for the nerve roots. Nerve roots are more resilient than the spinal cord, so injuries at this level tend to be less neurologically devastating.

15. How are spinal column injuries classified?

There are hundreds of classification systems for spinal trauma in general and injuries to certain vertebrae in particular. There is no widespread consensus as to which system to use. Mechanistic classifications divide injuries into groups based on the force that caused them. The groups are divided into grades to signal increasing severity.

16. What common force vectors cause spinal column injury?

When a car hits a tree, the seat belt holds the passenger back but inertia keeps the skull moving. An accident of this type imparts force to the cervical spine. A distraction vector, for example, lengthens the spinal column by tearing its ligaments. If the patient's head then hits the windshield, a compression vector shortens the vertebral column by fracturing its bones. Flexion (forward and lateral), extension, and rotation are the other major vectors. In reality, most injuries result from multiple simultaneous forces with one vector predominating.

17. What types of injuries are caused by compression-flexion moments?

MVAs or diving accidents often impart compression and flexion vectors to the spinal column. Early, the anterior column fails in compression. Later, the posterior and middle column ligaments fail in distraction. When the ligaments fail, the fractured level slides posteriorly over the underlying intact vertebra. These injuries are most common in the midcervical spine (C4-C5 and C5-C6).

Compression fractures represent early-stage injuries with no significant ligamentous failure and heal with 8 to 12 weeks of immobilization. Torn ligaments rarely heal without surgery. Therefore higher energy compression-flexion injuries require operative stabilization.

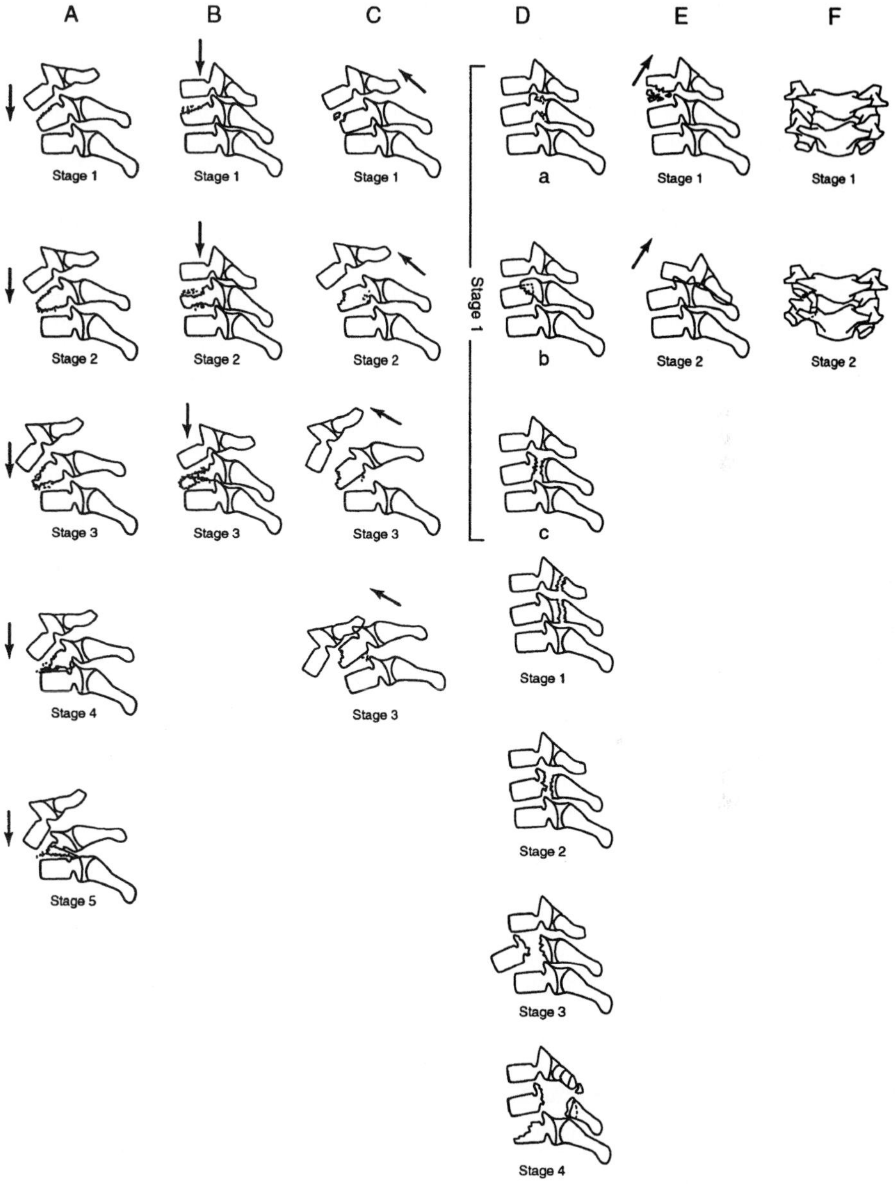

The Ferguson-Allen classification of cervical spine trauma. Spinal injuries are divided into subtypes based on the vector of force that produced them. Group A represents compressive flexion injuries of increasing severity. Group B includes types of vertical compression injuries. Distractive flexion injuries are part of group C. Group D represents compression extension patterns. The distractive extension patterns are found in group E, whereas lateral flexion injuries are shown in group F.

18. What is a flexion teardrop fracture?

The most severe flexion-compression injury—the flexion teardrop fracture—is the most devastating of all cervical spine injuries compatible with life. Most patients will have either anterior cord syndrome or a complete cord injury. The lateral radiograph demonstrates a large triangular fragment of anteroinferior vertebral body with marked kyphosis at the injured level leading to subluxation or dislocation of the facets. Complete disruption of the disk and all the ligaments at the level of injury leads to translation and rotation of the involved vertebrae. Surgical stabilization is usually required.

19. How are vertical compression injuries differentiated from compression-flexion injuries?

If an MVA or diving accident leads to a blow to the top of head rather than flexion, both the anterior and middle columns fail in compression (i.e., a **burst** fracture). With increasing force, vertebral arch fractures become more common. In cervical spine trauma, this is the only mechanism wherein the bony injury is more important than the ligamentous injury. The absence of ligamentous disruption allows some of these injuries to heal in a halo. In higher level injuries or those with neurologic injury, anterior decompression and fusion is recommended.

20. What is the most common type of cervical spine injury?

Distractive flexion injuries account for 61% of all subaxial spine injuries. In early stages, only the posterior ligaments fail (i.e., a flexion sprain). Later, the middle and, finally, the anterior columns fail. As the spine displaces, the superior end plate of the subjacent vertebra may compress, but this should not be confused with flexion-compression injuries. The key differences are marked kyphosis with mild bony collapse and displacement between the fractured vertebra and its *cranial* neighbor.

21. How are distractive flexion injuries treated?

Low-energy injuries disrupt only the posterior column, resulting in facet subluxation only. Collar immobilization allows complete healing. Increasing trauma leads to facet dislocation that merits reduction with skull tongs (Gardner-Wells tongs) followed by a posterior fusion to prevent late deformity, chronic pain, or worsening neurologic injury.

22. What are the characteristics of compressive extension injuries?

Accounting for almost 40% of cervical spine trauma, these injuries may result from a downward blow to the forehead. They may occur anywhere, but are concentrated at C6-C7. Most are stable. At higher energy levels, tension shear failure through the middle and anterior columns allows the superior vertebra to move *forward* on the subjacent vertebra, leaving the posterior elements behind. In injuries without displacement, halo immobilization yields acceptable healing rates. Injuries with translation are best treated with operative stabilization.

23. What is an odontoid fracture?

Also called the dens, the odontoid is a peg of bone extending from the body of C2 into the arch of C1. This unique geometry maintains stability while allowing significant rotation. In younger patients, odontoid fractures are associated with high-energy trauma. Patients report pain and a sense of instability; occasionally, the patient's presenting symptoms include holding the head with the hands. In children under age 7, the fracture passes through the growth plate and is treated with reduction and a halo or Minerva cast for 6 to 12 weeks.

In adults, dens fracture subtypes associated with poor healing and late instability have been identified. For example, the injuries through the cortical waist of the dens (type II fractures) have poor blood supply and a higher nonunion rate. Type III fractures pass through the cancellous bone of the C2 body and are more likely to heal. A trial of halo immobilization is attempted. However, in severely displaced injuries, early stabilization is recommended.

Recently, the significant cardiopulmonary and circulatory compromise engendered by halo-vest management in the elderly has led to increased emphasis on rigid, operative stabilization of dens fractures in these otherwise frail patients.

24. What is a hangman's fracture?

Also known as traumatic spondylolisthesis of the axis, a hangman's fracture represents a bilateral fracture of the C2 pars interarticularis. Because bilateral pars fractures enlarge the canal, neurologic injuries are rare. Minimally displaced injuries are immobilized in a Philadelphia collar. Displaced injuries benefit from reduction and halo immobilization. If significant subluxation of C2 on C3 is noted, a posterior stabilization procedure is required.

25. What is a Jefferson fracture?

A Jefferson bursting fracture (of the atlas) is a relatively uncommon injury, usually seen in the context of another spine injury, particularly an odontoid fracture or hangman's fracture. Classically, this injury encompasses bilateral fractures in both the anterior and posterior arches of the C1 ring. Most isolated Jefferson fractures heal in an orthosis. With increased loading, the fragments displace more widely. Beyond 5 to 8 mm lateral displacement, the transverse atlantal ligament ruptures or avulses, rendering the C1-C2 motion segment unstable. If the CT scan suggests bone avulsion, traction for reduction followed by halo immobilization may allow adequate healing. Rupture of the midsubstance of the ligament necessitates C1-C2 fusion. Minimally displaced or isolated single or double fractures through the C1 ring may be treated with a Philadelphia collar.

26. What is whiplash?

Whiplash is a poorly understood clinical syndrome in which seemingly inconsequential trauma leads to chronic neck pain. This injury complex, also called acceleration injury, cervical sprain syndrome, or soft tissue neck injury, usually follows a rear-end collision. Patients treated for whiplash are commonly involved in accident-related litigation. For some of these patients, economic incentives interfere with clinical improvement.

27. How is whiplash different from other cervical spine trauma?

Most cervical trauma results from contact force (e.g., striking the head on the dashboard, leading to an extension injury). Whiplash, on the other hand, results from inertial forces applied to the head. Anatomic structures including the sternocleidomastoid and longissimus colli muscles, intervertebral disk, facet capsule, and anterior longitudinal ligament have been implicated as pain generators.

28. Who tends to be susceptible to whiplash?

While there are 4 million rear-end collisions per year, only 1 million result in reported whiplash injuries. Of those involved in these injuries, 70% are women, usually between 30 and 50 years of age. The injury is more common in those with low physical activity jobs.

29. What are the typical symptoms of whiplash?

Most patients report neck pain and/or occipital headaches. These headaches can be dull, sharp, or aching and are usually worse with movement. The pain is associated with stiffness and often radiates to the head, arm, or between the scapulae. Some patients report vertigo, auditory or visual disturbances, hoarseness, temperature changes, fatigue, depression, and sleep disturbances. These symptoms are often provoked or exacerbated by emotion, temperature, humidity, or noise and have variably been attributed to cranial nerve and sympathetic chain disruption.

30. Describe the physical examination and radiologic signs of whiplash.

On examination, decreased range of motion and spasm are noted; however, other objective findings are absent. Similarly, various radiologic modalities have a poor correlation with symptoms. Often a loss of normal cervical lordosis is noted. Preexisting degenerative disease of the spine is associated with a worse prognosis in whiplash. An MRI scan usually appears normal and is rarely indicated.

31. What is the natural history of whiplash?

Symptom onset usually occurs within 2 days. Of patients diagnosed with whiplash, 57% recover completely in 3 months, and 8% remain so severely affected that they are unable to work. For the remaining 35% of patients, a partial recovery occurs. Maximum improvement is usually reached by 1 year.

32. How is whiplash treated?

The goal of treatment is to reengage patients in their normal activities as soon as possible. In mild cases, an immediate return to work is warranted. Otherwise, a 3-week respite to allow for pain control may be advised. Nonsteroidal antiinflammatory medications are usually recommended. Muscle relaxants and narcotics are not recommended. A collar should only be used for the first few days after the injury. The critical element in treatment is active mobilization. Short-arc active motion is used for pain and spasm. Gentle passive range of motion can be employed to counteract stiffness. After 48 hours, progression to active motion is suggested. After the acute pain subsides, proceed with isometric strengthening to tolerance. Other modalities are commonly employed, including traction, ultrasound, manipulation, massage, heat, and ice. If significant pain continues after 3 months, a multidisciplinary pain clinic approach has been found to be useful.

33. How are injuries to the thoracolumbar spine classified?

A number of classification schemes have been devised for the thoracolumbar spine. Some are descriptive; some are mechanistic. In general, however, the same principles apply as for the cervical spine. One useful classification, devised by Denis, divides injuries into major and minor types.

34. What might be considered a minor injury of the thoracolumbar spine?

Minor injuries account for 15% of thoracolumbar fractures. They include isolated fractures of the spinous and transverse processes, pars, and facets. They may be caused by direct trauma or violent muscular contraction in response to injury.

35. How are these minor injuries evaluated?

Obtain radiographs of the remainder of the spine to exclude other injuries. Then, further assess the affected level for subtle injury with axial CT slices. If the CT is negative, flexion-extension views are important to exclude dynamic instability. For example, a pars fracture may be the only plain film evidence of a flexion-distraction injury. Assuming these tests are negative, the patient can be mobilized without braces or restrictions, except as needed for the relief of symptoms.

36. What are the broad types of major injuries of the thoracolumbar spine?

Thoracolumbar Spine Trauma Classification of Denis

	Mechanism		
Fracture Type	**Anterior Column**	**Middle Column**	**Posterior Column**
Compression	Compression	None	None—distraction
Burst	Compression	Compression	None—compression
Seat belt	None—compression	Distraction	Distraction
Fracture-dislocation	Compression-rotation-shear	Distraction-rotation-shear	Distraction-rotation-shear

37. What are compression fractures, and how are they treated?

Compression fractures represent almost half of all major thoracolumbar spinal injuries. They result from a compression failure of the anterior column with the middle and posterior columns left intact. In younger patients with higher energy levels imparted to the spine, a full contact orthosis (such as a thoracolumbosacral orthosis [TLSO]) is recommended. For osteoporotic patients with lower energy trauma, a limited contact orthosis (such as a Cash or Jewett brace) may be appropriate. Increasingly, these injuries are being treated with percutaneous injection of bone cement (polymethyl methacrylate [PMMA]) either with (kyphoplasty) or without (vertebroplasty) balloon reduction of the deformity.

38. How is a burst fracture different from a compression fracture?

A burst fracture includes compression failure of the middle and posterior columns as well. This injury is associated with greater height loss of the anterior column, often with retropulsion of the middle column bone into the canal. A great deal of attention and controversy has been directed to what defines a stable and an unstable burst fracture. Therefore recommendations for treatment of given injuries are often variable. However, the angulation (kyphosis), loss of vertebral height, and canal encroachment as well as the presence or absence of neurologic deficit are evaluated. In general, a neurologically intact patient with little deformity is managed nonoperatively by use of an extension cast or TLSO. Unstable injuries, including those with posterior ligamentous disruption, neurologic deficit, or unacceptable deformities, are treated by surgical decompression and stabilization. This type of surgical procedure may be performed either with a direct, anterior decompression and strut graft fusion or with a posterior approach using indirect reduction techniques and screw stabilization.

39. What is a seat-belt injury?

Seen in belted passengers in an MVA without a shoulder harness, a seat-belt injury results from tension failure of the posterior and middle columns. The anterior longitudinal ligament is intact, but there may be compression failure of the anterior column. This injury may occur through bone or soft tissue. If it occurs through bone, it is termed a **Chance fracture.** Such bony injuries are treated nonoperatively with an extension cast or thoracolumbar spinal orthosis. Close follow-up is required to exclude progressive deformity. If significant soft tissue or ligamentous injury is involved, less predictable healing occurs with closed means, and a posterior stabilization procedure is recommended.

40. How are fracture-dislocations different from other types of thoracolumbar trauma?

In these injuries, all three columns fail and vertebral translation occurs, causing canal occlusion at the injury site. Therefore fracture-dislocations are associated with a high incidence of neurologic deficits. These injuries may be divided into subtypes based on the direction of translation: flexion-rotation, shear, and flexion-distraction. Almost all of these injuries require operative stabilization.

41. What are some complications associated with the surgical treatment of spinal trauma?

Implant displacement, which is most common after posterior instrumentation, is an important consideration in any patient describing increased pain or deformity. Such displacement is often related to poor bone quality, implant placement error, and noncompliance with brace/activity recommendations. Another common problem is postoperative wound infection. Increased drainage, redness, fever, and pain are signs of such an infection.

42. When may a spinal trauma patient be safely mobilized?

Mobilization is a critical issue in trauma patients and must be individualized. The benefits of immobilization in shielding the healing spine from excessive external loads are counterbalanced with the drawbacks, including increased muscular stiffness and weakness. In patients with polytrauma or neurologic injury, external bracing is burdensome and interferes with optimal rehabilitation.

Stable injuries are mobilized immediately with gentle, passive ROM. In these patients, modalities such as ice, heat, ultrasound, and massage appear helpful in symptomatic relief. A stretching and strengthening program is gradually added as pain levels decrease and motion increases. Unstable spinal column injuries will not tolerate early motion. In general terms, however, an injury with significant instability should be converted to a stable configuration by way of external bracing, surgery, or both.

A rigidly stabilized spine is often mobilized within 2 weeks. In injuries treated with less than rigid fixation or in those patients with poor bone quality or other factors compromising their fixation, 6 to 12 weeks of external orthosis wear is followed by the initiation of gentle, active ROM. Strengthening is instituted upon attainment of full and painless motion in patients for whom x-rays demonstrate no change in position of hardware or vertebral elements.

In patients with unstable injuries treated with nonoperative means, mobilization is started at times predicted by tissue healing. Therefore compression fractures through cancellous bone may tolerate mobilization at 4 weeks. On the other hand, cortical bone injuries (such as dens fractures) and injuries with a significant ligamentous component (burst fractures with severe collapse) will require 12 to 16 weeks of immobilization. Dynamic radiographs (flexion-extension views) are often useful to evaluate healing before aggressive rehabilitation.

43. Name other common postoperative medical problems to which spinal trauma patients are prone.

Deep venous thrombosis (DVT), pulmonary embolism, and pressure sores are very serious potential consequences of the immobilization required after major spinal injury. Pneumonia, pneumothorax, and other pulmonary problems are common as well. *Autonomic dysreflexia* is seen in patients with cervical and upper thoracic spinal cord injuries. In this disorder, bladder overdistention or fecal impaction causes an autonomic nervous system reaction leading to severe hypertension. The patient's presenting symptoms often include a pounding headache, anxiety, profuse head and neck sweating, nasal obstruction, and blurred vision. Treatment begins with immediate placement of a Foley catheter and rectal disimpaction. If the symptoms do not quickly resolve, medications are required.

44. What percentage of patients experience pain relief or functional improvement after kyphoplasty or vertebroplasty?

Good to excellent relief of pain is seen almost immediately after both kyphoplasty and vertebroplasty in 80% to 100% of patients. This pain relief persists over time. Vertebroplasty studies often report phone call follow-up of pain levels and have relatively little outcome data, but in studies of kyphoplasty, validated functional outcome instruments have demonstrated clinically and statistically significant improvements, including the SF-35 role physical and physical function subscales, Oswestry scores, and Roland-Morris scores.

45. What is the role of physical therapy in the status of osteoporotic patients following a vertebral compression fracture?

Osteoporotic patients are at risk for additional fractures. In particular, lifting while flexing or lifting overhead increases the risk of fracture. On the other hand, in the absence of weight-bearing, bones will continue to deteriorate. Increasingly, a rehabilitation program including gait and balance training and extensor muscle strengthening is being recommended in conjunction with a therapist-centered educational program about appropriate lifting techniques and back protection.

Bibliography

Allen BL Jr et al: A mechanistic classification of closed, indirect fractures and dislocations of the lower cervical spine, *Spine* 7:1-27, 1982.

An HS, Simpson JM: *Surgery of the cervical spine,* London, 1994, Martin Dunitz Ltd.

Coumans JV, Reinhardt MK, Lieberman IH: Kyphoplasty for vertebral compression fractures: 1-year clinical outcomes from a prospective study, *J Neurosurg Spine* 99(suppl 1):44-50, 2003.

d'Amato C: Pediatric spinal trauma: injuries in very young children, *Clin Orthop* 432:34-40, 2005.

Delamarter RB, Coyle J: Acute management of spinal cord injury, *J Am Acad Oorthop Surg* 7:166-175, 1999.

Denis F: The three column spine and its significance in the classification of acute thoracolumbar spinal injuries, *Spine* 8:8, 1983.

Grohs JG, Krepler P: Minimal invasive stabilization of osteoporotic vertebral compression fractures: methods and preinterventional diagnostics [in German], *Radiologe* 44:254-259, 2004.

Ledlie JT, Renfro M: Balloon kyphoplasty: one-year outcomes in vertebral body height restoration, chronic pain, and activity levels, *J Neurosurg* 98(suppl 1):36-42, 2003.

Levine AM et al, editors: *Spine trauma,* Philadelphia, 1998, Saunders.

Muller EJ et al: Management of odontoid fractures in the elderly, *Eur Spine J* 8:360-365, 1999.

Phillips FM et al: Early radiographic and clinical results of balloon kyphoplasty for the treatment of osteoporotic vertebral compression fractures, *Spine* 28:2260-2265 (discussion 2265-2267), 2003.

Rhyne A et al: Kyphoplasty: report of eighty-two thoracolumbar osteoporotic vertebral fractures, *J Orthop Trauma* 18:294-299, 2004.

Sliker CW, Mirvis SE, Shanmuganathan K: Assessing cervical spine stability in obtunded blunt trauma patients: review of medical literature, *Radiology* 234:733-739, 2005.

Slucky AV, Eismont FJ: Instructional course lecture. Treatment of acute injury of the cervical spine, *J Bone Joint Surg* 76-A:1882-1896, 1994.

Spivak JM, Vaccaro AR, Cotler JM: Thoracolumbar spine trauma I and II, *J Am Acad Orthop Surg* 3:345-360, 1995.

Truumees E: Osteoporosis of the spine. In Bono CM, Garfin SR, editors: *Orthopaedic surgery essentials: spine,* Philadelphia, 2004, Lippincott.

Truumees E, Hilibrand AS, Vaccaro AR: Percutaneous vertebral augmentation, *Spine J* 4:218-229, 2004.

Vaccaro AR, editor: *Orthopaedic knowledge update,* ed 8, Rosemont, Ill, 2005, AAOS.

White AA et al: Spinal stability: evaluation and treatment, *Instr Course Lect* 30:457-483, 1981.

Wood K et al: Operative compared with nonoperative treatment of a thoracolumbar burst fracture without neurological deficit: a prospective, randomized study, *J Bone Joint Surg (Am)* 85:773-781, 2003.

Chapter 61

Temporomandibular Joint

Sally Ho, PT, DPT, MS

1. What are the unique features of the temporomandibular joint (TMJ)?

The TMJ is divided by a fibrocartilage disk into an upper and a lower joint cavity. The movements of the joint are affected by the contacting tooth surfaces. The TMJ, functioning as one of a pair, must perform coordinated movements.

2. What is the incidence of TMJ dysfunction?

Fifty percent of the adult population suffers one sign of TMJ dysfunction at some time in their life. Population-based studies have reported 1% to 22% of the general population suffers severe TMJ dysfunction, depending on the criteria used. Women are affected 3 times as often as men. Approximately 40% of the population has clicks during daily function.

3. How does temporomandibular dysfunction (TMD) manifest clinically?

Clinical symptoms of TMD include pain in the masseter, temporalis, head, and neck area; headaches; dizziness; vertigo; earache or fullness; tinnitus; joint noise; toothache; and myofascial pain.

4. What is the anatomic attachment and the function of the disk?

Anteriorly, the disk is attached to the superior belly of the lateral pterygoid muscle. The posterosuperior portion of the disk is attached to the superior stratum, and the posteroinferior portion is attached to the inferior stratum. Medially and laterally, the disk is attached to the medial/lateral poles of the condylar head through the medial and lateral collateral ligaments. The disk protects and lubricates the articulating surfaces. It also accepts force that is exerted upon the TMJ.

5. Describe the innervation of the TMJ.

The anterior and medial regions of the TMJ are innervated by the deep temporal and masseteric nerves. The posterior and lateral regions of the TMJ are innervated by the auriculotemporal nerve. These three nerves arise from the mandibular division of the trigeminal nerve.

6. What are the kinematic movements within the TMJ?

During the first 11 to 25 mm of mouth opening, the mandibular condyle rotates anteriorly. From 25 mm to the end range of opening, the mandibular condyle translates anteriorly. However, some researchers believe that translation occurs from the beginning of the opening phase.

7. Describe the functional range and normal range of mouth opening.

The functional range of opening is measured by three fingers' width (or two knuckles' width) of the nondominant hand; the normal range is measured by four fingers' width (or three knuckles' width) of the nondominant hand. For men, the normal range of opening is between 40 and 45 mm; for women, the normal range of opening is between 45 and 50 mm.

8. What is the normal range of motion for lateral deviation and protrusion?

The normal range of motion for lateral deviation is usually one fourth of the normal opening. For example, if a person has a normal opening of 48 mm, the lateral deviation is expected to be 12 mm. The normal range of protrusion is approximately 5 mm.

9. Where are the center and axis of rotation of the TMJ?

Many researchers who support the hinge axis theory believe that in the first 20 mm of jaw opening, rotation occurs around a fixed center located in the head of the condyle. Other authors support the theory of the instantaneous center of rotation (i.e., the mean location is behind and below the condylar head, with the axis located outside the condyle). They think that the mandible undergoes both rotation and translation in varying degrees from the initiation of jaw opening.

10. What are the major elevators of the mandible?

The masseter, temporalis, and medial pterygoid muscles are the three major elevators of the mandible. The superior belly of the lateral pterygoid is active during the closing phase of the mouth, but its function is primarily for stabilization of the disk in relationship to the condylar head.

11. What are the depressors of the mandible?

The depressors of the mandible are the inferior belly of the lateral pterygoid, digastric, mylohyoid, geniohyoid, and stylohyoid muscles.

12. Describe the muscle function and kinematics of lateral deviation.

When the mandible deviates to one side, the muscles involved are the ipsilateral temporalis, the contralateral medial pterygoid, and the contralateral lateral pterygoid. Arthrokinematically, the ipsilateral condyle rotates and spins forward, downward, and medially, while the contralateral condyle translates horizontally toward the ipsilateral side.

13. What is the role of the lateral pterygoid in oral function?

Approximately 30% of the superior belly of the lateral pterygoid muscle attaches to the anteromedial portion of the articular disk. This superior belly is active during mandibular elevation, especially in the last phase of forceful chewing between molars. It helps to stabilize the disk and the condyle in a functional position. Spasm of the superior belly of the lateral pterygoid muscle can result in anterior displacement of the disk because of its anteromedial pull on the disk during contraction.

The inferior belly of the lateral pterygoid muscle inserts on the anterior surface of the condylar neck. When it contracts, the mandible depresses, protrudes, and deviates to the contralateral side.

Unilateral contraction of both bellies of the lateral pterygoid muscle produces effective contralateral deviation. Bilateral contraction of the lateral pterygoid muscle produces strong protrusion of the mandible.

14. How is pain arising from the retrodiskal pad differentiated from pain arising from muscular contraction?

Using a cotton roll, the patient bites down with the back molars. If pain decreases (because of decreased pressure on the retrodiskal pad caused by gapping the TMJ), the retrodiskal pad is involved. If pain increases, muscular or ligamentous involvement is indicated. Findings can be confirmed by asking the patient to bite down on the cotton roll with the contralateral molars. If pain increases on the ipsilateral side, then the retrodiskal pad is affected.

15. Define parafunctional habits.

Clenching, bruxing, biting nails, sucking on cheeks, chewing gum, and biting lips are examples of parafunctional habits. These nonfunctioning, repetitive movements can cause microtrauma to the soft tissue and the hard structure. Microtrauma may result in pain, spasm, altered mandibular dynamics, abnormal development, and TMJ dysfunction.

16. How does an anteriorly displaced disk present clinically?

A patient with an anteriorly displaced disk (ADD) usually has pain and limited opening with deviation to the involved side. An anteriorly displaced disk may produce a single click noise in the early stage, reciprocal opening and closing clicks when in the reducing phase (ADD with reduction), and absent joint noise in the late nonreducing phase (ADD without reduction). Crepitus may be heard in the late, arthritic phase.

17. What is an open lock?

An open lock is the inability to close the mouth when the condyle is locked in an open position. This usually happens after wide opening from yawning or a dental procedure. The most likely cause is an overstretched lateral pterygoid muscle or a posteriorly displaced disk.

18. Explain the significance of opening with a C curve or S curve.

Altered TMJ kinematics are often presented by mouth opening with deviation. A "C" curve usually indicates a capsular pattern, whereas an "S" curve indicates muscle imbalance. However, when joint noises, limited opening, and ipsilateral deflection are present simultaneously, disk displacement must be suspected.

19. Define myofascial pain disorder syndrome (MPDS).

MPDS is defined by pain syndromes that originate from the myofascial structure, characterized by trigger points that may cause local tenderness and referred pain. MPDS is the most prevalent cause of TMJ dysfunction. Its clinical manifestation includes headaches, face pain, neck pain, earache, tinnitus, and dizziness.

20. Describe the connection between TMD and forward-headed posture.

The tight suboccipital muscles caused by the habitual forward-headed posture rotate the cranium posteriorly; in compensation, the mandible either is depressed by gravity and the overstretched, lengthened masseter/temporalis muscles or is elevated by increased tension of the same muscles. This pattern sets off a chain reaction of imbalanced muscle tension and results in TMD.

Patients with TMD demonstrate a more forward-headed posture than patients without TMD. Generally, it is believed that approximately 85% of patients with TMD hold a forward-headed posture.

21. How is a closed lock treated?

Modalities such as ice, heat, electrical stimulation, ultrasound, soft tissue release, joint mobilization (if range permits), and self-stretching home exercise can relieve symptoms and improve opening range initially. Then the treatment program should be complemented with instruction about proper body mechanics and appropriate diet.

22. How should patients be instructed to carry out the home exercise program?

All head, neck, and TMJ exercises should include 6 repetitions 6 times per day. Exercises should be performed on a time-contingent basis (approximately every 2 hours, regardless of symptoms).

23. How can TMJ problems cause dizziness, headache, and ear pain?

The TMJ is innervated by the trigeminal nerve. The neurons from the trigeminal nerve (cranial nerve V) share the same neuron pool as the upper cervical nerves (cervical nerves 1, 2, and 3) and cranial nerves VII, IX, X, and XI. Consequently, all the afferent nerves converge and may affect each other's innervation. The spinal nucleus of the trigeminal nerve and the dorsal horns of the upper three cervical segments form the trigeminocervical nucleus. This area is considered the principal nociceptive center for the entire head and upper neck. Any pain in the TMJ area can be transmitted through the trigeminocervical nucleus to the head and neck area or perceived as pain arising from the head and neck area.

Patients with TMJ problems usually demonstrate forward-headed posture and suffer from cervical dysfunction. Tightness of the cervical musculature may compromise vertebrobasilar blood flow, which is one of the causes of dizziness. On the other hand, disturbances in the cervical column, whether it originates from muscles, ligaments, or joints, can interfere with tonic neck reflexes and also affect the function of the vestibular nuclei.

The auriculotemporal nerve (a branch of the trigeminal nerve) innervates the posterolateral region of the TMJ and also sends a few branches to innervate the tympanic membrane, external auditory meatus, and lateral surface of the superior auricle. Therefore any symptom that affects the auriculotemporal nerve also may cause earache or tinnitus.

24. What is the resting position of the tongue?

With the head and neck in neutral position, the tip of the tongue is placed lightly against the roof of the mouth (palate), not touching the back of the upper front teeth. Upper and lower lips are kept together and back molars are kept apart.

25. Discuss the roles of splints.

The **repositioning splint** is generally used to recapture the anteriorly dislocated disk and/or manage the disk-condyle discoordination. It should be worn continuously throughout the day and night except during oral cleaning or eating. The duration may last from a few weeks to several months, depending on progress in joint stability. The goal of the repositioning splint is to achieve the concentric position of the disk-condyle complex.

The resting splint is preferred when relaxation or balancing of soft tissue is desired. This type of splint can be worn during the day or only at night to offset the soft tissue reaction from nocturnal clenching/bruxing.

26. What imaging modalities are used to diagnose TMDs?

Plain radiography of the TMJ includes lateral transcranial, transpharyngeal, and transorbital projections. The lateral transcranial projection is used most often; it images the lateral one third to one half of the condyle and fossa but does not include the condylar neck. The transpharyngeal projection images the lateral and medial portions of the condyle; in combination with the transorbital projection, it images the condylar neck.

Panoramic radiography is a modified tomogram used to provide a comprehensive view of the dental and bony structures.

Arthrograms are used to identify soft tissue abnormalities (e.g., disk displacement, disk perforation, or retrodiskal inflammation). This technique involves the injection of a contrast medium into the joint space followed by static or dynamic imaging. Arthrography is the most sensitive technique for detecting soft tissue perforation; however, it is invasive and involves high levels of radiation exposure.

Magnetic resonance imaging (MRI) provides the most accurate information about the soft tissues of the TMJ. Disk position and disk condition can be identified with MRI. The use of dynamic MRI can reveal functional information of the joint studied.

27. Discuss the relationship between malocclusion and TMD.

Malocclusion used to be considered the major cause of TMD. Now it is widely accepted that multiple factors usually are involved. Epidemiologic research demonstrates absent or low correlation between occlusal factors and signs and symptoms of TMJ, indicating that occlusion plays a minor role in the cause of TMD.

28. What is the therapeutic outcome assessment in permanent TMJ disk displacement?

Literature review conducted by Kropmans et al. determined that all 24 outcome studies claimed the effectiveness of various interventions, including arthroscopic surgery, arthrocentesis, and physical therapy. Eleven papers compared different sets of interventions but none reported distinguishing effects on mouth opening, pain level, or functional impairment between arthroscopic surgery, arthrocentesis, and physical therapy. This result indicates physical therapy is as effective as surgical procedures in the management of TMJ disk displacement.

29. What evidence exists in the literature regarding the efficacy of physical therapy for TMD?

Wright and colleagues studied the usefulness of posture training for patients with TMD and proved that postural exercises can significantly decrease symptoms.

A randomized clinical trial conducted by Yuasa et al. reported that a combination of NSAIDs and physical therapy (mouth-opening exercise) for 4 weeks was effective as a primary treatment for patients with disk displacement without reduction and without osseous changes.

Gray et al. studied four methods of physical therapy (short-wave diathermy, mega pulse, ultrasound, and soft laser) for TMJ disorders. They found no statistically significant difference in success rate between any of the four methods tested. However, each individual method was significantly better than the placebo treatment.

A critique conducted by Feine et al. on the effect of physical therapy in the management of TMD concluded that TMJ patients are helped by reversible, noninvasive therapy, especially a general fitness exercise program.

30. What are the differential diagnoses of facial and TMJ pain?

Differential diagnoses include trigeminal neuralgia, migraine headaches, herpes zoster, parotid gland tumor, temporal arteritis, tooth abscess, and acoustic neuroma, to name a few.

31. Indicate the origin, insertion, function, and innervation of various masticatory musculature.

Name	Origin	Insertion	Function	Innervation
Masseter—superficial fibers	Zygomatic arch	Outer surface of mandibular ramus	Mandible elevation and protrusion	Masseteric nerve
Masseter—deep fibers	Zygomatic arch	Outer surface of coronoid process,	Mandible elevation and retrusion	Masseteric nerve

continued

Name	Origin	Insertion	Function	Innervation
		superior half of ramus		
Temporalis	Temporal fossa	Coronoid process	Mandible elevation, ipsilateral deviation, retrusion	Temporal nerve
Medial pterygoid	Medial surface of lateral pterygoid plate of palatine	Inner mandibular surface	Mandible elevation, protrusion, contralateral deviation	Medial pterygoid nerve
Lateral pterygoid—inferior head	Lateral surface of lateral pterygoid plate of palatine	Anterior surface of condylar neck	Mandible depression, protrusion, contralateral deviation	Branches of masseteric or buccal nerve
Lateral pterygoid—superior head	Infratemporal surface of sphenoid bone	Articular disk	Mandible elevation	Same as inferior head
Suprahyoids (digastric, mylohyoid, geniohyoid, stylohyoid)	Mandible	Hyoid bone	Depression and retraction of mandible when hyoid is fixed, or elevation of hyoid when mandible is fixed	Facial nerve (posterior digastric, stylohyoid) Mylohyoid nerve (anterior digastric, mylohyoid) First and second cervical nerves (geniohyoid)
Infrahyoids (sternohyoid, thyrohyoid, omohyoid)	Sternum, hyoid, upper scapula border	Hyoid bone	Stabilization of hyoid bone	First, second, and third cervical nerves

Bibliography

Bell WE: *Temporomandibular disorders,* ed 3, Salem, Mass, 1990, Year Book Medical Publishers.

Bogduk N: Cervical causes of headache and dizziness. In Grieve G, editor: *Modern manual therapy,* Edinburgh, 1986, Churchill Livingstone.

Bourborn B: Craniomandibular examination and treatment. In *Saunders' manual of physical therapy practice,* Philadelphia, 1995, WB Saunders.

Clark GT, Adachi NY, Doran MR: Physical medicine procedures affect temporomandibular disorders: a review, *J Am Dent Assoc* 121:151-162, 1990.

Feine JS, Widmer CG, Lund JP: Physical therapy: a critique, *Oral Surg Oral Med Oral Pathol Oral Radiol Endod* 83:123-127, 1997.

Friedman MH, Weisberg J: The temporomandibular joint. In Gould JA, Davies GJ, editors: *Orthopedic and sports physical therapy,* St Louis, 1985, Mosby.
Gray RJ et al: Physiotherapy in the treatment of temporomandibular joint disorder: a comparative study of four treatment methods, *Br Dent J* 176:257-261, 1994.
Gray RJM et al: Temporomandibular joint pain dysfunction: can electrotherapy help?, *Physiotherapy* 81:47-51, 1995.
Iglarsh ZA, Snyder-Mackler L: Temporomandibular joint and the cervical spine. In Richardson JK, Iglarsh ZA, editors: *Clinical orthopedic physical therapy,* Philadelphia, 1994, WB Saunders.
Katzberg RW, Westesson PL: *Diagnosis of the temporomandibular joint,* Philadelphia, 1993, WB Saunders.
Kraus SL: Influences of the cervical spine on the stomatognathic system. In Donatelli R, Wooden MJ, editors: *Orthopedic physical therapy,* New York, 1989, Churchill Livingstone.
Kraus SL: *Temporomandibular disorders: clinics in physical therapy,* ed 2, New York, 1994, Churchill Livingstone.
Kropmans TH et al: Therapeutic outcome assessment in permanent temporomandibular joint disk displacement, *J Oral Rehabil* 26:357-363, 1999.
McNeill C: Management of temporomandibular disorders: concepts and controversies, *J Prosthetic Dent* 77:510-522, 1997.
Neumann DA: Kinesiology of mastication and ventilation. In Neumann DA, editor: *Kinesiology of the musculoskeletal system,* St Louis, 2002, Mosby.
Okeson JP: *Management of temporomandibular disorders and occlusion,* ed 4, St Louis, 1998, Mosby-Year Book Inc.
Perry JF: The temporomandibular joint. In Norkin CC, Levangie PK, editors: *Joint structure and function: a comprehensive analysis,* ed 2, Philadelphia, 1992, FA Davis.
Wright EF, Domenech MA, Fischer JR Jr: Usefulness of posture for patients with temporomandibular disorders, *J Am Dent Assoc* 131:202-210, 2000.
Yuasa H, Kurita K: Randomized clinical trial of primary treatment for temporomandibular joint disk displacement without reduction and without osseous changes: a combination of NSAIDs and mouth-opening exercise versus no treatment, *Oral Surg Oral Med Oral Pathol Oral Radiol Endod* 91:671-675, 2001.

Section IX

The Sacroiliac Joint

Chapter 62

Functional Anatomy of the Sacroiliac Joint

M. Elaine Lonnemann, PT, DPT, MSc

1. Name the osseous structures of the pelvic ring.

The ilia, sacrum, coccyx, femora, and pubis are the osseous structures of the pelvic ring.

2. How is the sacroiliac joint classified?

The sacroiliac joint is part synovial and part syndesmosis.

3. Describe the composition of the articular surfaces of the sacroiliac joint.

The sacral articular cartilage resembles typical hyaline cartilage, and its thickness ranges from 1 to 3 mm. The iliac cartilage resembles fibrocartilage and is usually <1 mm in thickness.

4. What is the function of the sacroiliac joint?

The sacroiliac joint is the link between the axial skeleton and the lower appendicular skeleton and thus its main function is to transmit forces from the axial skeleton to the lower limbs and vice versa.

5. How does the orientation of the sacroiliac joint make it difficult to establish a specific axis of motion using conventional planes?

In general, the axes of motion lie in a transverse plane at the level of S2. However, motion and rotational axes at the sacroiliac joint have been found to vary considerably because of contour variations in the joint surfaces in both the frontal and the sagittal planes. Motion variations also may result from individual differences in ligamentous laxity.

6. Describe the mechanisms of stability in the sacroiliac joint in terms of form and force closure.

Form closure is a concept describing the congruity or interlocking mechanisms of the sacroiliac joint based on its osteology. Force closure is described as the mechanism by which the ligaments and muscles achieve stability within the joint.

7. Name and label the ligaments of the sacroiliac joint and explain their function in limiting joint movement.

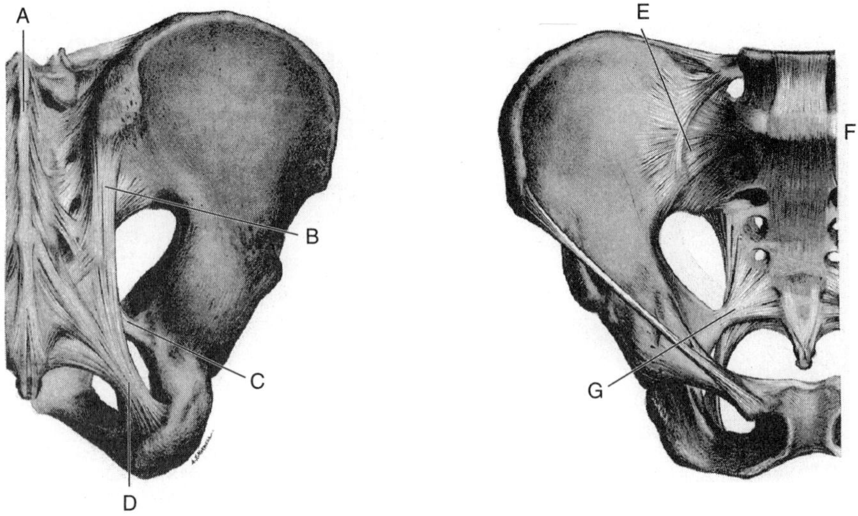

Interosseous sacroiliac ligament: binds the ilium to the sacrum (not pictured). Long and short posterior sacroiliac ligaments: the long ligaments prevent counterrotation of the ilium (B) whereas the short ligament (A) binds the ilium to the sacrum. Anterior sacroiliac ligament: prevents anterior displacement and diastasis of the joint (F). Sacrospinous (C and G) and sacrotuberous (D) ligaments: prevent nutation of the sacrum by anchoring it to the ischium. Iliolumbar ligament: prevents downward and anterior displacement of the ilium (E). *(From Gray H:* Anatomy of the human body, *ed 20, Philadelphia, 1918, Lea & Febiger.)*

8. Describe the attachments of the anterior sacroiliac and sacrospinous and sacrotuberous ligaments.

The anterior sacroiliac ligament covers the ventral aspect of the joint and extends from the sacral ala and anterior sacral surface to the anterior surface of the ilium beyond the margins of the joint. The sacrospinous ligament originates from the inferior lateral angle of the sacrum to the ischial spine of the ilium. The sacrotuberous ligament arises from the posterior superior iliac spine (PSIS), merges with the long posterior sacroiliac ligaments and the lateral margin of the sacrum (where it combines with the sacrospinous ligament), and attaches to the ischial tuberosity.

9. Which muscles contribute to the stability of the sacroiliac joint?

The muscles that cross the sacroiliac joint (SIJ) are designed to create movement of the lumbar spine or hip, as well as contribute to the stability of the sacroiliac joint. They are not prime movers of the sacroiliac joint. The adjacent muscles, including the quadratus lumborum, multifidus, erector spinae, gluteus minimus, piriformis, iliacus, and latissimus dorsi, contribute to the strength of the joint capsule and ligaments. Other muscles attaching to the pelvic girdle and contributing to the function of the sacroiliac joint include the abdominal muscles: internal and external obliques, rectus abdominis, and transversus abdominis. Also, the superficial layer of the thoracolumbar fascia attaches to the latissimus dorsi and gluteus maximus, thereby contributing to compression of the SIJ through its contraction.

10. Describe the innervation of the sacroiliac joint.

The posterior portion of the joint receives innervation from the lateral branches of the posterior primary rami of L4-S3. The anterior portion of the joint receives innervation from the L2-S2 segments.

11. What neurologic structures emerging from the sacrum innervate the pelvic region and lower limbs?

Nerve	Structures innervated
Tibial (L4-S3)	Medial hamstrings, adductor magnus, posterior compartment of leg, intrinsics of foot
Fibular (L4-S2)	Lateral hamstrings, lateral compartment of leg, EDB of foot
Pudendal (S2-S4)	External urethral and anal sphincters, levator ani, and skin of perineum, penis, clitoris
Superior gluteal (L4-S1)	Gluteus medius, gluteus minimus, tensor fasciae latae
Inferior gluteal (L5-S2)	Gluteus maximus
Nerve to obturator internus and superior gemellus (L5-S2)	Obturator internus, superior gemellus
Nerve to quadratus femoris and inferior gemellus (L4-S1)	Quadratus femoris and inferior gemellus
Posterior femoral cutaneous (S1-S3)	Skin on posterior thigh
Nerve to piriformis (S1-S2)	Piriformis muscle
Nerves to levator ani, coccygeus, exernal anal sphincter (S4)	Levator ani, coccygeus, and external anal sphincter; skin between anus and coccyx
Anococcygeal nerves (S4-C0)	Perianal skin

12. What are the anatomic differences between the male and the female pelvis?

The male pelvis is heavy and thick with large joint surfaces. The female pelvis is light and thin with small joint surfaces. The muscle attachments in the male pelvis are well-defined, whereas the female muscle attachments are rather indistinct. The male sacrum is long and narrow, whereas the female sacrum is short and wide.

13. What are the functional differences between the male and the female pelvis? How do they affect the sacroiliac joint?

In males the weight of the body is situated in a direct vertical position above the axis of support of the legs. The body weight in females falls behind the axis of support (upward through the acetabulum) so that the gravity vector tends to create a posterior rotation force on the pelvis. Morphologic changes in the joint surface appear earlier in men and are more extensive in regard to joint surface irregularities. Such changes may be a normal response to greater forces on the sacroiliac joints of men compared with women. The primary function of the sacroiliac joint in women is to increase the pelvic diameter during labor for vaginal delivery.

14. Describe the influence of hormones on the sacroiliac joint.

Relaxin, a hormone secreted by the corpus luteum, is present throughout pregnancy. The role of relaxin is to remodel collagen, thus creating ligamentous laxity in target tissues, including the pubic symphysis, in preparation for delivery. Relaxin is produced during the luteal phase of menstruation, at which time the endometrium of the uterus prepares for pregnancy (between ovulation and menses). The increased levels of relaxin may provoke symptoms in patients with mobility dysfunctions of the sacroiliac joint. Changes in progesterone levels also may affect the laxity of the joint.

15. Does motion occur at the sacroiliac joint?

Yes. Because of the synovial characteristics of the sacroiliac joint and the supporting anatomic studies, it is clear that some motion occurs at the sacroiliac joint.

16. Describe the amount of potential movement at the sacroiliac joint.

Minimal range of motion of the sacroiliac joint has been reported in studies with good methodology and reproducibility. Sturesson et al. used roentgen stereophotogrammetry of metal balls inserted into the sacrum and ilium and found 1 to 3 degrees or 1 to 3 mm of motion at the sacroiliac joint. Walheim and Selvik used a similar method at the symphysis pubis and found rotation did not exceed 3 degrees and translation did not exceed 2 mm.

17. Describe the possible movements of the sacrum and ilium (based on the osteopathic model).

Plane of Motion	Ilial Movement	Sacral Movement
Sagittal	Anterior and posterior rotation	Flexion (nutation), extension (counternutation)
Frontal	Superior and inferior translation	Side-bending
Transverse	External and internal rotation (outflare and inflare)	Rotation

18. Discuss the theoretical movements of the ilium and sacrum that may occur during trunk forward bending, backward bending, hip flexion, hip extension, and gait.

After about the first 60 degrees of trunk forward bending, the pelvis rotates anteriorly around the hip joints. The sacrum follows the lumbar spine to the extreme of flexion in both standing and sitting positions, when counternutation or backward nodding of the sacrum occurs. During trunk hyperextension of the spine, nutation of the sacrum occurs. With hip flexion, rotation of the ilium occurs in a backward direction, and the opposite occurs with hip extension. Inman studied walking and describes posterior iliac rotation during hip flexion through the swing phase, which is accentuated by heel contact and initial loading. During the loading response, the ipsilateral ilium begins to rotate anteriorly. The sacrum seems to rotate forward about a diagonal axis, creating torsion on the side of loading at midstance.

19. Describe the age-related changes in the sacroiliac joint.

During the first 10 years of life, the joint surfaces remain flat, but in the second and third decades the joints begin to develop uneven articular surfaces. By the third decade, the iliac surface has developed a convex ridge through the center of the joint surface with a corresponding ridge on the sacrum. By the fourth and fifth decades, the joint surfaces become yellowed and roughened with plaque formation and peripheral joint erosions. In all specimens, marked degenerative arthrosis is the rule by the fourth decade. Sacral osteophytes begin to form in the fourth decade at the joint margins. By the sixth and seventh decades, the osteophytes enlarge and begin to interdigitate across the joint surface. The joint surfaces become irregular with deep erosions that sometimes expose the subchondral bone. By the eighth decade, osteophyte interdigitation increases to the extent that some specimens exhibit true bony ankylosis. The joint surfaces demonstrate marked degenerative changes with diminished articular cartilage on both surfaces.

20. Why does the sacroiliac joint begin as a plane mobile joint and progress toward a plane stable joint?

In the non–weight-bearing infant, the sacroiliac joint is not required to provide stability. As the child progresses to weight-bearing movements, the sacroiliac joint undergoes a transformation into a stable interlocking joint that serves as a force transmission center from the spine to the lower limbs and vice versa.

21. Explain the standard views for radiographic evaluation of the sacroiliac joint and discuss the anatomic structures that are best visualized in each image.

Standard radiographic views of the sacroiliac joint include anteroposterior (AP) axial and right and left posterior obliques (RPO and LPO, respectively). In the AP view, the articular surfaces present as two radiolucent lines because they are superimposed on each other. The joints are assessed for symmetry and joint margin contour. In the posterior oblique view, the entire margin of the joint space can be visualized. Assessment from this view includes extent of joint width, location of bony margins, and degenerative or fibrous changes within the joint.

22. What is the incidence of sacralization?

The occurrence of sacralization is greater in men than women. Studies indicate an incidence of 15% to 30% in the general population. It is also more common than lumbarization. Studies tend to suggest a weak association between sacralization and low back pain.

23. What is the association between the cervical ribs and sacralization?

In a recent study of 1053 patients, 73% with cervical ribs had sacralization and 64% with sacralization had cervical ribs. The value of this information is that if a patient is determined to have either a cervical rib or sacralization, the clinician should be aware of the association, which may help with the differential diagnosis of musculoskeletal complaints.

24. What major vessels bifurcate slightly anterior to the sacroiliac joint?

The common iliac artery bifurcates into the internal and external iliac arteries. The gluteal muscles derive their arterial supply from the internal iliac arteries. Occlusion of the internal iliac can occur, which will cause ischemic pain in the gluteal region. Gluteal pain could be confused with sacroiliac pain; thus this information may be useful in the differential diagnosis of sacroiliac pain.

Bibliography

Bernard TN, Cassidy JD: The sacroiliac joint syndrome: pathophysiology, diagnosis and management. In Frymoyer JW, editor: *The adult spine: principles and practice,* New York, 1991, pp 2107-2130, Raven Press.
Bogduk N: *Clinical anatomy of the lumbar spine and sacrum,* ed 3, New York, 1997, Churchill Livingstone.
Bowen V, Cassidy JD: Macroscopic and microscopic anatomy of the sacroiliac joint from embryonic life until the eighth decade, *Spine* 6:620-628, 1981.
Fast A, Shapiro D, Ducommun EJ: Low-back pain in pregnancy, *Spine* 12:368-371, 1987.
Goldthwait JE, Osgood RB: A consideration of the pelvic articulations from an anatomical, pathological, and clinical standpoint, *N Engl J Med* 152:593-601, 1905.
Greenman P: *Principles of manual medicine,* ed 2, Philadelphia, 1996, Williams & Wilkins.
Hayne C: Manual transport of loads by women, *Physiotherapy* 67:226-231, 1981.
Inman VT, Ralston JH, Todd F: *Human walking,* Baltimore, 1981, Williams & Wilkins.
Kapandji IA: *The physiology of the joints,* Vol 3, New York, 1947, pp 54-71, Churchill Livingstone.

Lee D: *The pelvic girdle: an approach to the examination and treatment of the lumbo-pelvic-hip region,* Edinburgh, 1989, Churchill Livingstone.
MacLennan AH: The role of the hormone relaxin in human reproduction and pelvic girdle relaxation, *Scand J Rheumatol* 20:7-15, 1991.
Mckinnis L: *Fundamentals of orthopedic radiology,* Philadelphia, 1997, FA Davis.
Paquin JD et al: Biochemical and morphologic studies of cartilage from the adult human sacroiliac joint, *Arthritis Rheum* 26:887-895, 1983.
Paris SV: Anatomy as related to function and pain, *Orthop Clin North Am* 14:475-489, 1983.
Pool-Goudzwaard AL et al: Insufficient lumbopelvic stability: a clinical, anatomical and biomechanical approach to 'a-specific' low back pain, *Manual Ther* 3:12-20, 1998.
Sashin D: A critical analysis of the anatomy and the pathological changes of the sacroiliac joints, *J Bone Joint Surg* 12:891-910, 1930.
Sturesson B et al: Movements of the sacroiliac joints: a roentgen stereophotogrammetric analysis, *Spine* 14:162-165, 1989.
Vleeming A et al: Relation between form and function in the sacroiliac joint. I: Clinical anatomical aspects, *Spine* 13:133-135, 1990.
Vleeming A et al: The posterior layer of the thoracol-lumbar fascia: its function in load transfer from spine to legs, *Spine* 20:753-758, 1995.
Walheim GG, Selvik G: Mobility of the pubic symphysis: in vivo measurements with an electromechanic method and a roentgen stereophotogrammetric method, *Clin Orthop* 191:129-135, 1984.
Walker J: The sacroiliac joint: a critical review, *Phys Ther* 72:903-916, 1992.
Weisl H: The ligaments of the sacroiliac joint examined with particular reference to their function, *Acta Anat* 22:1-14, 1954.
Wilder DG, Pope MH, Frymoyer JW: The functional topography of the sacroiliac joint, *Spine* 5:575-579, 1980.

Chapter 63

Sacroiliac Dysfunction

M. Elaine Lonnemann, PT, DPT, MSc

1. How are pelvic girdle disorders classified from an impairment-based model?

Lee distinguishes three types of pelvic girdle disorders: (1) hypomobility with or without pain, (2) hypermobility with or without pain, and (3) normal mobility with pain.

2. What mechanisms typically injure the sacroiliac joint?

Activities that produce posterior torsion stress on the sacroiliac joint include heavy lifting, falls on the ischial tuberosity, vertical thrusts on the extended leg (such as a sudden, unexpected step off a curb), and persistent postures (such as standing on one leg, bowling, and kicks that miss the ball or target).

Activities that produce anterior torsion stress include golf swings and horizontal thrusts on the knee with the hip flexed (such as during a motor vehicle accident when the knee is suddenly thrust against the dashboard).

Repetitive strain to the sacroiliac joint can result from decreased extensibility of muscles associated with the pelvic girdle. Decreased extensibility of the hip flexor musculature can create a repetitive anterior torsion strain during gait. Decreased extensibility of the hamstrings can produce a repetitive posterior torsion strain.

3. When a patient's symptoms include sacroiliac dysfunction, are there certain activities that either aggravate or relieve the pain as supported by a base of evidence in physical therapy practice?

Evidence indicates that no aggravating or relieving factors are of value for the diagnosis of sacroiliac joint–related pain. Anecdotal evidence has supported walking, unilateral standing, sexual intercourse, climbing or descending stairs, sit-to-stand movements, and getting in and out of a car as activities that aggravate the sacroiliac joint. Rolling over in bed also may cause pain by gapping or compressing the involved joint.

4. Why is sacroiliac dysfunction more common in women aged 15 to 40 years?

Women tend to have smaller and flatter joint surfaces, which increase joint mobility. This may be exacerbated by hormonal changes caused by relaxin. The increase in mobility may lead to hypermobile conditions of the sacroiliac joint. The female patient usually presents when age-related changes in degenerative arthrosis are mild. Because the female's body weight falls behind the axis of support (through the acetabulum), the gravity vector tends to create a posterior rotation force on the pelvis that causes strain on the posterior ligaments of the sacroiliac joint.

5. Describe the pattern of pain referral from the sacroiliac joint, as mapped by injection.

The pain referral pattern from the sacroiliac joint has been described by Fortin and April as unilateral to the involved side in an area approximately 3 by 10 cm immediately inferior to the posterior superior iliac spine. Slipman found a similar pain pattern using intra-articular injection and reported the following pain patterns: 94% buttocks, 48% posterior thigh, 28% posterior lower leg, 13% foot/ankle, 14% groin, and 2% abdomen.

6. Has limitation in lumbar range of motion been determined to be a predictor of sacroiliac joint dysfunction?

No; Schwarzer and Maigne both assessed range of motion in patients with sacroiliac joint dysfunction and found no statistical significance for the use of decreased lumbar range of motion as an indicator of sacroiliac joint dysfunction.

7. Based on current literature, which appears to be more useful for evaluating the sacroiliac joint—assessment of anatomic symmetry or pain provocation?

Assessment of pain provocation is more useful because many asymptomatic patients have minor asymmetry.

8. Which pain provocation tests have good inter-rater reliability?

Laslett and Williams assessed the inter-rater reliability of seven provocation tests for the sacroiliac joint. Iliac compression, iliac gapping, posterior shear or thigh thrust, pelvic torsion right, and pelvic torsion left had inter-rater reliabilities of 78% to 94%. Potter and Rothstein examined the intertester reliability of 13 tests for sacroiliac joint dysfunction. They found that the iliac gapping and compression tests achieved good reliability at 90% and 70% agreement, respectively. All other tests in their study showed poor reliability when studied individually.

9. Which pain provocation tests have been found to be the most useful in terms of reliability, sensitivity, specificity, and validity?

- Compression
- Distraction
- Thigh thrust
- FABER (fixed abduction external rotation)
- Resisted hip abduction
- Sacral shear

10. Which four tests are used in a cluster to assess sacroiliac dysfunction?

- Standing flexion test
- Supine long-sitting test
- Sitting posterior-superior iliac spine palpation
- Prone knee flexion test

Positive results from at least three of the four tests improve the specificity and reduce the chance of false-positive findings. Cibulka et al. report 82% sensitivity, 88% specificity, 86% positive predictive value, and 84% negative predictive value for the cluster of tests. Individual sacroiliac tests can cause false-positive results because they have been found to be unreliable—with the exception of the iliac gapping and compression tests.

11. Describe the posterior shear or thigh thrust test.

This test is performed with the patient in a supine position. The therapist applies a gentle progressive posterior shearing stress to the sacroiliac joint through the femur by contracting the knee and pushing the thigh posterior with the hip flexed. Care must be taken to limit excessive hip adduction. This test assesses the ability of the ilium to translate independently on the sacrum. A painful reaction may be attributable to strain placed on the posterior elements of the joint.

12. Describe the right posterior rotation pelvic torsion provocation test.

Posterior rotation of the right ilium on the sacrum is achieved by flexion of the right hip and knee and simultaneous left hip extension with the patient in the supine position. Overpressure is applied through the right lower extremity to force the right sacroiliac joint to its end range. This provocation is sometimes called Gaenslen's test. A painful reaction may be reproduced by strain on the posterior elements as well as by joint irritability caused by movement within the joint.

13. Discuss the method and benefits of using injections to diagnose the sacroiliac joint as a cause of low back pain.

Diagnostic injections with a local anesthetic and contrast medium can be introduced precisely into the joint via fluoroscopy or computed tomography to assess relief or provocation of pain. A control block eliminates placebo effects. Thus relief of pain gives compelling evidence that the intra-articular sacroiliac joint dysfunction is the source. However, it should be noted that pain that arises from the surrounding ligaments or muscles would not be affected by this type of injection. This may give us a reason to question the guided double SIJ injection as the gold standard for validity testing.

14. What osteopathic classifications of sacroiliac dysfunction are described in clinical practice, and what are the clinical signs associated with each?

Diagnosis	Bony Landmarks	Leg Length Changes	Lumbar Scoliosis	Muscular/ Ligamentous Changes
Posterior iliac rotation (left)	Left PSIS inferior, ASIS superior	Left short	None	Increased piriformis and hamstring tone
Anterior iliac rotation (left)	Left PSIS superior, ASIS inferior	Left long	None	Increased psoas and rectus femoris tone
Iliac outflare (left)	Left ASIS lateral, PSIS medial	None	None	None
Iliac inflare (left)	Left ASIS medial, PSIS lateral	None	None	None
Iliac upslip (left)	Left ASIS and PSIS superior	Left short	None	Left sacrotuberous ligament is slack
Iliac downslip (left)	Left ASIS and PSIS inferior	Left long	None	Left sacrotuberous ligament is tense
Sacral torsion anterior (left on left)	Right sacral base deep, left ILA prominent	Left short	Convex right	Increased psoas and piriformis tone
Sacral torsion posterior (left on right)	Left sacral base prominent, left ILA prominent	Left short	Convex right	Increased psoas and piriformis tone
Unilaterally flexed sacrum (left)	Left sacral base deep, right ILA inferior	Left long	Convex left	Increased psoas and piriformis tone
Unilaterally extended sacrum (left)	Left sacral base prominent, left ILA superior	Left short	Convex right	Increased psoas and piriformis tone
Bilaterally flexed sacrum	Bilateral bases of sacrum deep	None	None	Increased psoas and piriformis tone
Bilaterally extended sacrum	Bilateral bases of sacrum prominent	None	None	Tight pelvic diaphragm

PSIS, Posterior superior iliac spine; *ASIS,* anterior superior iliac spine; *ILA,* inferior lateral angle.

15. Describe the objective position and mobility findings of sacral torsion dysfunction.

The sacrum is positioned in rotation with an anterior sacral base on one side and a posterior inferior lateral angle on the opposite side in either trunk flexion or trunk extension. Greenman describes these positions as either an anterior torsion (when tested with flexion) or a backward torsion (when tested with extension).

16. Describe the clinical signs and treatment of sacroiliac hypermobility.

Increased passive or active mobility of either the innominate or the sacrum presents with sacroiliac hypermobility dysfunction. Treatment may consist of therapeutic exercises for muscle imbalances, joint manipulation of neighboring hypomobilities in the lumbar spine or hips, patient education about reducing postural and functional stresses through positioning and normal movement for activities of daily and nightly living, and use of a sacroiliac binder. The use of a sacroiliac binder has been studied in cadavers and found to enhance pelvic stability.

17. What special test is good for determining sacroiliac laxity in postpartum patients?

- Mens et al. (1999) found that a positive active straight leg raise (ASLR) test is associated with increased SIJ mobility.
- Damen et al. found that the ASLR test and also the thigh thrust test are good for identifying postpartum patients who have SIJ laxity.

18. What may cause sacroiliac pain when mobility of the sacroiliac joint is normal?

- Mild sprain or strain injury
- Inflammatory disease
- Overuse of the adjacent articular or myofascial tissues

19. How can excellent diagnostic accuracy be achieved in the prediction of sacroiliac dysfunction?

Use of an evaluation to exclude pain of diskogenic origin in combination with use of three provocation tests has been shown to have excellent diagnostic accuracy for sacroiliac dysfunction.

20. What motor control strategies have been shown to be delayed in patients with a clinical diagnosis of sacroiliac joint pain?

Hungerford et al. found that the onset of contractions of the internal obliques, multifidus, gluteus maximus, and biceps femoris was significantly delayed compared to patients without pain during hip flexion while standing.

21. What common medical conditions affect the sacroiliac joint?

- Ankylosing spondylitis (AS) begins as inflammation involving the synovium of the sacroiliac joints. The ligaments are transformed to bone, beginning at the insertion point, which ends in bony fusion or ankylosis. The incidence varies with ethnic groups: AS is most common in Haida Indians (4.2 per 1000) and Caucasians (1 per 1000). It is more prevalent in males than females by a 3:1 ratio and is most common in males under the age of 40. Symptoms usually begin in the lumbar spine. Radiologic changes vary from blurring to complete obliteration of the joint margins, resulting in bony fusion of the sacrum to the ilium. AS often appears first with abnormal narrowing of the upper half of the sacroiliac joints.
- Reiter syndrome is precipitated by an infection in the genitourinary or gastrointestinal tract. Although the infection is not found within the joint, the organism causes reactive arthritis, which can cause sacroiliitis. Radiologic changes demonstrate erosions at the insertion points of ligaments.
- About 15% of patients with inflammatory bowel disease (Crohn's disease or ulcerative colitis) have sacroiliitis clinically. The radiologic changes resemble those in AS.
- Psoriatic spondylitis causes bone spur formation and partial bony ankylosis of the sacroiliac joints, often asymmetrically. Psoriasis affects 1.2% of the general population; 7% of patients with psoriasis may have arthritis.
- Other conditions that may affect the sacroiliac joint include rheumatoid arthritis, pyogenic infection, tuberculosis, brucellosis, gout, hyperthyroidism, Paget's disease, diffuse idiopathic skeletal hyperostosis, and osteitis condensans ilii.

22. What are the best imaging studies for diagnosing the cause of sacroiliac joint pain?

No specific imaging studies provide precise findings that are helpful in the diagnosis of sacroiliac joint pain. Computed tomography and MRI provide an unobstructed view of the joint and the ability to view the joint margins superiorly and inferiorly for osteophytes. However, they are predominantly used to exclude other causes of sacroiliac pain (tumor, spondyloarthropathies). Bone scans are helpful in determining stress fractures, infection, inflammation, and tumor.

23. What are the radiologic signs of pubic symphysis instability?

Instability of the pubic symphysis is suggested by radiographic findings of pubic symphysis separation >10 mm and vertical displacement >2 mm with the single leg stance.

24. Do sacroiliac braces provide pain relief?

They may provide pain relief. Biomechanical studies of sacroiliac motion while wearing a sacroiliac belt directly superior to the greater trochanter showed an approximately 30% decrease in sacroiliac joint motion in cases of peripartum instability. This stabilizing effect could be linked to pain reduction in patients considered to have greater than normal sacroiliac joint motion.

25. Do osseous positional changes occur following a high-velocity manipulation to the sacroiliac joint?

No. Radiographic stereophotogrammetric analysis before and after manipulation does not demonstrate positional changes of the sacrum and ilium.

26. What is prolotherapy, and is it effective in the treatment of sacroiliac joint pain?

Prolotherapy is a form of injection therapy. Sclerosing agents are injected into injured ligaments, which provokes a localized inflammatory reaction. Prolotherapy is proposed to stimulate regrowth of collagen, thus strengthening the ligaments and improving their elasticity and possibly function. Prolotherapy has been found to have superior results to sham injections for chronic nonspecific low back pain; however, its specific application to the sacroiliac joint has not been studied.

27. What are some other forms of medical treatment for sacroiliac joint pain?

- Nerve stimulators (implanted)—Partial pain relief has been reported with selective stimulation of sacral root 3.
- Viscosupplementation—Partial pain relief has been reported with intra-articular injection of hylan G-F 20.
- Radiofrequency neurotomy—Sixty-four percent of 14 patients with sacroiliac joint pain that underwent radiofrequency neurotomy demonstrated a >50% pain reduction at a 6-month follow-up visit.
- Arthrodesis—This is a very controversial treatment approach for idiopathic sacroiliac joint pain.

Bibliography

Alderink G: The sacroiliac joint: review of anatomy, mechanics, and function, *J Orthop Sports Phys Ther* 13:71-84, 1991.

Cibulka MT, Koldenhoff R: Clinical usefulness of a cluster of sacroiliac joint tests in patients with and without low back pain, *J Orthop Sports Phys Ther* 29:83-89, 1999.

Damen L et al: The prognostic value of asymmetric laxity of the sacroiliac joints in pregnancy-related pelvic pain, *Spine* 27:2820-2824, 2002.

Dreyfuss P et al: The value of medical history and physical examination in diagnosing sacroiliac joint pain, *Spine* 21:2594-2602, 1995.

Fortin JD et al: Sacroiliac joint: pain referral maps upon applying a new injection/arthrography technique, *Spine* 19:1475-1482, 1994.
Freburger JK, Riddle DL: Measurement of sacroiliac joint dysfunction: a multicenter intertester reliability study, *Phys Ther* 79:1134-1141, 1999.
Greenman P: *Principles of manual medicine,* ed 2, Philadelphia, 1996, William & Wilkins.
Hayne C: Manual transport of loads by women, *Physiotherapy* 67:226-231, 1981.
Helms C: *Fundamentals of skeletal radiology,* ed 2, Philadelphia, 1995, WB Saunders.
Huijbregts PA: Sacroiliac joint dysfunction: evidence-based diagnosis, *Orthop Division Rev* 18:32, 41-44, 2004.
Hungerford B, Gilleard W, Hodges P: Evidence of altered lumbopelvic muscle recruitment in the presence of sacroiliac joint pain, *Spine* 28:1593-1600, 2003.
Laslett M: The value of the physical examination in diagnosis of painful sacroiliac joint pathologies: comment, *Spine* 23:962-964, 1998.
Laslett M, Williams M: The reliability of selected pain provocation tests for sacroiliac joint pathology, *Spine* 19:1243-1249, 1994.
Laslett M et al: Diagnosing painful sacroiliac joints: a validity study of a McKenzie evaluation and sacroiliac provocation tests, *Aust J Physiother* 49:89-97, 2003.
Lee D: *The pelvic girdle: an approach to the examination and treatment of the lumbo-pelvic-hip region,* Edinburgh, 1989, Churchill Livingstone.
Maigne J et al: Results of sacroiliac joint double block and value of sacroiliac pain provocation tests in 54 patients with low back pain, *Spine* 21:1889-1892, 1996.
Mens J et al: The active straight leg raise test and mobility of the pelvic joints, *Eur Spine J* 8:468-473, 1999.
Mens J et al: Validity of the active straight leg raise test for measuring disease severity in patients with posterior pelvic pain after pregnancy, *Spine* 27:196, 2002.
Potter N, Rothstein J: Intertester reliability for selected clinical tests of the sacroiliac joint, *Phys Ther* 65:1671-1675, 1985.
Schwarzer AC et al: The sacroiliac joint in chronic low back pain, *Spine* 20:31-37, 1995.
Slipman CW et al: Sacroiliac joint pain referral zones, *Arch Phys Med Rehabil* 81:334-338, 2000.
Vleeming A et al: An integrated therapy for peripartum pelvic instability: a study of the biomechanical effects of pelvic belts, *Am J Obstet Gynecol* 166:1243-1247, 1992.

Section X

The Hip and Pelvis

Chapter 64

Functional Anatomy of the Hip and Pelvis

Teri L. Gibbons, PT, MPT, OCS

1. Describe the articular surfaces of the hip joint.

The hip joint is created by the acetabulum of the pelvis and the head of the femur. The acetabulum is a cup-shaped structure located laterally on the pelvis and formed by the fusion of the ilium, ischium, and pubis. Only a horseshoe-shaped portion of the acetabulum is covered with articular cartilage and contacts the head of the femur. The acetabular notch lies inferior to this cartilage and is bridged by the acetabular labrum, which also covers the entire periphery of the acetabulum. The acetabular fossa is thus nonarticular and contains a fat pad covered with synovial fluid. The acetabulum faces laterally, anteriorly, and inferiorly.

The head of the femur is covered completely by articular cartilage except for the fovea or central portion, which serves as the location for the ligamentum teres. The femoral head is circular and attaches to the shaft of the femur by the femoral neck. The femoral head faces medially, superiorly, and anteriorly.

2. How is the hip joint classified?

The hip joint is a diarthrodial, ball-and-socket joint with three degrees of movement: (1) flexion and extension occur in the sagittal plane around a coronal axis; (2) abduction and adduction occur in the frontal plane around an anteroposterior axis; and (3) internal and external rotation occur on the transverse plane around a longitudinal axis.

3. What is the angle of inclination of the femur?

It is the angle between (1) the axis of the femoral head and neck and (2) the axis of the femoral shaft in the frontal plane. It begins at approximately 150 degrees in infants and decreases to 125 degrees in adults and 120 degrees in elderly people. The angle is slightly smaller in women than in men because of women's increased pelvic width. Coxa valga (>150 degrees) is a pathologic increase in the angle of inclination, and coxa vara (<120 degrees) is a pathologic decrease.

4. What is the angle of torsion of the femur?

It is the angle between the axis of the femoral condyles and the axis of the head and neck of the femur in the transverse plane. The plane of the head and neck is anterior to the plane of the condyles. It is approximately 40 degrees in infants and decreases to approximately 12 to 15 degrees in adults. An increase in the angle of torsion is called anteversion, and a decrease is called retroversion.

5. How is the angle of torsion assessed clinically?

Femoral anteversion may be assessed using Craig's test (also called Ryder's method). The patient is prone with the knee flexed to 90 degrees. The leg is then rotated internally and externally until the greater trochanter is parallel to the table. The amount of anteversion is measured by the angle of the lower leg to the vertical.

6. What gender differences exist in the anatomy of the hip?

Acetabula are shallower in women than in men. The female pelvis is broader with a greater pubic arch angle. The difference in pelvic geometry creates a reduced tolerance for hip fractures in front-end motor vehicle collisions. The female femur is shorter, lighter, and thinner than the male femur with a smaller femoral head diameter and shorter bicondylar width. This creates a shorter moment arm for the gluteus medius in women and an increase in femoral head pressure. These differences in pelvic and femoral geometry can create a reduced tolerance for hip fractures in female patients.

7. Describe the joint capsule of the hip.

The joint capsule is a strong and dense structure that figures prominently in hip joint stability. It attaches proximally to the entire rim of the acetabular labrum and distally to the base of the neck of the femur. The joint capsule covers the head of the femur like a sleeve. It is thickest anterosuperiorly, where the most protection is needed. The posteroinferior attachment is thinner and loose.

8. Which ligaments contribute to the stability of the hip?

Two ligaments reinforce the hip anteriorly: (1) the iliofemoral ligament (or Y-shaped ligament of Bigelow), which is the stronger and checks hip hyperextension; and (2) the pubofemoral ligament, which checks hip abduction and extension. The ischiofemoral ligament is located posteriorly; its fibers tighten with hip extension. All of these ligaments are major contributors to stability in an upright standing posture. The ligamentum teres, which passes from the acetabular notch under the transverse acetabular ligament or labrum and attaches to the head of the femur at the fovea, does not add stability to the hip joint.

9. Describe the arthrokinematics of the hip joint.

The convex femoral head glides in a direction opposite to the movement on the concave acetabulum in an open-chain condition. In the more common closed-chain condition, the concave acetabulum moves in the same direction as the opposite side of the pelvis.

10. Describe the osteokinematics of the hip joint.

Movement of the femur is affected in most directions by the passive tension of two joint muscles. Passive range of motion is as follows:

- Flexion—120 to 135 degrees (90 degrees if the knee is extended because of tension of the hamstrings)
- Extension—10 to 30 degrees (limited by the rectus femoris if combined with knee flexion)
- Abduction—30 to 50 degrees
- Adduction—10 to 30 degrees
- External rotation—45 to 60 degrees
- Internal rotation—30 to 45 degrees

The normal end-feel for all directions of the hip is either tissue approximation or tissue stretch. The movements of the pelvis include anterior and posterior tilting, lateral pelvic tilt, and pelvic rotation.

11. Name the muscles that cross the hip joint.

- Flexors—iliopsoas, rectus femoris, tensor fascia latae, sartorius, pectineus, adductor brevis, adductor longus, and oblique fibers of adductor magnus
- Extensors—gluteus maximus, biceps femoris, semimembranosus, and semitendinosus
- Abductors—gluteus medius, gluteus minimus, tensor fascia latae, and upper fibers of gluteus maximus
- Adductors—adductor magnus, adductor longus, adductor brevis, pectineus, and gracilis

- External rotators—obturator externus, obturator internus, quadratus femoris, piriformis, gemellus superior, gemellus inferior, gluteus maximus, sartorius, and biceps femoris
- Internal rotators—gluteus minimus, tensor fascia latae, anterior fibers of gluteus medius, semitendinosus, and semimembranosus

12. What is inversion of muscle action?

Muscles that cross a joint with 3 degrees of freedom may have alternate or even opposite (inverted) actions than their classically described actions. The action of the muscle depends on joint position and has important implications for muscle stretching and resistive exercise.

13. Describe inversion of the flexor component of the adductor muscles.

All adductors of the hip are also flexors (except the adductor magnus) with the hip in neutral position. With flexion, the femur lies anterior to the origin of the muscle and the adductors become extensors. The adductor longus is a flexor to 70 degrees, the adductor brevis to 50 degrees, and the gracilis to 40 degrees, at which point they become extensors.

14. Describe inversion of muscle action for the piriformis.

With the hip in neutral position, the piriformis is primarily an external rotator and a weak flexor and abductor. At 60 degrees of flexion, the piriformis becomes primarily an abductor and medial rotator of the hip.

15. What is the iliocapsularis muscle?

- Origin—anteromedial hip capsule and the inferior border of the anterior inferior iliac spine
- Insertion—distal to the lesser trochanter

The iliocapsularis muscle may tighten the anterior hip capsule to increase stability of the femoral head. The muscle is a landmark during hip surgery in order to expose the anteromedial hip capsule and the psoas tendon interval.

16. What changes occur to the hip musculature following an above-knee amputation?

Amputation changes the geometry of most of the hip muscles because two-joint muscles become one-joint muscles. The cleaved muscles will atrophy 40% to 60% while intact muscles will atrophy up to 30%. If the iliotibial (IT) band is fixed, there is a risk of developing an abduction contracture. With IT band fixation, there is improved hip extension torque by the gluteus maximius to improve propulsion and avoid hip flexion contracture caused by the intact iliopsoas. To avoid an abduction contracture, the adductor magnus is fixated to, and across, the distal femur. When the quadriceps are fixated to the distal femur, the hip should be maximally extended to avoid flexion contracture.

The power generated during the stance phase of gait is reduced 50% in the prosthetic limb. The hip extensors become the primary energy absorbers because of the loss of energy absorption by the knee extensors. During the first 30% to 40% of the stance phase, the hip extensors maintain hip and knee extension to avoid buckling caused by quadriceps and hamstring absence. The intact limb increases hip extension and ankle plantar flexion power in order to clear the prosthetic limb for the swing phase.

17. Are there differences in the strength of hip musculature with versus without osteoarthritis (OA) of the hip?

Arokoski et al. found a significant reduction in isometric hip abduction (31%) and adduction (25%) strength in males with OA versus without. Hip flexion strength was lower (18% to 22%) in males with OA versus without. Hip extension strength was not significantly lower in men with OA versus without, but in those who had bilateral hip OA, the more deteriorated side was 13% to 22% weaker. The cross-sectional area of the hip and thigh musculature did not differ between groups.

18. Describe hip range of motion needed for common daily activities.

- Ascending stairs—40 to 67 degrees of flexion
- Descending stairs—36 degrees of flexion
- Sit to stand—104 degrees of flexion
- Tying shoe—110 degrees of flexion, 33 degrees of external rotation (crossing leg)
- Walking—20 to 40 degrees of flexion

19. Which muscles are active during two-legged erect stance?

None. Stability is maintained by the capsule and ligamentous support.

20. How much force is unloaded from the hip when a cane is used in the opposite hand?

A cane can decrease force loads by 40%. A single contralateral crutch can decrease loads up to 50%.

21. What structures pass through the sciatic notch?

- Vessels—superior gluteal artery and vein, inferior gluteal artery and vein, internal pudendal artery and vein
- Nerves—sciatic nerve, superior gluteal nerve, inferior gluteal nerve, posterior gluteal nerve, nerve to quadratus femoris, nerve to obturator externus
- Muscle—piriformis

22. Describe the blood supply to the femoral head.

- Extracapsular arterial ring—The extracapsular ring is formed posteriorly by a large branch of the medial femoral circumflex artery and anteriorly by the lateral circumflex femoral artery, which are branches of the femoral artery or the profunda femoris artery. The extracapsular ring supplies most of the head and neck of the femur. These arteries surround the neck of the femur and ascend along it, forming rings around the upper neck and subcapital sulcus. The medial circumflex artery branches into the lateral, superior, and inferior epiphyseal arteries, with the lateral epiphyseal artery supplying more than half of the femoral head.
- Ascending cervical branches—The ascending cervical arteries are formed by the lateral circumflex artery and travel into the joint capsule and run along the neck of the femur, deep to the synovial lining of the neck. They are at risk with any disruption of the capsule, as may occur in a femoral neck fracture.
- Artery of the ligamentum teres—The artery of the ligamentum teres contributes little, if any, significant supply to the femoral head.

23. Describe the anatomy of the trochanteric bursa.

A series of three bursae exist: (1) between the gluteus maximus and the gluteus medius tendon; (2) between the gluteus maximius and the greater trochanter; and (3) between the gluteus medius and the greater trochanter. Dunn et al. found that multiple bursae could exist and tended to be aquired with age because of excessive friction between the greater trochanter and the insertion of the gluteus maximus at the insertion into the fascia lata.

24. What is the ideal position for hip arthrodesis?

The ideal position for hip arthrodesis is 25 to 30 degrees of hip flexion in conjunction with neutral abduction and rotation.

25. What is the functional range of motion of the hip?

The functional ROM of the hip is flexion to 90 degrees, abduction to 20 degrees, and internal/external rotation from 0 to 20 degrees.

Bibliography

Arokoski MH et al: Hip muscle strength and muscle cross sectional area in men with and without hip osteoarthritis, *J Rheumatol* 29:2185-2195, 2002.

Daniels L, Worthingham C: *Muscle testing: techniques of manual examination,* ed 5, Philadelphia, 1986, pp 38-70, WB Saunders.

Dunn T, Heller CA, McCarthy SW: Anatomical study of the "trochanteric bursa", *Clin Anat* 16:233-240, 2003.

Jaegers SM, Arendzen JH, de Jongh HJ: Changes in hip muscles after above-knee amputation, *Clin Orthop Relat Res* 319:276-284, 1995.

Magee DJ: *Orthopedic physical assessment,* ed 4, Philadelphia, 2002, pp 607-655, WB Saunders.

Norkin CC, Levangie PK: *Joint structure and function: a comprehensive analysis,* ed 2, Philadelphia, 1992, pp 300-336, FA Davis.

Norkin CC, White DJ: *Measurement of joint motion: a guide to goniometry,* Philadelphia, 1985, FA Davis.

Robbins CE: Anatomy and biomechanics. In Fagerson TL, editor: *The hip handbook,* Boston, 1998, pp 1-37, Butterworth Heinemann.

Wang SC et al: Gender differences in hip anatomy: possible implications for injury tolerance in frontal collisions, *Annu Proc Assoc Adv Automot Med* 48:287-301, 2004.

Ward W: Anatomy of the iliocapsularis muscle: relevance to surgery of the hip, *Clin Orthop Relat Res* 374:278-285, 2000.

Chapter 65

Common Orthopaedic Hip Dysfunction

Teri L. Gibbons, PT, MPT, OCS

1. How are muscle strains classified?

- Grade I—little tissue disruption, low-grade inflammatory response; strength testing produces pain without loss of strength; no loss of range of motion (ROM)
- Grade II—some disruption of muscle fibers but not complete; strength and ROM decreased; pain significant
- Grade III—complete rupture with complete loss of strength of involved muscle; palpable or visible defect may be present

2. How do gluteus medius strains occur?

The most common cause is the seesaw action of the pelvis during running, although strains also are seen in swimmers. Leg length discrepancies may increase the risk of an abductor strain. Pain is commonly located just proximal to the attachment at the greater trochanter and is reproduced with resisted abduction. It can be confused with greater trochanteric bursitis, which is thought to be painless with resisted abduction, or the two can exist together.

3. What is "bald trochanter"?

It is the rupture and retraction of the gluteus medius and minimus tendons at their attachment to the greater trochanter as a result of interstitial or deep surface degeneration. It can present as chronic trochanteric bursitis and can be diagnosed with MRI. Treatment involves using a cane in the ipsilateral hand and taking NSAIDs to reduce symptoms. Surgical repair or debridement may be an option.

4. How do groin pulls occur?

Groin pulls are strains of the hip adductors, most commonly the adductor longus, and occur in sports that require quick acceleration or direction changes. They frequently are seen in ice hockey players, who may be predisposed to groin pulls because of lack of strengthening (specifically abduction to adduction strength ratio deficits) and stretching of the adductors, previous injury in that area, and lack of experience. A straddle stretch lengthens the muscle bilaterally but a unilateral stretch may give the athlete better control. Adductor strains also occur in football, rugby, swimming (breast stroke), cricket, bowling, and horseback riding. Most injuries are grades I and II; complete ruptures are rare.

5. What treatment is effective in treating groin pulls?

Passive physical therapy (massage, stretching, and modalities) has been found to be ineffective in treating groin pulls. However, an 8- to 12-week active strengthening program has proven effective in treating chronic groin strains and allows return to sport. The adductor muscles should be within 80% of the strength of the abductors in order to avoid reinjury. Tyler has developed a program emphasizing eccentric resistive exercise, balance training, core strengthening, and sport-specific movements, which has been supported throughout the literature.

6. When is surgery necessary to treat a groin pull?

If symptoms persist after 6 months of appropriate physical therapy, and other pathology is ruled out, adductor tenotomy can be performed. However, only 10% of athletes will return to their previous level of competition.

7. What is a "sports hernia"?

Although several theories exist, it is most probably an overuse syndrome. Various structures around the pelvis may be at fault. Shearing occurs across the symphysis pubis with strong hip movements and may create stress on the inguinal wall musculature. Structures in the pelvic floor, the insertion of the rectus abdominus, the insertion of the internal oblique muscles at the pubic tubercle, and the external oblique muscle aponeurosis have all been found to be structures which may be at fault.

8. What is the most frequently strained muscle in the body?

The hamstrings have this dubious honor. Injury commonly recurs and usually affects the proximal aspect of the muscle group near the origin at the ischial tuberosity. The mechanism of injury is a rapid, uncontrolled stretch or forceful contraction. A classic example of hamstring injury occurs in hurdlers because maximal hip flexion is accompanied by full knee extension. Proper warm-up and endurance training are important to avoid hamstring strains, which most often occur early or late in a sporting event. Most injuries are grade I or II. True grade III injuries are rare; an avulsion fracture of the ischial tuberosity is more common. Once a strain occurs, proper rehabilitation (improved muscle balance, stretching, proper education about warming up, endurance training, and coordination) is imperative to avoid reinjury. Croisier et al. trained 18 athletes with hamstring strain with specific isokinetic exercises to address their specific strength deficits (quadriceps/hamstring ratios, both concentrically and eccentrically). Of these 18 athletes, 17 improved their isokinetic profiles and returned to sport within 2 months. All 17 remained hamstring injury free at a 1-year follow-up. Although a reduction in strength in the injured hamstring has been found to be a predictor of reinjury, Sherry and Best found that a rehabilitation program needs to include progressive agility and trunk stabilization exercises in order to avoid reinjury. Sports with a high prevalence of hamstring strain include running, sprinting, soccer, football, and rugby.

9. How is hamstring length assessed?

1. 90/90-degree straight-leg raise—The patient is positioned supine with the hip flexed 90 degrees (either actively or passively). The knee is then actively extended from a starting position of 90-degree flexion toward full extension. The test is positive for hamstring tightness if the angle of knee flexion is >20 degrees.
2. Tripod sign—The patient sits with knees over the table in 90 degrees of flexion. The examiner passively extends the knee. The test is positive for hamstring tightness if the pelvis is forced into a posterior tilt.
3. Hamstring contracture test—The patient sits with the tested leg extended while the untested leg is held toward the chest. The patient is instructed to reach the arm ipsilateral to the test leg toward the toes. The test is positive for hamstring tightness if the patient cannot reach the toes while maintaining knee extension.
4. Straight-leg raising—The patient rests supine while the examiner passively raises the leg with the knee fully extended, and the angle of hip flexion is measured. This test has been found to be highly reliable, but does not differentiate between elastic and inelastic posterior hip structures.

The medial and lateral hamstrings can be differentiated with a manual muscle test. The semitendinosus and semimembranosus are isolated by positioning the patient in prone with the hip internally rotated and resisted knee flexion. The biceps femoris is isolated by positioning the patient prone with external rotation of the hip and resisted knee flexion. Hamstring tightness should be differentiated from radicular symptoms caused by the sciatic nerve or lumbar spine.

10. Are quadriceps strains common?

No. However, when they occur, they are usually the result of rapid deceleration from a sprint. The rectus femoris is the most commonly affected of the quadriceps muscles because of its two-joint action, but the vastus medialis and vastus lateralis also can be injured. Most damage occurs either in the middle of the thigh or approximately 8 cm from the anterior superior iliac spine for grade I and II strains. Strains are seen in soccer, weight lifting, football, sprinting, and rugby. Tight quadriceps, muscle imbalance between the two extremities, leg length discrepancy, and improper warm-up may be contributing factors.

11. How is rectus femoris length measured?

1. Thomas test or rectus femoris contracture test—The patient is positioned in supine with one knee flexed and held toward the chest. The opposite test leg is positioned so that the lower leg hangs off the edge of the table. If the test knee rests in less than 90 degrees of flexion, the test is considered positive for tightness of the rectus femoris. A positive result is indicated by the inability to rest the leg flat on the table and an increase in lumbar lordosis when the examiner

passively extends the knee by pushing the leg into the table. The Thomas test assesses tight hip flexors, which may be present with iliopectineal bursitis. To differentiate between soft tissue and joint restriction, contract-relax maneuvers can be applied at end ROM. If hip extension increases, the hip flexors are the tissue at fault. If the tested leg abducts as the opposite leg is flexed (J sign), tightness in the iliotibial band/tensor fasciae latae (ITB/TFL) is indicated. The Thomas test can detect statistical differences in ROM between the two extremities, and applying manual pressure at end range can provide the examiner with valuable information. Information gathered from the Thomas test has not been found to be reflective of dynamic movements of the pelvis during running.

2. Ely test—The patient is positioned prone. The examiner passively flexes the knee and watches for any hip flexion, which indicates a tight rectus femoris. The examiner should compare results with the other side and watch for reproduced symptoms that may be referred from the femoral nerve.

12. How are the oblique muscles injured?

The external obliques may become strained at their insertion on the iliac crest. Forceful contraction of the abdominals with the trunk laterally flexed is one mechanism of injury (most common in contact sports). The patient has pain with opposite side-bending as well as pain on palpation. Abdominal binders or taping may be necessary to protect the area once the player returns to sport after a period of rest.

13. Describe the treatment for muscle strain.

The length of time for each stage will depend upon the severity of the injury.

- Stage 1 (acute phase, first 24 to 72 hours)—Follow basic first-aid protocols of rest, ice, compression, and elevation (RICE). Nonsteroidal antiinflammatory drugs (NSAIDs) may be administered. Crutches may be required for severe strains.
- Stage 2 (reduction of acute symptoms, 2 to 7 days)—Use gentle ROM and isometric exercise with modalities to reduce pain and swelling as needed. Modalities may include ultrasound, hydrotherapy, and muscle stimulation. Gentle friction massage may help avoid adhesion of scarred muscle tissue.
- Stage 3 (pain-free isometrics)—Continue with stage 2 treatment as needed for pain, but begin pain-free isotonic and isokinetic exercise. Include stretching and aerobic activity with proper warm-up. Stretching should include static stretches as well as proprioceptive neuromuscular facilitation (PNF) techniques such as contract-relax, hold-relax, and contract-relax-contract. Sanders and Nemeth also suggest the use of ballistic stretching, which should follow static stretches and proper warm-up and involves only small movements in the last 10% of the available ROM.
- Stage 4 (ROM 95% of normal, strength 75% of normal)—Begin sport-specific exercise with emphasis on endurance and coordination activities. Jogging and running should be progressed gradually.
- Stage 5 (strength 95% of normal)—Return to sports with education for maintenance of proper warm-up, stretching, and strengthening program.

14. Describe trochanteric bursitis.

Women are more commonly affected because of the increased breadth of the pelvis. Although trochanteric bursitis occurs most commonly in middle-aged and elderly people, it is also seen in athletes, especially long distance runners. There are three trochanteric bursae. The first lies between the gluteus maximus and greater trochanter, the second between the gluteus maximus and gluteus medius tendon, and the third between the gluteus medius and greater trochanter.

Onset of disease caused by overuse is gradual, and the patient complains of aching over the trochanter and along the lateral thigh. In runners, a leg length discrepancy may precipitate the condition. Running on banked surfaces may focus more stress on one hip than on the other.

Runners who cross midline have an increased adduction angle, which may increase friction at the greater trochanter. Check for excessive wear of the lateral heel in running shoes. Trochanteric bursitis also is seen in cross-country skiing and ballet. Contact sports such as hockey, football, and soccer may cause bursitis because of direct blows to the lateral hip, which can produce excessive swelling as well as pain.

15. What are the symptoms of trochanteric bursitis?

The patient may complain of a "snapping" at the lateral hip if tightness of the iliotibial band (ITB) is a factor. Pain typically is provoked by ascending stairs and lying on the affected side. Pain also may radiate into the ipsilateral lumbar region. Stretching the gluteus maximus with full hip flexion, adduction, and internal rotation reproduces pain. Resisted testing of abduction may be painful as well as resisted hip extension and external rotation. Palpation is positive for tenderness over the posterior aspect of the greater trochanter.

16. How is trochanteric bursitis treated?

Initial treatment consists of rest, ice, and compression wraps, especially in traumatic cases. NSAIDs or local corticosteroid injections may be beneficial. Lying on the affected side should be avoided by changing pillow arrangement. Using pillows between the knees reduces the angle of hip adduction in the side-lying position. Stairs should be avoided. Ultrasound causes an increase in local circulation and may help to resolve the condition. Proper stretching of tightened structures is important; the tensor fasciae latae (TFL), gluteals, and hamstrings may be shortened. Strengthening exercise should correct muscle imbalances across the hip, especially focusing on the gluteals. Cold packs or ice massage help to reduce exercise-induced inflammation.

17. What is Ober's test?

The patient is positioned in a side-lying position with the tested hip facing upward. The untested leg is flexed at the hip and knee to stabilize the patient. The examiner firmly stabilizes the pelvis at the iliac crest to prevent side-bending of the trunk. The tested hip is extended maximally and adducted. Variations of this test include testing with the knee extended instead of flexed. Stretch on the ITB is increased with the knee extended. Hip internal and external rotation can be added. A positive test reproduces lateral hip pain or restriction in movement. This test is used to assess the length of the ITB/TFL and may be positive in patients with greater trochanteric bursitis. Both Ober's test and the modified Ober's test have been found to be a reliable method of testing ITB flexibility, but should not be used interchangeably as the modified test will produce significantly more hip adduction range than Ober's test.

18. How does iliopectineal/iliopsoas bursitis develop?

The iliopectineal bursa lies deep to the iliopsoas tendon anterior to the hip joint. Bursitis commonly results from osteoarthritis or rheumatoid arthritis. Other causes include overuse or direct trauma. Overuse can occur with sports such as weight lifting, rowing, uphill running, and competitive track and field. It occurs more commonly in women. An attachment of the bursae to the joint capsule is seen in 15% of cases. Hip joint pathology should be ruled out by checking for a capsular pattern of pain or restriction.

19. Describe the clinical findings in iliopectineal bursitis.

The onset of iliopectineal bursitis is insidious. Pain occurs at the anterior hip and groin with radiation in an L2 or L3 distribution. Lower abdominal pain may be present. The patient may ambulate with a psoatic gait in which the hip is externally rotated, adducted, and flexed during the swing phase. Passive hip flexion with adduction is painful, as is passive hip extension. Strength testing of the hip flexors may be painful and external rotation may be weak when tested with the hip flexed. Palpation elicits tenderness just lateral to the femoral artery at the femoral triangle. The patient may have a palpable snapping at the anterior hip as the involved hip is passively moved from a flexed position into abduction/external rotation, and then passively returned to neutral.

20. Describe the treatment for iliopectineal bursitis.

Sanders and Nemeth suggest that ultrasound and interferential current can be beneficial, as is gentle stretching of tightened structures, particularly the iliopsoas. External rotation strengthening has also been proposed, but no studies have verified its efficacy. Local corticosteroid injections may provide relief. Chronic cases may require release of the iliopsoas tendon. Radiographs may be useful to rule out bony pathology.

21. How does ischial tuberosity bursitis present? What is its treatment?

The involved bursa lies between the ischial tuberosity and gluteus maximus. Bursitis usually occurs in people with sedentary occupations or results from a direct fall onto the ischial tuberosity. Pain worsens with sitting and may refer to the posterior thigh; therefore it is important to rule out lumbar pathology. Palpation over the ischial tuberosity is painful. Hamstring stretching is painful. Hip extension may be reduced in the late stance phase of gait with a shortened stride on the affected side.

NSAIDs and rest are usually successful. The patient should avoid sitting or sit only on well-cushioned surfaces.

22. What is the sign of the buttock?

The patient is positioned in supine while the examiner performs a passive straight-leg raise test. If ROM is limited, the examiner flexes the patient's knee to see whether hip flexion range increases. If hip flexion increases, the test is negative, but the patient should be examined for sacroiliac, sciatic nerve, or lumbar pathology. A positive test shows no increased hip flexion and indicates pathology of the buttock, which may include ischial tuberosity bursitis. Other pathology should be ruled out, including neoplasm, abscess of the buttock, osteomyelitis, fractured sacrum, and septic bursitis.

23. How are contusions in athletes classified?

- Grade I—produces minimal discomfort and should not limit participation in competition
- Grade II—more painful and limits ability to perform at extremes of ROM or strength
- Grade III—more pain, swelling, and bleeding

24. What is a hip pointer?

A hip pointer is contusion of the lateral hip, which usually results from a blow to the iliac crest. In most cases, the TFL muscle belly is impacted and presents with hematoma; however, the injury may involve tearing of the external oblique at its iliac insertion, periostitis of the iliac crest, or contusion to the greater trochanter. Contact sports such as football, ice hockey, volleyball, soccer, wrestling, lacrosse, and rugby often produce hip pointers from impact with other players. Gymnasts may suffer this injury from impact with equipment. It can also result from a fall with any activity.

25. Describe the clinical findings of a hip pointer.

The injured athlete is immediately disabled by pain. The trunk is flexed forward and toward the side of injury because any side-bending or rotation of the trunk is extremely painful. Abrasion or swelling may be present over the iliac crest. Bruising may be immediately present or may become apparent a few days after injury. Pain is caused by any movement involving the muscles that attach to the iliac crest, including the gluteus maximus, gluteus medius, TFL, sartorius, quadratus lumborum, and transverse abdominals. The abdominals may be in spasm.

26. How are hip pointers treated?

Initial treatment is RICE. Crutches may be needed if the patient has pain with ambulation. NSAIDs should not be used until 48 hours after injury because their blood-thinning properties may lead to hematoma. Ice massage is recommended as often as 3 to 4 times per day or as pain levels dictate. Gradual stretching keeps the injured area from healing in a contracted position. All exercise should be kept pain-free, and pain-relieving modalities such as ultrasound, transcutaneous electrical nerve stimulation, heat, and ice may be used. Strengthening programs should include trunk and leg muscles. The athlete must try to prevent hip pointers in the future by maintenance of a flexibility program and wearing proper protective padding over the iliac crest. Return to sports is allowed in 1 week for grade I injuries; up to 6 weeks may be required for grade II and III injuries.

27. What tests are useful in the diagnosis of hip pointers?

Radiographs help to rule out iliac crest fracture or displaced epiphyseal fracture in athletes who have not reached skeletal maturity.

28. What is the mechanism for a quadriceps contusion? What are the clinical findings?

Usually a direct blow from another player is the cause. In football, contact may be made with a helmet, thigh, or padding. Quadriceps contusion also is seen in rugby, soccer, basketball, and ice hockey. The anterior thigh and lateral thigh are most commonly affected.

Pain occurs with ambulation. The patient is unable to flex and extend the knee fully and may not be able to perform an active straight-leg raise or isometric quadriceps contraction. A hematoma may be palpable.

29. How does treatment for a quadriceps contusion progress?

Initial RICE must be followed strictly for at least 48 hours. Crutches should be used for ambulation. For 48 hours the patient should be non–weight-bearing and immobilized in knee flexion to maintain motion. Then weight-bearing should progress once the patient has good quadriceps control and 90-degree pain-free range of motion. Patients should gradually begin passive ROM to avoid contracture. Ice, pulsed ultrasound, and high-voltage galvanic stimulation help to reduce pain and swelling. Patients should begin with isometric exercise and try to progress to straight-leg raises without a quadriceps lag. Massage should be avoided because it may increase hematoma. As patients progress toward pain-free ambulation, crutch use is discontinued and strengthening should progress gradually as pain allows. Return to sport can begin after full ROM and sport-specific training. There should be less than a 10% difference in strength between the injured and noninjured quadriceps before full return to sport.

30. What causes myositis ossificans?

Myositis ossificans may be a complication of quadriceps contusion and involves development of heterotropic bone in nearby muscle. Surgery or paraplegia also can cause myositis ossificans, or it may result from early treatment of a contusion with massage or heat, premature return to aggressive stretching or strengthening, or premature return to sport. About 7 to 10 days after injury, radiographs may show beginning ossification, which can progress to heterotropic bone in 2 to 3 weeks. Acute contusions should be monitored to watch for thigh and gluteal compartment syndromes.

31. How is myositis ossificans treated?

Early treatment consists only of rest. Weight-bearing is reduced with crutches. Once pain and swelling decrease and rehabilitation can begin, initial treatment is geared at gently regaining ROM.

Aggressive passive stretching should be avoided for 4 months after injury. Initially no strengthening takes place, but once swelling subsides, gentle isometrics can begin. NSAIDs or corticosteroids may be required to reduce persistent swelling. Once radiographs show that bony growth has subsided, gradual return to activity is progressed. One case study by Wieder showed possible resolution of the bony defect with iontophoresis with acetic acid followed by pulsed ultrasound.

32. Is surgery indicated for myositis ossificans?

Generally, no surgery is indicated. If the defect causes significant loss of function, surgery should be performed 9 to 12 months after injury when a bone scan shows no active calcification.

33. What is "snapping hip" syndrome? How is it treated?

Also known as coxa saltans, snapping hip can be internal, external, or intra-articular. The syndrome is characterized by reproduction of a snap or click at the hip with repetitive motion. Most commonly, the cause of external coxa saltans is snapping of the ITB or anterior fibers of gluteus maximus over the greater trochanter. Causes of internal coxa saltans include snapping of the iliofemoral ligaments over the femoral head, the suction phenomenon of the hip joint, and the movement of the iliopsoas tendon over the iliopectineal eminence or lesser trochanter. Intra-articular coxa saltans can be caused by the suction phenomenon of the hip joint, subluxation, a torn acetabular labrum, a loose body, synovial chondromatosis, and osteocartilaginous exostosis. The long head of the biceps tendon snapping over the ischial tuberosity can cause "snapping bottom." The syndrome is most common in female athletes, such as dancers, runners, gymnasts, and cheerleaders. The clicking in the hip is a greater complaint than pain.

Evaluation of which structure is causing the snap or click is made through palpation while the causative movement is reproduced. Treatment should progress toward alleviating muscle tightness or weakness that may contribute to the disorder. In general, modalities are not required because the condition is usually pain-free.

34. Define osteitis pubis.

Osteitis pubis is chronic inflammation of the symphysis pubis. It may occur after operations of the prostate or bladder or result from athletic activity such as soccer, race walking, running, fencing, weight lifting, hockey, swimming, and football. The mechanism of injury is repetitive stress of muscles with attachments at the symphysis pubis, such as the rectus abdominis, gracilis, and adductor longus. Pain in the groin or medial thigh is reproduced with palpation over one side of the symphysis pubis. Abdominal and adductor muscle spasm may accompany pain, and gait may be antalgic with movement adapted to reduce pain.

35. How is osteitis pubis diagnosed and treated?

Radiographs show loss of definition of bony margins with widening of the symphysis pubis. In chronic cases, the area may appear "moth-eaten." Bone scans are hot over the pubic symphysis. Treatment consists of rest and administration of NSAIDs with possible use of corticosteroid injections.

36. How does damage occur to the acetabular labrum?

It can occur in a dysplastic hip from changes in the congruency of the joint and abnormal joint stress. It can also occur in nondysplastic hips where labral microtearing, impingement, and cyst formation are precursors to arthritis. Dislocation can result in a labral tear. Anatomic variations in the proximal femur, such as a reduction in anteversion or head-neck offset, can lead to labral tears.

37. How can acetabular labral tears be identified?

- Fitzgerald's acetabular labral test—If passively moving the hip from flexion, adduction, and external rotation into extension, abduction, and internal rotation reproduces pain, with or without clicking, an anterior labral tear is suspected. If pain is reproduced by moving from extension, abduction, and internal rotation into flexion, adduction, and external rotation, a posterior labral tear is suspected. Fitzgerald found that 54 of 55 hips that tested positive also showed labral tears on MRI or arthrogram.
- Impingement provocation test—The patient is supine with the hip flexed to 90 degrees, adducted 25 degrees, and then maximally internally rotated. Pain indicates a possible torn labrum, acetabular rim, or snapping hip syndrome. This test has been found to be able to detect incomplete detaching tears of the posterosuperior portion of the acetabular labrum of dysplastic hips, but it does not correlate well with other arthroscopic findings of dysplastic hips.

38. How are acetabular labral tears treated?

Acetabular tears are treated by reduced weight-bearing using crutches and performing range of motion exercises for 4 weeks. If conservative treatment fails, surgery may be an option using open arthrotomy or arthroscopy. Fitzgerald found 13% of patients recovered when treated conservatively. Of those who underwent open arthrotomy or arthroscopic surgery, outcomes were improved if surgery was performed before damage occurred to the femoral head (which created unfavorable outcomes for approximately 12% of subjects).

39. Define piriformis syndrome.

Piriformis syndrome is pain in the buttock or posterior thigh and calf caused by inflammation or spasm of the piriformis muscle. Pain is referred in a sciatic distribution because of the close proximity of the piriformis to the sciatic nerve as the two exit the pelvis. Patients complain of pain with walking, ascending stairs, or trunk rotation.

40. How is piriformis syndrome assessed?

1. Frieberg test—The patient is positioned supine with the thigh resting against the table while the examiner applies passive internal rotation of the hip.
2. Pace test—The patient is positioned in a sitting position while the examiner resists hip abduction.
3. Piriformis test or FAIR test (**f**lexion, **a**dduction, **i**nternal **r**otation)—The patient is positioned in side-lying position with the tested leg facing upward. The test hip is flexed to 60 degrees with the knee flexed. The examiner stabilizes the hip at the iliac crest and passively moves the hip into adduction. A variation of this test is performed in the supine position; with the hip and knee maximally flexed, the examiner moves the hip into full adduction. EMG studies performed in the FAIR position have been found to identify patients who will respond to physical therapy intervention. The FAIR test has been found to have a sensitivity of 0.881 and a specificity of 0.832.
4. Beattie test—The patient is positioned side-lying as for the piriformis test. With the hip and knee flexed and the knee resting on the examining table, the patient actively externally rotates the hip by lifting the knee off the table and then holds the position.
5. Lee test—The patient is positioned in the supine hook-lying position (hip flexed 60 degrees with the foot flat on the table). The examiner resists hip abduction.

A positive result for any of these tests is reproduction of pain symptoms either occurring in the buttock or radiating along the sciatic nerve. Restricted mobility is also a positive finding. Further examination should rule out hip joint and lumbosacral pathology.

41. How is piriformis syndrome treated?

Modalities such as ultrasound or cold pack/ice massage can help to reduce pain and spasm. Fagerson suggests that massage or spray and stretch can help to reduce pain from trigger points in the muscle. Static stretching may be more beneficial than contract-relax if pain is caused by resisted external rotation of the hip. Modifications may be needed in the patient's base of support in the seated position. Crossing the legs should be avoided, and wallets should be removed from back pockets. Shock-attenuating insoles may help patients who spend a lot of time on their feet, especially on hard surfaces. Correction of leg length discrepancy with a heel lift reduces tension on the piriformis. NSAIDs may be necessary to reduce inflammation. Injection of botulinum toxin A in conjunction with physical therapy has also been found to be of benefit.

42. Define meralgia paresthetica.

Meralgia paresthetica is a nerve entrapment of the superficial branch of the lateral femoral cutaneous nerve as it exits through the femoral canal in the groin or next to the anterior sacroiliac spine (ASIS), where the nerve emerges from the pelvis. Paresthesia is referred along the anterolateral thigh. Common causes include tight-fitting garments such as a hip-pad girdle or a heavy tool belt, obesity, pregnancy, or direct trauma during contact sports.

43. How is meralgia paresthetica diagnosed and treated?

Tinel's sign may be positive medial to the ASIS or over the inguinal ligament. Sensory testing should be performed. Meralgia paresthetica is treated with rest. Symptoms typically subside in time; ultrasound and NSAIDs may help a persistent problem. Injection of corticosteroids or surgical nerve release may be required in severe cases.

44. What is hamstring syndrome?

In hamstring syndrome, the sciatic nerve becomes entrapped by adhesions in the proximal hamstrings, which result from repetitive strain. It is seen most commonly in hurdlers and sprinters, and pain may be worse with sitting or stretching or during sport. If conservative measures fail, surgical release of the adhesions may be successful.

45. How does the superior gluteal nerve become entrapped?

As the superior gluteal nerve passes between the greater sciatic notch and piriformis, it may become entrapped by compression of the muscle. Reduced internal rotation of the hip and anterior innominate rotation may be causative factors. Pain occurs in the gluteal area, and tenderness can be reproduced with palpation just lateral to the greater sciatic notch. Treatment is the same as for piriformis syndrome.

Bibliography

Anderson K, Strickland SM, Warren R: Hip and groin injuries in athletes, *Am J Sports Med* 29:521-533, 2001.

Cibulka MT, Threkeld J: The early clinical diagnosis of osteoarthritis of the hip, *J Orthop Sports Phys Ther* 34:461-467, 2004.

Croisier JL, Forthomme B, Namurois MH: Hamstring muscle strain recurrence and strength performance disorders, *Am J Sports Med* 30:199-203, 2002.

Eland DC et al: The "iliacus test": new information for the evaluation of hip extension dysfunction, *J Am Osteopath Assoc* 102:130-142, 2002.

Fagerson TL: Diseases and disorders of the hip. In Fagerson TL, editor: *The hip handbook,* Boston, 1998, pp 39-95, Butterworth Heinemann.

Fishman LM, Anderson C, Rosner B: BOTOX and physical therapy in the treatment of piriformis syndrome, *Am J Phys Med Rehabil* 81:936-942, 2002.

Fishman LM, Dombi GW, Michaelsen C: Piriformis syndrome: diagnosis, treatment, and outcome: a 10-year study, *Arch Phys Med Rehabil* 83:295-301, 2002.
Fitzgerald RH: Acetabular labrum tears: diagnosis and treatment, *Clin Orthop Relat Res* 311:60-68, 1995.
Hertling D, Kessler R: *Management of common muskuloskeletal disorders: physical therapy principles and disorders,* ed 2, Philadelphia, 1990, pp 272-297, JB Lippincott.
Iko K et al: Femoroacetabular impingement and the cam-effect, *J Bone Joint Surg* 83-B:171-176, 2001.
Johnston CA et al: Iliopsoas bursitis and tendinitis: a review, *Sports Med* 25:271-283, 1998.
Jones SL: Evaluation of the hip. In Fagerson TL, editor: *The hip handbook,* Boston, 1998, pp 97-159, Butterworth Heinemann.
Kendall FP et al: *Muscles: testing and function,* ed 5, Baltimore, 2005, pp 418-419, Lippincott Williams & Wilkins.
Klaue K, Durnin CW, Ganz R: The acetabular rim syndrome: a clinical presentation of dysplasia of the hip, *J Bone Joint Surg* 73-B:423-429, 1991.
LaBan MM, Weir SK, Taylor RS: 'Bald Trochanter' spontaneous rupture of the conjoined tendons of the gluteus medius and minimus presenting as a trochanteric bursitis, *Am J Phys Med Rehabil* 83:806-809, 2004.
Lee RY, Munn J: Passive moment about the hip in straight leg raising, *Clin Biomech* 15:330-334, 2000.
Lynch SA, Renstrom P: Groin injuries in sport: treatment strategies, *Sports Med* 28:137-144, 1999.
Magee DJ: *Orthopedic physical assessment,* ed 4, Philadelphia, 2002, pp 607-655, WB Saunders.
Nicholas SJ, Tyler TF: Adductor muscle strains in sport, *Sports Med* 32:339-344, 2002.
Reese NB, Bandy WD: Use of an inclinometer to measure flexibility of the iliotibial band using the Ober test and the modified Ober test: differences in magnitude and reliability of measurements, *J Orthop Sports Phys Ther* 33:362-330, 2003.
Sanders B, Nemeth WC: Hip and thigh injuries. In Zachazewski JE, Magee DJ, Quillen WS, editors: *Athletic injuries and rehabilitation,* Philadelphia, 1996, pp 599-622, WB Saunders.
Schache AG, Blanch PD, Murphy AT: Relation of anterior pelvic tilt during running to clinical and kinematic measures of hip extension, *Br J Sports Med* 34:279-283, 2000.
Sherry MA, Best TM: A comparison of 2 rehabilitation programs in the treatment of acute hamstring strains, *J Orthop Sports Phys Ther* 34:116-125, 2004.
Sim FH, Scott SG: Injuries of the pelvis and hip in athletes: anatomy and function. In Nicholas JA, Hershman EB, editors: *The lower extremity and spine in sports medicine,* vol 2, St Louis, 1986, pp 1119-1169, Mosby.
Suenga E et al: Relationship between the maximum flexion-internal rotation test and the torn acetabular labrum of a dysplastic hip, *J Orthop Sci* 7:26-32, 2002.
Wahl CJ et al: Internal coxa saltans (snapping hip) as a result of overtraining: a report of 3 cases in professional athletes with a review of causes and the role of ultrasound in early diagnosis and management, *Am J Sports Med* 32:1302-1309, 2004.
Weiker GG, Munnings F: Selected hip and pelvis injuries: managing hip pointers, stress fractures, and more, *Phys Sportsmed* 22:96-106, 1994.
Wieder DL: Treatment of traumatic myositis ossificans with acetic acid iontophoresis, *Phys Ther* 72:133-137, 1992.

Chapter 66

Fractures and Dislocations of the Hip and Pelvis

Teri L. Gibbons, PT, MPT, OCS

1. Describe the Garden classification of femoral neck fractures.

- Type I—incomplete
- Type II—complete, nondisplaced
- Type III—complete, displaced <50%
- Type IV—complete, displaced >50%

2. What are the treatment options for femoral neck fractures?

In older patients, Garden types I and II may be treated with three percutaneously placed pins. Types III and IV are treated with hemiarthroplasty because of disruption of the femoral head blood supply and high rates of osteonecrosis and nonunion. Patients with preexisting degenerative joint disease may benefit from total hip arthroplasty, although morbidity and mortality are slightly higher. Younger patients (<65) should undergo open reduction and internal fixation (ORIF), if possible, in an attempt to save the femoral head.

3. What is the difference between unipolar and bipolar hemiarthroplasties?

- Unipolar (Austin-Moore)—Only the femoral head is replaced; the native acetabulum is retained. This noncemented prosthesis is used primarily for bedridden and low-demand patients.
- Bipolar—The femoral head is replaced and snaps into a rotating polyethylene shell, which sits in the acetabulum. Bipolar prostheses attempt to reduce acetabulum wear. The superiority of bipolar prostheses has not been proved, although the dislocation rate is lower than with unipolar prostheses.

4. What preventive measures can elderly people take to avoid hip fractures?

Performing weight-bearing exercises, maintaining adequate calcium intake, decreasing caffeine consumption, cessation of smoking, elimination of household hazards (e.g., throw rugs), treatment of impaired vision, and hormonal implementation decrease hip fracture risk.

5. Describe the Evans classification of intertrochanteric (IT) hip fractures.

- Type I—Fracture line extends superiorly and laterally from the lesser trochanter.
- Type II—Fracture line extends inferiorly and laterally from the lesser trochanter.

Evans further divides the two types into stable and unstable patterns.

6. What are the treatment options for IT fractures?

IT fractures usually are treated surgically with a dynamic hip screw (lateral sideplate with sliding head screw) or an intramedullary device such as the Gamma nail (Howmedica, Rutherford, NJ). Both allow controlled fracture impaction. The Gamma nail may offer more stability for fractures with subtrochanteric extension. The choice of fixation is highly operator-dependent.

7. How successful are magnetic resonance imaging (MRI) and bone scans in detecting nondisplaced hip fractures?

Bone scans detect approximately 80% of fractures within 24 hours of injury. Sensitivity improves to nearly 100% at 3 days. MRI offers immediate, nearly 100% sensitivity in the detection of occult hip fractures.

8. Describe the mortality and morbidity rates associated with hip fractures.

MORTALITY RATE

- Approximately 10% to 30% in the first year after fracture. The mortality risk then returns to the prefracture rate.

MORBIDITY RATES

- Infection—2% to 17%
- Decubitus ulcers—20%
- Nonunion at IT—1% to 2%
- Nonunion at femoral neck—10% to 30%
- Fracture—3% to 4% (for hemiarthroplasty)
- Dislocation—1% to 10% (for hemiarthroplasty)
- Heterotopic ossification—25% to 40% (for hemiarthroplasty)
- Deep venous thrombosis—50% to 60%
- Pulmonary embolism—7%
- Mechanical failure—IT fractures, 12%

In 1990 there were an estimated 1.31 million new hip fractures, 740,000 deaths associated with hip fractures, and 4.48 million patients with disability from hip fracture.

9. Describe the treatment for isolated avulsion fracture of the greater and lesser tuberosities.

These rare fractures usually do well with limited bed rest and progression of weight-bearing and ambulation as tolerated. ORIF may be indicated for widely displaced fragments.

10. Define subtrochanteric (ST) femur fractures.

Fractures that occur within 5 cm distal to the lesser trochanter are termed ST femur fractures.

11. What is the recommended treatment for femoral shaft and ST femur fractures?

Fractures in children may be treated with immediate spica casts, traction, external fixation, or flexible nails. Older children and adults usually are treated with a locked intramedullary nail.

12. What rehabilitation considerations are important after hip fracture?

Capsular trauma is common with a hip fracture despite the lack of frank dislocation. Therefore hip precautions should be used even in patients with ORIF. Hemiarthroplasty allows immediate weight-bearing. Although the goal of ORIF is to allow immediate weight-bearing to tolerance, weight-bearing status should be based on the stability of the fracture pattern and fracture fixation.

13. Define the Morel-Lavale lesion.

The Morel-Lavale lesion is a closed degloving injury in which the subcutaneous tissue is separated from the underlying fascia. The avascular tissue then undergoes necrosis, resulting in accumulation of liquefied fat and hematoma. This injury is caused by significant blunt trauma that results in acetabular fracture and is at significant risk for infection.

14. What features distinguish a stable pelvis fracture from an unstable one?

Several classification systems attempt to identify which fractures of the pelvis are stable and may be treated nonoperatively and which fractures are unstable and require operative stabilization. Essentially the pelvis is a ring structure. Therefore a single break in the ring usually does not lead to pelvic instability, whereas double breaks (bony or ligamentous) may lead to vertical and/or rotatory instability. The posterior sacroiliac ligamentous complex is the single most important structure for pelvic stability. Fractures that lie entirely outside the ring (i.e., inferior pubic rami fractures) are stable.

15. What is a Malgaigne fracture?

Malgaigne fracture refers to a double vertical fracture of the pelvis, typically superior and inferior pubic rami fracture associated with an ipsilateral sacroiliac dislocation. The double fracture makes the hemipelvis unstable. Instability can lead to shortening of the hemipelvis and subsequent limb length discrepancy if left untreated.

16. What is the usual mechanism of injury for pelvis fracture?

Low-velocity injuries in older osteoporotic bone often result from lateral compression of the pelvis secondary to a fall. Patients often present with fracture to the superior and/or inferior pubic ramus. High-velocity trauma may result in fractures caused by lateral compression, anteroposterior compression, and vertical shear. These fractures tend to cause significant disruption of the pelvic ring and are therefore more likely to be unstable.

17. Describe the usual mechanism of injury for acetabular fractures.

Fractures of the acetabulum often occur when a direct force is transmitted from the proximal femur. When the hip is flexed (as in an automobile accident), the posterior wall fails. When the hip is extended (as in falls from a height), the anterior wall fails.

18. What are the long-term complications of unstable pelvic ring disruptions?

Chronic low back pain, sacroiliac pain, residual gait abnormalities, and leg length discrepancy are common complaints. Fewer than 30% of patients with >1-cm displacement of the pelvic ring are pain-free at 5-year follow-up.

19. Is physical therapy useful after hip fracture?

PT immediately after surgery is beneficial, based on functional independence measure (FIM) scores at 2 and 6 months postfracture. Home therapy programs, especially those including weight-bearing exercise, have been shown to provide improved strength, walking velocity, and sense of safety with ambulation. Postinjury levels of function are dependent more upon the age of the patient and their preinjury level of independence than the location of the fracture.

20. Does the rehabilitation site have an effect on recovery of function after hip fracture?

Patients treated in inpatient rehabilitation facilities had higher FIM motor outcome scores and were more likely to reach 95% of their prefracture FIM motor score by week 12 post–hospital discharge than those treated in skilled nursing facilities. Also, a significantly greater number of patients were discharged to home from the inpatient rehabilitation facility than the skilled nursing facility.

21. What are the effects of extended outpatient rehabilitation after hip fracture?

Binder et al. compared community-dwelling, frail, elderly patients in supervised physical therapy and exercise training versus home exercise. It was concluded that 6 months of outpatient rehabilitation that included progressive resistance training improved quality of life and reduced disability versus lack of improvement with low-intensity home exercise.

22. What are the differences in rehabilitation between men and women following hip fracture?

Although no differences in the rehabilitation process or outcomes of rehabilitation exist, there is a significant difference in mortality and morbidity. Men are at greater risk of developing a postsurgical complication than women. The risk of increased mortality and morbidity remains elevated for 1 to 2 years postfracture. Men are more susceptible to infections including septicemia and pneumonia than their female counterparts and are twice as likely as women to die within 2 years of hip fracture.

23. Does early mobility after hip fracture influence mortality?

A Finnish study found that patients who could not stand up, sit down, or walk within 2 weeks of hip surgery had the highest mortality rates at a 1-year follow-up. The authors recommend more intensive rehabilitation immediately after surgery. Suetta et al. found that early resistance training markedly reduced hospital length of stay. However, Lauridsen et al. found no significant reduction in time to discharge from rehabilitation with a more intensive program (3.6 hours per week versus 1.9 hours per week); this was probably attributable to a high dropout rate with the more intensive rehabilitation program.

24. Does neuromuscular stimulation to the quadriceps hasten return to mobility after hip fracture?

A study of British women found that neuromuscular stimulation, as part of a home-based rehabilitation program, provided faster return to mobility and a higher percentage of patients returned to preinjury indoor mobility levels by 13 weeks. Electrical stimulation has been found to increase functional muscle performance more than standard rehabilitation alone, but did not increase cross-sectional area of the quadriceps as resistance training did. Neuromuscular stimulation of the quadriceps versus placebo produced greater return to recovery of prefracture mobility in the stimulation group.

25. Is there a difference in home PT versus institutional treatment?

Once discharged from the hospital, home-based PT has been shown to yield better ambulation results within 5 visits than conventional institution-based rehabilitation for 1 month, following fixation of hip fracture.

26. What are the presenting symptoms of a patient with a hip dislocation?

Ninety percent of all hip dislocations are posterior secondary to the mechanism of dislocation and the weak posterior supporting capsule. The posterior hip dislocation can be differentiated clinically because the limb is flexed, adducted, and internally rotated. An anterior dislocation presents with the limb shortened, abducted, and externally rotated. Radiographs should be obtained to evaluate for fracture.

27. What is the postreduction treatment of traumatic hip dislocation?

After closed reduction, thorough neurovascular assessment continues for 24 hours. Patients may be placed in gentle traction for 24 to 48 hours. At that time gentle range of motion may begin. Weight-bearing restrictions continue to be a subject of debate, but in general patients without fracture may slowly begin progressive weight-bearing.

28. What complications are associated with hip dislocation?

- Osteonecrosis—1% to 17%; early reduction decreases the rate
- Degenerative joint disease—33% to 50%
- Sciatic nerve injury—8% to 19%; approximately 50% of patients recover spontaneously
- Femoral head fracture—7% to 68%

Bibliography

Binder EF et al: Effects of extended rehabilitation after hip fracture: a controlled, randomized trial, *JAMA* 292:837-846, 2004.
Browner BD et al: *Skeletal trauma,* ed 2, Philadelphia, 1998, WB Saunders.
Cornwall R et al: Functional outcomes and mortality vary among different types of hip fractures, *Clin Orthop Relat Res* 425:64-71, 2004.
Endo Y et al: Gender differences in patients with hip fracture: a greater risk of morbidity and mortality in men, *J Orthop Trauma* 19:29-35, 2005.
Heinonen M et al: Post-operative degree of mobilization at two weeks predicts one-year mortality after hip fracture, *Aging Clin Exp Res* 16:476-480, 2004.
Huittinen VM, Slatis P: Nerve injury in double vertical pelvic fractures, *Acta Chir Scand* 138:571-575, 1972.
Johnell O, Kanis JA: An estimate of the worldwide prevalence, mortality and disability associated with hip fracture, *Osteoporosis Int* 15:897-902, 2004.
Kusima R: A randomized, controlled comparison of home versus institutional rehabilitation of patients with hip fracture, *Clin Rehabil* 16:553-561, 2002.
Lamb SE et al: Neuromuscular stimulation of the quadriceps muscle after hip fracture: a randomized controlled trial, *Arch Phys Med Rehabil* 83:1087-1092, 2002.
Lauridsen UB et al: Intensive physical therapy after hip fracture: a randomized clinical trial, *Dan Med Bull* 49:70-72, 2002.
Lieberman D, Lieberman D: Rehabilitation following hip fracture surgery: a comparative sudy of females and males, *Disabil Rehabil* 26:85-90, 2004.
McLaren AC, Rorabeck CH, Halpenny J: Long term pain and disability in relation to residual deformity after displaced pelvic ring fractures, *Can J Surg* 33:492-494, 1990.
Munin MC et al: Effect of rehabilitation site on functional recovery after hip fracture, *Arch Phys Med Rehabil* 86:367-372, 2005.
Penrod JD et al: Physical therapy and mobility 2 and 6 months after hip fracture, *J Am Geriatr Soc* 52:1114-1120, 2004.
Rockwood CA et al: *Rockwood and Green's fractures in adults,* ed 4, Philadelphia, 1996, Lippincott-Raven.
Sherrington C, Lord SR: Home exercise to improve strength and walking velocity after hip fracture: a randomized controlled trial, *Arch Phys Med Rehabil* 78:208-212, 1997.
Sherrington C, Lord SR, Herbert RD: A randomized controlled trial of weight-bearing versus non-weight-bearing exercise for improving physical ability after usual care for hip fracture, *Arch Phys Med Rehabil* 85:710-716, 2004.
Suetta C et al: Resistance training in the early postoperative phase reduces hospitalization and leads to muscle hypertrophy in elderly hip surgery patients—a controlled, randomized study, *J Am Geriatric Soc* 52:2016-2022, 2004.
Wehren LE et al: Gender differences in mortality after hip fracture: the role of infection, *J Bone Miner Res* 18:2231-2237, 2003.

Chapter 67

Total Hip Arthroplasty

Mark A. Cacko, PT, MPT, OCS, and Jay D. Keener, MD, PT

1. How much force is placed across the hip during routine activities of daily living?

The force vectors created by contraction of the surrounding hip musculature are the primary determinant of hip joint reactive forces. The double-leg stance has been shown to create hip joint reactive forces of 1 times body weight compared with 2 to 3 times body weight for the single-leg stance. Walking produces hip joint reactive forces of 2 to 4 times body weight depending on the pace of gait. Stair-climbing produces forces of 3 to 4 times body weight on the hip joint in addition to significant torsional forces at the proximal femur. Simply elevating the pelvis to position a bedpan can produce hip joint reactive forces of 5 to 6 times body weight as a result of the required hip muscle contractions.

2. What are total hip precautions?

Instructions given to patients to help minimize the risk of postoperative hip dislocation are termed **total hip precautions**. The majority of hips that dislocate have a tendency to do so posteriorly. This usually occurs in positions of extreme hip flexion or hip flexion in combination with adduction and/or internal rotation. These hips tend to be stable in positions of extension, abduction, and external rotation. Most patients are instructed not to flex the hip greater than 90 degrees or adduct the leg across midline, especially during the first 6 weeks following surgery, while soft tissues are healing. Patients are instructed not to sleep on the affected hip and to keep pillows between their knees to prevent adduction of the hip.

3. What are different types of surgical approaches used for hip arthroplasty and how do they impact rehabilitation?

The most common approaches performed today are the anterolateral, direct lateral, and posterior. The anterolateral approach is performed by developing an interval between the tensor fascia lata and gluteus medius with either partial reflection of the medius or takedown of the greater trochanter to expose the underlying hip joint. After the components are placed, the gluteus medius is repaired or the greater trochanter is reattached. The posterior approach involves splitting of the gluteus maximus with takedown of the deep hip external rotators and conjoint tendon to expose the posterior aspect of the hip joint. After the components are placed, the posterior capsule and conjoint tendon are repaired. The anterolateral approach has been shown to have a lower rate of postoperative hip dislocation, as the posterior hip soft tissues are not violated. However, with this approach time is needed to allow the gluteus medius repair or greater trochanter osteotomy to heal, often restricting active hip abduction and full weight-bearing. The posterior approach preserves the integrity of the gluteus medius and greater trochanter and allows wide exposure of the hip and proximal femur often needed for revision surgery. Dementia, mental retardation, Parkinson's disease, stroke, or seizure disorders are relative contraindications to the posterior approach because of the greater potential for postoperative hip dislocation. Implications for rehabilitation include avoidance of active hip abduction exercises following anterolateral and direct lateral approaches for at least 6 weeks and more stringent adherence to total hip precautions following posterior hip approaches because of the potential for hip dislocation.

4. What are typical hip range of motion goals following total hip arthroplasty?

Range of motion following total hip arthroplasty usually advances rapidly. By the time of hospital discharge, patients should be able to extend to neutral and easily flex the hip to 90 degrees. Most patients will be able to achieve 110 to 120 degrees of hip flexion and will have the needed 160 degrees of combined hip flexion, abduction, and external rotation motion necessary to put on socks and shoes by 6 weeks after surgery.

5. You notice that a patient you are treating following total hip arthroplasty has developed increased calf swelling and localized tenderness. What should you do?

An increase in calf swelling, calf pain with dorsiflexion of the ankle, calf tenderness, and/or erythema are all potential signs of deep vein thrombosis (DVT) and should prompt the therapist to contact the physician as soon as possible. These findings warrant the immediate attention of the physician so that appropriate studies may be obtained. The development of DVT following total hip arthroplasty is very common despite the use of various types of DVT prophylaxis (aspirin, warfarin, heparin derivatives, and sequential compression devices). Even with preventive therapy, rates of postoperative DVT following total hip arthroplasty range from 10% to 20%. In spite of the high incidence of DVT, the rate of progression to fatal pulmonary embolism in unprotected patients is only 0.34%.

6. What are other typical complications associated with total hip arthroplasty?

There are several serious but relatively infrequent complications, including loosening/osteolysis, dislocation, periprosthetic fractures, sciatic nerve injury, heterotopic ossification, and infection. Dislocation following total hip arthroplasty is a multifactorial problem with reported rates ranging from 1% to 10%. The majority of dislocations occur within the first month following surgery. The prevalence of dislocation has been related to posterior surgical approaches, smaller prosthetic femoral head size, surgical technique, revision surgery, and patient compliance. Many dislocations can be treated conservatively with bracing and activity modification, particularly in the early postoperative period. Often, recurrent dislocation requires revision surgery. In a Mayo Clinic study of 19,680 hips, it was found that the incidence of dislocation was 1.8% at 1 year and 7% at 5 years and increased 1% every subsequent 5-year period. The incidence of dislocation also increased after revision surgery to between 9% and 21%. Of the patients who had a dislocation, 16% to 59% had recurrent dislocations. Nerve injuries occur approximately in 1% of primary total hip replacements and 6% of revisions. The rate of nerve injury is higher in females than males. Functional recovery occurs in approximately 80% of patients. Nerve injuries can increase with approximately 1.5 cm of limb lengthening, and if the limb is lengthened 4 cm, significant nerve injury will be seen in 28% of patients. The femoral nerve and the peroneal branch of the sciatic nerve are more likely to recover than injuries to the tibial branch or the entire sciatic nerve. Most patients who recover do so within 7 months, but recovery can continue for 2 to 3 years.

7. What are the outcomes following total hip arthroplasty?

Survivorship analysis in multiple studies has shown acetabular and femoral components lasting 15 to 20 years with acceptable rates of survivorship ranging from 85% to 95%. Pain relief and improved function correlate well with survivorship of components for most patients, with good to excellent results in 85% to 95% of patients at 15 to 20 years. Postoperative limp has been associated with takedown of the greater trochanter and hip abductor muscles. Thigh pain has been associated with uncemented femoral stems. It has been found that the strength of the muscles surrounding the operated hip joint was 84% to 89% of the strength of the uninvolved side in men, and 79% to 81% of the strength of the uninvolved hip in women. It was also found that significant residual muscle weakness persisted in the operated hip for up to 2 years following surgery. This persistent weakness could contribute to higher rates of component loosening. Physical therapy early in total hip arthroplasty does restore range of motion, but significant impairments in postural stability remain 1 year after surgery. It is recommended that muscle strengthening exercises be continued for at least 1 year after total hip arthroplasty (THA).

8. When can patients with THA resume sexual intercourse?

Out of 254 surgeons surveyed, 67% recommended return to normal sexual activity 1 to 3 months after total hip replacement surgery; 31% of the physicians permitted return to sexual intercourse in 4 weeks or less following surgery. In addition, the surgeons recommended that patients with hip revisions abstain from sexual activity for slightly longer time periods; because of the higher rate of reported instability, time is needed to allow for pericapsular and muscular healing. It was also recommended that extreme hip flexion, adduction, and internal rotation be avoided.

9. Can patients with total hip arthroplasties return to play tennis effectively? Do physicians recommend this?

The average return to tennis was 6.7 months (ranging between 1 and 12 months) when tennis was played approximately 3 times a week. National rating levels did not drop significantly—from 4.25 before surgery to 4.12 after surgery (with a range of 1 to 7). Before surgery, all patients had severe pain and stiffness while playing; this was decreased to 31% of patients after 1 year, and only 16% reported having pain at the time of the survey (which was a mean of 8 years following surgery). In a study of 28 physicians surveyed at the Mayo Clinic, 3 physicians approved of total hip replacement patients returning to tennis; 9 physicians approved only doubles tennis.

10. Can patients with total hip arthroplasties return to play golf effectively? Do physicians recommend this?

Most golfers returned within 3 to 4 months following surgery, while some returned at 4 weeks after surgery. According to hip society surgeons, the recommended average return to golf was 19.5 weeks, with a range of 12 to 52 weeks. On average, patients' handicaps increased by 1.1 strokes. Patients also noted increased drive length by 3.3 yards; 92% of patients reported no discomfort while playing golf, while only 6% noted having pain, but stated that this was decreased from preoperative levels. Golfers with a cementless hip prosthesis were recommended to decrease golfing activities for 6 to 8 months if they developed thigh pain while playing. Among doctors in the hip society, 69% requested that patients use a cart for the first year after THA. Of hip society surgeons, 96% permitted or did not discourage golf after total hip arthroplasty, and 68.3% did not discourage patients who had THA revisions from playing golf.

11. Does exercise before total hip arthroplasty improve outcomes?

Subjects that exercised before total hip replacement demonstrated progress that was 3 months ahead of that seen in the control group during early rehabilitation. The exercise group had two 1-hour supervised exercise sessions and also performed home exercises 2 times a week. The exercise group demonstrated greater stride length and gait velocity at 3 weeks after surgery. At 24 weeks postoperatively, in a 6-minute time test the exercise group was able to walk 549.7 meters, as opposed to 485.1 meters for the control group. Gait velocity was also faster in the exercise group at 24 weeks after surgery—1.57 meters per second, as compared to 1.36 meters per second in the control group. A gait velocity of 1.22 meters per second is the guideline used by city engineers who set traffic signal crossing times.

12. What is the postoperative weight-bearing status of a total hip arthroplasty patient?

Patients with cemented joint replacements can weight-bear as tolerated unless the operative procedure involved a soft tissue repair or internal fixation of bone. Patients with cementless or ingrowth joint replacements are put on partial weight-bearing or toe-touch weight-bearing for 6 weeks to allow maximum bony ingrowth to take place.

13. What types of patients are candidates for minimally invasive total hip arthroplasty? What are the outcomes with this procedure?

Patients that qualify for a mini-invasive total hip replacement have a lower average body mass index, are thinner and healthier, and have fewer medical comorbidities. Patients are typically between 40 and 75 years of age and usually do not have larger, muscular frames. Mini-invasive hip replacements reduce blood loss, transfusion requirements, postoperative pain, and hospital stays. Dislocation rates have been found to be between 2% and 10%, and 35% of those patients do not have a reoccurrence. Three times more patients ambulate on day 1 and 50% more patients meet all discharge criteria by day 3 with minimally invasive total hip arthroplasty: discharge criteria were ability to transfer, ambulate with assistive device, and negotiate stairs independently. The average time for patients to discontinue the use of crutches was 6 days, 9 days to walk independently without an assistive device, 10 days to resume activities of daily living, and 16 days average time to walk ½ mile. Patients were able to return to walking with no limp, secondary to insufficiency of the gluteus medius. Average return to driving was 6 days, as compared to between 4 and 12 weeks for THA patients.

14. What are the pros and cons of the different types of arthroplasty surfaces: metal-on-metal, ceramic-on-ceramic, and metal-on-polyethylene?

METAL-ON-METAL

- Pros—Metal-on-metal provides a strong material that resists bending, torsion forces, and fatigue, which allows it to carry a sufficient load. Metal-on-metal has an initial rapid wear period for the first 1 to 2 years, and after this has a lower and steadier wear. Metal has a 20 to 100 times lower wear rate than conventional polyethylene. Metal surfaces have been found to last over 2 decades. Wear rates have been found to be 25 to 35 μm/year for the first 3 years and then 5 μm/year thereafter, or $\approx 0.6 \text{ mm}^3$ of metallic wear debris per year, which is an order of magnitude less than that from metal-on-polyethylene.
- Cons—Metal-on-metal does produce metallic debris, which can be cytotoxic, altering the phagocytic activity of macrophages and leading to cell death. Metallosis and its effect on accelerating macrophage responses can damage the shell or femoral neck. There are elevated ion levels in the blood and urine, effects of which are unknown. Hypersensitivity responses in the immune system are found in 2 out of 10,000 replacements. There are also possible links to cancer because cobalt and chromium have been found to cause cancer in animals, but more research must be done on this. The coefficient of friction is approximately 2 to 3 times greater than that for polyethelene. Metal-on-metal replacements have higher cost, are heavier, and are stiffer.

CERAMIC-ON-CERAMIC

- Pros—Ceramic-on-ceramic is resistant to chemical and mechanical dissolution. Ceramic is hard, strong, and resistant to oxidation, and has high wettability. It has a low coefficient of friction and a scratch-resistant surface. Wear rates are 5 to 10 μm/year.
- Cons—Ceramic-on-ceramic is brittle, and there is risk of fracture to the femoral head and acetabular component. Chipping can also occur with impingement to the hip. There are a limited number of femoral head and neck lengths and sizes that are ceramic. There is accelerated wear with higher degrees of abduction of the acetabular component. Ceramics are also high in cost and have increased rates of acetabular component loosening.

METAL-ON-POLYETHYLENE

- Pros—Metal-on-polyethylene has low wear rates, costs less, and provides absence of oxidation. There is better adaptability and forgiving nature of the bearing surface. There is low friction, long-term stability, and low water absorption. Cross-linked polyethylene has been found to have better wear rates than standard polyethylene.
- Cons—Metal-on-polyethylene has a tendency to scuff the surface, wearing it away. Other cons with polyethylene are aging, creep, breakage, and abrasion. Polyethylene has a wear rate of ≈0.1 mm/year.

Bibliography

Amstutz HC et al: Prevention and treatment of dislocation after total hip replacement using large diameter balls, *Clin Orthop Relat Res* 429:108-116, 2005.

Barrack RL et al: Concerns about ceramics in THA, *Clin Orthop Relat Res* 429:73-79, 2004.

Berger RA et al: Rapid rehabilitation and recovery with minimally invasive total hip arthroplasty, *Clin Orthop Relat Res* 429:239-247, 2004.

Brand RA, Crowninshield RD: The effect of cane use on hip contact force, *Clin Orthop* 147:181-184, 1980.

Callaghan JJ et al: *The adult hip,* Philadelphia, 1998, Lippincott and Raven.

Dahm DL et al: Surgeons rarely discuss sexual activity with patients after THA: a survey of members of the American Association of hip and knee surgeons, *Clin Orthop* 428:237-240, 2004.

Harris WH: Etiology of osteoarthritis of the hip, *Clin Orthop* 213:21-33, 1986.

Harris, WH: Highly cross-linked, electron-beam-irradiated, melted polyethylene: some pros, *Clin Orthop Relat Res* 429:63-67, 2004.

Jackson-Trudelle E et al: Outcomes of total hip arthroplasty: a study of patients one year postsurgery, *J Orthop Sports Phys Ther* 32:260-267, 2002.

Magee DJ: *Orthopedic physical assessment,* ed 3, Philadelphia, 1997, WB Saunders.

Mallon WJ et al: Total joint replacement and golf, *Clin Sports Med* 15:179-190, 1996.

Mont MA et al: Tennis after total hip arthroplasty, *Am J Sports Med* 27:60-64,1999.

Pelligrini VD et al: Natural history of hip thromboembolic disease after total hip arthroplasty, *Clin Orthop* 333:27-40, 1996.

Pritchett JW: Nerve injury and limb lengthening after hip replacement: treatment by shortening, *Clin Orthop Relat Res* 418:168-171, 2004.

Rasul AT, Wright J: Precautions for patients to prevent hip dislocation after THR: www.emedicine.com/pmr/topic221.htm. Accessed April 13, 2004.

Silva M et al: Metal-on-metal total hip replacement, *Clin Orthop Relat Res* 430:53-61, 2005.

Snider RK: *Essentials of musculoskeletal care,* Rosemont, Ill, 1997, American Academy of Orthopedic Surgeons.

Wang AW et al: Perioperative exercise programs improve early return of ambulatory function after total hip arthroplasty: a randomized, controlled trial, *Am J Phys Med Rehabil* 81:801-806, 2002.

Warrick D: Death and thromboembolic disease after total hip replacement: a series of 1162 cases with no routine chemical prophylaxis, *J Bone Joint Surg* 77B:6-10, 1995.

Section XI

The Knee

Chapter 68

Functional Anatomy of the Knee

Turner A. "Tab" Blackburn, Jr., PT, MEd, ATC, and John Nyland, PT, EdD, SCS

1. What is a plica?

During embryonic development, the knee is initially divided into three separate compartments by synovial membranes. By the third or fourth month of fetal life, the membranes are resorbed, and the knee becomes a single chamber. If the membranes resorb incompletely, various degrees of separation may persist. These embryonic remnants are known as synovial plicae. Four types of synovial plicae of the knee have been described in the literature. The suprapatellar plica divides the suprapatellar pouch from the remainder of the knee. Rarely, this plica may imitate a suprapatellar bursitis or chondromalacia, and symptoms secondary to these conditions may be present. It courses from the anterior femoral metaphysis or the posterior quadriceps tendon to the medial wall of the joint. The mediopatellar plica is the most frequently cited cause of plica syndrome. It lies on the medial wall of the joint, originating suprapatellarly and coursing obliquely down to insert on the infrapatellar fat pad. This plica, sometimes known as a "shelf," lies in the frontal plane. The lateral synovial plica is rare and poorly documented. This wider and thicker plica is located along the lateral parapatellar synovium, inserting on the lateral patellar facet. The plica found to be the least symptomatic of all—the infrapatellar plica or ligamentum mucosum—is ironically the most commonly encountered plica. This plica is seldom, if ever, identified as the cause for plica syndrome. This bell-shaped remnant originates in the intercondylar notch, widens as it traverses the anterior joint space, and attaches to the infrapatellar fat pad. The capacity for this plica to block or obscure arthroscopic portal entry sites or interfere with visualization may be its only known significance.

2. Describe the symptoms of an irritated plica.

The exact symptoms will be determined by the location of the irritated plica. The most common symptom location is along the medial (inside) side of the knee. If the plica connects the patella to the femoral condyle, symptoms will mimic patellofemoral syndrome. The plica can refer pain to the medial meniscus and cause patients to describe pain "under the kneecap." It causes discomfort with prolonged sitting, prompting the term "moviegoer's sign" because the knee is less painful in extension. An irritated plica also may cause a "pseudo-locking" as the knee is extended and may "pop" beneath the patella or "snap" over the medial femoral condyle.

3. Describe patella-trochlear groove contact as the knee moves from full extension to full flexion.

Classic open kinetic chain or non–weight-bearing descriptions of patellofemoral tracking suggest that during the initial 20 degrees of knee flexion, there is no contact between the patella and femur. At 20 to 30 degrees of knee flexion, the distal third of the patella makes contact with the uppermost portion of the femoral condyles, with initial contact occurring between the lateral femoral condyle and the lateral patellar facet. At 45 degrees of knee flexion, the middle third of the patella contacts the femur. At 90 degrees of knee flexion, the proximal portion of the patella makes contact. Finally, at full flexion the odd facets of the patella make contact. In summary, as flexion angle increases, the contact area moves from proximal to distal on the femur and from distal to proximal on the patella. Additionally, femoral rotation creates increased patellofemoral contact pressures on the contralateral patellar facets, while tibial rotation creates increased patellofemoral contact pressures on the ipsilateral patellar facets.

4. Patella baja may result from adhesions caused by disruption of what bursa?

The infrapatellar bursa is located between the undersurface of the distal patella and the anterior proximal tibia. It can be violated in two types of surgery: (1) during distal extensor mechanism realignment when the surgeon medializes the tibial tuberosity; (2) during the harvesting of the central one third of the patella tendon for reconstruction of the anterior cruciate ligament (ACL). After the bursa is traumatized, bleeds, and heals, adhesions form.

5. What portion of the capsular ligament holds the menisci to the tibia?

The capsular ligament of the knee is often called the coronary ligament. Anatomically the fibers of the capsule run proximal to distal. The capsule originates on the femur and courses first to the outer edge of the meniscus and then to its distal attachment on the tibia. The two distinct ligaments proximal and distal to the menisci are called the meniscofemoral ligament and the meniscotibial ligament, respectively. The **meniscotibial portion** of the capsule secures the menisci to the tibial plateau. Injury to the meniscofemoral portion leads to a less stable meniscal tear. If the capsule tears completely, swelling may leave the knee joint completely, giving the appearance of a milder knee injury.

6. Describe the "lateral blow-out" sign of the knee.

Because the anterior lateral portion of the capsule, just lateral to the patella tendon, is quite thin, Hughston and others refer to it as the "lateral blow-out" sign. When swelling is present in the knee, this area bulges outward, especially when the knee is flexed. Patients often deduce that they have a torn lateral meniscus.

7. Discuss the role of the posterior oblique ligament.

The posterior oblique ligament (POL) is the predominant ligamentous structure on the posterior medial corner of the knee joint. The POL is located at the posterior one third of the medial capsular ligament, attaching proximally to the adductor tubercle of the femur and distally to the tibia and posterior aspect of the joint capsule. The POL plays a small role in preventing posterior translation of the tibia on the femur because the posterior cruciate ligament (PCL) is so overpowering. The main role of the POL is to control anterior medial rotatory instability and to provide static resistance to valgus loads when the knee moves into full extension. When an athlete makes a side-step cut, the POL contributes to keeping the pivot leg from opening in valgus, possibly acting in synergy with semimembranosus muscle activation. It also helps to prevent excessive tibial external rotation and femoral internal rotation.

8. What important function does the arcuate complex provide?

Each step at heel strike with the knee near full extension exerts tremendous force across the posterior lateral knee. The arcuate complex (posterior one third of lateral supporting structures including the lateral collateral ligament, the arcuate ligament, and the extension of the popliteus) helps to control internal rotation of the femur on the fixed tibia during closed kinetic chain function (or external rotation of the tibia on the femur during open kinetic chain function).

9. How does the anatomic arrangement of the ACL dictate its function?

The major functions of the ACL are (1) to stop recurvatum of the knee to control internal rotation of the tibia on the femur during open kinetic chain or non–weight-bearing function (external rotation of the femur on the fixed tibia during closed kinetic chain or weight-bearing function) and (2) to stop anterior translation of the tibia on the femur during open kinetic chain or non–weight-bearing function (posterior translation of the femur on the tibia during closed kinetic chain or weight-bearing function). This action stops the pivot-shift phenomenon. Therefore the position of the ACL in extension of the knee elevates it against the intercondylar notch, acting like a "yard arm" to provide strength to the ligament and prevent recurvatum. Internal rotation of the tibia on the femur causes the ACL to tighten. The two main bundles of the ACL are the anterior medial and posterior lateral bundles. The posterior lateral bundle becomes more taut in extension, and the anterior medial bundle becomes more taut in flexion. This arrangement allows the ACL to control the pivot-shift through the complete knee flexion-extension range of motion. Innovative surgical techniques have been developed to reconstruct individual ACL bundles to improve control of combined internal tibial torque and valgus torque; however, evidence regarding the implications of these techniques on improved patient function is currently lacking.

10. What is the function of the PCL?

The major function of the PCL is to stop posterior translation of the tibia on the femur during open kinetic chain or non–weight-bearing function or anterior translation of the femur on the fixed tibia during closed kinetic chain or weight-bearing function. Its femoral and tibial attachments in the central knee joint enable it to be an ideal passive decelerator of the femur. The PCL is composed of three bundles, which allow some portion of the ligament to be taut throughout the range of motion. When the knee is in full extension, the posterior medial bundle of the PCL is most taut. Even when all of the other ligaments have been resected, the knee maintains some stability to varus and valgus forces when the posterior medial PCL bundle is intact. As the knee moves into flexion, the anterior lateral bundle becomes more taut. When the femur moves into external rotation during closed kinetic chain or weight-bearing function or when the tibia moves into internal rotation during open kinetic chain function, the PCL becomes tauter.

11. What is the function of the iliotibial band? How does it contribute to the integrity of the knee?

The iliotibial band (ITB) inserts at Gerdy's tubercle or the lateral tibial tubercle. In this location it changes its function from extensor to flexor as the knee flexes at approximately 30 degrees. At near full extension, the ITB, through the action of the tensor fascia lata muscle, adds force to extend the knee. Once past 30 degrees, the tendon slips behind the horizontal axis of the knee, providing force for flexion. A portion of the ITB is the iliotibial tract. It has attachments into the linea aspera, which are very strong and help to prevent the pivot-shift. Traditionally, surgeons have used it with certain techniques to substitute for an ACL-deficient knee (ITB tenodesis). In combination with the muscles of the pelvic deltoid, the ITB and its fascial attachments contribute to composite lower extremity postural control during locomotion.

12. How does the ITB affect the pivot-shift test of the knee?

The ITB plays an integral role in the pivot-shift test. As the knee flexes in the pivot-shift test, the ITB shifts posteriorly. The ACL and the middle one third of the lateral capsular ligament normally prevent the tibia and femur from shifting. However, in their absence, the pull of the ITB allows the shift to occur, with the tibia moving posteriorly and the femur anteriorly.

13. Describe the anatomic reasons for patellar instability.

A high Q-angle (intersection formed by lines drawn from the anterior superior iliac spine to the center of the patella and from the center of the patella to the tibial tuberosity; normally 13 degrees in males and 18 degrees in females) predisposes the patella to sublux laterally. With the addition of a loose retinaculum, patella alta, and a weak or dysplastic vastus medialis obliquus muscle, the patella can easily sublux in the first 30 degrees of knee flexion. With a flattened lateral femoral condyle, the patellofemoral joint becomes unstable, even though the patella is seated in the trochlear groove.

14. Describe how patella alta can lead to patellar tendinitis.

One of the roles of the knee extensor mechanism is to keep the femur from sliding forward on the tibia (dynamic back-up to the PCL). When a person decelerates, the knee is flexed and the patella should be in the trochlear groove. If patella alta is present, the patella may not be in the groove, thus increasing stress on the patellar tendon.

15. Describe the anatomy of articular cartilage.

The superficial layer or tangential zone is composed of densely packed, elongated cells that contain 60% to 80% water. It is the thinnest articular cartilage layer and has the highest collagen content arranged at right angles to adjacent bundles and parallel to the articular surface. This layer has the greatest ability to resist shear stresses and serves to modulate the passage of large molecules between synovial fluid and articular cartilage. The superficial layer is the first to show changes with osteoarthritis. Next is the transitional layer with its rounded, randomly oriented chondrocytes (articular cartilage producing cells). The design of this layer reflects the transition from the shearing forces of the superficial layer and the more compressive forces of the deep articular cartilage layers. The radial layer is the largest articular cartilage layer. It is known for vertical columns of cells that anchor the cartilage, distribute loads, and resist compression. The calcified cartilage layer contains the tidemark layer (boundary between calcified and uncalcified cartilage). The tidemark layer is composed of a thin basophilic line of decalcified articular cartilage separating hyaline cartilage from subchondral bone.

16. Describe the arterial blood vessels of the knee.

Branches of the popliteal artery split and form a genicular anastomosis composed of the superior medial and lateral genicular arteries and the inferior medial and lateral genicular arteries. These vessels combine to give the ACL such a plentiful blood supply that a torn ACL results in generous bleeding and hemarthrosis of the knee after injury. The middle geniculate artery supplies the PCL.

17. Do the cruciate ligaments really cross?

From their tibial attachment sites at the anterior (ACL) and posterior (PCL) intercondylar areas, the cruciate ligaments cross before they attach to the lateral and medial femoral condyles, respectively. The cruciate ligaments also twist upon themselves during knee flexion and extension.

18. Describe the alignment of the femur and tibia during weight-bearing.

The weight-bearing line or mechanical axis of the femur on the tibia is normally biased slightly toward the medial side of the knee, creating a 170- to 175-degree angle between the longitudinal axis of the femur and tibia, which is opened laterally. If this alignment is altered by degenerative changes, fracture, or genetic conditions, excessive stress is placed on either the medial or the lateral tibiofemoral joint compartment. Tibial varum or femoral valgus (angle greater than 170 to 175 degrees) leads to increased medial compartment stress, whereas femoral varum or tibial valgus (angle less than 170 to 175 degrees) leads to increased lateral compartment stress.

19. Are there differences between female and male knee joint anatomy and biomechanics?

No particular anatomic or biomechanic knee joint characteristic is unique to either gender. However, females tend to have a wider pelvis, greater femoral anteversion, more frequent evidence of a coxa varus–genu valgus hip and knee joint alignment with lateral tibial torsion, a greater Q-angle (18 degrees versus 13 degrees), more elastic capsuloligamentous tissues, a narrower femoral notch, and smaller diameter cruciate ligaments.

20. What is the normal amount of tibial torsion and how does the physical therapist measure it clinically?

Tibial torsion can be measured by having the patient sit with their knees flexed to 90 degrees over the edge of an examining table. The therapist then places the thumb of one hand over the prominence of one malleolus and the index finger of the same hand over the prominence of the other malleolus. Looking directly down over the end of the distal thigh, the therapist visualizes the axes of the knee and of the ankle. These lines are not normally parallel but instead form a 12- to 18-degree angle because of lateral tibial rotation.

21. Which meniscus is most commonly injured and why?

Meniscal injuries most commonly occur at the medial meniscus. While both menisci are prone to injury, the medial meniscus is at greater injury risk for both isolated and combined injury in the young athlete because of its adherence to the medial collateral ligament. In addition to transverse plane rotatory knee joint loads, any direct blows to the lateral aspect of the knee while the foot is planted may lead to injury at both the medial collateral ligament and the medial meniscus. Additionally, as a result of generally greater medial compartment weight-bearing loads during gait, the medial meniscus is more prone to degenerative tears as we age. The lateral meniscus is more often injured in combination with noncontact anterior cruciate ligament injury.

22. What is the function of the popliteus musculotendinous complex?

The popliteus musculotendinous complex functions as a kinesthetic monitor and controller of anterior-posterior lateral meniscus movement—for unlocking and internally rotating the knee joint during flexion initiation, and for balance or postural control during single-leg stance. Increased popliteus activity during tibial internal rotation with concomitant transverse plane femoral and tibial rotation lends support to the theory that it withdraws and protects the lateral meniscus, prevents forward dislocation of the femur on the tibia, and provides an equilibrium adjustment function. Popliteus activation may be most essential during movements performed in midrange knee flexion, when capsuloligamentous structures are unable to function optimally. The anatomic location, biomechanic function, muscle activation, and kinesthesia characteristics of the popliteus musculotendinous complex suggest that it warrants greater attention during the design and implementation of lower extremity injury prevention and functional rehabilitation programs.

Bibliography

Basmajian JV, Lovejoy JF: Functions of the popliteus muscle in man, a multifactorial electromyographic study, *J Bone Joint Surg* 3A:557-562, 1971.

DeLee JC, Drez D: *Orthopaedic sports medicine, vol 2,* Philadelphia, 1994, WB Saunders.

Gerlach UJ, Lierse W: Functional construction of the superficial and deep fascia system of the lower limb in man, *Acta Anat* 139:11-25, 1990.

Harner CD: Double bundle or double trouble?, *Arthroscopy* 20:1013-1014, 2004.

Hughston JC et al: Classification of knee ligament instabilities, *J Bone Joint Surg* 58A:159-179, 1976.

Kelly MA, Insall JN: Historical perspectives of chondromalacia patellae, *Orthop Clin North Am* 23:517-521, 1992.

Lee TQ, Morris G, Csintalan RP: The influence of tibial and femoral rotation on patellofemoral contact area and pressure, *J Orthop Sports Phys Ther* 33:686-693, 2003.

Magee D: *Orthopedic physical assessment,* ed 4, Philadelphia, 2002, WB Saunders.

Nyland J et al: Anatomy, function, and rehabilitation of the popliteus musculotendinous complex, *J Orthop Sports Phys Ther* 35:165-179, 2005.

Powers CM et al: Patellofemoral kinematics during weight-bearing and non-weight-bearing knee extension in persons with lateral subluxation of the patella: a preliminary study, *J Orthop Sports Phys Ther* 33:677-685, 2003.
Yagi M et al: Biomechanical analysis of an anatomic anterior cruciate ligament reconstruction, *Am J Sports Med* 30:660-666, 2002.
Yasuda K et al: Anatomic reconstruction of the anteromedial and posterolateral bundles of the anterior cruciate ligament using hamstring tendon grafts, *Arthroscopy* 20:1015-1025, 2004.

Chapter 69

Patellofemoral Disorders

Terry R. Malone, PT, EdD, ATC, and
Andrea Lynn Milam, PT, MSEd

1. What is the Q-angle?

The Q-angle is measured by extending a line through the center of the patella to the anterior superior iliac spine and another line from the tibial tubercle through the center of the patella. The intersection of these two lines is the Q-angle; the normal value for this angle is 13 to 18 degrees. Men tend to have Q-angles closer to 13 degrees while women usually have Q-angles at the high end of this range. Because the Q-angle is a measure of bony alignment, it can be altered only through bony realignment surgical procedures. Despite the common opinion among clinicians that excessive Q-angle is a contributing factor to patellofemoral (PF) pain, it has not been shown to be a predictive factor in the outcome of patients with PF pain undergoing rehabilitation.

2. What is the tubercle-sulcus angle?

A measurement similar to the Q-angle, the tubercle-sulcus angle is reported to be a more accurate assessment of the quadriceps vector. It is measured with the patient sitting and the knee at 90 degrees of flexion. The tubercle-sulcus angle is formed by a line drawn from the tibial tubercle to the center of the patella, which normally should be perpendicular to the transepicondylar axis.

3. What may cause an increase in the Q-angle?

Excessive femoral anteversion, external tibial torsion, genu valgum, and subtalar hyperpronation can contribute to an increase in the Q-angle. When these conditions are found together, a patient is often said to have malicious or "miserable" malalignment syndrome.

4. What anatomic structures encourage lateral tracking of the patella?

Bony factors, such as a dysplastic patella, patella alta, or a shallow intercondylar groove, can contribute to lateral tracking of the patella. Soft tissue structures, such as a tight lateral retinaculum

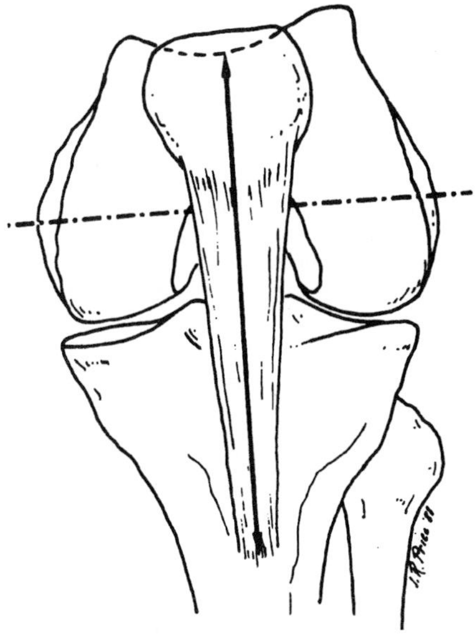

A normal tubercle-sulcus angle at 90 degrees of knee flexion. A line from the tibial tubercle to the center of the patella should be perpendicular to the transepicondylar axis. *(From Kolowich PA et al: Lateral release of the patella: indications and contraindications,* Am J Sports Med *18:359-365, 1990.)*

or a tight iliotibial band (which has a fibrous band that extends to the lateral patella), can encourage lateral tracking of the patella.

5. Define patella alta.

Patella alta refers to a cephalad position of the patella. Usually it is diagnosed by radiography and by determining the ratio between the length of the patellar tendon and the vertical length of the patella (Insall-Salvati ratio). The length of the patellar tendon is determined by measuring the distance between the inferior pole of the patella and the most cephalad part of the tibial tubercle. The normal ratio is 1:1. If the ratio is >1:3, the patient has patella alta. Patients with patella alta are more susceptible to patellar instability because the patella is less able to seat itself in the intercondylar groove.

6. What is the function of the vastus medialis oblique (VMO) muscle?

In their classic cadaver study of quadriceps function, Lieb and Perry reported that the primary function of the VMO is to counter the pull of the vastus lateralis and thus prevent lateral subluxation of the patella. They concluded that the ability of the VMO to contract and maintain patellar alignment throughout the full range of active knee extension enhanced the ability of the vastus lateralis to produce knee extension. Furthermore, when acting without the other quadriceps muscles, the VMO produced no knee extension.

7. How is chondromalacia classified?

The four types of chondromalacia are based on arthroscopic appearance:
- Type I—patellar surface intact; softening, swelling, "blister" formation
- Type II—cracks and fissuring in surface but no large cavities
- Type III—fibrillation; bone may be exposed; "crab-meat" appearance
- Type IV—crater formation; underlying bone involvement

8. How is PF pain classified?

Merchant classified patients according to five different etiologic factors: (1) trauma, (2) PF dysplasia, (3) idiopathic chondromalacia patellae, (4) osteochondritis dissecans, and (5) synovial plicae. These categories were subdivided into 38 subcategories. Others have classified patients with PF pain according to radiologic findings. A simple classification scheme that helps to determine treatment was proposed by Holmes and Clancy. The three major categories are PF instability, PF pain with malalignment, and PF pain without malalignment. In addition, Wilk et al. proposed a classification system that focuses on the underlying anatomic cause and presenting symptoms. The four major "rehabilitation" categories associated with this system require the clinician to recognize instability, tension, friction, and compression disorders and the specific protocols for their appropriate treatment.

9. Describe treatment based on the classification scheme of Holmes and Clancy.

Patellofemoral instability includes patients with patellar subluxation or dislocation—either recurrent or a single episode. First-time or infrequent subluxations and dislocations are treated with rehabilitation. Patients who continue to have problems after exhaustive therapy often require surgery.

PF pain without malalignment includes a number of diagnoses, such as osteochondritis dissecans of the patella or femoral trochlea, fat pad syndrome, patellar tendinitis, bipartite patella, prepatellar bursitis, PF osteoarthritis, apophysitis, plica syndrome, and trauma (e.g., quadriceps or patellar tendon rupture, patella fracture, contusion). Most patients are treated conservatively with physical therapy, including quadriceps strengthening, lower extremity stretching, and treatment of potential contributing factors.

PF pain with malalignment includes patients with increased Q-angles, tight lateral retinaculum, grossly inadequate medial stabilizers, patella alta or baja, and dysplastic femoral trochlea. Such patients often are treated with surgery only after an exhaustive trial of rehabilitation.

10. Describe the classification scheme of Wilk et al.

Category	Affected Anatomic Area	Presenting Symptoms	Examination	Treatment
Instability (hypermobile patella)	Ligamentous structures (passive) or insufficient musculature (active)	Patellar instability (subluxation/ dislocation)	Integrity of static patellar restraints Medial and lateral patellar glides	Avoid terminal knee extension Suggest exercise from 90° to 30° Use external support braces (taping, late buttress brace, pain-free ROM) Open- and closed-chain exercise
Tension (overload of muscle, tendon, or tendon-bone junction)	Muscle, tendon, or tendon-bone junction Commonly related conditions: jumper's knee,	Pain with eccentric actions, particularly maximal efforts	Palpation of inferior patellar pole, patellar ligament, and insertion of patellar ligament onto tibial	Open- and closed-chain eccentric exercise emphasized Pyometrics Stretch tight opposing muscles Physical agents and

continued

Category	Affected Anatomic Area	Presenting Symptoms	Examination	Treatment
	patellar tendonitis, and Osgood-Schlatter disease		tuberosity	electromodalities
Friction (soft tissue rubbing)	Friction points under sliding tissues Commonly involved structures: ITB, plica, fat pad	Pain with repetitive loaded flexion-extension	Observation of activity that replicates pain Palpation of structures associated with common friction syndromes	Avoid repeated flexion and extension exercises Exercise in pain-free ROM; exercise above and below painful ROM
Compression (articular and periarticular compression)	Articular surfaces	Osteoarthritis, pain with function under load	Compression testing of PF joint via special clinical tests or functional movements that apply compressive loads to PF joint Radiographic and other imaging studies helpful	Key is to increase quadriceps function to assist in absorbing weight-bearing loads Exercise in pain-free ROM in unloaded environment (pool)

ITB, Iliotibial band; *ROM,* range of motion.

11. How can the system of Wilk et al. be applied to common anterior knee pain disorders?

General Name/Disorder	Treatment Category
Lateral patellar compression syndrome	Compression
Global patellar pressure syndrome	Compression
Patellar instability	Instability
Patellar trauma (depends on structure)	Compression or friction
Osteochondritis dissecans	Compression
Articular defect	Compression or friction
Suprapatellar plica	Friction

continued

continued

General Name/Disorder	Treatment Category
Fat pad irritation	Friction or compression
Medial retinacular pain	Friction
Medial patellofemoral ligament	Friction or instability
Iliotibial band syndrome	Friction
Bursitis	Friction or compression
Muscle strain	Tension
Tendinosis/tendinitis	Tension
Osgood-Schlatter disease (apophysitis)	Tension

12. What is lateral pressure syndrome?

Lateral pressure syndrome, which can result in PF pain, is caused by a tight lateral retinaculum that pulls and tilts the patella laterally, increasing pressure on its lateral facet. Treatment includes stretching of the lateral retinaculum, such as medial glides and tilts. It is also beneficial to stretch the distal iliotibial band. McConnell advocates quadriceps strengthening exercises with a medial glide of the patella with patellar taping. If rehabilitation is not successful, a lateral retinacular release often is performed.

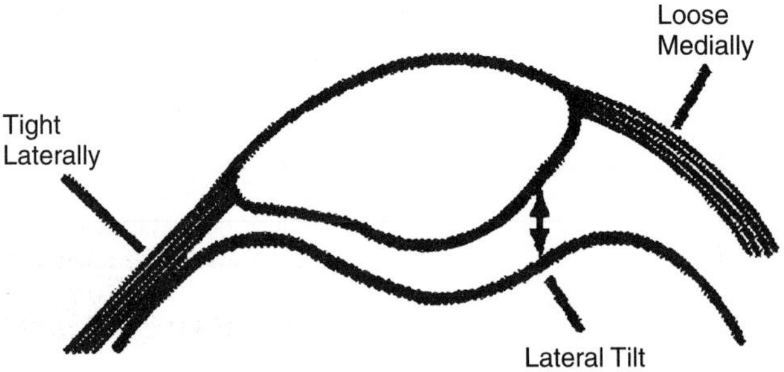

In lateral pressure syndrome, the tight lateral retinaculum causes a lateral tilt of the patella and may stretch the medial retinaculum. *(From Wilk KE et al: Patellofemoral disorders: a classification system and clinical guidelines for nonoperative rehabilitation,* J Orthop Sports Phys Ther *28:307-322, 1998.)*

13. Define bipartite patella.

Bipartite patellas still have an intact ossification center, most commonly at the superolateral pole. They are present in about 2% of adults and usually are asymptomatic. An anteroposterior radiograph of the bipartite patella may be mistaken for a fracture by the inexperienced eye. Extremely active people may irritate or disrupt this epiphyseal plate, causing PF pain. This area also can become painful after direct trauma to the patella. A bone scan may assist the clinician in diagnosing symptomatic disruption of the bipartite patella.

14. What is the difference between Osgood-Schlatter disease and Sinding-Larsen–Johansson disease?

Osgood-Schlatter disease is apophysitis of the tibial tubercle, and Sinding-Larsen–Johansson disease is apophysitis of the distal pole of the patella. Both occur during adolescence.

15. Can a leg length discrepancy contribute to PF pain?

Few authors describe the precise relationship between PF pain and leg length. However, the typical compensations that can result from leg length discrepancy theoretically may contribute to PF pain. Functional shortening of the longer lower extremity may involve excessive subtalar pronation, genu valgus, forefoot abduction, and/or walking with a partially flexed knee. All of these situations can distort PF mechanics.

16. Since articular cartilage is aneural, what tissues around the PF joint cause PF pain?

Normally, healthy articular cartilage absorbs stress across the PF joint. However, when the cartilage is not healthy, stresses are transferred to the subchondral bone, which is highly innervated. Subchondral bone is often thought to be the source of pain arising from the PF joint. Other structures around the PF joint also can cause peripatellar pain, including the infrapatellar fat pad, medial plica, bursa, and distal iliotibial band.

17. Define Hoffa's disease.

Hoffa's disease (fat pad syndrome) manifests as pain and swelling of the infrapatellar fat pad, usually from direct trauma to the anterior knee. Tenderness often is present at the anteromedial and anterolateral joint lines and on either side of the patellar tendon. A large fat pad also may become entrapped between the anterior articular surfaces of the knee with forced knee extension.

18. How is Hoffa's disease treated?

Treatment normally begins with protection of the anterior knee, particularly during activities where repetitive contusion may occur. Local physical agents such as ice or ultrasound also may be used. Quadriceps strengthening should be performed to prevent weakness or atrophy resulting from disuse.

19. Describe the mechanism for pain stemming from the medial plica.

The medial plica is a crescent-shaped, rudimentary synovial fold extending from the quadriceps tendon to around the medial femoral condyle and ending in the fat pad. The medial plica can be injured with a direct blow to the knee or through overuse activities such as repetitive squatting, running, or jumping. Inflammation and edema can lead to stiffening and contracture of the plica. Contracted tissue running repetitively over the medial femoral condyle can cause pain and even erosion of the articular surface of the medial femoral condyle.

20. How is plica syndrome diagnosed?

Patients with plica syndrome have similar complaints as those with PF joint pain. Pain is aggravated by running, squatting, jumping, and prolonged sitting with the knee flexed. The most frequent clinical sign is tenderness located one finger's breadth medial to the patella. The fold is often palpable, especially when the knee is flexed and the plica is stretched across the medial femoral condyle. Techniques designed to assess the presence of plica syndrome include the stutter test, Hughston's plica test, and the mediopatellar plica test, but their sensitivity and specificity have not been studied. However, magnetic resonance imaging (MRI) is reported to have a sensitivity and specificity of up to 95% and 72%, respectively.

21. Define housemaid's knee.

Housemaid's knee is the layman's term for prepatellar bursitis. This injury occurs when the prepatellar bursa is subjected to blunt trauma or repetitive microtrauma over the anterior knee, often found in individuals who work on their knees (carpenters or gardeners). Swelling in the prepatellar bursa occurs almost immediately and varies from slight to severe. Treatment consists of protecting the area from further trauma, applying ice, administering antiinflammatory medications, and performing exercises to maintain range of motion and strength.

22. Describe the mechanism for patellar dislocation.

The typical mechanism is external rotation of the tibia combined with valgus stress to the knee. Frequently this is actually the result of internal rotation of the femur over the tibia with the tibia thus becoming externally rotated and valgus associated with knee positioning. This is often related to strong quadriceps activation. Patellar dislocation also may result from blunt trauma that pushes the patella laterally.

23. What population is more susceptible to patellar dislocations?

Patellar dislocations occur more frequently in women than in men. Patellar dislocations typically affect the adolescent population, with the frequency of their occurrence decreasing with age. Patients with patellar dislocation often experience recurrent episodes, especially adolescent patients.

24. What is the rate of repeat dislocation?

Reports in the literature on the rate of repeat dislocation vary. Repeat dislocation rates among first-time dislocations treated with immobilization are 20% to 43%. The rate depends to a significant degree on the presence of congenital predisposing factors such as PF dysplasia.

25. Can hip weakness contribute to PF pain?

From initial contact to mid-stance, the hip rotates internally. The external rotators must control this motion eccentrically. If the external rotators are weak, they may not decelerate internal rotation effectively. The result is excessive hip internal rotation, which functionally increases the Q-angle and encourages additional contact pressures between the lateral patellar facet and the lateral portion of the trochlear groove. Powers has proposed as an analogy for this movement the alteration of a train track under the train.

Hip extension weakness also can contribute to PF pain. During a weight-bearing activity such as climbing stairs, the hip and knee extensors work together to elevate the body. People with weak hip extensors may recruit the knee extensors to a greater degree, thus creating greater PF joint reaction force. By itself this reaction force may not cause a problem; in association with malalignment, however, it may contribute to PF pain.

Several researchers have increasingly examined hip weakness as either a result or a cause of patellofemoral pain syndromes. Proximal strengthening is now often a significant part of clinical protocols, but well-defined clinical trials with specific reliable outcome measures are needed for definitive care.

26. What criteria are used to assess patellar instability?

1. Static approach—If the examiner can glide the patella laterally >50% of the total patellar width over the edge of the lateral femoral condyle, the patella is said to be unstable.
2. Dynamic technique—The examiner observes patellar tracking as the patient moves from approximately 30 degrees of flexion to complete extension. If the patella makes an abrupt lateral movement at terminal extension, it may be considered unstable. This finding also is called a "J" sign because the patella follows the path of an inverted "J."

27. Are radiologic studies useful?

Routine radiologic studies can show the depth of the intercondylar groove, level of congruence of the PF joint, presence of patella alta or baja, and patellar tilt. When instability is the focus, these tests are helpful as significant structural abnormality may limit the success of conservative measures.

28. What views are best to examine the PF joint?

The Merchant view provides an excellent view of the PF joint. The radiograph is shot with the patient in supine position with the legs over the edge of the exam table and the knees in approximately 45 degrees of flexion. The x-ray beam is aligned parallel to the femoral condyles. From this view, the clinician can see the shape of the articular surface of the patella and femoral condyles, PF joint space, medial and lateral facets, and degree of medial or lateral tilt of the patella.

29. Define the congruence angle.

The congruence angle is measured from a Merchant's view and provides information about patellar position. A normal congruence angle is ± 6 degrees (see figure). Other studies have shown the normal congruence angle to be –6 degrees in men and –10 degrees in women. CT scans delineate this better than radiographs and higher values tend to be associated with patellar subluxation.

30. Is MRI a useful tool to assess patients with PF pain?

With arthroscopy as the gold standard, McCauley et al. found that MRI had a sensitivity of 86%, specificity of 74%, and accuracy of 81%. The accuracy of MRI in identifying patients with chondromalacia patellae is excellent (accuracy of 89%) for identifying stage III or IV chondromalacia and poor for identifying stage I or II chondromalacia patellae.

31. Does strengthening of the quadriceps help patients with PF pain?

Almost all rehabilitation programs for patients with PF pain include some type of quadriceps strengthening exercises. Natri et al. examined 19 factors to determine the best predictors of positive outcome with quadriceps strength being the single best predictor of outcome. According to Natri et al., the smaller the difference in quadriceps strength between the affected and the unaffected extremity, the better the resultant outcome. Bennett and Stauber reported that a few weeks of concentric/eccentric quadriceps strength training within a pain-free range of motion obliterated an eccentric strength deficit and provided pain relief in patients with PF pain. Thomee compared 12-week isometric and eccentric quadriceps training programs in the rehabilitation of patients with PF pain and found significant increases in vertical jump height, knee extension torque, and activity level and decreases in pain for both groups. A recent review of the literature examining evidence for rehabilitation efficacy in these patients demonstrates good evidence for the positive impact of pain-free strengthening but limited support for ancillary interventions.

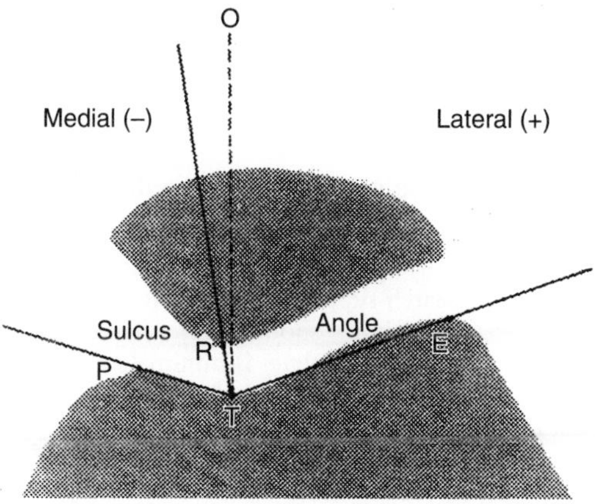

The congruence angle is formed by line TO and TR. A normal value is ±6 degrees. *(From Merchant AC: Classification of patellofemoral disorders,* Arthroscopy *4:235-240, 1988.)*

32. Do all patients need to perform aggressive quadriceps strengthening exercises?

The answer can be found by examining the classification schemes for PF pain. Patients should be treated specifically, depending upon the particular problem. In patients with patellar instability, aggressive quadriceps strengthening in the safe parts of the range of motion is a key component of rehabilitation. Patients with global patellar pressure syndrome may have a primary flexibility problem. Although quadriceps strengthening exercises are included in the rehabilitation program, stretching and mobility exercises are the main emphasis.

33. Does electromyographic (EMG) biofeedback strength training help patients with PF pain?

Few studies support the use of biofeedback training in the rehabilitation of patients with PF pain. Early research suggested a statistically significant increase in recruitment of the VMO compared with the vastus lateralis after 3 weeks of biofeedback training. The increase of 6%, however, is unlikely to be clinically meaningful. Ingersoll and Knight found that terminal knee extension exercises without EMG biofeedback resulted in a more lateral patellar position than performing the same exercises with VMO EMG biofeedback. The preponderance of the literature supports EMG biofeedback as an adjunct rather than as a primary focus.

34. What are the advantages of non–weight-bearing exercises for patients with PF pain?

Traditional non–weight-bearing strengthening exercises, such as seated knee extension, offer many advantages to patients with PF pain. Of primary importance, the knee joint and the quadriceps work independently during non–weight-bearing exercises. The only muscle group that can perform knee extension in the non–weight-bearing position is the quadriceps. Other muscle groups cannot substitute for weak or pain-inhibited quadriceps. Thus a maximal strengthening stimulus is provided for the quadriceps. In addition, ROM can be carefully controlled. Strengthening in a limited range can be easily achieved with most equipment. Finally, the amount of resistance also can be easily controlled with non–weight-bearing quadriceps strengthening.

35. What are the disadvantages of non–weight-bearing exercises?

Non–weight-bearing strengthening is nonfunctional. The quadriceps muscles do not work in isolation during normal activities. Strengthening in the non–weight-bearing position does not train the lower extremity muscle groups to work together in synchrony. In addition, in an exercise such as seated knee extension, the quadriceps are working maximally at end-range extension—the position at which the PF joint is most unstable. If the patient has PF instability and/or quadriceps imbalance that directs the patella laterally, the patella may easily track abnormally in complete extension.

36. What are the advantages of weight-bearing exercises for patients with PF pain?

The primary advantage is that the weight-bearing position is the position of function for the knee joint. An exercise such as the lateral step-up allows the quadriceps to train in synchrony with other muscle groups to complete the activity. Although the research supporting this concept is sparse, the law of specificity of training suggests this type of training should lead to the greatest improvement in functional performance. In addition, quadriceps activity is minimal as the knee approaches terminal extension. Therefore minimal quadriceps activity in the least stable position of the PF joint does not encourage lateral tracking of the patella. This advantage is especially important if the patient has patellar hypermobility or muscle imbalance that encourages lateral tracking.

37. What is the main disadvantage of weight-bearing exercises?

In the weight-bearing position, other muscle groups, specifically the hip extensors and soleus muscle, can contribute to knee extension force. Therefore patients with weakness or pain inhibition of the quadriceps may rely on other muscles to perform the knee extension. The result is insufficient stimulus for the quadriceps and minimal strength gains.

38. Are open-chain or closed-chain exercises better for a patient with PF pain?

Clinicians should focus on interventions that enable pain-free actions and target the underlying "cause" with an appropriate protocol (instability, tension, friction, compression). Integration of both open and closed activities appears optimal whenever possible.

39. Can the VMO be strengthened in isolation?

This question is highly controversial. Some studies support the concept of preferential recruitment of the VMO. The VMO is more active than the vastus lateralis during hip adduction. Laprade et al. reported that the VMO is more active than the vastus lateralis with tibial internal rotation. It remains questionable whether the differences are clinically significant. Many studies do not support the concept of selective recruitment of the VMO over the vastus lateralis.

40. Is it better to perform quadriceps strengthening in a specific part of the knee's range of motion?

The answer may depend on the patient's specific problem. If lateral tracking or patellar instability is a concern, the patient should avoid strengthening in the last 40 degrees, where the patella is not well seated in the intercondylar groove. If lateral tracking or patellar instability is not a problem, strengthening in the range of 0 to 90 degrees is generally safe. At the other end of the spectrum, extreme amounts of knee flexion (>90 degrees) result in higher PF joint reaction forces and should be avoided.

41. Tightness of which muscles can contribute to PF pain?

Tightness of several musculotendinous groups has been implicated as a contributing factor to PF pain, including the gastrocnemius-soleus group, hamstrings, and iliotibial band. Inflexible plantar flexors may not allow full ankle dorsiflexion, which may result in a compensatory increase in subtalar pronation. This increase may encourage lateral tracking of the patella. Hamstring inflexibility is thought to cause an increase in quadriceps contraction to overcome the passive resistance of the tight hamstrings. The result is an increase in PF joint reaction force and quadriceps fatigue as well as a decrease in dynamic patellar stabilization. Finally, the distal iliotibial band has fibers that attach to the lateral retinaculum. Tightness of the distal iliotibial band may encourage lateral tracking of the patella. The distal portion of the iliotibial band can be stretched by performing medial glides of the patella with the hip adducted. Patellar taping also provides a prolonged passive stretch to the retinacular tissues.

42. Should physical modalities be a part of the rehabilitation program?

Ice can be an effective modality to decrease pain and inflammation in patients with patellofemoral pain syndrome. In patients with inhibition of the quadriceps resulting from pain or effusion, electrical stimulation may aid in quadriceps muscle reeducation. It should be noted that the modalities are used to facilitate a second intervention rather than serving as independent treatments in the vast majority of rehabilitation programs.

43. Is patellar taping an effective treatment adjunct?

Patellar taping is thought to improve "functional" patellar alignment and decrease pain to allow the patient to perform rehabilitation exercises more effectively. Many studies report a decrease in pain or an increase in knee extension moment with patellar taping. Whether the taping actually alters patellar position is controversial and is likely to be minimal if present. Taping has the advantage over bracing because it can be customized to fit the patient's specific patellar alignment problem. However, the reliability of patellar orientation assessment has been poor. The majority of tape use is probably associated with attempting to provide a medial pull (taping lateral to medial) on the "patella."

44. Is bracing beneficial for the patient with PF pain?

Early reports suggested decreased PF pain in 93% of patients who used an elastic sleeve brace with a patella cutout and lateral pad. Shellock et al. used MRI to demonstrate centralization of the patella with a patellar realignment brace during active movement. Bracing generally is thought to "more likely" be beneficial in patients with patellar instability than in patients with patellar compression syndromes.

45. How is a patellar tendon strap supposed to alleviate PF pain?

No well-controlled studies have evaluated the efficacy or mechanics of the patellar tendon strap. One study reported success in 16 of 17 patients who used an infrapatellar strap. The proposed mechanism for the success of the strap was that it displaced the patella upward and slightly anteriorly. In addition, it was proposed that compression of the patellar tendon altered PF mechanics. Theoretically, elevation of the patella may slightly diminish PF joint reaction force, and compression of the patellar tendon may reduce excessive lateral movement of the tibial tubercle during tibial external rotation. Therefore, although the patellar tendon strap has been shown to provide pain relief, there are limited data available on its mechanism of action.

46. What is the relationship between foot mechanics and PF pain?

Two studies have demonstrated a relationship between foot posture and PF pain. Powers et al. found that patients with PF pain had an increase in rearfoot varus compared with controls without PF pain. Klingman et al. used radiographic analysis to show that orthotic posting of the subtalar joint in patients with excessive foot pronation results in less lateral displacement of the patella. These data indicate relationships but not necessarily "cause and effects." Further research is required for definitive implications.

47. Are foot orthotics beneficial for patients with PF pain?

Many clinicians treating patients with PF pain provide anecdotal support for using orthotics. The clinician must treat the patient according to the classification of PF pain. If abnormal foot mechanics are suspected as an etiologic factor, orthotics may play a role in treatment. Eng and Pierrynowski showed that patients treated with soft orthotics and exercise had better 8-week outcomes than patients treated with an exercise program alone.

48. When are distal realignment surgical procedures indicated?

Three disorders may require distal realignment procedures: PF instability, PF arthritis, or infrapatellar contracture syndrome. Criteria for considering realignment for each of these categories are outlined below.

PF INSTABILITY

- Three-quadrant medial patellar glide
- Tubercle sulcus angle >0 degrees
- Patella alta combined with generalized ligamentous laxity and flat trochlear groove

PF ARTHRITIS

- Significant PF chondromalacia or arthritis combined with PF instability indicates the need for anterior and medialization of the tibial tubercle.

INFRAPATELLAR CONTRACTURE SYNDROME

- If after lateral release and debridement of the fat pad and infrapatellar tissues there is no change in patellar height, a proximal advancement of the tibial tubercle is indicated.

49. What are the long-term results of nonsurgical management of PF disorders?

Patients generally respond well to nonsurgical intervention. The long-term success rate is 75% to 85%. Multiple outcome studies support the importance of strengthening as the primary activity demonstrating efficacy. Hence the first line of attack is an appropriate rehabilitation program, but the clinician must recognize that some patients require surgical intervention.

Bibliography

Bennet JG, Stauber WT: Evaluation and treatment of anterior knee pain using eccentric exercise, *Med Sci Sport Exerc* 18:26-30, 1986.

Bolgla L, Malone T: Exercise prescription and patellofemoral pain: evidence for rehabilitation, *J Sport Rehabil* 14:72-88, 2005.

Eng JJ, Pierrynowski MR: Evaluation of soft orthotics in the treatment of patellofemoral syndrome, *Phys Ther* 73:62-70, 1993.

Ernst GP, Kawaguchi J, Saliba E: Effect of patellar taping on knee kinetics of patients with patellofemoral pain syndrome, *J Orthop Sports Phys Ther* 20:661-667, 1999.

Fulkerson JP: *Disorders of the patellofemoral joint*, ed 3, Baltimore, 1997, Williams & Wilkins.

Holmes SW, Clancy WG: Clinical classification of patellofemoral pain and dysfunction, *J Orthop Sports Phys Ther* 28:299-306, 1998.

Hughston JC, Walsh WM, Puddu G: *Patellar subluxation and dislocation*, Philadelphia, 1984, WB Saunders.

Ingersoll C, Knight K: Patellar location changes following EMG biofeedback or progressive resistance exercises, *Med Sci Sport Exerc* 23:1122-1127, 1991.

Jee WH et al: The plica syndrome: diagnostic value of MRI with arthroscopic correlation, *J Comput Assist Tomogr* 22:814-818, 1998.

Klingman RE, Liaos SM, Hardin KM: The effect of subtalar joint posting on patellar glide position in subjects with excessive rearfoot pronation, *Phys Ther* 25:185-191, 1997.

Laprade J, Elsie C, Brouwer B: Comparison of five isometric exercises in the recruitment of the vastus medialis oblique in persons with and without patellofemoral pain syndrome, *J Orthop Sports Phys Ther* 27:197-204, 1998.

Lieb FJ, Perry J: Quadriceps function: an anatomical and mechanical study using amputated limbs, *J Bone Joint Surg* 50A:1535-1548, 1968.

McCauley TR, Recht MP, Disler DG: Clinical imaging of the articular cartilage in the knee, *Semin Musculoskelet Radiol* 4:293-304, 2001.

McConnell J: The management of chondromalacia patellae: a long term solution, *Aust J Physiother* 32:215-223, 1986.

Merchant AC: Classification of patellofemoral disorders, *Arthroscopy* 4:235-240, 1988.

Natri A, Kannus, Jarvinen M: What factors predict the long-term outcome in chronic patellofemoral pain syndrome? A 7-yr prospective follow-up study, *Med Sci Sports Exerc* 30:1572-1577, 1998.

Powers CM: Patellar kinematics part I and II, *Phys Ther* 80:956-976, 2000.

Powers CM, Maffucci R, Hampton S: Rearfoot postures in patients with patellofemoral pain, *J Orthop Sports Phys Ther* 22:155-160, 1995.

Shellock FG et al: Effect of a patellar realignment brace on patellofemoral relationships: evaluation with kinematic MR imaging, *J Magn Reson Imag* 4:590-594, 1994.

Thomee R: A comprehensive treatment approach for patellofemoral pain syndrome in young women, *Phys Ther* 77:1690-1703, 1997.

Tomisch DA et al: Patellofemoral alignment: reliability, *J Orthop Sports Phys Ther* 23:200-208, 1996.

Wilk KE et al: Patellofemoral disorders: a classification system and clinical guidelines for nonoperative rehabilitation, *J Orthop Sports Phys Ther* 28:307-322, 1998.

Chapter 70

Meniscal Injuries

Janice K. Loudon, PT, PhD, ATC

1. Describe the anatomy of the meniscus.

The menisci are wedges of fibrocartilage located on the articular surface of the tibia. The outer portion of the meniscus is thick and convex, whereas the inner portion is thin and concave. The menisci are composed of cells and an extracellular matrix of collagen, proteoglycans, glycoproteins, and elastin. The collagen content is 90% type I collagen with the remaining 10% consisting of collagen types II, III, V, and VI. The collagen fibers are oriented circumferentially, which helps to transmit compressive loads. Cell types are fibroblastic in the outer third, chondrocytes in the inner third, and fibrochondrocytic in the middle third. The menisci are attached to the tibia at their anterior and posterior horns. The medial meniscus is more C-shaped, whereas the lateral meniscus is more O-shaped.

2. What structures attach to the medial meniscus?

- Joint capsule
- Deep medial collateral ligament (MCL)
- Coronary ligament of patella
- Meniscopatellar fibers from lateral border
- Semimembranosus tendon

3. Is the meniscus avascular?

No. The outer third of the meniscus is supplied by the branches of the geniculate arteries. The anterior and posterior horns are vascular, but the posterolateral corner of the lateral meniscus has no blood supply. The outermost third is called the red-red zone, the middle third the red-white zone, and the inner third the white-white zone. Healing is greatest at the outermost third and decreases with inward progression because of diminished blood supply.

4. List the functions of the meniscus.

- Helps to transmit loads across the tibiofemoral joint by increasing the contact surface area.
- Viscoelastic properties add to shock-absorbing capacity.
- Serves as secondary restraint to tibiofemoral motion by improving joint fit.
- Helps with roll and glide of tibiofemoral arthrokinematics.
- May assist in nutrition and lubrication of the joint.

5. How important are the menisci in transmitting loads across the knee joint?

The medial and lateral menisci are responsible for carrying 50% to 60% of the compressive load across the knee. At 90 degrees of knee flexion, the percentage of the load borne by the menisci increases to 85%.

6. Do the menisci move with knee joint motion?

Yes. The lateral meniscus is more mobile because of its slacker coronary ligament. It does not attach to the lateral collateral ligament (LCL), whereas the medial meniscus attaches to the deep portion of the MCL. The lateral meniscus translates approximately 11 mm versus 5 mm for the medial meniscus. The menisci move posteriorly with knee flexion and anteriorly with extension. External rotation of the tibia is accompanied by anterior translation of the lateral meniscus and posterior translation of the medial meniscus.

7. What is the most common mechanism of meniscal injury?

The patient describes a turning or twisting maneuver of the leg in weight-bearing. Most acute meniscal injuries are associated with ligamentous injury. Additionally, the meniscus may become injured while rising from a squatting position because of excessive compression of the posterior horn in association with an anterior translation of the menisci.

8. Which meniscus is more commonly injured?

Tears of the medial meniscus are more common than tears of the lateral meniscus.

9. What are the signs and symptoms of a meniscal tear?

The patient complains of symptoms such as catching or locking of the knee joint, pain with twisting of the knee, and tenderness along the joint line. In addition, swelling may be present (usually 24 hours after injury), especially with activity. Some patients complain of a "giving-way" sensation secondary to instability. A locked knee that will not fully extend usually indicates a large bucket-handle tear.

10. Describe the most common meniscal tears.

Meniscal tears are classified as longitudinal, vertical (transverse), or horizontal. Bucket-handle tears are classified as longitudinal tears that eventually separate and may cause locking of the joint. The parrot-beak tear is a pedunculated tag tear located on the posterior horn.

11. Describe the clinical test for a meniscal tear.

The McMurray test is the classic manipulative test for meniscal tear. The patient lies supine with the knee in full flexion. The tibia is rotated, internally (lateral meniscus) and externally (medial meniscus), while valgus stress is applied and the knee is extended. A positive test is a painful "pop" over the joint line. The McMurray test has a sensitivity of 26% and a specificity of 94%.

12. What other tests are available? List their sensitivities and specificities.

Sensitivities and Specificities of Common Meniscal Tests

Clinical Test/Sign	Sensitivity (%)	Specificity (%)
Joint-line tenderness	85	30
Apley test	16	80
Pain at end-range flexion	51	70
Extension block	44	86

13. Describe the Steinmann point tenderness test.

The Steinmann test is designed to evaluate meniscal tears. It is performed with the patient sitting and the knee flexed. A tender point along the medial or lateral joint line is located, the knee is either flexed or extended a few degrees, and the tender joint line is palpated again. If joint-line tenderness moves posteriorly as knee flexion increases or anteriorly as the knee is extended, meniscal injury is indicated rather than capsular ligament pathology.

14. What is the most common surgical management of meniscal injury?

Arthroscopic examination followed by partial meniscectomy or meniscal repair is the most typical surgical management of meniscal injury.

15. When is surgery indicated for meniscal tears?

- Symptoms of joint-line catching and pain, effusion, locking, and/or giving way that interfere with daily function
- Failure to respond to conservative measures of physical therapy in the form of strengthening

16. Why is a total meniscectomy not preferred for patients with a meniscal tear?

Total meniscectomy results in premature degenerative arthritis of the knee, causes a 50% to 70% reduction in tibiofemoral contact area, and increases contact pressure by 200% to 235%. Partial meniscectomy increases contact pressure by 50% to 60%. Therefore partial meniscectomy is preferred.

17. What is the usual time frame for return to function after partial meniscectomy?

Usually 2 to 6 weeks are required before return to function. Patients ambulate with crutches immediately after surgery and with no restriction in range of motion. Rehabilitation progresses rapidly.

18. When is a meniscal repair indicated?

Meniscal repair is preferable to partial meniscectomy for salvaging the tibiofemoral joint. There are four basic surgical approaches: open, inside-out sutures, outside-in sutures, and arthroscopic with implantable devices.

Indications for repair are peripheral nondegenerative longitudinal tears <3 cm. Short tears of 1 to 2 cm have better success rates, and young patients seem to have the best outcomes.

19. What are contraindications for meniscal repair?

Tears greater than 3 cm do not seem to heal following surgery; transverse tears, even in the periphery, do not seem to heal. In addition, flap tears, radial tears, cleavage tears, or vertical tears with secondary lesions that extend into the avascular inner two thirds of the meniscus are not candidates for meniscal repair, except in teenagers.

20. What is a fibrin clot?

The fibrin clot is placed at the site of meniscal injury to form a wound hematoma, which facilitates repair because the majority of the menisci is avascular. The exogenous fibrin clot is morphologically similar to the reparative tissue in the vascular area of the meniscus.

21. Describe rehabilitation after meniscal repair.

Guidelines for rehabilitation include weight-bearing as tolerated in a drop-lock brace in full extension for 4 to 6 weeks, full range of motion in 4 weeks, and restricted loaded flexion for the first 4 weeks. Full weight-bearing without an extension brace is not recommended before the fourth week after surgery because compressive and torsional stresses may exceed the strength capacity of the meniscal repair. Patients usually return to activity 3 to 6 months after repair. After meniscectomy, rehabilitation is quicker. Weight-bearing as tolerated is started immediately, and range of motion is progressed as tolerated and should reach preinjury levels by 3 weeks. Twisting activities are limited for the first 2 weeks.

Phase	Goals	Treatment
Protection	Decrease pain and swelling Improve quadriceps function	RICE Active assisted range of motion Quadriceps sets Straight leg raises Ambulation (with crutches as needed)
Moderate protection	Improve range of motion Normalize gait Improve muscle strength Improve flexibility	Stationary bike Load-limited squats Gait training Aerobic conditioning (UBE, swimming) Stretching (as needed) Ice/electrical stimulation
Early functional	Restore normal range of motion Improve muscle strength, power, and endurance Improve proprioception Improve conditioning	Closed kinetic chain exercise Single-leg balance BAPS
Late functional	Return to function (sport/work)	Closed kinetic chain exercise Functional exercises (squats, stair-climbing, running) Sport-specific exercise

RICE, Rest, ice, compression, elevation; *UBE,* upper body ergometer; *BAPS,* biomechanical ankle platform system.

22. What is a meniscal transplant?

For patients with total meniscectomies, a meniscal transplant from a cadaveric specimen may help to salvage the joint. Meniscal transplantation is a fairly new technique; long-term outcome is unknown.

23. What is a meniscal cyst? Where is it likely to occur?

Meniscal cysts are ganglion-like formations secondary to central degeneration of the meniscus. They may occur on either meniscus but are more common on the lateral meniscus at the midportion or posterior one third. The patient may be asymptomatic or complain of a dull ache on the side of the cyst (medial versus lateral). Localized extra-articular swelling may be present and is proportional to the patient's activity level.

24. What is a diskoid meniscus?

It is a congenital deformity in the shape of the meniscus and is more commonly found in the lateral than medial meniscus. The abnormality affects the contact stresses and mobility of the menisci. The diskoid meniscus may cause symptoms of pain, effusion, or snapping. Partial meniscectomy may be required to create a more normal cartilage.

25. How accurate is magnetic resonance imaging (MRI) in detecting a meniscal tear?

MRI has a fair accuracy rate for detecting medial (88%) and lateral (88%) meniscal tears. According to Gelb et al., MRI has a sensitivity of 82% and a specificity of 87% for an isolated meniscal lesion.

26. Do surgically repaired menisci appear normal on MRI after 10 years?

A 13-year follow-up study of asymptomatic patients that underwent a previous surgical repair of the meniscus demonstrated abnormal MRI signals even though the meniscus had a stable union. These abnormalities at the site of repair represent edematous scar tissue, not the failure to heal.

27. What is meniscal repair using a bioabsorbable screw or arrow?

This is a relatively new technique that uses an all-inside device. All-inside devices for meniscal repair are attractive because they do not require additional incision or arthroscopic knot-tying. An arrow or screw is inserted across the torn meniscus to bring the torn edges together and stabilize the tear. Some of the more recent devices have been designed to allow tensioning of the construct after insertion. This approach is less time-consuming and has similar pullout strength to that of sutures used in a standard meniscal repair.

28. What are the outcomes of meniscal repair using a bioabsorbable screw or arrow?

Long-term studies are not available; however, short-term outcomes (12 to 24 months) are encouraging. In general, Lysolm scores postoperatively range from 80 to 90 and failure occurs in 7% to 10% of the repairs. Surgical complications and infections are minimal. A recent study demonstrated a 28% failure rate with postoperative complications, such as chondral scoring, fixator breakage, and postoperative joint-line irritation.

29. If a meniscal repair fails, can it be repaired a second time?

Yes; a case series of 14 patients that underwent a second repair had a success rate of approximately 72% after a 7-year follow-up.

Bibliography

Anderson AF: Clinical diagnosis of meniscal tears: description of a new manipulation test, *Am J Sports Med* 14:291, 1986.

Arnoczky SP, Warren RF: Microvasculature of the human meniscus, *Am J Sports Med* 10:90-95, 1982.

Arnoczky SP, Warren RF: The microvasculature of the meniscus and its response to injury: an experimental study in the dog, *Am J Sports Med* 11:131-141, 1983.

Arnoczky SP, Warren RF, Spivak J: Meniscal repair using an exogenous fibrin clot, *J Bone Joint Surg* 70A:1209-1217, 1988.

Cavanaugh JT: Rehabilitation following meniscal surgery. In Engle RP, editor: *Knee ligament rehabilitation,* New York, 1991, Churchill Livingstone.

Clark CR, Ogden JA: Development of the menisci of the human knee joint, *J Bone Joint Surg* 65A:538-547, 1983.

Fairbank TJ: Knee joint changes after meniscectomy, *J Bone Joint Surg* 30B:664-670, 1948.

Gelb HJ et al: Magnetic resonance imaging of knee disorders, *Am J Sports Med* 24:99-103, 1996.

Gray JC: Neural and vascular anatomy of the menisci of the human knee, *J Orthop Sports Phys Ther* 29:23-30, 1999.

Kelly MA et al: Imaging of the knee: clarification of its role, *Arthroscopy* 7:78-82, 1991.
Kurzweil PR, Tifford CD, Ignacio EM: Unsatisfactory clinical results of meniscal repair using the meniscus arrow, *Arthroscopy* 21:905, 2005.
Rosenberg TD et al: Arthroscopic meniscal repair evaluated with repeat arthroscopy, *Arthroscopy* 2:14-20, 1986.
Stone KR, Rosenberg T: Surgical technique of meniscal transplantation, *Arthroscopy* 9:234-237, 1993.
Voloshin I et al: Results of repeat meniscal repair, *Am J Sports Med* 31:874-880, 2003.
Walker PS, Erkman PJ: The role of the menisci in force transmission across the knee, *Clin Orthop* 109:184, 1975.

Chapter 71

Ligamentous Injuries of the Knee

Eric Wint, PT, OCS

1. What ligaments of the knee can be disrupted by a hyperextension force?

The first stop to recurvatum is the anterior cruciate ligament (ACL). As the knee extends, the intercondylar shelf comes in contact with the ACL in mid-stance, tearing the ligament in a mop-end tear. The result is an isolated ACL tear. The patient shows a positive Lachman's test. If the anterior lateral capsule is weak, the patient demonstrates positive pivot-shift and anterior drawer tests with the tibia in neutral. The diagnosis is anterior lateral rotary instability.

2. Which ligament of the knee may be disrupted by a motor vehicle accident in which the tibial tuberosity strikes the dashboard?

The posterior cruciate ligament (PCL) is the ligament affected in this type of injury. The dashboard drives the tibia posteriorly until the patella and distal end of the femur reach the dashboard and stop the posterior movement. The result is an isolated PCL injury. Clinical testing indicates the loss of "step down" but no other instability. The diagnosis is straight posterior instability.

3. Which ligament may be injured by a crossover cut maneuver?

The ACL is subjected to severe internal rotation stresses. The middle one third of the lateral capsule assists the ACL in controlling internal rotation and varus stress. If the knee pops back into hyperextension during the cut, the potential for ACL injury is high.

4. Which structures of the knee can be injured during a side-step cut maneuver with valgus force?

A side-step maneuver stresses the medial side of the knee as the lead leg steps to the side, the plant knee flexes, and the femur rotates internally as the tibia rotates externally. Valgus stress is applied across the medial side of the knee joint. The medial collateral ligament (MCL) or tibial collateral ligament resists the valgus force. The middle one third and posterior one third of the MCL provide the first resistance to rotation. If the force continues, the medial meniscus may be torn because of the stress across the meniscofemoral and meniscotibial ligaments. On the lateral side, the lateral meniscus may be impinged and damaged. Further force damages the ACL; if even more force is applied, the patella may dislocate, tearing the raphe of the vastus medialis obliquus (VMO).

5. How might an occult osteochondral lesion be associated with an ACL rupture and where is it commonly found?

Johnson et al. found that as many as 80% of all ACL disruption injuries have an associated osteochondral lesion. Lateral compartment chondral lesions associated with ACL ruptures are a result of the abnormal anterior and rotary translation of the tibia during common ACL mechanisms of injury. This lesion or "bone bruise" is commonly found in one of two locations: the lateral femoral condyle at the sulcus terminalis (anatomic junction between the tibiofemoral articular surface and the patellofemoral articular surface) or the posterolateral tibial plateau.

6. How might an occult osteochondral lesion associated with an ACL rupture affect long-term outcomes?

Sixty percent of patients with a documented osteochondral lesion at the time of ACL rupture demonstrated persistent MRI evidence of osteochondral defect and symptom sequelae at 5.5 years' follow-up. A significant percentage of patients who have immediate ACL reconstruction develop degenerative changes in the surgical knee within 5 to 10 years. Osteochondral lesions may be the event that predisposes the knee joint to this postsurgical degenerative osteoarthritis.

7. What is a Segond fracture?

A Segond fracture is an avulsion fracture of the anterolateral margin of the lateral tibial plateau, associated with ACL tears. The fracture is distinguished by a "lateral capsular sign" on radiographs and considered pathognomonic for ACL tears. The mechanism of injury is abnormal internal rotation stress of the tibia that causes abnormal tension on the central portion of the lateral capsular ligament, resulting in the avulsion.

8. Does research consistently support the use of bone-patellar tendon-bone graft versus hamstring tendon graft for ACL reconstruction?

No. Bone-patellar tendon-bone (BPTB) grafts and double/quadruple hamstring tendon (HT) grafts, using the semitendinosus and gracilis, continue to be the most widely used autologous grafts. Neither graft tissue has consistently been shown to be superior for ACL reconstructions. The incidence of postsurgical instability is not significantly different between BPTP and HT grafts; however, BTBP grafts are more likely to result in reconstructions with normal Lachman and pivot-shift testing, fewer incidences of reinjury postsurgically, and fewer cases of significant postsurgical flexion loss. On the other hand, research demonstrates that HT grafts have fewer incidences of patellofemoral crepitus, less kneeling pain, and fewer incidences of significant residual extension loss.

9. Which ACL graft is better—allograft or autograft?

Autografts are better. Allografts may transmit infections and are a bit looser and less stiff. Allografts are an acceptable alternative, especially in patients who do not put extreme stress on the knee. The patellar tendon graft is the most commonly used, but it is associated with patellofemoral morbidity. The quadriceps tendon graft appears to have all of the benefits of the patellar tendon graft without patellofemoral morbidity, but it is less commonly used. The hamstring graft is being used more frequently. Many believe that it has all of the benefits of the patellar tendon graft and few disadvantages.

10. What is the incidence of ACL injury in females versus males and what are the anatomic, physiologic, and neuromuscular risk factors that could be responsible for a higher percentage of female athletes sustaining ACL tears than male athletes?

Female athletes are 2.4 to 9.5 times more likely to sustain an ACL injury than male athletes. The following risk factors have been proposed:

ANATOMIC RISK FACTORS

- Less muscle mass per total body weight
- Greater joint hyperextension
- Greater joint rotational laxity
- Increased femoral internal rotation (IR), causing valgus stress at the knee
- Increased valgus stress at the knee secondary to increased Q-angle
- Increased femoral anteversion, causing increased valgus positioning at the knee
- Increased foot pronation, causing increased tibial internal rotation and valgus positioning at the knee
- Smaller diameter ACL housed in smaller intracondylar notch, although no consensus as to the role of notch size in ACL injury
- Smaller skeletal size

PHYSIOLOGIC RISK FACTORS

- Although there is no consensus in the literature, there have been studies correlating menstruation with ACL tears in women. Estrogen and progesterone receptor sites have been reported in human ACL cells. It has been proposed that levels of these hormones may have deleterious effects on the tensile strength of the ACL.

NEUROMUSCULAR RISK FACTORS

- Increased electromechanical delay (elapsed time between neuroactivation of the muscle and actual force generated secondary to increased extensibility of the musculotendinous unit)
- Contraction of quadriceps rather than hamstrings, which are supportive to the ACL, in response to anterior tibial translation
- Tendency for females to land from a jump and perform cutting activities in a more upright position with increased trunk, knee, and hip extension

11. What is the effectiveness, if any, of ACL prevention programs for female athletes?

A recent study by Madelbaum et al. shows as much as an 88% decrease in incidence of ACL injury at 1-year follow-up and a 74% reduction of ACL injury at 2-years follow-up after sports-specific prevention training for a sample of over 1000 female soccer players. However, literature is scarce that describes which regimens are most effective and the long-term outcomes after training.

12. What is the epidemiology of ACL tears in the United States?

Tears of the ACL have been estimated to occur in 1 out of 3000 to 3500 people in the United States each year. As a result, as many as 100,000 ACL reconstructions are performed annually. The incidence of ACL injury in females is 2.4 to 9.5 times greater than in males. Reinjury of the ACL reconstruction graft is 12% to 15% in males and 25% to 30% in females. About 70% of all ACL injuries are a result of sports participation: 10% to 15% of ACL injuries occur in soccer, 10% to 13% in skiing, 9% to 15% in football, 9% to 10% in baseball, and 8% to 15% in basketball. Sixty-one percent occur in the 15- to 29-year-old age-group and 23% in the 30- to 44-year-old age-group. About 70% of all ACL injuries are a result of noncontact mechanisms, and 47% of all severe knee ligamentous injuries involve the ACL (single tear).

13. Define anteromedial rotary instability. Which clinical tests are positive for this type of instability?

The classic mechanism of injury for anteromedial rotary instability is the football "clip." The slightly flexed knee is forced into valgus while the tibia externally rotates. The structures that usually are disrupted are the MCL, posterior oblique ligament, middle third of the capsular ligament, and ACL. The Lachman test, anterior drawer test, and valgus stress test at 20 to 30 degrees are positive.

14. Define anterolateral rotary instability. Which clinical tests are positive?

The classic mechanism of injury for anterolateral rotary instability is noncontact deceleration on a planted foot. The slightly flexed knee is forced into varus while the tibia internally rotates. The structures that usually are disrupted are the ACL, LCL, iliotibial band (ITB), and possibly the arcuate complex in the posterior lateral corner of the knee. The pivot-shift test is positive.

15. Define posterolateral rotary instability. Which clinical tests are positive?

A varus blow from the anterior direction on a slightly flexed knee with the foot planted may result in posterolateral rotary instability (PLRI). The soft tissues involved in a PLRI are the arcuate complex (LCL, posterior oblique ligament, and popliteus tendon). The reverse pivot shift, the posterior lateral drawer sign, the external rotation recurvatum test, and Loomer's PLRI test may be positive.

16. Define straight medial knee ligament instability. Which clinical tests are positive?

If the knee receives a valgus blow in extension, the PCL, MCL, and middle one third of the capsular ligaments may be disrupted. In addition, the medial meniscus is pulled apart, and the lateral meniscus is compressed. Laxity noted with valgus stress test in extension indicates disruption to the PCL in addition to the MCL damage.

17. Define straight lateral knee ligament instability. Which clinical tests are positive?

If the knee receives a varus blow in extension, the PCL, LCL, ITB, tract fibers, and middle one third of the capsular ligaments may be disrupted. In addition, the lateral meniscus is pulled apart, and the medial meniscus is compressed. Functionally the patient has difficulty on heel strike as the knee shifts laterally. Laxity noted with the varus stress test in extension indicates disruption to the PCL in addition to the LCL damage.

18. Why is there no such thing as posterior medial rotary instability?

Following the logic of the other rotary instabilities, a posterior medial rotary instability would be increased internal rotation of the tibia on the femur. Internal rotation of the tibia on the femur is controlled by the ACL and PCL. Therefore if the posterior medial corner is damaged, the cruciate ligaments stop the instability. By definition, posterior medial rotary instability cannot exist. If the PCL is torn, the patient has straight instability.

19. How accurate is a clinical exam for ACL injury?

A well-trained clinician can diagnose an ACL tear with the use of his or her hands and perhaps a knee arthrometer. Lachman's test is approximately 95% sensitive. Sensitivity decreases in larger patients. The pivot-shift is pathognomonic of ACL rupture, but false-positive rates approach 30%. The prone alternate Lachman test may be significantly more sensitive (78%) than the anterior drawer (59%) or the standard Lachman test (28%) in patients with large thighs.

20. What is the healing rate of a patellar tendon autograft?

Original animal studies indicate 18 to 24 months. The patellar tendon autograft is almost 100% stronger than the ACL. Newer research indicates that it takes 4000 N to rupture the patellar tendon graft.

21. Do ACL tears require surgery?

Approximately 33% of ACL injuries require surgery immediately and another 33% require surgery after reinjury. Some authors believe that a "capsularly dominant" knee may function well if only the ACL is torn. The ACL and PCL are extrasynovial. When their sheaths are torn, they are subjected to the strong phagocytic action of synovial fluid. Although they have an excellent blood supply, the ligaments do not heal even when the ends are approximated by surgery.

22. In an open-chain active extension motion, where does maximal stress fall on the ACL?

In open-chain knee extension exercise, anterior translation of the tibia on the femur puts stress on the structures that restrict motion. The force is highest at 20 degrees of knee flexion (beginning at 45 degrees) and diminishes to very little force at full extension, when the quadriceps compresses only the tibia and femur.

23. Do open- and closed-chain exercises put equal amounts of stress on the ACL?

In vitro strain gauge studies indicate that closed-chain squats and open-chain knee extensions put almost equal amounts of strain on the ACL. If resistance is increased in either type of exercise, the strain increases.

24. Can an independent, home-based rehabilitation program be successful for the postsurgical ACL reconstruction patient who is unable to attend skilled physical therapy sessions?

A home-based program can be an effective alternative to supervised rehabilitation. No significant statistical differences in long-term outcomes have been found between groups who participated in home-based rehabilitation and those who participated in physical therapy in a clinical setting (provided there is ample monitoring of outcomes at regular intervals and attention paid to any warning signs by the physician and/or physical therapist). Studies suggest that for an athlete or patient who will be returning to a demanding, active lifestyle, phase III and phase IV of the ACL rehabilitation process, involving more advanced physical demands such as cutting and plyometric loading, had better outcomes when supervised by a skilled clinician. Other similar research suggests that there are higher dropout rates and lower patient satisfaction rates among patient groups performing a home-based program.

25. What criteria are used for the diagnosis of ACL tears with joint arthrometry?

- Absolute translation >10 mm (at 20 lb)
- Bilateral differences >3 mm

If both criteria are met, arthrometry is 99% sensitive for ACL injury.

26. How accurate is magnetic resonance imaging (MRI) in detecting ACL injury?

Sensitivity is 95% to 100%, and specificity is approximately 50%. MRI is 90% accurate for an acute rupture <24 hours old. This is less accurate than a physical exam.

27. How strong are ACL grafts?

A 10-mm-wide bone-patella-bone (BPB) graft can be 1½ times as strong as the normal ACL. Double-looped hamstring/gracilis grafts are 1½ to 2 times as strong as the native ACL.

28. What are the common guidelines for activities after ACL reconstruction?

- 50% of quadriceps strength for jogging
- 65% of quadriceps strength for sports agility
- 80% of quadriceps strength for full return to sports

29. What are the outcomes of ACL repair?

About 88% to 95% of patients have a stable knee at 5-year follow-up, and 80% to 92% return to full previous level of play. Of patients with BPB grafts, 10% to 40% have some anterior knee pain with average quadriceps strength losses of 10%. Patients with hamstring grafts have a lower incidence of anterior knee pain (approximately 6%).

30. Describe the grading system for collateral ligament injuries.

- Grade 1—<5-mm joint-line opening with stress
- Grade 2—5- to 10-mm joint-line opening with stress
- Grade 3—>10-mm joint-line opening with stress

31. Compare third-degree injury of the ACL with third-degree injury of the medial compartment ligaments of the knee.

Complete and even partially torn ACLs progress to complete demise over time. Complete rupture of the medial compartment ligaments with 1+ or 2+ anterior medial rotary instability heals to almost normal stability without surgical intervention.

32. What is the most commonly used graft for a PCL reconstruction?

Achilles tendon allograft is the most popular graft site for both acute (43%) and chronic (50%) PCL reconstructions. Other grafts used to lesser degrees are bone-patellar tendon-bone autografts, hamstring tendon autografts, quadriceps tendon autografts, and anterior/posterior tibialis allografts.

33. Describe the treatment for MCL injuries.

Grades 1 and 2 are treated nonsurgically with immobilization for 48 hours, followed by gentle ROM and progression of exercise as tolerated. Grade 3 injuries are treated similarly, but surgery may be indicated if residual instability or stiffness occurs.

34. Testing for medial knee instability in a 10-year-old boy after a valgus injury demonstrates a pathologic opening of the medial compartment using a valgus stress test. What should be the primary diagnosis?

In a prepubescent individual, primary diagnostic thought should be an epiphyseal plate injury rather than an MCL sprain, as would be suspected in an adult. The reasoning is two-fold: (1) The MCL is much stronger than the physes in a younger person, making it more prone to failure in a valgus stress injury mechanism. (2) An epiphyseal injury is a much more serious injury in a young person than an MCL injury. An epiphyseal injury may require more aggressive medical treatment than an MCL sprain. An MCL sprain is often treated conservatively and therefore less of a long-term functional threat if initially misdiagnosed.

Bibliography

Beard JD, Dodd CA: Home or supervised rehabilitation following anterior cruciate ligament reconstruction: a randomized controlled trial, *J Sports Phys Ther* 27:134-143, 1998.

Beynnon BD et al: The measurement of elongation of anterior cruciate ligament grafts in-vivo, *J Bone Joint Surg* 76A:520-531, 1994.

Beynnon BD et al: Anterior cruciate ligament strain behavior during rehabilitation exercises in-vivo, *Am J Sports Med* 23:24-34, 1995.

DeLee JC, Drez D: *Orthopaedic sports medicine, vol 2,* Philadelphia, 1994, WB Saunders.

Fischer DA et al: Home based rehabilitation for anterior cruciate ligament reconstruction, *Clin Orthop* 347:194-199, 1998.

Fleming BC et al: Anterior cruciate ligament strain during an open and closed chain exercise: an in vivo study, *Am J Sports Med* 25:235-240, 1997.

Good ES et al: Biomechanics of the knee-extension exercise, *J Bone Joint Surg* 66A:725-733, 1984.

Gotling RS, Huie G: Anterior cruciate ligament injuries: operative and rehabilitative options, *Phys Med Rehabil Clin North Am* 11:895-915, 2000.

Holm I et al: Effect of neuromuscular training on proprioception, balance, muscle strength, and lower limb function in female athletes, *Clin J Sports Med* 14:88-94, 2004.

Hughston JC et al: Classification of knee ligament instabilities, *J Bone Joint Surg* 58A:159-179, 1976.

Johnson DL et al: Articular cartilage changes seen with MRI-detected bone bruises associated with acute ACL rupture, *Am J Sports Med* 26:409-414, 1998.

Madelbaum BR et al: Effectiveness of a neuromuscular and proprioceptive training program in preventing anterior cruciate ligament injuries in female athletes, *Am J Sports Med* 33:1003-1101, 2005.

Magee D: *Orthopedic physical assessment,* ed 3, Philadelphia, 1997, WB Saunders.

Margheritini F et al: Posterior cruciate ligament injuries in the athlete: an anatomical, biomechanical, and clinical review, *Sports Med* 32:393-408, 2002.

Oates KM et al: Comparative injury rates of uninjured, anterior cruciate ligament-deficient and reconstructed knees in a skiing population, *Am J Sports Med* 27:606-612, 1999.

Paterno MV et al: Neuromuscular training improves single limb stability in young female athletes, *J Orthop Sports Phys Ther* 34:305-316, 2004.

Schenck RC Jr et al: A prospective outcome study of rehabilitation programs and anterior cruciate ligament reconstruction, *Arthroscopy* 13:285-290, 1997.

Shelbourne DK, Davis TJ: Evaluation of knee stability before and after participation in a functional sports agility program during rehabilitation after anterior cruciate ligament reconstruction, *Am J Sports Med* 27:156-161, 1999.

Chapter 72

Total Knee Arthroplasty

Mark A. Cacko, PT, MPT, OCS, and Jay D. Keener, MD, PT

1. Is the patella typically resurfaced at the time of total knee arthroplasty (TKA)? What are the outcome differences?

Most surgeons advocate resurfacing the patella, especially in the presence of patellar chondromalacia, rheumatoid arthritis, and obesity. The decision of whether or not to resurface the patella has been investigated in several randomized trials. Some studies have shown no difference in subjective performance (ascending or descending stairs) or the incidence of anterior knee pain between resurfaced and nonresurfaced groups with short-term follow-up. Some studies have shown decreased pain and improved extensor mechanism strength in nonresurfaced compared to resurfaced groups. However, several authors have documented persistent anterior knee pain requiring repeat operation for patellar resurfacing following knee arthroplasty.

2. What type of patient should use a continuous passive motion (CPM) machine following total knee arthroplasty?

Although many patients will gain knee flexion range of motion quicker with the use of a CPM machine, some studies show that there is no long-term difference in range of motion between patients using a CPM machine and those that did not at 6 weeks and 1 year following surgery. Furthermore, CPM machine use has been associated with increased postoperative blood loss in patients when used immediately following surgery. Continuous passive motion has been shown to be of no protective benefit for the prevention of postoperative deep venous thrombosis.

3. How are knee braces used following total knee arthroplasty?

Many patients are placed into a knee immobilizer or a hinged knee brace locked in full extension immediately following surgery. The brace is used to facilitate terminal knee extension motion and to support the knee during weight-bearing activities. The brace is taken off for dressing changes and while performing exercises. The decision to remove the brace or unlock the hinges and allow motion is often left to the therapist. Factors such as available knee range of motion and quadriceps control should be considered when weaning the patient from the brace. Some authors advocate minimal or no bracing after surgery if quadriceps control is good and the patient can maintain full extension range of motion immediately following surgery.

4. What is the weight-bearing status of most patients following total knee arthroplasty?

Most total knee arthroplasty components are placed using cement fixation. Cement fixation is stable immediately, allowing most patients to bear weight as tolerated on the involved lower extremity. Uncemented components generally rely on bone ingrowth into the component, which usually is present to some degree within 6 weeks following surgery. For this reason, patients with uncemented components usually have a restricted weight-bearing status during this period, most commonly 25% to 50% of full weight-bearing.

5. What are the common knee range of motion goals following total knee arthroplasty?

Most patients who are able to achieve 75 degrees of knee flexion at the time of discharge will have at least 90 degrees of knee flexion at 1 year after surgery. The amount of knee flexion needed to perform various activities of daily living has been shown to range from 50 degrees while walking, to 80 to 90 degrees for stair-climbing, to 100 to 110 degrees for activities such as rising from a chair or tying a shoe. Most orthopaedists consider 105 to 110 degrees the best long-term goal for knee flexion that will optimize patient function.

6. Describe a common progression of strengthening exercises following total knee arthroplasty.

Patients generally begin a program of isometric exercises for the quadricep, gluteal, and hamstring muscles on postoperative day 1. Once the ability to recruit the often-silent quadriceps muscle is evident, patients begin short-arc quadriceps isotonic exercises. The patient is allowed to begin active assistive and active knee flexion and extension exercises during the inpatient setting. Resistance in the form of ankle weights or a Thera-Band is usually implemented before discharge as well. It is important to incorporate strengthening exercises of the hip and ankle musculature into the rehabilitation program. The preoperative evaluation often shows relative deficits in upper extremity strength that should be addressed, as these are now weight-bearing joints in patients relying on a walker or crutches for ambulation. Patients should be comfortable in performing these exercises on their own at the time of hospital discharge.

7. How do you know when a patient is ready to be weaned from the knee immobilizer or brace while ambulating?

There are no hard and fast rules that dictate when a patient can be weaned from knee support. The ability to perform a straight leg raise with no extensor lag often indicates enough quadriceps strength to control the knee while ambulating. For most patients this is present between weeks 3 and 5 postoperatively with adequate rehabilitation.

8. What are the indications for manipulation of the knee joint for motion following total knee arthroplasty?

In general, manipulation is reserved for the most recalcitrant cases of range of motion restriction following knee replacement. However, manipulation can be a valuable adjunct for many patients. Many practitioners do not manipulate to gain extension range of motion. Patients with an inability to achieve full extension are generally braced in extension as much as possible, and therapy is focused accordingly, including aggressive patellar mobilizations once the postoperative dressing is removed. Manipulation is generally reserved for patients having difficulty gaining flexion motion. Timing of manipulation becomes an issue and is somewhat controversial. Manipulation is commonly performed from the second week to the 3-month postoperative period as the soft tissues continue to mature. Some studies have shown that patients tend to return to premanipulation motion in the long-term. Many believe the beneficial effects of knee manipulation are less when performed more than 3 months after surgery. Indwelling epidural analgesia may help maintain range of motion. Physical therapy is focused upon immediate aggressive range of motion exercises to keep the gains in range of motion obtained at the time of manipulation.

9. You notice that a patient you are treating following knee arthroplasty has developed increased calf swelling and localized tenderness. What should you do?

An increase in calf swelling, calf pain with dorsiflexion of the ankle, calf tenderness, and/or erythema are all potential signs of deep vein thrombosis and should prompt the therapist to contact the physician as soon as possible. Deep vein thrombosis (DVT) following total knee arthroplasty is very common despite the use of various types of DVT prophylaxis (aspirin, warfarin, heparin derivatives, and sequential compression devices). Rates of postoperative deep vein thrombosis, despite preventive therapy, range from 10% to 57% of patients following total knee arthroplasty, while the incidence of fatal pulmonary embolism in unprotected patients is only 0.19%. The reliability of physical examination findings for the detection of a deep vein thrombosis is notoriously inaccurate.

10. What is the difference between a posterior cruciate substituting and a posterior cruciate retaining knee replacement? How do they affect rehabilitation?

Posterior cruciate substituting systems require removal of both cruciate ligaments at the time of surgery. Knee stability is obtained through a design that allows the tibial intercondylar eminence to articulate within the femoral intercondylar box during knee flexion, thus preventing posterior translation of the tibia in relation to the femur. Posterior cruciate retaining designs spare the posterior cruciate ligament, allowing the ligament to retain its functional purposes. Clinical trials have demonstrated excellent results with both design types. Posterior cruciate retaining devices have the theoretical advantage of maintaining the proprioceptive function of the ligament. Additionally, posterior femoral rollback facilitated by the posterior cruciate ligament during knee flexion potentially allows greater knee flexion range of motion and improves the mechanical advantage of the quadriceps mechanism. One study has shown improved knee kinematics while ascending stairs in patients with posterior cruciate retaining knee replacements versus those with substituting designs. Proponents of posterior cruciate substituting designs cite greater ease of surgery, the greater ability to correct deformities, and, most importantly, potentially decreased polyethylene wear rates as advantages of these designs. Rehabilitation protocols are generally identical for both design types. Because of the rare reports of posterior knee dislocation in cruciate-substituted knees, some studies advocate avoidance of resistant hamstring strengthening in positions of extreme knee flexion.

11. What are other complications associated with total knee arthroplasty?

There are many complications that are relatively uncommon, including peroneal nerve palsy (0.5%), vascular injury (0.03% to 0.2%), infection (1% to 5%), periprosthetic fracture, extensor mechanism dysfunction, wound healing complications, and arthrofibrosis. Peroneal nerve palsy is a serious complication that may have permanent consequences upon ankle strength and control. The prevalence of peroneal nerve palsy after total knee arthroplasty has been reported to be around 0.5%. The development of nerve palsy has been associated with several risk factors, including preoperative valgus knee alignment, preoperative knee flexion contracture, and epidural anesthesia for postoperative pain control. In many instances, nerve function will return if diagnosed early and treated accordingly. The extensor mechanism is the most common source of continued post-operative knee pain and can be related to patella fracture, patellar tracking problems, parapatellar soft tissue impingement, and failure of patellar components. Arthrofibrosis relates to scar tissue formation in and around the knee, resulting in restriction of range of motion. This is treated with manipulation, aggressive physical therapy, and arthroscopic release of scar tissue. Infection is a dreaded complication following total knee arthroplasty, with reported rates of 1% to 5% depending upon the patient population. Risk factors include revision surgery, delays in wound healing, skin ulcers, rheumatoid arthritis, and, in some studies, urinary tract infections and diabetes mellitus. Early infections can sometimes be treated with debridement and antibiotics while later infections often require removal of components.

12. What are the outcomes of total knee arthroplasty?

Outcomes following total knee arthroplasty are excellent in appropriately selected patients. Most clinical studies following total knee arthroplasty report survival rates between 80% and 95% for the tibial and femoral components at 10 to 15 years' follow-up. Approximately 10% of patients will have pain local to the patellofemoral joint. Up to 94% survival rates of tibial and femoral components at 18 to 20 years have been reported following cemented posterior stabilized total knee arthroplasty, with overall survival rates of 90% when patellar revisions were included. Lower rates of success have been demonstrated in certain well-defined patient populations. It is found that the greatest amount of improvement is seen within the first 3 to 6 months after surgery, with more gradual improvements occurring up to 2 years after surgery. Walking speeds for patients with total knee arthroplasties were found to be 13% and 18% slower at normal and fast speeds, as compared to subjects without knee pathology. Stair-climbing was compromised by 43% to 51% with patients following total knee replacement as compared to other subjects. Men with total knee arthroplasty were 37% to 39% weaker and women were 28% to 29% weaker in their knee extensors as compared to healthy individuals.

13. What are the indications for unicompartmental knee arthroplasty (UKA)?

- Greater than 60 years old
- Arthritis limited to one compartment of the knee
- Patient who is not overweight or a heavy-demand laborer
- Knee ROM >90 degrees with less than a 5-degree flexion contracture
- Angular deformity <10 degrees
- A functional ACL

14. What are the outcomes of UKA?

UKA may be converted to TKA with somewhat less difficulty than a proximal tibial osteotomy. Augmentation with metal wedges is required in approximately 20% of the cases, and pain relief and function are similar to those for primary TKA. Unicompartmental knee replacements are less invasive, preserve the bone stock, are more cost-effective, and have faster recovery times. Survivorship at 10 years after surgery for patients ≤55 years has been reported to be 87.5% to 96%, and patients ≥60 years have survivorship rates of 94% to 98%. Average range of motion is 114 to 125 degrees after UKA. Patients have shown a loss of torque of approximately 30% in extension and flexion at 60 to 180 degrees/sec of isokinetic testing compared to individuals without knee pathology. Patients with UKAs showed no significant difference with regard to proprioceptive testing as compared to normal controls. Unicompartmental knee replacements also preserve normal knee kinematics, which are significantly changed in total knee replacements. A common cause of failure that would lead to revision is progression of arthritis at the patellofemoral joint and the contralateral compartment. Progression of arthritis to the lateral compartment can result from slight overcorrection into valgus, and better results are found when the knee is slightly undercorrected. It has been found that neutral to slight valgus is the optimal alignment for unicompartmental knee arthroplasty for anterior medial osteoarthritis. Overcorrection can shift the mechanical axis to the unreplaced compartment.

15. What are the indications for proximal tibial osteotomy?

- Less than 60 years old
- Arthritis limited to one compartment of the knee
- Patient who is not overweight or a heavy-demand laborer
- Knee ROM >90 degrees
- Varus angle deformity of 10 to 15 degrees
- Flexion contracture <15 degrees
- Enough strength to successfully use walker or crutches

16. What are the outcomes of proximal tibial osteotomy?

Typically there is ≈73% survivorship at 10 to 14 years, thus significantly delaying TKA for the appropriately chosen patient. Good to excellent results are slightly lower after conversion to TKA (63%) versus primary TKA (88%).

17. Can a patient kneel after total knee arthroplasty?

Two studies found that 64% and 82% of subjects tested were able to kneel after at least 6 months following surgery with minimal to no pain (rated 0 to 4 out of 10). Range of motion was a mean of 114 degrees in patients who could kneel comfortably, and was 110 degrees for subjects who could not kneel comfortably. Forces through the femoral component are similar in kneeling as compared to those of walking and standing. Most patients avoid kneeling secondary to third-party advice in order to protect the prosthesis. Scar pain and back-related problems were also factors in limiting kneeling ability.

18. Can patients with total knee arthroplasty return to playing tennis? Do doctors recommend this?

Subjects returned to playing tennis approximately 5.9 months after surgery (range between 1 and 10 months). The average national tennis player rating level before surgery was 4.35 as compared to 4.26 after surgery (range 1 to 7). Subjects noted that court speed deficiencies disappeared as quickly as 6 months after surgery (range between 1 and 12 months). Two subjects in the study needed revision but they were also playing 5 times a week, while the rest of the subjects were playing approximately 3 times a week. In a survey of surgeons, 21% believed that patients could return to playing singles tennis; 45% allowed doubles tennis only.

19. Can patients with total knee arthroplasty return to playing golf? Do doctors recommend this?

Surgeons' recommendation for return to golf was approximately 3 months, and to begin slowly. One study allowed for patients to start chipping and putting as soon as they demonstrated good balance and were no longer using assistive devices. A total of 77% of physicians have suggested that patients use a golf cart. Approximately 84% to 90% of patients reported having no discomfort while playing golf, and 34.9% had mild pain after golfing. Patients did note that pain was increased if their replacement was on their lead knee. In two different studies, 93% and 92% of surgeons did not discourage patients from golfing.

20. Does following an exercise program before total knee replacement surgery improve outcome?

Studies have found no significant difference between groups who followed an exercise program before surgery and a control group that did not exercise. It was found that preoperational levels of pain and function are the best predictors of pain and function at 6 months following surgery. These studies did have poor patient compliance, however. Implementing a strengthening program before surgery did improve patients' general confidence, increased knee strength, augmented thigh muscle strength, and improved endurance after surgery. Patients with poor preoperational functional levels did not attain the same level of function at 2 years following surgery.

21. What is a rotating platform total knee arthroplasty?

A mobile-bearing rotating platform total knee replacement consists of a dual-surface articulation between a polyethylene insert and a metallic femoral tibial tray. The tibial tray has a conical cavity that articulates with the central cone of the one-piece polyethylene insert. This design increases articulation conformity, decreases polyethylene wear, and minimizes the shear stress at the tibial tray-bone cement interface. Rotating platforms provide unlimited axial rotation but with limited anterior, posterior, medial, and lateral translation of the femoral polyethylene insert. This was designed to approximate the kinematics of a natural knee. Dislocation rates were found to range between 0.5% and 4.65%, and usually occurred in the early stage of total knee replacement between 6 days and 2 years, although late dislocation has also been known to occur. Dislocation rates are higher in those patients with a preoperative valgus deformity and greater age at surgery. Average range of motion has been determined to be between 107 and 115 degrees of knee flexion. Survival rates have varied from 89.5% at 12 years, to 92.1% at 15 years, to 97.7% at 20 years. There has been no superiority found from a mobile-bearing rotating platform total knee replacement as compared to a fixed total knee arthroplasty.

Bibliography

Ackerman IN, Bennel KL: Does pre-operative physiotherapy improve outcomes from lower limb joint replacement surgery? A systematic review, *Aust J Physiother* 50:25-30, 2004.

Andriacchi TP et al: The influence of total knee replacement design on walking and stair climbing, *J Bone Joint Surg* 64A:1328-1336, 1982.

Ayers DL et al: Common complications of total knee arthroplasty, *J Bone Joint Surg* 79A:278-311, 1997.

Barrack RL et al: Resurfacing the patella in total knee arthroplasty: a prospective randomized double-blind study, *J Bone Joint Surg* 79A:1121-1131, 1997.

Collier MB et al: Proprioceptive deficits are comparable before unicondylar and total knee arthroplasties, but greater in the more symptomatic knee of the patient, *Clin Orthop Relat Res* 423:138-143, 2004.

Daluga D: Knee manipulation following total knee arthroplasty. Analysis of prognostic variables, *J Arthroplasty* 6:119-128, 1991.

Deyle GD et al: Effectiveness of manual physical therapy and exercise in osteoarthritis of the knee: a randomized control trial, *Ann Intern Med* 132:173-181, 2000.

Esler C: Manipulation of total knee replacements. Is the flexion retained?, *J Bone Joint Surg* 81B:27-29, 1999.

Felson DT et al: The epidemiology of knee osteoarthritis; results from the Framingham Osteoarthritis Study, *Semin Arthritis Rheum* 20(suppl 1):42-50, 1990.

Fuchs S et al: Muscle strength in patients with unicompartmental arthroplasty, *Am J Phys Med Rehabil* 83:650-654, 2004.

Huang CH et al: Long-term results of low contact stress mobile-bearing total knee replacements, *Clin Orthop Relat Res* 416:265-270, 2003.

Jones CA et al: Determinants of function after total knee arthroplasty, *Phys Ther* 83:696-706, 2003.

Keating EM et al: Use of lateral heel and sole wedges in treatment of medial osteoarthritis of the knee, *Othop Rev* 22:921-924, 1993.

Khaw FM et al: The incidence of fatal pulmonary embolism after knee replacement with no prophylactic anticoagulation, *J Bone Joint Surg* 75B:940-942, 1993.

Lotke PA et al: Blood loss after total knee replacement. Effects of tourniquet release and continuous passive motion, *J Bone Joint Surg* 73A:1037-1040, 1991.

Mallon WJ et al: Total joint replacement and golf, *Clin Sports Med* 15:179-190, 1996.

Mont MA et al: Tennis after total knee arthroplasty, *Am J Sports Med* 30:163-166, 2002.

Naudie D et al: Medial unicompartmental knee arthroplasty with the Miller-Galante prosthesis, *J Bone Joint Surg* 86A:1931-1935, 2004.

Palmer SH et al: Ability to kneel after total knee replacement, *J Bone Joint Surg* 84B:220-222, 2002.

Sorrells RB et al: Uncemented rotating-platform total knee replacement: a five to twelve-year follow-up study, *J Bone Joint Surg* 86A:2156-2162, 2004.

Thompson NW et al: Dislocation of the dislocating platform after low contact stress total knee arthroplasty, *Clin Orthop Relat Res* 425:207-211, 2004.

Walsh M et al: Physical impairments and functional limitations: a comparison of individuals 1 year after total knee arthroplasty with control subjects, *Phys Ther* 78:248-258, 1998.

Yashar AA et al: Continuous passive motion with accelerated flexion after total knee arthroplasty, *Clin Orthop* 345:38-43, 1997.

Chapter 73

Knee Fractures and Dislocations

Robert "Cliff" Hall, PT, MS, SCS

PATELLAR FRACTURES

1. List, in order of frequency of occurrence, the five types of patellar fractures.

- Transverse
- Comminuted or stellate
- Vertical
- Osteochondral
- Polar (apical or basal)

2. List the two major mechanisms of injury that result in patellar fractures.

- Direct trauma (blow or fall) to the patella with significant articular cartilage damage
- Indirect force (jumping) resulting in a displaced or transverse fracture

3. When is nonsurgical treatment indicated for a patellar fracture?

- Minimal displacement (<2 to 3 mm)
- Intact extensor mechanism
- Minimal articular step-off (1 to 2 mm)

4. Describe the course of conservative treatment for patellar fractures.

- Aspiration of hematoma and full extension in a long-leg cylinder cast or brace for 3 to 6 weeks
- Quadriceps set and straight-leg raises with return to weight-bearing as tolerated
- Gradual progression of active knee flexion and strengthening after cast removal
- Progression of closed-chain exercises (e.g., biking) at 6 weeks, with goal of return to full ROM and strength at 12 weeks

5. What are the common sequelae of patellar fractures?

The typical sequelae of patellar fractures is the following: patellofemoral arthritis, instability, decreased knee range of motion (ROM), quadriceps weakness, and difficulty with stairs, downhill walking, and kneeling.

6. How is a bipartite patella differentiated from a fracture?

On radiographs a bipartite patella shows well-rounded, smooth margins and usually has one fragment in the superolateral position. Bipartite patellas occur in 0.05 to 2% of the population and are bilateral in 43% of the cases.

7. Describe the outcomes for nonoperative treatment of nondisplaced patellar fractures.

Most patients have full ROM and return to normal quadriceps strength without patellofemoral problems. Complications, such as nonunion or patellofemoral problems, occur in <2% of cases. Patient satisfaction has been reported as high as 95% or greater.

8. What are the outcomes for open reduction and internal fixation (ORIF) of patellar fractures?

Good to excellent results (return to full function within 6 to 9 months) are reported in 70% to 80% of all cases. Fair to poor results are reported in 20% to 30% of cases, and loss of the extensor mechanism is reported in 20% to 49% of cases. In one study, late displacement occurred in 7.4% of cases. Refracture has been reported in 5%. Prolonged immobilization (>8 weeks) increases the likelihood of poor results.

9. By what mechanism does the tension-banding technique stabilize patellar fractures?

The wires are placed in such a fashion that with knee flexion (increased quadriceps tension) the tension in the wires increases to intensify compression of the fragments and facilitate fracture healing.

10. How does rehabilitation differ between patients with nondisplaced fractures and patients with severely comminuted fractures?

Nondisplaced fractures are treated with knee immobilization in full extension, early weight-bearing as tolerated, and isometric quadriceps exercises with a gradual increase in active assisted ROM at 4 to 6 weeks. Severely comminuted fractures with ORIF are treated like nondisplaced fractures but require partial weight-bearing for the first 6 weeks and a gradual increase in active assisted ROM at 3 to 6 weeks (with demonstration of stable fixation). All other patients with ORIF may begin active assisted ROM at 1 to 2 weeks.

11. What are the outcomes for patellectomy?

Good to excellent outcomes have been reported in 22% to 85% of cases and fair to poor outcomes in 14% to 60%. Loss of quadriceps strength has been reported at around 50% decrease in peak torque. As a result, rehabilitation and return to function may be prolonged up to 6 to 8 months or longer.

12. At what age does a quadriceps tendon rupture typically occur? How do patients present?

Eighty percent of quadriceps tendon ruptures occur in patients older than 40 years. The mechanism of injury is forced knee flexion with maximal quadriceps contraction. Presentation includes intense pain, inability to walk, swelling, palpable defect, and hemarthrosis. Patients usually seek immediate medical attention.

13. How is a quadriceps tendon rupture treated? What is the expected outcome?

Repair is often primary anastomosis, with the knee immobilized in full extension for a minimum of 6 weeks, followed by 6 months of rehabilitation for full recovery. Acute repairs usually result in good recovery of ROM and strength sufficient for activities of daily living. A 20% decrease in quadriceps strength was reported in 50% of patients in one case series. Late repairs are at risk for significant extension deficit.

14. At what age does a patellar tendon rupture typically occur? How do patients present?

Patellar tendon ruptures most commonly occur in people younger than 40 years with a history of patellar tendonitis or steroid injections. Other pathogenesis includes long-standing tendonopathy, mucoid degeneration, and tendolipomatosis. Tendon ruptures are associated with high-energy trauma. Presentation is similar to that of a quadriceps tendon rupture, with a palpable defect and superiorly displaced patella.

15. What is the incidence of repeat patellar tendon rupture following surgical repair?

The rerupture rate of patellar tendon rupture repairs is reported at less than 10%.

16. How are patellar tendon ruptures repaired? What is the expected outcome?

Ligament is sutured to bone, and the knee is immobilized in full extension for 6 to 8 weeks with <50% weight-bearing. Earlier repairs have better outcomes than late repairs. Complications include decreased knee flexion and patella baja.

DISTAL FEMORAL FRACTURES

17. What is the typical direction of displacement for a supracondylar distal femoral fracture? Why?

The distal fragment is flexed by the gastrocnemius, causing posterior displacement and angulation. The pull of the quadriceps and hamstrings causes the femur to shorten.

18. How are closed supracondylar fractures treated after reduction?

A cast brace is used for 6 to 8 weeks. If displaced and not reducible, supracondylar fractures may require ORIF. Skeletal traction is used less often.

19. What are the primary goals of operative treatment of distal femoral fractures?

- Anatomic reduction of joint surfaces
- Rigid fixation
- Restoration of limb length
- Early knee motion

20. What injuries are commonly associated with distal femoral fractures?

- Ipsilateral hip fracture or dislocation
- Peroneal nerve injury
- Vascular injury
- Damage to the quadriceps apparatus

21. Describe the age distribution of distal femoral fractures.

The age distribution is bimodal: (1) young males have a higher incidence of high-energy trauma and intra-articular damage, and (2) elderly women have a higher incidence of low-energy trauma with fractures secondary to osteopenia.

22. What are the indications and contraindications for operative and nonoperative treatment of distal femoral fractures?

- Operative indications—**absolute:** displaced intra-articular fractures, open fractures, neurovascular injury, ipsilateral lower extremity fractures, and pathologic fractures; **relative:** isolated extra-articular fractures and severe osteoporosis
- Operative contraindications—preexisting infection, marked obesity, comorbid conditions, poor bone quality, and systemic infections
- Nonoperative indications—nondisplaced or incomplete fractures, impacted stable fractures in elderly osteopenic patients, significant underlying medical disease (cardiac, pulmonary, neurologic), advanced osteoporosis, selected gunshot wounds, and nonambulatory patients

23. Why is fat embolism such a concern with femoral fractures?

The pathogenesis of fat embolism is a subject of conjecture and controversy. Most investigators agree that the bone marrow is the source of the fat. Fat embolism is associated more often with intramedullary instrumentation of the femur than with fracture. Fat embolism typically occurs in high-energy tibial or femoral fractures among patients between the ages of 20 and 40. Embolism is also common among elderly patients (60 to 80 years old) with low-energy hip fractures.

24. What are the outcomes for low profile minimally invasive plating for distal femoral fractures?

ROM averages 1 to 109 degrees, 93% heal without bone grafting, nearly all maintain fixation, malreduction occurs in approximately 6%, and infection occurs in 3% of patients.

25. How do distal femoral fractures present in children? What is the incidence of distal femoral fractures in children? What are the common mechanisms of injury?

Presenting symptoms for distal femoral fractures in children include inability to weight-bear, maintaining the knee in flexion, gross deformity, and occasionally neurovascular compromise. Salter-Harris type II fractures are the most common category of distal femoral fractures in children (54%), with physeal fractures accounting for 1% to 6% of all physeal injuries in children.

Mechanisms of injury include indirect varus or valgus stress, breech birth, and minimal trauma in conditions that weaken the growth plate (osteomyelitis, leukemia, myelodysplasia).

26. Describe the nonoperative treatment of nondisplaced and displaced distal femoral fractures in children.

- Nondisplaced fractures are treated with a long-leg cast or hip spica cast for 4 to 6 weeks.
- Displaced Salter-Harris type I and II fractures are treated with closed reduction with traction and gentle manipulation, followed by immobilization with or without percutaneous pinning. The position of immobilization depends on the direction of the displacement.
- Displaced Salter-Harris type III and IV fractures are treated with open anatomic reduction.

27. What are the indications for ORIF of distal femoral fractures in children?

Irreducible Salter-Harris type II fractures, unstable reductions, and Salter-Harris type III and IV fractures are all candidates for ORIF.

28. What complications are associated with distal femoral fractures in children?

- Acute—peroneal nerve palsy (3%) from traction or attempts at reduction, recurrent displacement, and popliteal artery injuries (<2%) associated with hyperextension injuries

- Late—angulation deformity (19% to 24%), leg length discrepancy (24% to 30%), knee stiffness (16%), avascular necrosis (rare), and nonunion (rare)

PROXIMAL TIBIAL FRACTURES

29. What are the general types of proximal tibial fractures?

- Extra-articular—tibial spine, tibial tubercle, and subcondylar
- Articular—condylar, bicondylar, and comminuted
- Intra-articular—epiphyseal

30. What kind of condylar fractures are often seen in elderly people?

Insufficiency fractures of the medial tibial condyle are often found in the elderly. Varus deformity on exam usually indicates a depression or split-depression fracture (more common).

31. What injuries are associated with condylar fractures?

Meniscal injuries occur in up to 50% of all condylar fractures and ligamentous injuries in 30%. Peroneal nerve neurapraxia and popliteal artery injury are also associated injuries.

32. Which tibial condyle is fractured more frequently? Why?

The lateral condyle is fractured 70% to 80% more often because of weaker trabeculation, valgus orientation of the knee, and valgus-directed external forces.

33. Describe conservative treatment of nondisplaced condylar fractures.

- Early passive exercise to maintain mobility and strength without weight-bearing; weight-bearing delayed until the fracture heals (6 to 12 weeks)
- Non–weight-bearing cast immobilization (long-leg foot-groin cast, 5 degrees of flexion) for 3 to 6 weeks, followed by 2 to 4 weeks of non–weight-bearing rehabilitation, with progressive weight-bearing from 9 to 16 weeks
- Traction with passive exercise for 6 weeks, followed by non–weight-bearing at about 12 weeks; return to full weight-bearing when tissue healing is evident
- Cast bracing with initial non–weight-bearing and progressive weight-bearing for up to 12 weeks; full weight-bearing when tissue healing is evident

34. Describe the outcomes of low profile minimally invasive plating for proximal tibia fractures.

Approximately 91% heal without major complication, some malalignment occurs in 10%, need for hardware removal occurs in 5%, and infection is seen in 4%. Mean final ROM is approximately 1 to 122 degrees, with full weight-bearing allowed an average of 12.6 weeks postoperatively.

35. Traumatic avulsions of the tibial tubercle are seen most often in what age-group? Describe the mechanism and rate of injury for proximal tibial physeal fractures in children.

Traumatic avulsions of the tibial tubercle are most often seen in young patients. Injury results from a strong quadriceps contraction with a slight degree of knee flexion. The sustained or sudden force disrupts either the tibial apophysis or the proximal tibial epiphysis.

Proximal tibial physeal fractures account for 3% of all physeal injuries. Hyperextension forces the metaphysis posteriorly. Salter-Harris type II fractures are most common (35%).

36. How are proximal tibial physeal fractures in children treated?

- Types I and II are treated with closed reduction followed by immobilization.
- Types III and IV are treated with closed reduction, percutaneous pinning, and immobilization with an above-the-knee cast in 10 to 20 degrees of flexion for 6 to 8 weeks.

37. What complications are associated with proximal tibial physeal fractures?

Vascular compromise occurs in 5% to 7% of cases, angular deformity in 28% of cases, and leg length discrepancy in 19% of cases.

38. Describe the weight-bearing progression for the various fractures about the knee.

Weight-Bearing Status of Knee Fractures

	Surgical Fixation			*Nonoperative Treatment*		
Fracture	**NWB**	**PWB**	**FWB**	**NWB**	**PWB**	**FWB**
Patella	—	Immediate	6 weeks	—	Immediate	As tolerated
Distal femur	—	Immediate	12 weeks	—	2-3 weeks	8 weeks
Proximal tibia	2-4 weeks	9 weeks	16 weeks*	4-6 weeks† 12-16 weeks‡	—	Dependent on healing

NWB, Non–weight-bearing; *PWB,* partial weight-bearing; *FWB,* full weight-bearing.
*Based on signs of healing.
†Minimally displaced fractures.
‡After traction.

KNEE DISLOCATIONS

39. In addition to neurovascular injuries, knee dislocations are likely to result in injuries to what ligaments?

Both cruciate ligaments and at least one of the collateral ligaments are likely to be injured.

40. How does disruption of a popliteal artery after knee dislocation present? Describe the emergent treatment.

Disruption of a popliteal artery presents with absent or decreased distal pulses and signs of ischemia. The artery must be repaired within 8 hours of injury to avoid limb amputation. If timing allows, a vascular surgeon may elect to perform an arteriogram to rule out an intimal tear. In clinically ischemic legs, however, the surgeon may proceed directly to open exploration and repair.

41. Should repair of ligament tears be acute or delayed in knee dislocations?

This issue is somewhat controversial. Some authors advocate acute repair of arterial structures with delayed repair of ligamentous structures to allow better healing of vascular repairs. Others advocate acute repair of both vascular and ligamentous structures with limited early motion, depending on the extent of the vascular repair. The literature slightly favors acute ligamentous repair, because early motion results in fewer postoperative complications.

PATELLAR DISLOCATIONS AND SUBLUXATIONS

42. What are the anatomic characteristics of typical patients with patellar dislocations?

Genu valgum
Shallow lateral femoral condyle
Elongated patellar tendon
Deficient vastus medialis
Lateral insertion of patellar tendon
Shallow patellar groove
Deformed patella
Pes planus
Increased Q-angle
Ligamentous laxity

43. What type of fracture is frequently associated with acute patellar dislocations?

Osteochondral fractures of the medial facet of the patella have been reported in up to 66% of all patellar dislocations. Osteochondral fractures of the lateral femoral condyle are also common.

44. What are the two main mechanisms of patellar dislocation and subluxation?

- Direct trauma or blow to the patella with the knee in slight flexion
- Powerful quadriceps contraction combined with slight flexion and external rotation of the tibia on the femur

45. Describe the typical conservative course of treatment for a first-time patellar dislocation.

The course of treatment for first-time patellar dislocation is as follows: in the absence of osteochondral fracture, 6 weeks of brace immobilization in full extension; progressive weight-bearing as tolerated; early quadriceps isometrics, with straight leg raising (SLR) as pain allows; passive pain-free ROM progressing to full active ROM and aggressive closed-chain strengthening at 6 weeks.

A 44% recurrence rate has been reported after nonoperative treatment of first-time dislocations.

46. What are the indications for surgery with a patellar dislocation?

- First-time dislocation with significant osteochondral fracture
- First-time dislocation with inadequate or unstable reduction
- Recurrent dislocation not responding to nonoperative treatment
- Disruption of the medial patellofemoral ligament on magnetic resonance imaging

47. What are the indications and contraindications for lateral retinacular release?

- Indications—intractable patellofemoral pain with lateral tilt, lateral compression syndrome, persistent subluxations, patellar dislocations
- Contraindications—patellofemoral pain without lateral tilt, advanced patellofemoral arthrosis, lateral hypermobile patella, normal tracking patella, patella subluxation and dislocation with significant extensor mechanism malalignment

48. What is the typical progression of rehabilitation following a lateral retinacular release?

Weeks 1-2	Weeks 3-5	6 Weeks
Weight-bear as tolerated	Full weight-bearing	Sport-specific activities
Early AROM 1°-115°	Full AROM	Functional/isometric eval
Multi-angle isometrics	Closed-chain exercises	Brace for activity
Patella mobilization	Aerobic reconditioning	Agility drills
Control pain/swelling	Isometric strength eval	

Summarized from Table 1, p 327, in Mangine RE et al: Postoperative management of the patellofemoral patient, *J Orthop Sports Phys Ther* 28:323-335, 1998.

49. What is the average recurrence rate after lateral retinacular release for recurrent patellar dislocation?

Published studies show a recurrence rate of as much as 5%, with a range of 14 to 48 months of follow-up.

50. What degree of tubercle-sulcus angle (Q-angle at 90 degrees) indicates potential patellar instability?

A tubercle-sulcus angle <10 degrees indicates potential patellar instability.

51. What radiographic view is used to assess patellar malalignment?

The Mercer-Merchant patellar view at 45-degree knee flexion angle is used to assess patellar malalignment.

52. What are the outcomes of medial retinacular repair with lateral retinacular release for acute patellar dislocation?

Good to excellent results have been reported in 81% to 91% of cases, with <2% redislocation rates.

Bibliography

Aglietti P, Buzzi R: Fractures of the femoral condyles. In Insall JN, editor: *Surgery of the knee,* New York, 1993, pp 983-1034, Churchill Livingstone.

Aglietti P, Buzzi R: Fractures of the tibial plateau. In Insall JN, editor: *Surgery of the knee,* New York, 1993, pp 1035-1084, Churchill Livingstone.

Brotzman SB, Wilk KE, editors: *Clinical orthopaedic rehabilitation*, ed 2, Philadelphia, 2003, pp 346-350, Mosby.

Carpenter J, Kasman R, Mathews L: Fractures of the patella, *J Bone Joint Surg* 75A:1550-1561, 1993.

Cole PA, Zlowodzki M, Kregor PJ: Treatment of proximal tibia fractures using the less invasive stabilization system: surgical experience and early clinical results in 77 fractures, *J Orthop Trauma* 2004:528-535, 2004.

Helfet D, Novak K: The management of fractures of the tibial plateau, *Int J Orthop Trauma* 1:148, 1991.

Hsu K et al: Traumatic patellar tendon ruptures: a follow-up study of primary repair and a neutralization wire, *J Truama* 36:658-660, 1994.

Magee DL: Knee. In *Orthopedic physical assessment,* Philadelphia, 1997, pp 506-571, WB Saunders.

Mangine RE et al: Postoperative management of the patellofemoral patient, *J Orthop Sports Phys Ther* 28:323-335, 1998.

Markmiller M, Konrad G, Sudkamp N: Femur-LISS and distal femoral nail for fixation of distal femoral fractures: are there differences in outcome and complications?, *Clin Orthop Relat Res* 426:252-257, 2004.
Reid DC: Bursitis and knee extensor mechanism pain syndromes. In *Sports injury assessment and rehabilitation,* New York, 1992, pp 399-401, Churchill Livingstone.
Reilly JP: Tibial plateau fractures. In Scott WN, editor: *The knee,* St Louis, 1994, pp 1369-1392, Mosby.
Rockwood CA et al, editors: *Rockwood and Green's fractures in adults,* Vol 2, ed 4, Philadelphia, 1996, pp 1919-2178, Lippincott-Raven.
Scheinberg RR, Bucholz RW: Fractures of the patella. In Scott WN, editor: *The knee,* St Louis, 1994, pp 1393-1403, Mosby.
Simon RR, Koenigsknecth SJ: *Emergency orthopedics: the extremities,* ed 2, Norwalk, Conn, 1987, pp 234-387, Appleton & Lange.
Stanitski CL, Paletta GA Jr: Articular cartilage injury with acute patellar dislocation in adolescents: arthroscopic and radiographic correlation, *Am J Sports Med* 26:52-55, 1998.

Chapter 74

Nerve Entrapments of the Lower Extremity

John S. Halle, PT, PhD, and David G. Greathouse, PT, PhD, ECS

1. In what order are sensory fibers normally lost after nerve injury?

- Two-point discrimination
- Light touch
- Pinprick

2. Are motor fibers or sensory fibers the first to show electrophysiologically measurable signs of entrapment?

Compression and subsequent ischemia affect large fibers more than small fibers, and fibers situated peripherally in the fascicle are more susceptible than centrally located fibers. Some researchers have documented that sensory nerve function is affected before motor function, whereas others have observed the opposite. Because sensory decrements are observed by the patient before subtle motor changes, the most prominent clinical sign is usually sensory. The largest fibers, irrespective of type, are affected first; both motor and sensory function need to be evaluated as part of the physical examination.

3. What constitutes compression of a peripheral nerve?

An abridged list of factors that determine the impact of compressive force on peripheral nerves includes:

- Manner in which the compressive force is applied
- Type of underlying surface
- Whether the nerve passes through or is contained within an unyielding compartment
- Location and size of individual fibers and neural connective tissue
- Magnitude and duration of the compressive trauma

Nerves with increased amounts of connective tissue tend to be more resistant to compressive trauma, and nerves exposed to either long-lasting or high-magnitude compression demonstrate a greater degree of dysfunction. Epineurial blood flow is reduced at 20 mm Hg. Axonal transport is decreased at 30 mm Hg. Paresthesias occur at 30 to 40 mm Hg, and complete axonal blockade may occur at 50 mm Hg. Ischemia and motor blockade occur at pressures >60 mm Hg.

4. Describe the negative effects of compression on nerve function.

- Endoneurial stasis of circulation caused by retrograde effects from the epineurial venule circulation
- Anoxia of the endothelial cells of the endoneurial capillaries
- Loss of integrity of the endothelial capillary tight junctions secondary to anoxia, resulting in increased vascular permeability
- Leakage of fluid and proteins from the endoneurial capillaries into the endoneurial space, resulting in edema
- Increased endoneurial fluid pressure
- Antegrade and retrograde axonal transport systems also may be affected; low-pressure compressions most common type with entrapment injuries

5. What nerve entrapments are found in the lower extremity?

- Meralgia paresthetica—The lateral cutaneous nerve of the thigh (lateral femoral cutaneous nerve) is compressed about the anterior superior iliac spine as it passes under the inguinal ligament.
- Femoral nerve entrapment—The femoral nerve is a mixed nerve that can be entrapped in the anterior abdominal wall as it passes under the inguinal ligament or in the femoral triangle.
- Obturator nerve entrapment—The obturator nerve, although not usually compromised, is a mixed nerve that can become entrapped in the obturator foramen and as it passes through the obturator externus.
- Saphenous nerve entrapment—The saphenous nerve is a cutaneous nerve that can become entrapped in the distal thigh as it passes through the adductor canal. It is the distal extension of the femoral nerve.
- Piriformis syndrome—The sciatic nerve can become entrapped as it passes through the piriformis muscle.
- Common fibular (peroneal) neuropathy—Both the superficial and the deep fibular nerve branches can become compressed as they pass around the fibular head.
- Fibular neuropathy (superficial branch)—The superficial fibular nerve can be compressed as it passes through the deep fascia of the anterolateral leg to become subcutaneous.
- Fibular neuropathy (deep branch)—Compression can affect the deep fibular nerve in the anterior compartment.
- Ski boot syndrome (anterior tarsal tunnel syndrome)—The deep fibular (peroneal) nerve can become entrapped at the ankle, most commonly as a result of tight-fitting shoes.
- Tarsal tunnel syndrome—The medial and/or lateral plantar nerve can be compressed at the ankle.
- Sural nerve compression—The purely cutaneous sural nerve can be compressed as it passes through the deep investing fascia of the leg or by an extrinsic source such as tight boots.

6. How does meralgia paresthetica present clinically? Describe its pathogenesis.

Presenting symptoms typically include altered or absent sensation over the lateral aspect of the mid-thigh. Other sensory symptoms may include burning pain, dull ache, itching, and tingling over the cutaneous nerve field supplied by the lateral cutaneous nerve of the thigh (lateral femoral cutaneous nerve). The nerve is purely cutaneous and becomes superficial to supply the skin of the lateral thigh about 10 cm distal to the inguinal ligament. No loss in motor function should occur with isolated involvement of this nerve, apart from possible guarding secondary to pain with hip extension, which may increase symptoms.

7. Describe the cause and prognosis of meralgia paresthetica.

The cause may be tight clothing (tight underwear or tight jeans), pendulous abdomen, or rapid increase in weight. A variant in the normal path of exit from the pelvis also may increase the likelihood of entrapment. The prognosis is good in the vast majority of patients when the predisposing cause has been identified and removed. The peak incidence occurs during middle age, when progressive weight gains are also frequently observed. The incidence is equivalent on both right and left sides; symptoms may occur intermittently over a period of years, either unilaterally or bilaterally. Other forms of treatment include injection of an anesthetic agent with or without a corticosteroid in the area of suspected involvement.

8. What causes femoral nerve entrapment?

The femoral nerve can become compressed anywhere along its course by such diverse factors as tumors, psoas abscesses, lymph node enlargement, hematoma, or penetrating trauma. The nerve also can be compressed at the inguinal ligament or stretched when it is subjected to excessive hip abduction and external rotation (e.g., during vaginal deliveries). Weakness in knee extension and possibly hip flexion, because of the involvement of the rectus femoris, may be noted. Sensation may be affected on the medial aspect of the knee and the anterior aspect of the thigh, which are supplied by the saphenous branch of the femoral nerve and the anterior cutaneous nerve of the thigh, respectively.

9. How does an obturator nerve entrapment present?

Obturator nerve entrapments are rare. When they occur, they usually are associated with acute trauma attributable to an event such as childbirth, pelvic trauma, or surgery. The adductor muscles supplied by the obturator nerve may be weakened, and sensation may or may not be decreased in the middle portion of the medial thigh. Problems noted by the patient include pain in the region of the inguinal ligament, instability of the lower extremity during gait, and atrophy of the adductor muscles.

10. What clinical manifestations are associated with entrapment of the saphenous nerve?

Before passing through the adductor hiatus, the saphenous nerve pierces the tough connective tissue layer between the sartorius and gracilis muscles to supply the skin of the anteromedial knee, medial leg, and medial side of the foot as distally as the metatarsal phalangeal joint. In some cases, the nerve also may pass through the sartorius muscle. The possible site of entrapment at this location is the point where the nerve passes through the thick connective tissue of the investing fascia and undergoes a sharp angulation. It is also possible to have a second site of entrapment as the infrapatellar branch of the saphenous nerve passes through the sartorius tendon. In this case, symptoms are restricted to the infrapatellar region.

The most common complaint is knee pain, which may or may not be associated with sensory changes in the distribution of the saphenous nerve. Vigorous palpation at the point where the nerve pierces the subsartorial canal may reproduce the patient's symptoms. Treatments range from injection of an anesthetic with or without corticosteroid to surgical decompression.

11. List four sites of potential fibular nerve entrapment.

- In the popliteal space behind the knee
- At the fibular head
- In the anterior compartment of the leg (as the deep fibular nerve)
- In the lateral compartment of the leg (as the superficial fibular nerve)

The common fibular nerve is the most commonly injured nerve in the lower extremity.

12. Describe the clinical presentation of compression of the superficial sensory fibular nerve.

Approximately at the junction between the middle and distal third of the leg, the purely cutaneous continuation of the superficial sensory fibular nerve passes through the deep fascia to become subcutaneous. At this site, the fascia may be tough or restrictive, creating a potential point of entrapment. The terminal extensions of the superficial fibular nerve are the medial and lateral cutaneous branches, which supply the distal two thirds of the anterolateral leg and the dorsum of the foot, apart from the web space between the great and second toes. Symptoms are present along the distribution supplied by the nerve—over the distal leg and dorsum of the foot. Common injuries, such as an inversion sprain of the ankle, may stress this nerve at the point where it passes through the fascial opening.

13. Describe the clinical presentation of a deep fibular nerve injury.

Once the nerve has left the region of the fibular head and entered the anterior compartment, it is relatively protected and rarely entrapped, apart from problems associated with the anterior compartment. Anatomically, a compartment is created with the tibia medially, the fibula laterally, the interosseous membrane posteriorly, and a tough fascial layer anteriorly. Insults that involve this compartment can affect deep fibular nerve or anterior tibial artery function or muscle tissue directly. Examples range from anterior tibialis strain (shin splints: a mild form of anterior compartment syndrome) to muscle inflammation secondary to prolonged exercise, direct trauma to the leg, snake bites, or arterial bleeding. Significant increases in pressure are treated with fasciotomy—an incision of the anterior fascia of the leg.

14. Describe the tarsal tunnel.

The tarsal tunnel can be anatomically described as an anterior tarsal tunnel and a posterior tarsal tunnel. The more common and traditional use of the term tarsal tunnel syndrome relates to the nerve and vascular structures that may be compromised in the posterior tarsal tunnel. The anterior tarsal tunnel (ATT) is located anterior to the talotibial and talonavicular joints where the deep fibular (deep peroneal) nerve and dorsal pedis artery pass beneath the inferior extensor retinaculum of the ankle. The posterior tarsal tunnel (PTT) or tibiotalocalcaneal tunnel is posterior to the medial malleolus of the tibia. The tibial nerve usually branches into its four divisions—medial plantar, lateral plantar, medial calcaneal, and inferior calcaneal nerves—within the confines of the PTT. In the PTT, the posterior tibial artery usually branches into the medial plantar, lateral plantar, and medial calcaneal arteries.

15. What is anterior tarsal tunnel syndrome?

Anterior tarsal tunnel syndrome (ATTS), also known as ski boot syndrome, is caused by compression of the deep fibular nerve (DFN) as it passes deep to the inferior extensor retinaculum. ATTS is also seen in runners and soccer players that wear tight-fitting shoes, compressing the nerve in the region of the anterior ankle. After the deep fibular nerve passes through the ATT, it will provide motor function to the extensor digitorum brevis (EDB) and extensor hallucis brevis (EHB) and sensation to the web space between the great and second toes. The most common presentation involves only the sensory component; numbness and tingling are identified in the web space between the great and second toes. However, both motor and sensory fibers may be involved, in which case weakness may be identified in the EDB and EHB. Electrophysiologic testing, including sensory and motor nerve conduction studies of the DFN and needle EMG studies of the EDB and EHB, can be used to identify involvement of the distal aspect of the deep fibular nerve. Clinically, this nerve is sometimes compromised after repeated ankle sprains.

16. What is posterior tarsal tunnel syndrome?

The posterior tarsal tunnel (PTT) is the region where the muscular, vascular, and nerve structures of the posterior compartment of the leg continue into the foot, passing between the medial malleolus and calcaneus in a tunnel created by the flexor retinaculum. In 90% of individuals, the tibial nerve splits into the medial plantar, lateral plantar, medial calcaneal, and inferior calcaneal nerves while still within the posterior tarsal tunnel. The medial calcaneal branch of the tibial nerve may bifurcate in this region, but its origin is highly variable and may occur proximal to, within, or distal to the PTT. Thus entrapment of the nervous structures in this region may affect the medial plantar nerve, lateral plantar nerve, medial calcaneal branch, or inferior calcaneal branch, or any combination of these nerves. Symptoms involving the plantar nerves include pain, burning, and paresthesias, often in the distribution of one or both plantar nerves.

17. Is tarsal tunnel syndrome a common problem? What branch of the plantar nerve is preferentially involved?

The diagnosis of posterior tarsal tunnel syndrome (PTTS) is not particularly easy because there are no hallmarks of the disorder. An area of potential controversy is the actual extent of the posterior tarsal tunnel (PTT). Some clinicians refer only to the region under the flexor retinaculum as the PTT. Others refer to the entire region from the flexor retinaculum proximally to the metatarsophalangeal joint distally as the PTT. Both methods of describing the posterior tarsal tunnel are accepted although electrophysiologic testing of these structures may specifically demonstrate involvement of the individual plantar or calcaneal nerves. Sensory nerve conduction is the most sensitive electrodiagnostic examination for possible compromise of the medial plantar nerve, lateral plantar nerve, or calcaneal nerve in the region of the ankle or foot.

The medial plantar nerve may be involved more frequently than the lateral plantar nerve, although the overall incidence of plantar neuropathies is relatively low. Steinitz et al. reported an incidence rate of 0.58% (51) after 8727 electromyographic examinations, similar to the 0.5% incidence found by Oh. Because repetitive pronation or foot hypermobility may stress the medial plantar nerve in activities such as jogging or jumping, the constellation of symptoms associated with medial plantar neuropathy has been called "jogger's foot." Determination of the extent of nerve involvement is an electrodiagnostic challenge that requires detailed examination and meticulous technique.

18. What causes entrapment of the sural nerve?

In general, passage through the fascia of the leg is not a common site of entrapment; thus sural nerve compressions are relatively rare. When an entrapment occurs, it usually is associated with factors such as a ganglion cyst, tight combat boots, or stretch injury. An important clinical point is that the sural nerve is often evaluated when generalized polyneuropathy is suspected. A decrease in nerve conduction velocity in this nerve as well as other major nerves of the leg (e.g., tibial and deep peroneal) suggests polyneuropathy.

19. How sensitive and specific is electrophysiologic testing?

Most of the work investigating sensitivity and specificity in electrophysiologic testing has been conducted in the upper extremities, with values of greater than 85% sensitivity and 95% specificity reported for entrapments of the median nerve at the wrist. Other researchers have found for the median nerve that the composite electrophysiologic measures for sensitivity range between 49% and 84%, with specificity values of 95% or higher reported. Assuming that these values can be applied to lower extremity entrapments, they indicate that while the electrophysiologic tests are quite good, they are not perfect. False-positive electrophysiologic findings have been reported, and the clinician using the information derived from these examinations must also consider the patient's clinical presentation and clinical evaluation.

20. Are there regions of the lower extremity that have a tendency to generate electrophysiologic "false positives"?

Yes. Recent research identified that 21% of patients have abnormal needle electromyographic (EMG) results that suggested denervation, when examining the abductor hallucis intrinsic muscle of the foot. These abnormal electrophysiologic findings additionally appeared to increase with age, being most noticeable in individuals over the age of 60. A second muscle examined, the fibularis (peroneus) tertius, also demonstrated positive findings in normal subjects over the age of 60, but at a much lower rate of 9%. The reasons for these findings and the anecdotal reports of spontaneous abnormal EMG in the foot are unclear, but the findings may be associated with the fact that we ambulate on some of the intrinsic muscles of the foot, or that these muscles and their vascular and nerve supplies are restricted by structures such as shoes.

Other studies have demonstrated a much more conservative prevalence of only 2% when examining foot intrinsics in normal subjects. Regardless of the cause, false positives are possible and relatively common with EMG of the small muscles of the foot.

Bibliography

Akyuz G et al: Anterior tarsal tunnel syndrome, *Electromyogr Clin Neurophysiol* 40:123-128, 2000.

American Association of Electrodiagnostic Medicine: Practice parameters for electrodiagnostic studies in carpal tunnel syndrome—summary statement, *Muscle Nerve* 16:1390-1391, 1993.

Boon A, Harper C: Needle EMG of abductor hallucis and peroneus tertius in normal subjects, *Muscle Nerve* 27:752-756, 2003.

Dillingham T: Electrodiagnostic approach to patients with suspected radiculopathy, *Phys Med Rehabil Clin North Am* 13:567-588, 2002.

Dumitru D: Reaction of the peripheral nervous system to injury. In Dumitru D, editor: *Electrodiagnostic medicine,* Philadelphia, 1994, pp 341-384, Hanley & Belfus.

Dumitru D, Diaz C, King J: Prevalence of denervation in paraspinal and foot intrinsic musculature, *Am J Phys Med Rehabil* 80:482-490, 2001.

Dumitru D, Zwarts M: Focal peripheral neuropathies. In Dumitru D, Amato A, Zwarts M, editors: *Electrodiagnostic medicine,* Philadelphia, 2002, pp 1043-1126, Hanley & Belfus.

Fritz J, Wainner R: Examining diagnostic tests: an evidence-based perspective, *Phys Ther* 81:1546-1564, 2001.

Jablecki C, Andary M, So Y: Literature review of the usefulness of nerve conduction studies and electromyography for the evaluation of patients with carpal tunnel syndrome, *Muscle Nerve* 16:1392-1414, 1993.

Jablecki C et al: Second AAEM literature review of the usefulness of nerve conduction studies and needle electromyography for the evaluation of patients with carpal tunnel syndrome, *Muscle Nerve* June 11, 2002.

Kimura J: *Electrodiagnosis in diseases of nerve and muscle,* Philadelphia, 1978, FA Davis.

Kuntzer T: Carpal tunnel syndrome in 100 patients: sensitivity, specificy on multi-neurophysiological procedures and estimation of axonal loss of motor, sensory and sympathetic median nerve fibers, *J Neurol Sci* 20:221-229, 1994.

Netter F: *Atlas of human anatomy,* ed 3, Teterboro, NJ, 2003, Icon Learning Systems.

Oh S: Nerve conduction in focal neuropathies. In Oh S, editor: *Clinical electromyography: nerve conduction studies,* Baltimore, 1993, p 496, Williams & Wilkins.

Portney L, Dumitru D: Validity of measurements. In Portney L, Watkins M, editors: *Foundations of clinical research: applications to practice,* Englewood, NJ, 2000, pp 79-110, Prentice Hall Health.

Steinitz E, Singh S, Saeed M: Diagnostic tests help clarify tarsal tunnel mystery, *Biomechanics* 10:43, 1999.

Section XII

The Foot and Ankle

Chapter 75

Functional Anatomy of the Foot and Ankle

Jeffrey E. Balazsy, MD, and Joseph A. Brosky, Jr., PT, MS, SCS

1. What are the major anatomic divisions of the bones of the foot?

The rear foot (tarsus) consists of the talus and calcaneus. The midfoot (lesser tarsus) consists of the navicular, cuboid, and cuneiforms (lateral, medial, and intermediate). Distal to the midfoot are the metatarsals and phalanges. The foot also may be divided into medial and lateral columns. The medial column is the talus, navicular, cuneiforms (lateral, medial, and intermediate), and metatarsals 1 to 3 with their respective phalanges. The lateral column consists of the calcaneus, cuboid, and metatarsals 4 to 5 with their respective phalanges.

2. What are the four muscular layers, from superficial to deep, on the plantar aspect of the foot?

FIRST LAYER (3 MUSCLES)

- Abductor hallucis
- Flexor digitorum brevis (FDB)
- Abductor digit minimi (ADM)

SECOND LAYER (2 MUSCLES)

- Quadratus plantae
- Lumbricals

The *tendons* of the flexor hallucis longus and the flexor digitorum longus, which are considered extrinsic foot muscles located in the leg, also pass through this layer.

THIRD LAYER (3 MUSCLES)

- Flexor hallucis brevis (FHB)
- Adductor hallucis
- Flexor digit minimi brevis (FDMB)

FOURTH LAYER (2 MUSCLES)

- Plantar interossei (3 muscles; PAD = Plantar ADduct)
- Dorsal interossei (4 muscles; DAB = Dorsal ABduct)

The *tendons* of the peroneus longus and tibialis posterior, which are considered extrinsic foot muscles located in the leg, also pass through this layer.

3. Describe the axis of movement and range of motion (ROM) of the foot and ankle.

	Talocrural	Subtalar	Midtarsal	Tarsometatarsal
ROM	PF: 0°-50° DF: 0°-20°	IN: 0°-35° EV: 0°-15°	IN: 0°-20° EV: 0°-10°	PF: 0°-15° DF: 0°-3°
Axis	80° from vertical (10° up from horizontal), 84° from longitudinal reference of foot	40°-45° superior from horizontal reference, 15°-18° medially from longitudinal reference (sagittal plane)	15° superior from horizontal reference, 9° to midline for IN/EV	Similar to subtalar joint

PF, Plantar flexion; *DF,* dorsiflexion; *IN,* inversion; *EV,* eversion; *ROM,* range of motion.

4. How much ankle ROM is typically required for normal gait?

Approximately 6 to 10 degrees of dorsiflexion and 20 to 30 degrees of plantar flexion are required for normal gait.

5. How much subtalar ROM is required for normal gait?

A total of 4 to 6 degrees of inversion/eversion is required for normal gait.

6. What is the correct terminology to use when referring to or describing foot and ankle motion?

It is correct to use the suffix "-us" or "-ed" when describing or referring to a position (e.g., supinatus or pronated), and "-ion" and "-ing" when describing or referring to motion (e.g., supination or pronating).

7. Define pronation and supination in relation to the rear foot.

Pronation and supination are the triplane motions in the subtalar joint, the so-called universal joint of the lower extremity. In closed kinetic chain gait (i.e., weight-bearing, foot planted on the ground), pronation occurs at heel strike or initial contact and through the loading response during gait. Internal rotation of the lower leg produces talar adduction and plantar flexion relative to the calcaneus, and the calcaneus everts. This process occurs during the first 25% of the stance phase of gait, as the foot approaches and adapts to the ground.

Supination during closed kinetic chain gait occurs from the start of the midstance phase of gait (foot flat) until the end of stance (toe-off). This process occurs as the lower leg starts to rotate externally, leading to talar abduction (dorsiflexion relative to the calcaneus), and the calcaneus inverts. In open kinetic chain gait (i.e., non–weight-bearing, foot off the ground), the talus is relatively fixed in the ankle mortise, and supination/pronation occurs through the subtalar joint by movement of the calcaneus and foot around the subtalar joint axis of motion. In supination, the calcaneus and foot move through a combination of inversion, adduction, and plantar flexion in relation to the fixed talus. In pronation, the calcaneus moves through eversion, abduction, and dorsiflexion relative to the fixed talus.

8. Explain the windlass mechanism of the foot.

The windlass mechanism refers to the seemingly simple maneuver of dorsiflexion of the toes of the foot, most specifically related to passive hallux extension that produces a medial longitudinal arch through hindfoot supination. The plantar fascia and intrinsic foot musculature are supinators around the subtalar joint axis of motion. Hence dorsiflexion of the digits produces supination, which creates the medial longitudinal arch of the foot through reciprocal midtarsal joint motion.

9. What are the common arches of the normal foot?

There are four primary arches of the normal foot supported by myoligamentous structures. The two longitudinal arches are the medial longitudinal arch (MLA) and the lateral longitudinal arch (LLA). The MLA is formed by the medial columnar structures of the calcaneus, the talus, the navicular, the three cuneiforms, and metatarsals 1, 2, and 3. The LLA is formed by the calcaneus, the cuboid, and metatarsals 4 and 5. The two transverse arches are the proximal transverse arch (formed by the bony structures of the navicular, the three cuneiforms, and the cuboid) and the distal transverse arch (formed by the heads of the five metatarsals).

10. What is pes planus?

Pes planus (congenital flatfoot) describes a foot that exhibits no longitudinal arch and an ankle that is everted (valgus). It can be classified as rigid or flexible. A rigid flatfoot is often associated with a tarsal coalition or a vertical talus, and a flexible flatfoot is considered a normal variant. Pes planus is normal in children up to 6 to 7 years of age. A rigid flatfoot is always flat, but a flexible flatfoot appears normal when non–weight-bearing, but becomes flat when standing. If a flexible flatfoot is asymptomatic, no treatment is warranted, but if symptomatic, then stretching and arch supports are often incorporated. If the deformity is rigid, then the underlying cause (e.g., tarsal coalition, vertical talus) must be addressed.

11. What is pes cavus?

Pes cavus refers to a high arch foot. This can be a benign condition that merely describes a foot type exhibiting an abnormally high arch or can be related to muscle imbalances in the immature foot, although it is important to rule out the possibility of underlying neuromuscular disease (such as Charcot-Marie-Tooth disease) The presentation is typically an 8- to 10-year-old child who complains of ankle pain, habitually toe-walks, and exhibits tight tendo Achilles and limited ankle dorsiflexion. A clinical workup may be needed that includes radiographs, EMG/NCS, and MRI of the spine to rule out occult neuromuscular disease. Treatment may include bracing/ankle-foot orthoses (AFOs), osteotomies, and tendon transfers.

12. What is the ideal position for ankle fusion (e.g., arthrodesis)?

The ideal position for ankle arthrodesis is neutral dorsiflexion (slight plantar flexion if heeled shoes are preferred, e.g., women), slight valgus (0 to 5 degrees), and external rotation of approximately 5 to 10 degrees.

13. What percentage of weight does the fibula bear?

The fibula supports approximately 12% to 17% of the axial load.

14. What is Fick's angle?

Normally when an individual stands, the posture of the foot assumes a slight toe-out position, and this angle, approximately 12 to 18 degrees in the adult (5 degrees in children), is sometimes referred to as Fick's angle.

15. Describe the function of the deltoid ligament.

The deltoid or medial collateral ligament of the rear foot consists of a superficial and a deep ligament complex. The superficial deltoid ligament consists of the ligament attachment to the distal tibia (medial malleolus) with insertions onto the navicular, sustentaculum tali, and talus. These ligament fibers are vertically oriented and therefore prevent excessive rear-foot eversion in the frontal plane. The deep deltoid ligament consists of relatively transversely oriented fibers deep to the superficial band from the medial malleolus anteriorly and posteriorly along the medial body of the talus. Thus it resists excessive transverse plane rotation (abduction) of the talus. The deltoid ligament may be sprained under excessive loading of the ankle and rear foot in eversion or may avulse a portion of the medial malleolus as part of an ankle fracture (four components: tibionavicular, tibiocalcaneal, anterior tibiotalar, and posterior tibiotalar).

16. What are the lateral collateral ligaments of the ankle and rear foot?

The lateral collateral complex of rear-foot and ankle ligaments consists of the anterior and posterior talofibular ligaments and the calcaneofibular ligament. The anterior talofibular ligament and calcaneofibular ligaments are most commonly sprained in inversion ankle injuries. The horizontally oriented anterior talofibular ligament and the more vertically oriented calcaneofibular ligaments provide reciprocal stability to the rear foot. In a plantar-flexed position of the ankle, the anterior talofibular ligament (flat, fan-shaped capsular ligament) is the primary stabilizer to rear-foot inversion. In a dorsiflexed position, the cordlike calcaneofibular ligament is the stabilizer to rear-foot inversion.

17. Define Lisfranc's ligament.

Lisfranc's ligament is the plantar tarsometatarsal ligament spanning the medial cuneiform to the base of the second metatarsal. In fractures and dislocations of Lisfranc's joint, this ligament commonly avulses a fragment of bone from the plantar medial base of the second metatarsal.

18. What is the "spring ligament"?

The spring ligament is the calcaneonavicular ligament, which extends from the plantar aspect of the sustentaculum tali to the navicular. It provides support to the plantar head of the talus and talonavicular joint and is a primary static stabilizer reinforcing the medial longitudinal arch.

19. What is the bifurcate ligament?

The bifurcate ligament is y-shaped and originates from the anterior floor of the sinus tarsi and anterior process of the calcaneus. It extends and divides distally into two distinct bands that attach to the cuboid laterally and navicular medially. This ligament provides important stability to the rear foot.

20. Define Chopart's and Lisfranc's joints.

Chopart's joint is the midtarsal joint, which consists of the talonavicular and calcaneocuboid joints. Lisfranc's joint is the tarsometatarsal joint, which consists of the three cuneiforms and metatarsals 4 and 5.

21. How does the weight-bearing surface of the ankle change after syndesmotic injury of the ankle?

Mortise widening resulting in a 1-mm lateral shift of the talus decreases the weight-bearing surface of the talus by 40%, a 3-mm shift by >60%, and a 5-mm shift by approximately 80%. Increased contact pressures lead to early degenerative joint disease.

22. Why is the anterior talus subject to impingement?

The anterior talus is 2.5 mm wider than the posterior talus. With dorsiflexion, the space available in the anterior mortise is decreased. This space can be further compromised by osteophytes, scar tissue, or overly compressed open reduction and internal fixation (ORIF) to the syndesmosis after ankle fracture. The compression/distraction of the (talocrural joint) ankle joint that occurs with normal walking may be important for normal lubrication of the joint.

23. What is the sinus tarsi?

The sinus tarsi is a funnel-shaped opening in the rear foot between the talus and calcaneus. It is widest anterolaterally and narrows as it passes posteromedially between the talus and calcaneus, separating the anterior and middle facets of the subtalar joint from the posterior facet. The narrow posteromedial section of this space often is called the tarsal canal. Through this area pass the interosseous talocalcaneal ligament and the major blood supply to the body of the talus (the anastomosis between the artery of the tarsal canal and the artery of the tarsal sinus).

24. What are the contents of the tarsal tunnel?

From superficial to deep, the contents of the tarsal tunnel can be remembered by the mnemonic Tom, Dick, And Very Nervous Harry:

Tom = posterior Tibial tendon
Dick = flexor Digitorum longus
And Very Nervous = posterior tibial Artery, Vein, and Nerve
Harry = flexor Hallucis longus

25. Describe the structure of the tarsal tunnel.

The tunnel is bounded by the distal tibia (medial malleolus) anteriorly and the Achilles tendon posteriorly; it is roofed by the flexor retinaculum (laciniate ligament). The flexor retinaculum divides into fibrous (septae) bands that separate the contents of the tarsal tunnel into individual compartments.

26. List the five nerves that cross into and supply the motor and sensory fibers to the foot.

1. Sural nerve (posterolaterally)
2. Superficial peroneal nerve (anterolaterally)
3. Deep peroneal nerve (anteriorly, travels with the dorsalis pedis artery)
4. Saphenous nerve (anteromedially, as the long continuation of the femoral nerve distally)
5. Posterior tibial nerve (posteromedially, as it divides to supply the foot distally as the medial and lateral plantar nerves)

27. Define porta pedis.

The porta pedis is the anatomic opening into the plantar aspect of the foot beneath the belly of the abductor hallucis muscle. Through this opening pass the medial and lateral plantar nerves and arteries/veins distally from the tarsal tunnel into the foot. The porta pedis is a potential site for compression of the plantar nerves and may also be a cause of heel pain.

28. What structure is referred to as "freshman's nerve"?

The plantaris tendon, which often appears like a nerve to new dissectors of the human cadaver, is referred to as "freshman's nerve." However, its location; flat, firm appearance; and consistency reveal that it is tendon. It travels deep to the gastrocnemius and superficial to the soleus to lie medial to the Achilles tendon, where it attaches onto the medial aspect of the posterior calcaneal tuberosity.

29. What is meant by an "accessory bone" of the foot?

An accessory bone is a small ossicle or bone that separates from the normal bone (most commonly caused by fracture or a secondary ossification center). Accessory bones are more frequently found in the foot than anywhere else in the body. The most common are the os trigonum (from the posterior talus), the os tibiale externum (from the navicular tuberosity), the bipartite medial cuneiform (superior/inferior), the os vesalianum pedis (tuberosity of the base of the fifth metatarsal), the os sustentaculi (sustentaculum tali), and the os supranaviculare (dorsum of talonavicular joint).

30. Describe the function of the sesamoids.

The sesamoids are located beneath the head of the first metatarsal. The two functions of the sesamoids are (1) to transfer loads through the soft tissues to the metatarsal head and (2) to increase the lever arm of the flexor hallucis brevis to aid in push-off.

31. What is the "master knot of Henry"?

The "master knot of Henry" is a fibrous band on the plantar aspect of the foot adjoining the flexor digitorum longus and flexor hallucis longus tendons in the second layer.

32. What is the effect of an increasing hallux valgus on plantar flexion force at push-off?

A hallux valgus angle of 40 degrees decreases push-off strength of the great toe by 78%. Adding a 30-degree pronation deformity decreases the plantar flexion strength to 5% of normal.

33. What is Toygar's triangle?

On the lateral radiograph of the foot and ankle, Toygar's triangle is the hypodense radiographic triangle bordered by the more radiodense Achilles tendon posteriorly, the superior border of the calcaneus at its base, and the posterior border of the mid-to-distal tibia. When the triangle is not apparent on the lateral radiograph, the usual cause is accumulation of fluid along the tarsal tunnel, which may suggest inflammation from ankle, subtalar joint, or retrocalcaneal bursitis. The triangle may be obliterated completely by hematoma or swelling around an Achilles tendon rupture.

34. What are the normal forces (relative to body weight) acting on the ankle joint during functional activities such as walking, running and jumping?

Compressive forces during normal walking are 1 to 1.2 times body weight, running 2 times body weight, and jumping (from a height of about 24 inches) 4 to 5 times body weight.

35. How many muscles attach to the talus?

None. One of the unique features of the talus is that there are no musculotendinous attachments to it.

36. What is metatarsus adductus?

This refers to one of the most common pediatric foot disorders and describes the position of the forefoot in varus and adduction. It is often associated with intrauterine position, and clinically presents with a "kidney bean" appearance depicting the nature of the deformity, and an in-toeing gait. Most will resolve with normal development, minor shoe modifications, or serial casting; rarely is surgical intervention (e.g., midfoot osteotomy) required.

37. What is the function of the interossei and lumbrical muscles?

The dorsal interossei (DAB, four muscles) are abductors of the toes, while the plantar interossei (PAD, three muscles) perform adduction of the toes. The combined primary actions of the lumbricals and interossei are plantar flexion of the metatarsophalangeal joints and extension at the proximal interphalangeal and distal interphalangeal joints.

38. Describe the functional anatomy of the anterior talofibular ligament.

Bone is less dense at the fibular attachment, but the enthesis fibrocartilage is more prominent. Fibrocartilage is present at the site where the ligament wraps around the lateral talar articular margin in the plantar-flexed and inverted foot, likely as a result of compression in this region. Avulsion fractures are less common at the talar end because the bone is more dense here and stress is dissipated away from the talar enthesis by the fibrocartilaginous character of the ligament near the talus.

39. What is the relationship between metatarsal length and midfoot arthrosis?

Patients with midfoot arthrosis have a significantly higher ratio of second metatarsal to first metatarsal length as compared to controls. Studies have shown the functional length of the second metatarsal was 18.6% greater than the first metatarsal in the arthrosis group, as compared to 4.1% for the control group.

Bibliography

Davitt JS et al: An association between functional second metacarpal length and midfoot arthrosis, *J Bone Joint Surg Am* 87:795-800, 2005.

Kapandji IA: *The physiology of the joints,* vol 2, New York, 1987, Churchill Livingstone.

Kumai T et al: The functional anatomy of the human anterior talofibular ligament in relation to ankle sprains, *J Anat* 200:457-465, 2002.

Magee DJ, editor: *Orthopedic physical assessment,* ed 4, Philadelphia, 2002, Saunders-Elsevier Science.

Mizel MS, Miller RA, Scioli MW, editors: *Orthopaedic knowledge update—foot and ankle II,* Rosemont, Ill, 1998, American Academy of Orthopedic Surgeons.

Nordin M, Frankel VH, editors: *Basic biomechanics of the musculoskeletal system,* Philadelphia, 1989, Lea & Febiger.

Rockwood CA et al, editors: *Fractures in adults,* Philadelphia, 1996, Lippincott-Raven.

Thompson JC: *Netter's concise atlas of orthopaedic anatomy,* Teterboro, NJ, 2002, Icon Learning Systems.

Chapter 76

Common Orthopaedic Foot and Ankle Dysfunctions

Susan Mais Requejo, PT, DPT, and
Stephen F. Reischl, PT, DPT, OCS

1. What is the difference between Achilles tendonitis and Achilles tendonosis?

True tendonitis is an inflammatory process of the midsubstance of the tendon. This can be caused by overuse activities or be related to a specific disease process such as rheumatic diseases. Therefore a thorough medical history including knowledge of the patient's activity level is necessary. The signs of inflammation are pain on palpation, swelling, warmth, and pain on active contraction of the muscle-tendon complex. Passive stretching may also induce pain.

Achilles tendonosis is the pathologic condition of the tendon beyond the inflammatory stage, when the tendon has failed to heal. The patient may report mild pain with their desired level of activity, and it may progress to limiting their activity considerably. There may be an appearance of thickening of the tendon, but this is not swelling related to the inflammation. Most patients will report a failure of NSAIDs to provide relief. MRI findings may show signal changes inside the tendon. In addition, high-resolution ultrasound and Doppler recording can identify this pathology more clearly. The tendon may have hyperechoic areas indicating disorganization of the collagen fibers. There have been multiple studies confirming the phenomenon of neovascularization—the attempt of the tendon to heal by bringing blood vessels to the damaged areas. It is speculated that nerve fibers that accompany these new blood vessels are the source of long-term pain experienced in these patients.

2. What areas of the Achilles complex need to be palpated?

In addition to differentiating Achilles tendonosis and tendonitis, it is important to discriminate between pain in the midsubstance of the tendon versus pain in the myotendinous junction and the insertion of the tendon. Patients may have pain at the attachment of the Achilles tendon to the calcaneus caused by an inflamed retrocalcaneal bursa. Pain or symptoms at the myotendinous junction are often related to muscular strain.

3. What is the treatment for Achilles tendonitis?

In the inflammatory phase, modalities are used to reduce edema and pain. In addition, the use of medication may relieve symptoms. It is necessary to unload the tendon with heel lifts and activity modification for healing to occur. Studies have shown that heel lifts of ½ inch have resulted in a decrease in the EMG activity of the calf during walking. Once the inflammatory process is resolved, a program of "reloading" the muscle-tendon complex can be accomplished with return to activities.

4. What is the treatment for Achilles tendonosis?

The initial intervention is rest and adequate unloading of the tendon. The patient must understand that tendons "heal" very slowly, and this process will take months to accomplish. Frequently, heel lifts of ½ inch either in shoes or attached to the outer sole reduce symptoms. It is the responsibility of the physical therapist to assess the function of the entire lower extremity to identify if there are other impairment findings in the lower extremity (hip/knee weakness, flexibility issues) that may have contributed to the cause of the tendon dysfunction.

5. What is the evidence for the use of eccentric exercise in Achilles tendonosis?

Once the therapist determines the period of rest needed for the tendon, a program of reloading the tendon can be started. Alfredson and others have confirmed that following a program of 12 weeks of eccentric loading, patients improved significantly in function and had reduced pain. The program consisted of a heavy-load eccentric workout of 3 sets of 15 calf-lowering exercises. In addition, Ohberg, using high-definition ultrasound, confirmed improvements in the structure of the tendon following this eccentric type of loading program.

6. What are the common rupture sites of the Achilles tendon complex?

The most common site is a complete midsubstance rupture of the Achilles tendon. This area, 2 to 6 cm proximal to the insertion site, is most susceptible to injury because it is hypovascular. The second most common site is the musculotendinous interface, followed by the rare avulsion of the tendon from the bone. An incomplete rupture of the Achilles tendon also can evolve from chronic tendonosis.

7. Describe the typical patient with Achilles tendon rupture.

The typical patient is over age 40 and engages in a physical activity or sport. Predisposing factors include advanced age, weekend athletes, history of tendonitis or tendonosis, and loss of flexibility in the Achilles tendon.

8. How is an Achilles tendon rupture diagnosed?

The gold standard is the Thompson test. The patient is positioned prone with the foot hanging off the table. The examiner squeezes the widest girth of the calf. Lack of plantar flexion indicates a complete rupture. In a negative test with the tendon intact, the ankle involuntarily plantar-flexes. The patient most likely will be unable to perform a heel rise while standing and will likely have a palpable deformity at the tendon.

9. Compare the outcomes of conservative and surgical treatments for complete Achilles tendon rupture.

The optimal treatment for complete Achilles disruption is highly controversial. Cetti et al. randomized 111 patients with acute rupture into groups of operative (56 patients) and non-operative treatment (55 patients). Ruptures recurred in 3 patients in the operative group and 7 in the nonoperative group. The operative group had a significantly higher rate of return to sport at the same level (57%) than the nonoperative group (29%) as well as better ankle movement and a lesser degree of calf atrophy. The authors concluded that operative treatment was more favorable, but nonoperative treatment is an acceptable alternative.

The major advantage of nonoperative treatment is reduced risk of infection from surgery, but because of the higher risk of recurrent rupture, competitive athletes and active people may be better candidates for surgery.

10. Describe the treatment protocol after surgical repair of Achilles tendon rupture.

The most common protocol after surgery is immobilization in a cast with the foot in slight plantar flexion for 6 to 8 weeks. Weight-bearing is at the discretion of the surgeon. After the cast is removed, the patient progresses to a heel lift in the shoe. Therapy focuses on progressive plantar flexion strengthening. Dorsiflexion stretching should be avoided until 4 months postoperatively. A reasonable goal is full plantar flexion strength with 20 single-leg heel raises by 6 months. The patient should be able to run by 7 to 9 months and return to full activity by 10 to 12 months.

11. Describe an accelerated program for patients undergoing surgical repair of the Achilles tendon.

A more aggressive protocol is used in patients who receive a type of suturing that results in stronger repair. The patient is immobilized for 72 hours, followed by early active range of motion exercises. The patient uses a posterior splint for 2 weeks and then ambulates in a hinged orthosis. Six weeks after surgery, the patient can fully bear weight, and progressive resistive exercises are initiated. Mandelbaum reported that with this technique ankle strength was 35% of the opposite side by the third month. All patients returned to preinjury activity levels at a mean of 4 months (range: 3 to 7 months) after repair. By 12 months, there were no significant differences in ankle motion, isokinetic strength, or endurance compared with the uninvolved side.

12. Describe symptoms for tarsal tunnel syndrome.

Pain in the area of the tarsal tunnel or into the foot is the most commonly reported symptom. Some patients also may complain of paresthesia in the foot.

13. What factors may contribute to tarsal tunnel syndrome?

Mechanical factors (such as foot pronation) may cause compression of the tibial nerve and its branches in this location. Trauma to the lower leg—from fracture, sprain, or other soft tissue injury—may also lead to increased swelling. The abnormal swelling of the lower leg may cause compression on the nerve in this closed space. In addition, more proximal pathology may be associated with tarsal tunnel syndrome. A thorough review of systems is essential in identification of tarsal tunnel syndrome. Rheumatic disease may also cause swelling around the nerve or a peripheral neuropathy can present with similar symptoms; both should be ruled out. For example, patients with other nerve lesions such as a lumbar spine pathology may also have concomitant symptoms in the area of the tarsal tunnel. In closer proximity to the tarsal tunnel is the soleus hiatus, where the tibial nerve can be compressed as it is surrounded by a fibromuscular tunnel.

14. What objective tests should be performed in identifying a patient with tarsal tunnel syndrome?

While clinical diagnosis of tarsal tunnel syndrome often lacks objectivity and consistency, the following tests may be helpful to identify impairments. Gait analysis is necessary to observe if abnormal pronation is present, which may place increased tension on the nerve. Palpation of pulses should be assessed to exclude ischemia as a cause of pain. Neurologic exam can be performed using reflexes and myotomal testing to assist in differential diagnosis of a more proximal neurologic pathology. Sensory testing using vibration, sharp/dull touch, and light touch is helpful to distinguish distribution related to the tibial nerve and its course versus a dermatomal distribution or stocking/glove-type distribution of a neuropathic condition. A positive Tinel sign may be sensitive for tarsal tunnel syndrome, but not specific. Both slump testing and the lower limb tension tests may be helpful. Because symptoms are in the more distal portion of the lower extremity, it has been advocated that the lower limb tension test sequence starts at the distal aspect and moves proximally, different from the more traditional proximal to distal addition of sensitizing movements.

15. What is posterior tibialis tendon dysfunction (PTTD)?

PTTD is a progressive degeneration of the posterior tibial tendon and is the most common cause of painful and debilitating acquired flatfoot deformity in adults. The dysfunction is often progressive and may result in collapse of the plantar arch associated with tendon rupture. Before rupture, the tendon undergoes attenuation and degeneration, resulting in frequent episodes of debilitating pain.

16. What are the signs and symptoms typically seen with PTTD?

Johnson and Strom described the progressive clinical stages of posterior tibial tendon dysfunction. In stage I the patient has mild swelling and medial ankle pain but no deformity. There is mild weakness and the length of the tendon is normal; however, degeneration is present. A patient may be able to perform a single heel rise, but this movement is painful. Stage II is progressive flattening of the arch, with an abducted midfoot. In this stage the tendon is ruptured or functionally incompetent. The foot is still flexible, and the patient is unable to perform a single heel rise. In stage III all of the signs of stage II occur; however, the hindfoot deformity becomes fixed. Myerson added stage IV for those patients who progressed to valgus tilt of the talus in the ankle mortise, leading to lateral tibiotalar degeneration.

17. What causes PTTD?

Age-related degenerative changes, preexisting tenosynovitis, and, less frequently, acute traumatic rupture are all potential causes of PTTD. Medical factors linked with PTTD include hypertension, obesity, diabetes, steroid exposure, and inflammatory arthritides. Another predisposition is a critical area of hypovascularity in the tendon posterior and distal to the medial malleolus.

18. Describe the clinical presentation of PTTD.

Patients with stages I and II most often complain of gradual pain and swelling on the medial aspect of the ankle and onset of flatfoot deformity. Pain is elicited by palpation of the posterior tibial tendon and often by resistance of plantar flexion and inversion. Flattening of the longitudinal arch often is seen with weight-bearing. In the later stages, the patient also may have pain laterally because of impingement of the fibula or lateral talar process by the anterior process of the calcaneus.

Tendon function is evaluated by ability to perform a heel rise. Inability to invert the calcaneus is often present, and repeated heel rise is difficult without pain and/or fatigue. In stage II and beyond, heel rise is often not possible. Subtalar motion may be limited, depending on severity. In the later stages of PTTD, forefoot abductus deformity may be present, and a forefoot varus relative to the rear foot may become fixed.

19. What is the best evidenced-based treatment for PTTD?

Initially, immobilization and rest of the tendon are necessary to prevent excessive pronation and to decrease demand on the posterior tibialis. Techniques include taping to support the arch, custom-made foot orthotics, a custom-made ankle-foot orthosis, or even complete immobilization with a cast or walking boot. Calf stretching with both the knee straight and flexed should be implemented. After immobilization, progressive strengthening in the pain-free range of the posterior tibialis as well as strengthening of the foot intrinsics is beneficial. Using the evidence-based medicine gained from Achilles tendonosis, eccentric training of the tibialis posterior should be the method of strengthening, and clinically has been shown to be beneficial. Kulig and colleagues have clearly demonstrated that the best exercise to selectively and effectively train the tibialis posterior is resisted foot adduction with the foot in contact with the floor, in a windshield wiper type of motion. In addition, the use of an arch support or orthoses during this exercise will recruit the tibialis posterior more effectively.

20. What causes peroneal tendon subluxation?

Both the longus and brevis tendons are at risk for subluxation or dislocation from the fibular retromalleolar sulcus. The most frequent cause is a skiing injury, but subluxation has been reported in several other sports (e.g., soccer, football, basketball, tennis, gymnastics). The most commonly described mechanism is sudden, forceful passive dorsiflexion of the everted foot with sudden, strong reflex contraction of the peroneal muscles. The injury also has been described with forced inversion, which also causes sudden contraction of the peroneals.

21. How is peroneal tendon subluxation diagnosed?

An acute subluxating peroneal tendon frequently is misdiagnosed as an ankle sprain. The patient usually describes a traumatic injury with lateral swelling and ecchymosis, which often are associated with popping or snapping sounds. Often patients with a subacute condition also have sprained the lateral collateral ligaments. Most patients complain of pain behind the fibula and above the joint line, which differentiates it from the pain of a lateral ankle sprain. The patient's presenting symptoms usually include swelling and tenderness posterior to the lateral malleolus. Provocative tests should be done but may not be helpful in the acute setting. Dislocation of the peroneal tendon is evident during a stress test of inversion. Testing is done by resisting eversion with a dorsiflexed ankle.

22. Summarize the differential diagnosis for heel pain.

POSTERIOR HEEL PAIN

- Retrocalcaneal bursitis
- Haglund's deformity ("pump bump")
- Achilles tendonitis or tendonosis
- Calcification within the Achilles tendon
- Referred pain from a soleus muscle trigger point
- Radiculopathy of S1

PLANTAR HEEL PAIN

- Inflammation or microtrauma of the plantar fascia
- Entrapment neuropathy of the tibial nerve or branches
- Fat pad atrophy
- Heel spur
- Stress fracture
- Tarsal tunnel syndrome
- Systemic problems (Reiter syndrome, rheumatoid arthritis, gout; more common bilaterally)
- Radiculopathy of S1

23. What is plantar fasciitis?

Plantar fasciitis is defined as pain on the plantar surface of the foot, arising from the insertion of the plantar fascia. Pain may arise from one or more of the following structures: subcalcaneal bursa, fat pad, tendinous insertion of the intrinsic muscles, long plantar ligament, medial calcaneal branch of the tibial nerve, or nerve to abductor digiti minimi. True plantar fasciitis is characterized by progressive pain with weight-bearing as well as pain with the first few steps upon rising from a sitting position.

24. What is the best treatment for plantar heel pain?

Limited evidence has been found supporting using topical corticosteroids administered via iontophoresis, wearing night splints), stretching the plantar fascia, and wearing soft shoe inserts. Using the best evidenced-based medicine and clinical experience, the following interventions are recommended for treatment of plantar heel pain:

- Patient education and decreasing the stress to the involved tissues—patients should be educated that the pain can likely last up to 6 to 9 months. Patients need to decrease the stress to the tissue immediately. This can be achieved by resting the tissue with taping of the arch, using a heel cushion, decreasing activity levels, managing weight, and wearing temporary or permanent foot orthoses (in chronic cases).
- Tissue mobilization—primarily addresses adverse neurodynamics of the tibial nerve, active calf stretching, and calf soft tissue mobilization
- Joint mobilization—increases dorsiflexion with talocrural glides

- Strengthening the muscles that support the arch—posterior tibial, peroneal, and intrinsic muscles

25. How can adverse neurodynamics cause plantar heel pain, and why do patients feel better with neural mobilization?

Heel pain can result from local mechanical entrapment of the medial calcaneal branch of the tibial nerve or the nerve to the abductor digiti minimi. The nerve may be painful secondary to intraneural adhesions, compression, or scarring inside the axons. Chronic irritation may cause reduced microcirculation, decreased axonal transport, and altered mechanics, resulting in a painful cycle. In addition, the nerve is a continuum with multiple sites of potential compression that may result in a double-crush phenomenon, exacerbating the pain. It is hypothesized that sliding between the neural tissue and interface tissue can decrease adhesions and promote healing. Neural tissue can shorten and lengthen and has considerable remodeling capabilities. Restoring normal neural mobility appears to be important in abolishing symptoms.

26. Describe the common cause and usual management of heel pain in children.

Calcaneal apophysitis of the os calcis (Sever's disease) is related to activity. The child usually complains of pain with running or jumping as well as tenderness over the insertion of the Achilles tendon. The patient should be referred to a physician. Radiographs are useful for diagnosis when pain has been prolonged and recalcitrant. Treatment should include decreased activity guided by the child's symptoms, foot taping, or, in severe cases, immobilization with a brace. A heel lift or improved shoe wear also helps to reduce the traction pull on the tendinous apophyseal attachment. The key is to restore heel cord flexibility.

27. Summarize the differential diagnosis for pain in the lateral aspect of the ankle after inversion sprain.

- Osteochondral fracture of the talus
- Distal fibula fracture
- Avulsion fracture of the fifth metatarsal
- Jones fracture (metaphyseal-diaphyseal junction of the fifth metatarsal)
- Peroneal tendon injury
- High ankle sprain of the anteroinferior tibial fibular ligament
- Peroneal or sural nerve irritation
- Cuboid subluxation
- Achilles tendon injury
- Subtalar joint ligament injury

28. Which radiographic stress views are commonly used in the diagnosis of ankle sprains?

Anterior drawer stress radiographs and talar tilt stress radiographs are most commonly performed to document the degree of ankle instability. In clinical practice, however, routine use of stress radiography for assessment of grade II and grade III ankle sprains is debatable.

Anterior talar translation >6 mm in the involved ankle or a difference >3 mm between the injured and uninjured side indicates rupture of the anterior talofibular ligament (ATFL). A talar tilt >10 degrees indicates tears in both the ATFL and calcaneofibular ligament (CFL). Some researchers believe that both the anterior drawer stress test and the inversion test should be used to improve the reliability of the stress radiography tests.

29. How common are the various ankle sprains?

Brostrom reported that 65% of ankle sprains involved complete rupture of the ATFL and 20% had combined injury to the ATFL and CFL. Isolated injury to the posterior talofibular ligament (PTFL) was rare; isolated injury to the CFL was not found. The anteroinferior tibiofibular ligament (high ankle sprain) was injured in 10% of patients and the deltoid in only 3%. In grade III sprains, the anterior deltoid ligament may be involved through the plantar flexion component of the injury.

30. When are radiographs warranted for ankle injuries?

The Ottawa ankle rules are highly sensitive for determining which patients require radiographs after ankle trauma. Bone tenderness in the posterior half of the lower 6 cm of the fibula or tibia or over the navicular or fifth metatarsal increases the risk for fracture. Another indication for radiographs is inability to bear weight immediately after injury or within 10 days of injury.

31. What is the best method for measuring ankle swelling?

Both the figure-of-eight tape measure and volumetric immersion are valid measurements of swelling. The figure-of-eight tape measure is a simple method to track rate and amount of progress during rehabilitation. The patient should be in a long sitting position with the distal one third of the leg off the plinth in a plantar-flexed position. The tape measure surrounds the most superficial aspect of the malleoli and then travels around the foot medially over the superficial aspect of the navicular and laterally over the cuboid bone to meet at the dorsum of the foot, resulting in a figure-of-eight pattern.

32. What are the guidelines for return to activities and sports after ankle sprains and what is the best evidence to prevent recurrent sprains?

Although each patient should be treated individually, suggested criteria for return to sport after an ankle sprain include:

- Full range of active and passive motion at the ankle
- No limp with walking
- Strength equal to 90% of the uninvolved side
- Single-leg hop, high jump test, and 30-yard zig-zag test at least 90% of the uninvolved side
- Ability to reach maximal running and cutting speed

Coordination/balance training and bracing have been proven to help reduce future ankle sprains. It is also necessary to strengthen all of the muscle of the lower extremity. For example, if the hip abductors are weak, one may compensate with lateral trunk lean, which causes the center of mass to deviate laterally, potentially creating an inversion force to the ankle and hindfoot.

33. What disorders may cause chronic pain after an ankle sprain?

- Tension neuropathy of the superficial peroneal nerve—Inversion sprains may stretch the superficial peroneal nerve and lead to chronic pain localized to the dorsum of the foot. Compression is found most often at the site where the nerve exits the deep fascia of the anterior compartment of the leg. Pain most often is localized to the anterolateral ankle and radiates to the anterior foot. It can be reproduced by plantar flexion and reduced by dorsiflexion. Careful physical exam and local nerve blocks are most helpful in correct diagnosis.
- Anterior or lateral soft tissue impingement—The hypertrophied synovial tissue or scarring of the ATFL can become entrapped in the joint during dorsiflexion. Entrapment is most severe in the anterolateral gutter of the ankle. A less common cause of pain is talar impingement by the anteroinferior tibiofibular ligament. Bassett and Spear hypothesized that after severe sprain, the ATFL has increased laxity, which causes the talar dome to protrude more anteriorly. During dorsiflexion the distal fascicle of the anteroinferior tibiofibular ligament may cause impingement on the talus. Management requires removal of the fascicle.

- Cuboid subluxation—This fairly common but often unrecognizable condition has been reported in the literature. Most commonly the cuboid is subluxated in the plantar direction and requires dorsal manipulation. The peroneals are often weak as a result of the displaced bone.

34. What is a syndesmotic ankle sprain?

Injury of the anterior and posterior inferior tibiofibular ligaments and damage to the interosseous membrane are known as a high ankle sprain. The common mechanism is external rotation of the tibia on a planted foot. High ankle sprains are common in football and baseball. They must be differentiated from routine lateral ankle sprains. Patients have tenderness and swelling over the anterior distal leg and may have swelling and ecchymosis on both sides of the ankle. External rotation of the foot while the leg is stabilized creates pain at the syndesmosis. The squeeze test is pain elicited distally over the syndesmosis with compression of the tibia and fibula at mid calf level.

It may be critical to rule out concurrent fracture of the fibula. Patients with a syndesmotic sprain should be referred to an orthopaedic surgeon. Complete diastasis of the syndesmosis should be evaluated by radiograph, and instability may require surgery. The syndesmotic sprain typically produces longer disability than the more routine ankle sprain.

35. What are shin splints?

"Shin splints" is not a specific diagnosis. The evidence is clear that shin splint pain has many different causes from tibial stress fractures to compartment syndrome. It is preferable to describe shin splint pain by location and etiology, for example, lower medial tibial pain resulting from periostitis or upper lateral tibial pain caused by elevated compartment pressure.

36. What is the most common cause of tibial overuse syndromes?

Tibial overuse injuries are a recognized complication of chronic, intensive, weight-bearing exercise or training commonly practiced by athletic and military populations. The most common tibial overuse injuries are anterior stress syndrome and posterior medial stress syndrome.

37. Why is anterior tibial stress syndrome (shin splints) often associated with runners?

Reber et al. using fine-wire EMG, identified that during running the tibialis anterior muscle increased in activity and fired above the fatigue threshold for 85% of the time. This may account for the high number of fatigue-related injuries to the tibialis anterior muscle seen in runners.

38. What is the cause of posterior medial tibial stress syndrome?

Beck and Osternig identified that the soleus, the flexor digitorum longus, and the deep crural fascia were found to attach most frequently at the site where symptoms of medial tibial stress syndrome occur. These data contradict the contention that the tibialis posterior contributes more to this particular condition. Therefore specific modalities and stretching to these muscles should be beneficial.

39. What is the best treatment for shin splints?

Generally, the most effective treatment is considered to be rest, often for prolonged periods. In a recent review of the literature, Thacker et al. found limited evidence for the use of shock-absorbent insoles, foam heel pads, heel cord stretching, and alternative footwear as well as graduated running programs among the military. They did identify the most encouraging evidence for effective prevention of shin splints was the use of shock-absorbing insoles.

40. Define sinus tarsi syndrome.

The sinus tarsi is an oval space laterally between the talus and the calcaneus and continuous with the tarsal tunnel. The sinus tarsi and tarsal canal are filled with fatty tissue, subtalar ligaments, an artery, a bursa, and nerve endings. Tenderness in the tarsal sinus indicates disruption or dysfunction of the subtalar complex. Chronic ankle sprains have been cited as a common cause of sinus tarsi syndrome. Arthroscopic reports indicate scarring and synovial inflammation in the lateral talocalcaneal recess.

41. Define tarsal coalition.

In this structural abnormality, a fibrous or osseous bar abnormally spans two of the tarsal bones, most commonly the talocalcaneal or calcaneonavicular joint. It most often occurs in the early teenage years, and slight trauma or growth-plate ossification may provoke pain. Typically the pain is unrelenting. Common findings are loss of rear-foot motion and concomitant rigid pes planus. A talocalcaneal coalition is difficult to identify on radiographs; magnetic resonance imaging or computed tomography may be required. Treatment focuses initially on rest followed by treatment to increase flexibility and decrease stiffness. Surgery may be necessary to resect the bar; extreme cases may require fusion.

42. What are hallux rigidus and hallux limitus, and what is the best treatment?

Hallux limitus is restriction in metatarsophalangeal (MTP) extension. Normal walking requires 65 degrees of extension during terminal stance. Hallux rigidus is further loss of motion characterized by the development of osteoarthritis, as evidenced by spurring or loss of joint space. Common problems associated with these two disorders include trauma to the forefoot, congenital variations in the head of the first metatarsal, and a dorsiflexed first ray.

Conservative management includes MTP joint mobilization after early trauma, sesamoid mobilization, and strengthening of the MTP flexors. In more chronic cases, treatment is focused on decreasing the force to the MTP by using a stiff-soled shoe or external metatarsal bar or by orthotic modifications such as a metatarsal bar and full contact orthoses.

43. Describe the normal mobility of the first ray. How is it assessed clinically?

The first metatarsal should lie in the same plane as the lesser metatarsals. Normal mobility is assessed with stabilization of the lateral four toes while the examiner's other hand applies dorsal or plantar force on the first metatarsal. Motion in plantar and dorsal directions should be equal, and during dorsal testing the inferior aspect of the first metatarsal should reach the plane of the lesser metatarsals.

44. What is the consequence of a hypomobile first ray?

Patients with a hypomobile first ray present with callus formation under the first metatarsal and hallux, suggesting shear and compressive forces. The problems result from inability of the first ray to dorsiflex with weight acceptance, which causes increased plantar pressure under the first ray. Patients report pain with walking, primarily at the end of stance, and with passive extension as well as decreased range of motion in dorsiflexion of the first MTP joint.

45. Describe the windlass mechanism. How can abnormal mechanics lead to pathology?

From midstance to terminal stance in gait, full body weight is transferred to the metatarsal heads. As a result, the MTPs extend and activate the windlass mechanics, tightening the tissues on the plantar aspect of the foot and elevating the arch.

Dorsal movement of the navicular results in plantar flexion of the first ray. Plantar flexion of the first ray allows the phalanges to glide, resulting in dorsiflexion of the first MTPs. If plantar flexion of the first ray is not achieved, dorsiflexion cannot occur at the MTPs and the windlass mechanism is lost. This leads, in turn, to loss of the structural stability of the foot. If the foot remains excessively pronated for any number of reasons, the windlass loses its effect. The loss of the windlass mechanism may result in the following clinical pathologies:

- Joint laxity of the metatarsals
- Metatarsalgia
- Formation of hallux valgus

46. Describe hammertoes. How are they treated?

A hammertoe is MTP extension with proximal interphalangeal (PIP) flexion, which may be a flexible or fixed deformity. Pain often results from a callus on the dorsum of the PIP and under the metatarsal head. Hammering of the second toe often is accompanied by a hallux valgus deformity. Treatment includes stretching of the dorsal extrinsics in a position of ankle plantar flexion and MTP extension, strengthening of the intrinsics, and wearing a deeper shoe.

47. Define claw toes. How are they treated?

Claw toe is also an extension deformity of the MTP joint with concomitant flexing or "clawing" of the toe at both the proximal and distal interphalangeal joints. The claw toe results from muscle imbalance in which the active extrinsics are stronger than the deep intrinsics (lumbricals, interosseus) and may indicate a neurologic disorder. It is commonly seen with high arches (cavus foot). Stretching, as with the hammertoe, is often successful with flexible deformities, and shoes should avoid unnecessary pressure.

48. What is sesamoiditis?

Active people may develop a problem in the two small bones (sesamoids) that lie in the tendon of the flexor hallucis brevis muscle under the first MTP joint. The medial digital plantar nerve also runs in close proximity to the medial sesamoid and can be irritated. Patients with an inflamed sesamoid find it quite painful to ambulate. They have palpable pain at the first MTP joint, pain on extension of the great toe, and often swelling at the head of the first metatarsal. The differential diagnosis should include fracture of the sesamoid and bipartite medial sesamoid.

49. How is sesamoiditis differentiated from metatarsalgia?

Metatarsalgia refers to an acute or chronic pain syndrome involving the metatarsal heads. Pain also prevents extension at the MTP joint and is provoked by gait. The various causes include overuse, anatomic misalignment, foot deformity, and degenerative changes. A cavus foot, which places more weight on the distal end, is commonly seen with this disorder. Metatarsalgia of the first MTP joint often results from a traumatic episode or degenerative arthritis. Patients should be screened for a hallux valgus rigidus as well as sesamoiditis.

50. In general, what is the best conservative treatment for forefoot disorders?

- Change pressure under the tender area with a metatarsal pad or cut-out under orthoses.
- Change ill-fitting shoes.
- Improve MTP flexion and IP extension by strengthening intrinsics with manual and weight-bearing exercises.
- Maintain correct arch position by strengthening in an arched or short-foot position.

51. Where is the most common site of a neuroma? Describe the symptoms of a neuroma.

Neuromas are found most commonly in the third web space between the third and fourth metatarsals. Neuromas at the first and fourth web spaces are rare. Patients complain of deep burning pain and may have paresthesia extending into the toe. The main symptom is pain in the plantar aspect of the foot, which is increased by walking and relieved by rest. The neuroma is secondary to irritation of the intermetatarsal plantar digital nerve as it travels under the metatarsal ligament. Pain often is elicited with MTP extension, which tightens the ligament and compresses the nerve.

52. How is a neuroma diagnosed?

Palpation in the interspace as opposed to over the joint should provoke the patient's pain. A positive Mulder's sign is also indicative of a neuroma; this test is positive when pain is reproduced or a click or pop is heard. The metatarsal squeeze test can also indicate the presence of a neuroma; in this test, compression of the foot from the medial and lateral directions while palpating the plantar aspect often reproduces the pain.

53. What is the suggested treatment for neuromas?

Traditional treatment includes shoe modification (specifically a wider toe box), use of metatarsal pads, steroid injection, and, in chronic unrelenting cases, referral for surgical neurectomy. Neurodynamics also should be assessed and treated because the nerve may be compressed more proximally as well as locally.

54. How is the level of protective sensation tested?

The Semmes-Weinstein microfilament test is a simple, inexpensive, and effective method for assessing sensory neuropathy in patients at risk for developing foot ulcers. Patients unable to feel the nylon filament with a 10-gram bending force are diagnosed with loss of protective sensation. They benefit from protective footwear and a foot care education program.

Bibliography

Alfredson H et al: Heavy-load eccentric calf muscle training for the treatment of chronic Achilles tendinosis, *Am J Sports Med* 26:360-366, 1998.

Bassett FHD, Speer FP: Longitudinal rupture of the peroneal tendons, *Am J Sports Med* 21:354-357, 1993.

Beck BR, Osternig LR: Medial tibial stress syndrome. The location of muscles in the leg in relation to symptoms, *J Bone Joint Surg* 76A:1057-1061, 1994.

Bonnin M, Tavernier T, Bouysset M: Split lesions of the peroneus brevis tendon in chronic ankle laxity, *Am J Sports Med* 25:699-703, 1997.

Cetti R et al: Operative versus nonoperative treatment of Achilles tendon rupture: a prospective randomized study and review of the literature, *Am J Sports Med* 21:791-799, 1993.

Chandler TJ: Iontophoresis of 0.4% dexamethasone for plantar fasciitis, *Clin J Sports Med* 8:68, 1998.

Cornwall MW, McPoil TG: Plantar fasciitis: etiology and treatment, *J Orthop Sports Phys Ther* 29:756-760, 1999.

DiGiovanni BF et al: Tissue-specific plantar fascia-stretching exercise enhances outcomes in patients with chronic heel pain. A prospective, randomized study, *J Bone Joint Surg* 85A:1270-1277, 2003.

Fallat L, Grimm DJ, Saracco JA: Sprained ankle syndrome: prevalence and analysis of 639 acute injuries, *J Foot Ankle Surg* 37:280-285, 1998.

Geideman WM, Johnson JE: Posterior tibial tendon dysfunction, *Phys Ther* 30:68-77, 2000.

Gerber JP et al: Persistent disability associated with ankle sprains: a prospective examination of an athletic population, *Foot Ankle Int* 19:653-660, 1998.

Johnson KA, Strom DE: Tibialis posterior tendon dysfunction, *Clin Orthop* 239:196-206, 1989.

Johnston EC, Howell SJ: Tendon neuropathy of the superficial peroneal nerve: associated conditions and results of release, *Foot Ankle Int* 20:576-582, 1999.

Kulig K et al: Selective activation of tibialis posterior: evaluation by magnetic resonance imaging, *Med Sci Sports Exercise* 36:862-867, 2004.

Lentell G et al: The contributions of proprioceptive deficits, muscle function, and anatomic laxity to functional instability of the ankle, *J Orthop Sports Phys Ther* 21:206-215, 1995.

Mandelbaum BR, Myerson MS, Forster R: Achilles tendon ruptures: a new method repair, early range of motion, and functional rehabilitation, *Am J Sports Med* 23:392-395, 1995.
Myerson MG et al: Posterior tibial tendon dysfunction: its association with seronegative inflammatory disease, *Foot Ankle* 9:219-225, 1989.
Ohberg LR et al: Eccentric training in patients with chronic Achilles tendinosis: normalized tendon structure and decreased thickness at follow up, *Br J Sports Med* 38:8-11 (discussion 11), 2004.
Pfeffer GP et al: Comparison of custom and prefabricated orthoses in the initial treatment of proximal plantar fasciitis, *Foot Ankle Int* 20:214-221, 1999.
Pugia ML et al: Comparison of acute swelling and function in subjects with lateral ankle injury, *J Orthop Sports Phys Ther* 31:384-388, 2001.
Reber LJ et al: Muscular control of the ankle in running, *Am J Sports Med* 21:805-810 (discussion 810), 1993.
Safran MR, O'Malley D Jr, Fu FH: Peroneal tendon subluxation in athletes: new exam technique, case reports, and review, *Med Sci Sports Exercise* 31(7 suppl):S487-S492, 1999.
Safran MR et al: Lateral ankle sprains: a comprehensive review. Part 1: Etiology, pathoanatomy, histopathogenesis, and diagnosis, *Med Sci Sports Exercise* 31:S429-S437, 1999.
Thacker SB et al: The prevention of shin splints in sports: a systematic review of literature, *Med Sci Sports Exercise* 34:32-40, 2002.

Chapter 77

Fractures and Dislocations of the Foot and Ankle

Todd R. Hockenbury, MD

1. How are ankle fractures classified?

Ankle fractures are described by the number of malleoli involved:

- Single malleolar fracture is a lateral or medial malleolar fracture.
- Bimalleolar fracture is a fracture of both the medial malleolus and the lateral malleolus.
- Trimalleolar fracture is a fracture of the lateral malleolus, medial malleolus, and posterior aspect of the distal tibial articular surface.

There are two major classification systems for ankle fractures: the Weber/AO classification and the Lauge-Hansen classification (more complex). Fractures are classified in order to dictate treatment, simplify communication between medical personnel treating the fracture, and predict outcome.

The Weber/AO classification is the simplest method to classify ankle fractures:

- Weber A—below the level of the syndesmosis
- Weber B—at or near the level of the syndesmosis; 50% have disruption of the syndesmosis
- Weber C—above the level of the syndesmosis; >50% have disruption of the syndesmosis

The four Lauge-Hansen classes are (the first term in parentheses refers to the foot position and the second term describes the external force applied to the ankle):

- Supination-Adduction (SA, 10% to 20%)

- Supination-External Rotation (SER, 40% to 75%)
- Pronation-Abduction (PA, 5% to 20%)
- Pronation-External Rotation (PER, 5% to 20%)

2. What are the indications for surgical treatment of an ankle fracture?

- Intra-articular displacement of the distal tibial surface of 2 mm or more requires surgical intervention.
- Distal tibiofibular ligament rupture causing widening of the ankle mortise is an indication for surgery.
- Any injury that causes two breaks in the ankle joint "ring" requires surgery. The ankle is a hinge joint in which the malleoli are connected to the talus through the collateral ligaments. Bimalleolar fractures are inherently unstable and require surgical stabilization. A fibular fracture combined with a deltoid ligament tear is a bimalleolar equivalent fracture and also requires surgery.
- Any fracture that allows the talus to shift laterally or medially in the mortise is treated surgically.

Ankle fractures that involve only one malleolar disruption and do not disturb the stability of the ankle mortise are treated nonoperatively; the patient wears a short-leg walking cast or fracture boot for 4 to 6 weeks.

3. Describe the radiographic views and alignment guides used in assessing ankle fractures.

ANTEROPOSTERIOR VIEW
- Tibiofibular clear space should be <5 mm
- Tibiofibular overlap should be >10 mm

LATERAL VIEW
- Assess joint line, talus, calcaneus, and posterior tibial fracture

MORTISE VIEW
- Tibiofibular line should be continuous
- Talocrural angle—normally 8 to 15 degrees or within 2 to 3 degrees of opposite side
- Talar tilt—0 ± 1.5 degrees; talus may tilt upward to 5 degrees in a normal ankle with inversion stress
- Medial clear space—normally equal to the superior clear space (should be <4 mm)
- Tibiofibular overlap should be >1 mm

SPECIALIZED STRESS VIEWS
- Mortise view with inversion stress—talar tilt is normally <5 mm; twofold difference from uninjured ankle is abnormal; tear >10 to 15 degrees indicates tear of the anterior talofibular ligament (ATFL) and calcaneofibular ligament (CFL)
- Lateral view with anterior drawer—anterior talar shift >8 to 10 mm indicates ATFL tear

4. Describe the complications and outcomes of ankle fractures.

Potential complications after open reduction and internal fixation (ORIF) include nonunion (about twice as common in diabetic patients), malunion, wound breakdown (2% to 3%), infection (2%), reflex sympathetic dystrophy, and arthritis (10% in anatomic reductions, 90% with malreduction).

5. Describe other fracture patterns around the ankle.

- Maisonneuve—pronation-external rotation fracture with fracture of the proximal fibula
- Curbstone—isolated posterior malleolus fracture
- Le Fort-Wagstaffe—anterior fibular avulsion, supination-external rotation injury
- Tillaux-Chaput—anterior tibial avulsion

- Pronation-dorsiflexion fracture—fracture of anterior articular surface
- Nutcracker fracture—avulsion fracture of the navicular with comminuted compression fracture of the cuboid
- Pilon—high-energy compression fracture through tibial plafond (≈50% develop arthrosis or other major complication; ≈26% require fusion)

6. What is the Hawkins classification of talar neck fractures?

Talar neck fractures usually result from hyperdorsiflexion injury, as in a motor vehicle accident or fall from a height. Hawkins classified the different types of fracture patterns as follows:

- Type I—vertical nondisplaced talar neck fracture
- Type II—displaced fracture with subluxation or dislocation of the subtalar joint
- Type III—type II with talotibial dislocation
- Type IV—type III with talonavicular dislocation

7. Describe the treatment and outcomes for talus fractures.

Treatment is usually surgical in light of problems with late displacement and prolonged immobilization. The risk of avascular necrosis (AVN) increases with Hawkins type (type I = 0% to 13%, type II = 20% to 50%, type III = 20% to 100%). Approximately 40% to 90% of patients suffer late arthritis.

8. What is Canale's view?

This radiographic view provides optimal visualization of the talar neck. The radiograph is taken with the foot in maximal plantar flexion and pronated at 15 degrees; the x-ray tube is directed 15 degrees cephalad to the vertical.

9. What radiographic views and lines are used to evaluate calcaneal fractures?

- Broden's view—foot in neutral and leg internally rotated 30 to 40 degrees. Views are angled 10, 20, 30, and 40 degrees cephalad. Broden's view allows visualization of the posterior facet but has largely been replaced by CT scan.
- Bohler's angle—first line from anterior calcaneus to highest posterior articular surface and second line from posterior articular surface to posterior tubercle. The normal angle is 25 to 40 degrees. A decreased angle indicates posterior facet collapse.
- Angle of Gissane—formed by the two cortical struts, one along the posterior facet and the other to the anterior process of the calcaneus. The normal angle is approximately 140 degrees. An increased angle indicates posterior facet collapse.

10. What are the outcomes of calcaneal fractures?

Surgical treatment generally provides better outcomes than nonoperative treatment. Nonoperative treatment includes casting and strict non–weight-bearing for 6 to 8 weeks, followed by progression of weight-bearing. Surgical treatment is ORIF. Complications include arthritis, peroneal impingement (10% to 20%), widening of heel, decreased dorsiflexion, weak plantar flexion, leg length discrepancy, wound dehiscence, and sural nerve injury. Approximately 65% of patients are limited in vigorous or sports activities, 50% are able to ambulate over any surface, and 40% are unable to return to previous employment.

11. How is a bipartite sesamoid distinguished from a sesamoid fracture?

Bipartite sesamoids occur in 10% to 30% of the population and may be easily confused with an acute fracture. Bipartite sesamoids are bilateral in 85% of cases, have smooth sclerotic borders, and exhibit no callus after several weeks of immobilization.

12. What is a pilon ankle fracture and how is it treated?

A pilon fracture is an intra-articular fracture of the distal tibia produced by dorsiflexion and/or axial loading forces. The term *pilon* refers to the talus as the pestle driving into the mortar-like ankle mortise, producing a fracture of the weight-bearing surface of the tibia.

The Ruedi-Allgower classification describes pilon fractures as follows:

- Type I—nondisplaced
- Type II—displaced
- Type III—displaced with joint surface comminution and impaction

The recommended treatment of displaced fractures is surgery. In low-energy fractures without significant soft tissue energy and swelling, ORIF is indicated 10 to 14 days after soft tissue swelling subsides.

13. What complications can occur following pilon fractures?

The most frequent complication following pilon fracture treatment is posttraumatic arthritis (50% to 70%). Other complications include wound healing problems, dehiscence, nonunion, malunion, and pin tract infections. In type III fractures, the goal is often to achieve soft tissue healing and sufficient bony healing of the metaphyseal bone to allow fusion at a later date.

14. What common fractures are frequently misdiagnosed as ankle sprains?

- Talar osteochondral fracture (a divot fracture involving bone and cartilage usually from the anterolateral or posteromedial talar dome)
- Lateral talar process fracture
- Anterior calcaneal process fracture
- Posterior talar process fracture
- "Flake fracture" of the posterior distal fibular rim, indicating a tear of the superior peroneal retinaculum and peroneal tendon dislocation
- Navicular fracture
- Lateral or medial malleolar fracture

15. What is the pathophysiology of stress fractures of the foot?

A stress or fatigue fracture is a break that develops in bone after cyclical, submaximal loading. In states of increased physical activity, bone is resorbed faster than it is replaced, which results in physical weakening of the bone and the development of microfractures. With continued physical stress these microfractures coalesce to form a complete stress fracture. Middle-aged and older adult patients with osteoporosis, diagnosed with a T score of lower than −2.5 on dual photon spectrometry (DXA scan), are also at risk for stress fractures. Amenorrheic athletes are predisposed to stress fractures; amenorrhea is present in up to 20% of vigorously exercising women and may be as high as 50% in elite runners and dancers.

16. What are common locations for stress fractures of the foot?

Common locations for foot stress fractures are the metatarsals, calcaneus, and navicular. Distal tibial stress fractures and lateral malleolar fractures are less common. Symptoms of stress fracture are localized pain and swelling with weight-bearing of insidious onset. A thin sclerotic line may be seen in a stress fracture of metaphyseal bone. Although initial radiographs may be negative, a technetium bone scan is positive as early as 48 to 72 hours after onset of symptoms.

17. Describe the Sanders' classification of calcaneal fractures.

Any displaced calcaneal fracture should be evaluated with a CT scan to determine the degree of posterior facet displacement and comminution. The Sanders' classification uses CT scanning in the coronal plane to describe the number of posterior facet fragments and their location. Sanders classifies an extra-articular fracture as a type I. A posterior calcaneal facet fracture with two pieces is a type II; a fracture with three pieces is a type III; and a fracture with four pieces is a type IV. Using this system, Sanders has reported results of ORIF of displaced intra-articular fractures by fracture type: 73% of type II fractures had a good or excellent result, 70% of type III fractures had a good or excellent result, and only 9% of type IV fractures had a good or excellent result.

18. What injuries are commonly associated with calcaneal fractures?

The calcaneus is the most fractured tarsal bone. Approximately 75% of calcaneal fractures are intra-articular. Approximately 10% of patients have associated fractures of the spine, 25% have extremity injuries, 10% are bilateral, and 5% are open.

19. How are calcaneal fractures treated?

- Nondisplaced fracture—Six weeks of splinting, elevation, non–weight-bearing, and early motion typically yield excellent results.
- Open calcaneal fractures—Immediate operative debridement, intravenous antibiotics, and splinting are the course of treatment. No internal fixation or limited percutaneous fixation is used in open fractures because of the significant risk of wound dehiscence, infection, chronic osteomyelitis, and amputation. Contraindications include insulin-dependent diabetes mellitus, neuropathy, vascular dysfunction, venous stasis, and localized dermatitis. Relative contraindications include cigarette smoking, poor bone quality, and older or inactive patients.

20. What are expected outcomes after calcaneal fractures?

Young, active patients with closed noncomminuted fractures are potential candidates for ORIF through an extensile lateral L-shaped incision. Surgery is performed 10 to 21 days after fracture to allow time for edema reduction. Type II and III fractures have shown good to excellent results in 70% to 85% of patients following this protocol. This compares favorably to 40% to 60% acceptable results following nonoperative management. A splint is used postoperatively until wound healing is documented; then early motion is begun. Weight-bearing is delayed for 8 to 10 weeks.

21. What fractures of the foot are at risk for avascular necrosis and why?

In the foot the bones at risk for AVN are the talus and the navicular. The talus is 60% to 70% articular cartilage and has no tendinous attachments. Most of the talar body blood supply enters the undersurface of the talar neck and flows posteriorly. The talus is at particular risk for osteonecrosis with displaced fractures of the talar neck. The weakened bone of the osteonecrotic segment of the talar dome may then collapse, causing pain and arthritis in the ankle and subtalar joints. In some instances, talar osteonecrotic segments will heal spontaneously over a course of 2 to 3 years in a process known as "creeping substitution," in which the dead bone is resorbed and replaced by live bone. The large articular surface area of the navicular also limits blood supply to the dorsal and plantar aspects. Blood perfusion is diminished to the central third of the navicular. AVN with late partial collapse of the navicular is common in comminuted navicular fractures.

22. What is a Lisfranc joint injury?

The Lisfranc joint, or tarsometatarsal joint, consists of the articulations between the five metatarsals, three cuneiforms, and cuboid. Stability is enhanced by the archlike configuration of the joint in the coronal plane and by the dorsal and plantar tarsometatarsal and intermetatarsal ligaments. The recessed second metatarsal base is connected to the medial cuneiform by the important Lisfranc ligament. Most Lisfranc injuries occur by forceful external rotation and pronation of the foot. A fall onto a maximally plantar-flexed foot can cause dorsal displacement of the metatarsals. Direct crushing injuries are less frequent causes of Lisfranc injury.

23. What are the classification patterns and treatment for Lisfranc injuries?

Lisfranc injuries are classified into three injury patterns:

- Homolateral—All metatarsals are displaced in the same direction.
- Divergent—Metatarsals are displaced in both sagittal and coronal planes in differing directions.
- Isolated—One or more metatarsals are separated from the remaining Lisfranc complex.

An anatomic reduction is required for the best result. Despite anatomic fixation, some patients will develop posttraumatic arthritis requiring fusion at a later date. Fifty percent of patients will have some long-term disability.

24. What is a Jones fracture?

A Jones fracture is a fracture of the fifth metatarsal base at the metaphyseal-diaphyseal junction. Because this fracture occurs in a watershed area of blood supply, these fractures are notorious for delayed unions and nonunions. Acute, nondisplaced fractures are treated with 4 to 6 weeks of non–weight-bearing cast immobilization followed by protected weight-bearing in a fracture boot until complete healing occurs. Delayed union and nonunions are treated with percutaneous intramedullary screw fixation. Acute, displaced fractures are treated with open reduction and internal fixation. Avulsion fractures of the metatarsal tuberosity proximal to the fourth to fifth articulation predictably heal with a weight-bearing fracture boot or hard-soled shoe. Intra-articular fractures displaced more than 2 to 3 mm may require surgery in high-demand patients.

25. What is Charcot neuroarthropathy?

A Charcot or neuropathic arthropathy is a process of chronic, noninfective, painless joint destruction. Charcot first described this condition associated with tabes dorsalis in 1868. Approximately 0.1% to 0.5% of diabetic patients will develop a neuroarthropathic joint. Two theories explain the development of a Charcot joint. The neurotraumatic theory states that decreased protective sensation and cumulative mechanical trauma lead to fracture and joint destruction. The neurovascular theory states that a neurally initiated vascular reflex leads to increased resorption by osteoclasts. Studies have shown increased osteoclastic activity without a concomitant increase in osteoblastic bone formation in the feet of diabetic patients.

The presenting symptoms of a Charcot foot include the spontaneous onset of a warm, swollen foot associated with no pain or vague pain. The midfoot is most commonly involved followed by the hindfoot and ankle. The midfoot will lose its arch over time and the forefoot will dorsiflex and abduct, producing a rocker-bottom foot deformity. The patient is then predisposed to plantar ulceration of the prominent plantar arch. The ankle will develop a significant varus or valgus deformity with eventual corresponding pressure ulceration over the prominent malleolus.

Early radiographs may show osteopenia with intact joints. Later radiographs will show fractures, joint subluxation or dislocation, bone destruction and fragmentation. The following clinical and radiographic stages of Charcot joints have been described:

- Stage 0—neuropathic patient with a history of sprain or fracture
- Stage 1—inflammatory stage with edema, hyperemia, erythema, and bone fragmentation on x-ray
- Stage 2—reparative stage with less swelling and erythema; radiographs show new bone formation at site of fracture and dislocation
- Stage 3—consolidation phase with resolution of swelling; radiographs show bony healing of fractures and dislocations

26. How are talar fractures classified?

Fractures of the talus are characterized by location. The different types of fractures are talar body fractures, fractures of the lateral talar process, fractures of the posterior talar process, osteochondral fractures of the talar dome, and talar neck fractures. Any of these fractures may be misdiagnosed as an ankle sprain.

Hawkins and Canale have classified talar neck fractures as four types:

- Type I—nondisplaced vertical fracture of talar neck
- Type II—displaced talar neck fracture with subluxation or dislocation of the subtalar joint
- Type III—displaced talar neck fracture with dislocation of both subtalar and ankle joints
- Type IV—type III fracture with talonavicular subluxation or dislocation

27. How are talar fractures treated?

Type I fractures of the talar neck are treated with immobilization for 3 months. Type II to IV fractures are treated with closed reduction. If an acceptable reduction is achieved, non–weight-bearing cast immobilization is used for 3 months. In the case of displaced fractures, which are irreducible, open reduction and screw fixation is indicated. Outcomes related to talar fractures treated with ORIF have demonstrated an incidence of osteoarthritis of up to 100%, osteonecrosis 50%, and nonunion 12%.

28. What is Hawkins sign?

Hawkins sign is the appearance of talar dome subchondral atrophy or lucency on the ankle AP view at 6 to 8 weeks following talar fracture. This indicates that the talar body is vascular and excludes the diagnosis of osteonecrosis. If the talar body appears more dense and sclerotic than the surrounding bone, then osteonecrosis is present.

29. How are osteochondral talar dome fractures classified?

Osteochondral talar dome fractures or talar osteochondritis dessicans lesions are believed to be caused by trauma, although idiopathic avascular necrosis may also be a factor. Location in the talar dome is either posteromedial or anterolateral. The classic Brendt and Harty classification is based on plain radiographic appearance and is most commonly used to classify these lesions:

- Type I—compression of subchondral bone
- Type II—incomplete fracture
- Type III—complete, nondisplaced fracture
- Type IV—completely detached, displaced fragment

These lesions are best evaluated by CT scan or MRI. More recent CT classifications include subchondral cystic lesions in the talar dome.

30. How are osteochondral talar dome fractures treated?

Initial treatment is immobilization of nondisplaced acute lesions (types I to III); type IV fractures require surgery. Ankle arthroscopy allows inspection and treatment of the lesion with removal of loose cartilage or bone and drilling of the subchondral bone to stimulate growth of fibrocartilage. In cystic lesions with intact articular cartilage, drilling and bone grafting can be achieved through the talar body. For lesions larger than 1 cm^2, drilling is inadequate to restore cartilage coverage of the lesion, and osteochondral grafting taken from the ipsilateral femoral condyle or from allografts is indicated.

31. What is compartment syndrome of the foot and how is it diagnosed?

When a foot is subjected to significant blunt trauma, crush injuries, or high-energy fracture, swelling occurs that leads to increased compartment pressure. Pressures greater than 30 to 40 mm Hg for longer than 8 hours result in permanent muscle injury, loss of sensation, and muscle contractures.

The foot has five muscle compartments—medial, central, lateral, interosseous, and calcaneal. Classic signs of compartment syndrome are swelling, pain out of proportion to injury, pain on passive stretch of toes, and paresthesias or sensory loss. Loss of pulse or poor capillary refill is not a sign of compartment syndrome, but of vascular compromise. Definitive diagnosis is made by measurement of compartment pressures using a hand-held pressure monitor. This is accomplished surgically through two longitudinal dorsal forefoot incisions and one medial midfoot incision. Wounds are left open for later secondary closure or skin grafting.

Bibliography

Al-Shaikh RA et al: Autologous osteochondral grafting for talar cartilage defects, *Foot Ankle Int* 239:381-389, 2002.

Arntz CT, Veith RG, Hansen ST: Fractures and fracture dislocations of the tarsometatarsal joint, *J Bone Joint Surg* 70A:174, 1988.

Charcot J-M: Sur quelques arthropathies qui paraissant depende d'une lesion du cerveau de la moelle epininiere, *Arch Physiol Norm Pathol* 1:161-178, 1868.

DiGiovanni CW: Fractures of the navicular, *Foot Ankle Clin North Am* 9:25-63, 2004.

Eisele SA, Sammarco GJ: Fatigue fractures of the foot and ankle in the athlete, *J Bone Joint Surg* 75A:290-298, 1993.

Etter C, Ganz R: Long term results of tibial plafond fractures treated with open reduction and internal fixation, *Arch Orthop Trauma Surg* 110:277-283, 1991.

French B, Tornetta P 3rd: Hybrid external fixation of tibial pilon fractures, *Foot Ankle Clin* 5:853-871, 2000.

Giannini S, Vannini E: Operative treatment of osteochondral lesions of the talar dome, *Foot Ankle Int* 25:168-175, 2004.

Gough A et al: Measurement of markers of osteoclast and osteoblast activity in patients with acute and chronic diabetic Charcot neuroarthropathy, *Diabetic Med* 14:527-531, 1997.

Hawkins LG: Fractures of the neck of the talus, *J Bone Joint Surg* 52A:991-1002, 1970.

Lauge-Hansen N: Fractures of the ankle: 2. Combined experimental-surgical and experimental-roentgenolgic investigations, *Arch Surg* 60:957-985, 1950.

Lauge-Hansen N: Fractures of the ankle: 5. Pronation dorsiflexion fractures, *Arch Surg* 67:813-820, 1953.

Lindvall E et al: Open reduction and stable internal fixation of isolated, displaced talar neck and body fractures, *J Bone Joint Surg* 86A:2229-2234, 2004.

Manoli A II: Compartment syndromes of the foot: current concepts, *Foot Ankle* 10:340-344, 1990.

Myerson MS et al: Fracture dislocations of the tarsometatarsal joints: end results correlated with pathology and treatment, *Foot Ankle* 6:225, 1986.

Ruedi TP, Allgower M: Fractures of the lower end of the tibia into the ankle joint, *Injury* 1:92-99, 1969.

Rutledge EW, Templeman DC, Souza LJ: Evaluation and treatment of Lisfranc fracture-dislocation, *Foot Ankle Clin* 4:603-615, 1999.

Sanders R: Intra-articular fractures of the calcaneus: present state of the art, *J Orthop Trauma* 6:252-265, 1992.

Sangeorzan BJ et al: Displaced intrarticular fractures of the tarsal navicular, *J Bone Joint Surg* 71A:1504-1510, 1989.

Tornetta P, Silver S: Calcaneal fractures, *Foot Ankle Clin* 4:571-585, 1999.

Chapter 78

Foot Orthoses and Shoe Design

David Tiberio, PT, PhD, OCS, and
James Robin Hinkebein, PT, OCS, ATC

1. Define the subtalar neutral position. Why is it important?

The subtalar neutral position is the position in which the head of the talus is aligned with the navicular. Radiographically it is defined as the position where the joint lines of the talonavicular joint and the calcaneocuboid joint are continuous. The subtalar joint (STJ) neutral position is used by clinicians to evaluate the amount of pronation and supination on either side of neutral position as well as to assess the foot for structural deformities. STJ neutral position also is used during weight-bearing assessment to evaluate foot structure and to determine how far from neutral the patient is functioning.

2. How is subtalar neutral position determined?

Other than radiographic analysis, there are two common clinical methods: (1) Divide the total amount of heel eversion (pronation)/inversion (supination) into thirds. The position one third from maximal pronation or two thirds from maximal supination is subtalar neutral. (2) Palpate "congruency" at the talonavicular joint. This procedure is based on creating the talonavicular alignment described above. The head of the talus is palpated on its medial and lateral aspects. Then the foot is moved between a pronated and a supinated position until the examiner feels talonavicular alignment or "congruency."

3. How reliable and valid are these methods?

Concerns have been raised about the validity of the first method. The inter-rater reliability of the second method is poor to moderate. Intra-rater reliability is much higher and may allow each clinician to develop a repeatable method for his or her own use. The reliability of the second method appears to be positively related to examiner experience.

4. What is the primary goal of a foot orthosis?

The primary goal of a foot orthosis is to make the STJ function around neutral position and to facilitate pronation during the initial part of stance and supination during the latter part of stance.

5. Does the subtalar joint function around neutral position?

This well-accepted principle of foot function has recently been questioned as a result of research about human locomotion. Two independent research groups found that the STJ demonstrates the predicted pronation/supination pattern but usually functions in a pronated position. Pierrynowski and Smith found that the STJ usually was pronated during stance. McPoil and Cornwall demonstrated that the STJ did not reach a supinated position before heel rise and that it had a tendency to function around the relaxed standing position. Despite this recent evidence, the principle of finding the cause of abnormal motion and reducing abnormal motion by treating the cause has not changed.

6. Do orthotics actually control motion?

Many studies demonstrate no effect, whereas others document significant reduction in STJ motion. Possible reasons for contradictory findings are errors in methodology, measurement of shoe motion instead of bone motion, differences in the composition and type of orthoses, and the patient's need for foot orthoses based on foot structure. This last factor is extremely important. If a patient has no need for foot orthoses and is functioning optimally, it is not unreasonable to expect that he or she will try to negate the effect of the orthoses. A recent study using intracortical pins demonstrated that the effects of medial foot orthoses on reducing motion were "small" and "subject-specific."

7. Why do orthotics function best in the clinical setting?

Elimination of symptoms requires a reduction in the stress on the symptomatic tissue. Stress may result from the amount, speed, or timing of STJ motion. Alteration in any of these three variables may reduce the stress below the symptomatic threshold or to a level that allows healing. The studies that demonstrate the greatest effect of orthoses are performed with patients instead of subjects. If foot orthoses are designed for a specific patient, considering the function of the entire lower extremity as well as foot structure, the chance for resolution of symptoms is maximized.

8. How do foot orthoses control motion?

Motion at the STJ occurs in all three planes but primarily in the frontal and transverse planes. Pronation and supination are a single motion; therefore if you control one plane of motion, you control all planes of motion. For this reason, a medial (varus) motion, which reduces the amount of eversion in the frontal plane, also reduces the motions in the other planes.

9. When can a foot orthosis "increase" motion?

When a patient has a rigid forefoot valgus, pronation of the STJ may be blocked when the medial side of the forefoot contacts the ground. A foot orthosis that includes a forefoot valgus post allows proper lateral-to-medial loading of the forefoot, minimizing the effect of the forefoot valgus; it also allows the STJ to pronate.

10. Are exercises more beneficial than a foot orthosis?

There is no universal answer to this question. Exercises to strengthen muscles within the foot have been employed for many years. More recently, functional exercises involving the more proximal joint of the lower extremity, as well as trunk exercises, have been employed to treat symptoms caused by excessive tissue stress. Clinical judgments must be made whether to use exercise, foot orthoses, or both in providing the most efficacious care to patients.

11. Are there any clinical tests to help make this decision?

One functional test addresses the question of whether exercise can be effective without foot orthoses. With the patient standing relaxed, he/she is asked to look and rotate the trunk in the transverse plane as far as possible. This trunk rotation should cause a reaction at the STJ. When the trunk is rotated to the right, the right STJ should supinate and the left STJ should pronate. If the foot does not react, it probably indicates that the feet are dictating lower extremity function, and that exercise alone may not be sufficient. The use of foot orthoses is not precluded if the feet do react.

12. What is the significance of heel eversion in a relaxed standing position?

Eversion of the calcaneus past a vertical position indicates that the rear foot is compensating for another structure because the calcaneus is resting in a less-than-optimal position for its own stability. Reasons include eversion to bring a forefoot varus deformity to the ground, compensation for a severely tight calf group by pronating to unlock the MTJ, functional shortening of a long leg, and transverse plane problems in the spine, pelvis, and hip that cause the leg to rotate internally.

13. Why do some patients stand with most of the weight on the outside of the feet?

The patient may be in a supinated position to compensate for a rigid forefoot valgus. The STJ may be held supinated to avoid pain (e.g., plantar fasciitis). However, the foot may not actually be supinated because a foot with cavus architecture looks similar. To distinguish between supinated position of the STJ and architecture, place the STJ in neutral position and assess the compensation from neutral to relaxed position.

14. What types of symptoms can be caused by a rigid plantar-flexed first ray?

Symptoms of plantar fasciitis, sesamoiditis, and hallux limitus or rigidus can be caused by a rigid plantar-flexed first ray. If the plantar-flexed first ray creates a forefoot valgus, the patient may suffer from chronic ankle sprains, lateral knee pain, central patellofemoral pain, and low back pain.

15. In what situation does the heel evert very little while the STJ pronates excessively?

In patients with a more vertical inclination of the STJ axis, the frontal plane component (eversion) decreases and the transverse plane component of pronation increases. Because clinicians usually assess and measure only the frontal plane component, the amount of STJ pronation is underestimated. High inclination angles are associated with a high-arch foot. In many cases, this type of foot requires more rear-foot varus posting than indicated by minimal heel eversion. A deep heel on the orthotic shell also may enhance control of the predominantly transverse plane motion.

16. Why does a rear foot with a varus position fail to pronate at the STJ during weight-bearing?

Ligamentous or osseous structures may restrict the STJ motion. A rigid forefoot valgus may prevent use of available pronation. In addition, a patient with pain or limited hip internal rotation may voluntarily prevent pronation.

17. With restricted calcaneal motion caused by limited STJ pronation, would there ever be a case for posting the heel medially?

Using a medial (varus) wedge when there is insufficient pronation would seem to be contraindicated. However, the patient may develop symptoms at end range, or may avoid end range by voluntarily limiting pronation. In these cases, a medial wedge that prevents the STJ from reaching end range but does not limit the beneficial pronation can be very effective at eliminating symptoms.

18. Can a foot that pronates excessively lack enough pronation?

When a foot has a large forefoot and/or rear-foot varus deformity, all the motion may be used just to get the foot to the ground. During locomotion this would be seen as excessive pronation. With the foot on the ground, any attempt to pronate further, for example, in order to jump, would be blocked. For the function of jumping, this abnormally pronated foot does not have enough pronation.

19. Can a foot that relaxes close to STJ neutral be abnormal and require orthotic intervention?

A foot that has a rear-foot varus and a rigid forefoot valgus has a tendency to relax in STJ neutral position during weight-bearing. The rear-foot varus wants the STJ to pronate, but the forefoot valgus does not allow pronation. Orthotic posting is required in the rear foot and forefoot for normal functioning during gait. Specifically, an orthosis with a rear-foot varus post and a forefoot valgus post is indicated. The forefoot valgus post allows more normal pronation, but the rear-foot varus post prevents excessive pronation.

20. What is the difference between forefoot varus and forefoot supinatus?

Traditionally, forefoot varus is described as a single-plane (inversion) bony deformity, whereas forefoot supinatus is described as a triplane soft tissue contracture. Assessment of joint mobility and symmetry of motion may distinguish between the two conditions. The orthotic treatment differs because the soft tissue supinatus may resolve, but the varus will not.

21. Are posting strategies different in children?

Most children pronate more than adults. As the calcaneus and talus endure developmental derotations, the pronation decreases. In designing orthoses for children with rear-foot and forefoot varus deformities, it is probably better to post the rear foot more aggressively and to use smaller forefoot posts in the hope that the forefoot varus will decrease. Except for special circumstances, the concept of treating the cause of the pronation does not change.

22. What is the role of the arch of the orthotic shell?

The arch of the shell plays an important role in capturing the inclination angle of the calcaneus and the architecture of the foot to optimize the effects of corrective posts. The arch of the shell usually does not serve as the primary corrective component. In most patients the decrease in arch height is not the cause of pronation but rather a result of STJ pronation. If the shell is used as the primary corrective component, it may need to be fabricated from a more flexible material to be tolerated by the patient.

23. What is an extended forefoot post?

In most orthoses, the shell ends behind the metatarsal heads. Therefore the forefoot posting exerts its influence on the metatarsal shafts. Some orthoses are fabricated with a flexible post that extends under the metatarsal heads. This type of post may be more effective because it exerts its influence directly under the metatarsal heads, but it is much more difficult to fit in certain shoes.

24. How does function improve with a first ray cut-out?

Propulsion occurs off the medial side of the foot. As the heel rises from the ground, the first metatarsophalangeal (MTP) joint dorsiflexes (up to 70 degrees). The first metatarsal must plantar flex to allow normal MTP dorsiflexion. If the patient has a rigid plantar-flexed first ray, excessive weight-bearing under the first metatarsal head may prevent plantar flexion of the first metatarsal. The first ray cut-out increases weight-bearing under the second metatarsal head and provides room for requisite plantar flexion of the first metatarsal.

25. What is the cause of exacerbated symptoms when a first ray cut-out is used to treat a patient with a plantar-flexed first ray and hallux limitus or rigidus?

Although the first ray cut-out is likely to improve mechanics to the first MTP joint, the dorsal spurring and limitation of motion may have reached the point where increased motion causes more impingement.

26. What problems may be associated with insufficient rear-foot varus posting with a substantial forefoot varus post?

If the rear foot pronates excessively, the MTJ is "unlocked" (mobile). The forefoot post becomes less effective at reducing motion and may actually cause the MTJ to collapse (the forefoot inverts and dorsiflexes relative to the rear foot).

27. Why would a patient with a large rear-foot and forefoot varus complain that they are sliding off the lateral side of the orthosis?

Many patients with severe pronation gradually acquire a shortening of the calf muscles. Dorsiflexion at the MTJ compensates for loss of ankle dorsiflexion. One objective of the orthosis is to stabilize the MTJ. When walking with the orthosis, the patient lacks sufficient ankle dorsiflexion and therefore attempts to pronate on top of the orthosis, producing the feeling of sliding. This compensation also may cause blisters under the shaft of the first metatarsal.

28. How does the forefoot adjust to a large degree of rear-foot posting?

The mobility of the MTJ allows the medial side of the forefoot to reach the ground with a moderate amount of rear-foot posting. At some point the rear-foot posting exceeds the ability of the MTJ to compensate, and the posting creates a pseudo-forefoot varus. The foot must pronate more to bring the medial side of the foot to the ground, creating a new problem.

29. Why should the midtarsal joint be considered when designing an orthosis?

Motion between the rear foot and forefoot occurs at the MTJ. The ability of the MTJ to compensate for surface irregularities, foot deformities, and orthotic posts depends on the amount of available motion. The amount of available motion is a function of the position of the STJ and general flexibility characteristics. Midtarsal joint mobility may influence the magnitude of both rear-foot and forefoot posts, depending on the particular posting strategies of individual clinicians.

30. What is the difference between a Thomas heel and a sole wedge?

A Thomas heel is a standard heel with an anteromedial extension $\frac{1}{2}$ inch longer than a standard heel. A Thomas heel is commonly used on the medial side of the foot to give added leverage for support under the sustentaculum tali and to stabilize motion as the foot goes from heel strike to foot flat. A sole wedge, which most frequently is tethered medial to lateral, is inserted with the highest part on the anteromedial corner and with a medial thickness of $\frac{1}{8}$ to $\frac{5}{16}$ inch, depending on the biomechanical correction needed. A wedge not only stabilizes motion but also may shift weight from one side of the shoe to the other. If even more control is needed, a sole wedge may be added beyond the heel. Because a forefoot sole wedge used alone may cause increased MTJ motion during toe-off, caution should be used.

31. Why do orthotics relieve Morton's neuroma?

The first metatarsal is supposed to bear 60% of the weight at toe-off in the gait cycle. With excessive or abnormal pronation at toe-off, the hallux assumes a more dorsiflexed position and the lesser metatarsals bear more weight than they are designed to sustain. Relative varus of the forefoot causes excessive STJ pronation at toe-off, thus creating a mobile lever at push-off instead of a rigid lever. Thus the medial longitudinal and transverse arches of the foot are compromised severely, causing compression of the interdigital nerves, most commonly the third and fourth nerves. A biomechanical orthosis addresses the faulty mechanics, and a metatarsal pad placed proximal to the involved metatarsal heads elevates the metatarsal shafts, taking pressure off of the interdigital nerves. The apex of the metatarsal pad should be placed between the affected metatarsals.

32. What is the function of an external metatarsal or rocker bar?

External metatarsal bars significantly change the dynamics of the gait cycle and require increased patient balance; therefore they should be used only as a secondary treatment option. The function of the metatarsal bar is to delay and decrease loading of the metatarsal heads during gait as well as to decrease early MTP joint extension as the foot moves from midstance to toe-off. The bar is placed at an apex point proximal to all five metatarsal heads and thus shifts foot pressure proximally.

33. List common problems with foot orthotics and their possible causes.

- Arch pain or blisters on plantar foot surface—Probably the arch or medial posting is too high and needs to be lowered, or the patient did not follow the break-in procedure of increasing wear by 1 hour per day for a 2-week period.
- Sensation of rolling to the outside of the foot—This sometimes may be normal because the medial longitudinal arch is not accustomed to weight-bearing. However, it also may indicate that the medial post is too high, that the orthotic shell is too rigid for the patient's foot type, or that the orthotic is not on a level plane on the insole.
- Sensation that the heel is coming out of the shoe—Wearing a shoe that has a low throat and heel quarter or using an orthotic that is too thick or slick may cause this sensation.
- Symptoms persist—Reevaluate biomechanics and determine whether more correction is necessary.
- Pain or blisters under metatarsal heads—Ensure that all rigid shell materials end slightly proximal to the metatarsal heads.
- Lateral foot pain—The most common causes of lateral foot pain are rolling motions over the lateral shell of the orthosis from a medial forefoot post that is too high or compression forces causing pain because of a forefoot valgus post that is too high.

34. What are the seven basic styles of footwear?

Although there are thousands of different shoe fashions in the world, there are only seven basic footwear styles: (1) The moccasin was originally a crudely tanned piece of leather that cradled around the foot and was secured with rawhide thongs. (2) The sandal originally used thongs to attach the sole or slab to the foot. (3) The mule was the original slipper or indoor shoe. Centuries after its development, a heel was attached to create a fashion shoe. (4) The clog is a platform-like piece of wood or other unyielding material on which the foot rests with an open heel. (5) The boot originally was developed for horseback riders by providing a low shoe with separate leggings. (6) The pump is a thin-soled slip-on shoe, originally worn by pre-Elizabethan English carriage footmen, who "pumped" the carriage brakes with their feet. (7) The Oxford, originally introduced in England in 1640, is defined by the use of laces to secure the upper shoe.

35. What are the effects on the foot and body of wearing high-heeled shoes?

In a normal standing position, approximately 50% of the weight is borne by the rear foot and 50% by the forefoot. A 2-inch heel shifts weight distribution: 10% is borne through the rear foot and 90% through the forefoot. With a flat-soled shoe, the angle between the body's weight line and the horizontal is 90 degrees. With a 2-inch heel, the angle is changed to 70 degrees. Thus the body must compensate by changing joint position and muscle functions of the feet, ankles, hips, and spine to maintain erect position. Furthermore, a 1-inch heel tilts the pelvis forward 5 degrees and a 2-inch heel 20 degrees. High-heeled shoes also force the knees to stay in relative knee flexion throughout the gait cycle. Finally, the chronic wearing of high-heeled shoes causes muscle imbalances such as shortening of the Achilles tendon. This decreases the calf muscles' mechanical advantage to develop power, causing loss of the natural heel-to-toe gait pattern and necessitating muscle compensations from the rest of the lower quadrant.

36. How should the shoe be checked for improper wear?

A normal sole is worn just laterally to the center of the heel, bisecting the sole and running medially toward the ball and great toe of the foot. Check the heel first to see that it is worn slightly lateral of center, indicating that the heel is supinated at heel strike. Next check the counter, making sure that it is firm and positioned perpendicular to the sole and has not migrated medially or laterally. A medially migrated counter or one that leans inward may indicate increased pronation during gait. Check the stability and flexibility of the sole by grasping the shoe from heel and toe; then twist and bend the shoe. The normal shoe should provide stability through the midfoot and shank area but flexibility at the toe break and forefoot. The front quarters should have a slight crease from the first MTP to the fifth MTP. An oblique crease may indicate a shoe that is too long or a condition such as hallux rigidus. The front quarter also should be perpendicular to the sole without medial or lateral migration. A front quarter that has migrated laterally is also an indication of an increased pronation response as the foot excessively abducts in the transverse plane. Finally, check the arch and midsole to make sure that the arch of the foot is not collapsing over the sole.

37. How can the patient ensure proper shoe fit?

- Fit a shoe only after you have been active so that your foot size and shape are typical.
- Allow ½ inch between the longest toe and the end of the toe box to ensure proper toe-off.
- The widest part of the shoe should coincide with the widest part of the forefoot.
- The shoe should be snug along the instep; therefore the dimensions from the heel to the ball of the foot and the shoe instep should be equal.
- The quarter, vamp, and toe box of the shoe should not gap excessively, nor should they allow the toes to wiggle freely.
- The heel counter should be rigid and should fit snugly around the heel of the foot, limiting excessive heel motion and slippage.
- Purchase a shoe that was designed for your foot type and that is immediately comfortable. Do not try to "break in" your shoes; they will probably break you.

38. What is the leading cause of diabetic foot ulcers? What are the appropriate recommendations for therapeutic footwear?

Most diabetic ulcers result from peripheral neuropathy, which leads to an insensate foot. The insensate foot is unable to recognize increased shear and pressure forces that cause skin breakdown and ulceration. Skin breakdown is most common over the exposed metatarsal heads, which bear most of the weight during walking. Once the ulcer has healed, therapeutic shoe wear is essential to prevent recurrence. Several research studies have shown that patients who return to normal footwear have a recurrence rate of 90%, whereas those who use modified shoes and orthosis have a recurrence rate of 15% to 20%. Therapeutic footwear should fulfill the following objectives:

- Redistribute and relieve high-pressure areas such as the metatarsal heads by using an accommodative total contact orthosis.
- Provide shock absorption by decreasing vertical load forces.
- Reduce shear by decreasing horizontal movement of the foot in the shoe.
- Accommodate deformities such as loss of fatty tissue or ligamentous support.
- Stabilize and support flexible deformities toward a more normal or neutral position while accommodating rigid deformities.
- Reduce painful joint motion or stress.

39. What is a last?

A **last** is a three-dimensional positive model or mold from which the upper and lower aspects of the shoe are constructed. There are two basic last types: a straight last and an inwardly curved last. The forefoot and rear foot are in neutral alignment with a straight last, whereas a curved last is angled medially at the forefoot. In general, the straighter the last, the greater the stability and control the shoe will have; the curved last is more mobile during the gait cycle.

40. Describe the anatomy and construction of the shoe.

The upper portion of the shoe includes the quarter, counter, vamp, throat, toe box, and top lining. The quarter is a horseshoe-shaped material that cradles the heel of the foot. The counter is a rigid piece of material surrounding the heel posteriorly to stabilize motion. Shoes often include an extended medial heel counter to limit midfoot motion in the overpronator. The vamp is the portion of the shoes that covers the dorsum of the foot to the upper ball of the foot. The throat is the line that connects the proximal portion of the vamp and distal portion of the quarter. The two most common styles are Blucher and Balmoral. The Blucher style is designed for a wider forefoot; the front edges of the quarter are placed on top of the vamp and not sewn together, yielding more room at the throat and instep. In the Balmoral style, the quarter panels are sewn together on the back edge of the vamp. The toe box then covers the end of the toes and refers to the depth of the toe region.

The sole of the shoe includes the outsole, midsole, innersole, and shankpiece. The outsole is the portion of the shoe that contacts the ground. Important outsole properties should include stability, flexibility, durability, and traction. The outsole is made of various materials, depending on the function of the shoe. Outsoles are typically made of leather or a synthetic material. Shank-pieces are commonly used in dress and orthopaedic shoes to provide rigidity to the midsection of the shoe. The shankpiece helps to reduce the twisting or torsion of the forefoot in relation to the rear foot as well as provides support for the midfoot region. The shank refers to the portion of the shoe from the heel to the metatarsal heads. In athletic shoes, the midsole replaces the use of the shank. The midsole is made of differing materials, depending on individual needs. For example, the overpronator may benefit from an athletic shoe that uses a dual-density midsole. A dual-density midsole uses a softer durometer material on the lateral side to decrease the lever arm ground reaction forces at heel strike and decrease the rate of pronation. The medial side of the midsole is made of a more dense or firmer durometer material to decrease the magnitude of pronation. The innersole attaches the upper part of the shoe to the soling and acts as a smooth filler for the foot to rest upon.

41. What are the three basic types of athletic shoe construction?

The three basic types are board-lasting, slip-lasting, and combination-lasting. In board-lasting the upper shoe is glued to a rigid fiberboard; the board-lasted shoe provides stability and motion control. A slip-lasted shoe is sewn together at the center of the sole, much like a moccasin, and is then cemented to the midsole. It affords little stability but significant flexibility. Finally, a combination-last is used to provide rear-foot stability and forefoot flexibility. The rear portion of the foot is board-lasted and the forefoot is slip-lasted.

42. What is a rocker sole?

A rocker sole is used to facilitate a heel-to-toe gait pattern while reducing the proportion of internal energy of the foot and ankle for the gait cycle. The toe of the shoe is curved upward to simulate dorsiflexion and allow the metatarsal heads to move through a decreased range of motion at toe-off. Ground reaction forces also are reduced on the ankle because the take-off point is moved posteriorly. In addition, a rocker sole may be used to reduce pressure on specific areas of the foot, such as the heel, midfoot, metatarsals, and toes. Two of the more common types of rocker soles include the forefoot rocker sole and the heel-to-toe rocker sole. A forefoot rocker sole reduces shock at toe-off by placing the apex of the rocker sole just proximal to the metatarsal heads. A forefoot rocker provides stability at midstance but unloads the forefoot at toe-off. A heel-to-toe rocker sole uses a rocker at both the posterior aspect of the heel and just proximal to the metatarsal heads. This type of rocker sole is able to dissipate ground reaction forces at heel strike and increase propulsion at toe-off.

43. What is the effect of a foot orthotic on quality of life and pain in patients with patellofemoral pain syndrome?

Quality evidence surrounding the use of foot orthotics for patients suffering from patellofemoral pain is limited. Definitive conclusions regarding the reduction of pain and increased quality of life are difficult to draw. However, the literature does seem to weakly support the use of orthotics (custom-made and generic) as a treatment for patellofemoral pain syndrome caused by abnormal biomechanical foot function.

44. What are the proposed mechanisms by which a foot orthotic has a positive effect on pain and function in patients with patellofemoral knee pain?

Some of the most common theories on how foot orthotics decrease knee pain and increase function in patients with patellofemoral knee pain include the following: (1) reduction of lower limb internal rotation; (2) reduction in Q-angle; (3) decrease in laterally directed soft tissue tension forces of the vastus lateralis, iliotibial band, and patellar tendon; and (4) reduction in lateral patellofemoral contact forces.

45. Does the use of a foot orthotic reduce the incidence of lower limb stress reactions in younger, active adults?

It appears the use of a shock-absorbing orthotic can reduce the incidence of lower limb stress reactions, especially in military recruits. The best designed insert is still not agreed upon; however, more important is the comfort and the ability of the wearer to tolerate the foot orthotic. Thus the use of a shock-absorbing orthotic as a preventative measure may be a wise choice for those participating in activities that often cause stress reactions of the lower limbs (e.g., running, walking—especially in boots).

46. Does the type of prophylactic foot orthosis have any effect on the incidence of lower limb overuse injuries?

The limited research in this area suggests that there is not a significant difference in overuse injury rates based on the type of orthotic used (soft custom, soft prefabricated, semirigid biomechanical, and semirigid prefabricated). Because there is no significant difference between the various types of orthotics, little justification for prescribing custom prophylactic orthotics exists.

47. Does the use of prophylactic foot orthoses have any effect on the incidence of low back pain in active individuals?

It appears the use of a foot orthotic may not reduce the incidence of weight-bearing–induced low back pain in military recruits with no prior history of low back pain. Thus the use of an orthotic (custom soft or semirigid biomechanical) as a preventative measure does not appear to be of any benefit.

Bibliography

Crawford F, Thomson C: Interventions for treating plantar heel pain, *Cochrane Database Syst Rev 3*, CD003674, 2005.

D'hondt NE et al: Orthotic devices for treating patellofemoral pain syndrome, *Cochrane Database Syst Rev* CD002267, 2002.

Ekenman I et al: The role of biomechanical shoe orthoses in tibial stress fracture prevention, *Am J Sports Med* 30:866-870, 2002.

Finestone A et al: A prospective study of the effect of foot orthoses composition and fabrication on comfort and the incidence of overuse injuries, *Foot Ankle Int* 25:462-466, 2004.

Fuller EA: A review of biomechanics of shoes, *Clin Podiatr Med Surg* 11:241-258, 1994.
Gross MT: Lower quarter screening for skeletal malalignment: suggestions for orthotics and shoe wear, *J Orthop Sports Phys Ther* 21:389-405, 1995.
Gross MT, Foxworth JL: The role of foot orthoses as an intervention for patellofemoral pain, *J Orthop Sports Phys Ther* 33:661-670, 2003.
Hunter S, Dolan MG, Davis JM: *Foot orthotic in therapy and sport,* Champaign, Ill, 1995, Human Kinetics.
Janisse D: *Introduction to pedorthics,* Columbia, Md, 1998, Pedorthic Footwear Association.
Johnston LB, Gross MT: Effects of foot orthoses on quality of life for individuals with patellofemoral pain syndrome, *J Orthop Sports Phys Ther* 34:440-448, 2004.
Luther LD, Mizel MS, Pfeffer GB: *Orthopedic knowledge update: foot and ankle,* Rosemont, Ill, 1994, American Academy of Orthopedic Surgeons.
McPoil TG, Cornwall MW: The relationship between subtalar joint neutral position and rearfoot motion during walking, *Foot Ankle* 15:141-145, 1994.
Michaund TM: *Foot orthoses and other forms of conservative foot care,* Baltimore, 1993, Williams & Wilkins.
Milgrom C et al: A controlled randomized study of the effect of training with orthoses on the incidence of weight bearing induced back pain among infantry recruits, *Spine* 30:272-275, 2005.
Northwestern University Medical School, Prosthetic-Orthotic Center: *Management of foot disorders: theory and clinical concepts,* Chicago, 1998, Northwestern University.
Northwestern University Medical School, Prosthetic-Orthotic Center: *Management of foot disorders: technical theory and fabrication,* Chicago, 1998, Northwestern University.
Picciano AM, Rowlands MS, Worrell T: Reliability of open and closed kinetic chain subtalar joint neutral positions and navicular drop test, *J Orthop Sports Phys Ther* 18:553-558, 1993.
Pierrynowski MR, Smith SB: Rear foot inversion/eversion during gait relative to the subtalar joint neutral position, *Foot Ankle Int* 17:406-412, 1996.
Smith-Orrichio K, Harris BA: Inter-rater reliability of subtalar neutral, calcaneal inversion and eversion, *J Orthop Sports Phys Ther* 12:10-15, 1990.
Stacoff A et al: Effects of foot orthoses on skeletal motion during running, *Clin Biomech* 15:54-64, 2000.
Tiberio D: Pathomechanics of structural foot deformities, *Phys Ther* 68:1840-1849, 1988.

Index

C

J

O

Q

R

S